Statistics for Industry and Technology

Series Editor

Advances in Statistical Methods for the Health Sciences

*Applications to Cancer and AIDS Studies,
Genome Sequence Analysis,
and Survival Analysis*

Jean-Louis Auget
N. Balakrishnan
Mounir Mesbah
Geert Molenberghs
Editors

Birkhäuser
Boston • Basel • Berlin

Jean-Louis Auget
UFR of Pharmaceutical Sciences
1 rue Gaston Veil
44035 Nantes Cedex 1
France

N. Balakrishnan
Department of Mathematics and Statistics
McMaster University
1280 Main Street West
Hamilton, Ontario L8S 4K1
Canada

Mounir Mesbah
Laboratoire de Statistique Théorie et Appliquée
Université Pierre et Marie Curie
175 rue de Chevaleret
75013 Paris
France

Geert Molenberghs
Center for Statistics
Hasselt University
Agoralaan–Building D
3590 Diepenbeek
Belgium

Mathematics Subject Classification: 62K99, 62L05, 62N01, 62N02, 62N03, 62P10, 62P12

Library of Congress Control Number: 2006934773

ISBN-10: 0-8176-4368-0   e-ISBN-10: 0-8176-4542-X
ISBN-13: 978-0-8176-4368-3   e-ISBN-13: 978-0-8176-4542-7

Printed on acid-free paper.

9 8 7 6 5 4 3 2 1

www.birkhauser.com   (Ham)

Contents

Preface   xix

Contributors   xxi

List of Tables   xxix

List of Figures   xxxv

PART I: PROGNOSTIC STUDIES AND GENERAL EPIDEMIOLOGY

1 Systematic Review of Multiple Studies of Prognosis:
   The Feasibility of Obtaining Individual Patient Data   3
   D. G. Altman, M. Trivella, F. Pezzella, A. L. Harris,
   and U. Pastorino

   1.1 Introduction   3
   1.2 Systematic Review Based on Individual
       Patient Data   5
   1.3 A Case Study: Microvessel Density in Non-Small
       Cell Lung Cancer   6
       1.3.1 Identifying studies (data sets) and obtaining
             the data   7
       1.3.2 Checking the data   9
       1.3.3 MVD measurements   11
       1.3.4 Meta-analysis   12
   1.4 Discussion   12
       1.4.1 Systematic review of prognostic studies using
             individual patient data   13
       1.4.2 The need for higher-quality prognostic studies   14
   References   16

2 On Statistical Approaches for the Multivariable
   Analysis of Prognostic Marker Studies   19
   N. Holländer and W. Sauerbrei

   2.1 Introduction   19

2.2 Examples: Two Prognostic Studies in
     Breast Cancer   20
2.3 Statistical Methods   21
     2.3.1 Regression models   21
     2.3.2 Classification and regression trees (CART)   22
     2.3.3 Formation of risk groups   23
2.4 Results in the GBSG-2 Study   23
     2.4.1 Regression models – standard applications   23
     2.4.2 Regression models – the MFP-approach   25
     2.4.3 Summary assessment – implication of the
           modelling strategy   25
     2.4.4 Application of classification and regression trees   28
2.5 Formation and Validation of Risk Groups   30
2.6 Discussion   32
References   35

3 Where Next for Evidence Synthesis of Prognostic Marker Studies? Improving the Quality and Reporting of Primary Studies to Facilitate Clinically Relevant Evidence-Based Results   39

*R. D. Riley, K. R. Abrams, P. C. Lambert, A. J. Sutton,
and D. G. Altman*

3.1 Introduction and Aims   40
     3.1.1 Prognostic markers and prognostic marker studies   40
     3.1.2 The need for formal evidence syntheses of
           prognostic marker studies   40
     3.1.3 Aims of this chapter   41
3.2 Difficulties of an Evidence Synthesis of Prognostic
     Marker Studies   42
     3.2.1 Poor and heterogeneous reporting   42
     3.2.2 Poor study design and problems clarifying study
           purpose   44
     3.2.3 Little indication of how to implement markers in
           clinical practice   45
     3.2.4 Small sample sizes   46
     3.2.5 Publication bias, selective within-study reporting,
           and selective analyses   46
     3.2.6 Lack of appreciation or validation of previous
           findings   48
3.3 What Improvements Are Needed in Primary Prognostic
     Marker Studies?   49
3.4 Evidence Synthesis Using Individual Patient Data Rather
     than Summary Statistics   51

3.5 Discussion   54
References   55

PART II: PHARMACOVIGILANCE

**4 Sentinel Event Methods for Monitoring
Unanticipated Adverse Events**   **61**
P. A. Lachenbruch and J. Wittes

4.1 Introduction   61
4.2 Examples   63
4.3 Usual Approaches to Monitoring Safety   64
4.4 Methods for Sentinel Events   66
    4.4.1 Constant follow-up time   66
    4.4.2 Censoring at a fixed calendar time   68
4.5 Methods for Sentinel Event Rates   71
4.6 Bayesian Models   72
4.7 Summary   73
References   74

**5 Spontaneous Reporting System Modelling for the
Evaluation of Automatic Signal Generation
Methods in Pharmacovigilance**   **75**
*E. Roux, F. Thiessard, A. Fourrier, B. Bégaud,
and P. Tubert-Bitter*

5.1 Introduction   76
5.2 Methods   78
    5.2.1 Spontaneous reporting system modelling   78
    5.2.2 Exposure to the drug (T_i) 79
    5.2.3 Events' relative risk (RR_{ij}) 79
    5.2.4 Reporting probability (p_{ij}) 80
    5.2.5 Data generation process   84
5.3 Application   84
    5.3.1 Values of the model parameters   84
    5.3.2 Application of the empirical Bayes method   86
5.4 Results   86
5.5 Discussion   88
5.6 Conclusion   89
References   90

PART III: QUALITY OF LIFE

**6 Latent Covariates in Generalized Linear Models:
A Rasch Model Approach**   **95**
K. B. Christensen

6.1 Introduction   95
6.2 Generalized Linear Mixed Models   96
  6.2.1 Latent regression models   97
6.3 Interpretation of Parameters   98
6.4 Generalized Linear Models with a Latent Covariate   98
  6.4.1 Model   99
  6.4.2 Interpretation of parameters   99
  6.4.3 Parameter estimation   100
6.5 Example   101
  6.5.1 Latent covariate   102
  6.5.2 Job group level effect of the latent covariate   103
6.6 Discussion   104
References   105

7 Sequential Analysis of Quality of Life Measurements with the Mixed Partial Credit Model

7 Sequential Analysis of Quality of Life Measurements with the Mixed Partial Credit Model   **109**
V. Sébille, T. Challa, and M. Mesbah

7.1 Introduction   110
7.2 Methods   111
  7.2.1 The partial credit model   111
  7.2.2 Estimation of the parameters   112
  7.2.3 Sequential analysis   112
  7.2.4 The Z and V statistics   112
  7.2.5 Traditional sequential analysis   113
  7.2.6 Sequential analysis based on partial credit
        measurements   113
  7.2.7 The sequential probability ratio test and
        the triangular test   115
  7.2.8 Simulation design   115
7.3 Results   116
7.4 Discussion   121
7.5 Conclusion   122
Appendix   122
References   123

8 A Parametric Degradation Model Used in Reliability, Survival Analysis, and Quality of Life   **127**
M. Nikulin, L. Gerville-Réache, and S. Orazio

8.1 Introduction   127
8.2 Degradation Process   129
8.3 Estimation Problem   130
8.4 Linear MVUE for a 131
8.5 Solution of the Optimizatio Problem   132

8.6 Estimation of σ^2 and θ_0 132
References   134

9 Agreement Between Two Ratings with Different Ordinal Scales   139
S. Natarajan, M. B. McHenry, S. Lipsitz, N. Klar, and S. Lipshultz

9.1 Introduction   139
9.2 Notation and Model   142
9.3 Examples and Interpretation   144
9.4 Discussion   147
References   147

PART IV: SURVIVAL ANALYSIS

10 The Role of Correlated Frailty Models in Studies of Human Health, Ageing, and Longevity   151
A. Wienke, P. Lichtenstein, K. Czene, and A.I. Yashin

10.1 Introduction   151
10.2 Shared Frailty Model   153
10.3 Correlated Frailty Model   155
10.4 Correlated Gamma Frailty Model   156
    10.4.1 Swedish breast cancer twin data   157
    10.4.2 Parametric and semiparametric models   158
    10.4.3 Correlated gamma frailty model with covariates   159
    10.4.4 Cure-mixture models   160
10.5 Discussion   163
References   164

11 Prognostic Factors and Prediction of Residual Survival for Hospitalized Elderly Patients   167
M. L. Calle, P. Roura, A. Arnau, A. Yáñez, and A. Leiva

11.1 Introduction   167
11.2 Cohort Description and Follow-Up   168
11.3 Multistate Survival Model   171
    11.3.1 Predictive process   173
11.4 Discussion   176
References   177

12 New Models and Methods for Survival Analysis of Experimental Data   179
G. V. Semenchenko, A. I. Yashin, T. E. Johnson, and J. W. Cypser

12.1 Introduction   179

12.2 Semiparametric Model of Mortality in Heterogeneous
Populations Influenced by Exogenous Interventions   180

    12.2.1 The heterogeneous mortality model   180

    12.2.2 Changes in the baseline hazard and frailty
distribution   181

    12.2.3 Semiparametric representation of the model   183

    12.2.4 Interpretation of parameters   184

12.3 One Example of the Model Application to the Analysis of
Poststress Survival Data   187

    12.3.1 Heat shock of different duration applied to
populations of nematodes *Caenorhabditis elegans*   187

    12.3.2 Technical details   188

    12.3.3 Results of fitting the model to the data   188

12.4 Discussion   190

References   191

13 Uniform Consistency for Conditional Lifetime Distribution Estimators Under Random Right-Censorship   195

P. Deheuvels and G. Derzko

13.1 Introduction and Results   195

    13.1.1 Notation and statement of the problem   195

    13.1.2 Definition of the estimators and uniform
consistency   198

13.2 Proofs   203

    13.2.1 Construction of the estimators   203

    13.2.2 A useful auxiliary result   206

    13.2.3 Concluding comments   208

References   208

14 Sequential Estimation for the Semiparametric Additive Hazard Model   211

L. Bordes and C. Breuils

14.1 Introduction   211

14.2 Example and Numerical Study   213

14.3 Assumptions and Theoretical Results   215

14.4 Technical Tools   220

    14.4.1 Complete convergence, Anscombe condition,
and exponential inequality   220

    14.4.2 Technical results   221

References   222

15 Variance Estimation of a Survival Function with Doubly Censored Failure Time Data **225**
C. Zhu and J. Sun

15.1 Introduction   225
15.2 Preliminaries   227
15.3 Variance Estimation   228
    15.3.1 Simple bootstrap method   228
    15.3.2 Generalized Greenwood formula   229
    15.3.3 Imputation methods I and II   230
15.4 Numerical Results   231
15.5 Concluding Remarks   233
References   234

PART V: CLUSTERING

16 Statistical Models and Artificial Neural Networks: Supervised Classification and Prediction Via Soft Trees **239**
A. Ciampi and Y. Lechevallier

16.1 Introduction   240
16.2 The Prediction Problem: Statistical Models and ANNs   241
    16.2.1 Generalized linear models as ANNs   243
    16.2.2 Generalized additive models as ANNs   245
    16.2.3 Classification and regression trees as ANNs   246
16.3 Combining Prediction Models: Hierarchy of Experts   248
16.4 The Soft Tree   250
    16.4.1 General concepts in tree construction   251
    16.4.2 Constructing a soft tree from data   252
    16.4.3 An example of data analysis   253
    16.4.4 An evaluation study   256
16.5 Extending the Soft Tree   257
16.6 Conclusions   259
References   260

17 Multilevel Clustering for Large Databases **263**
Y. Lechevallier and A. Ciampi

17.1 Introduction   263
17.2 Data Reduction by Kohonen SOMs   265
    17.2.1 Kohonen SOMs and PCA initialization   266
    17.2.2 Binning of the original data matrix using a
        Kohonen map   266
    17.2.3 Dissimilarity for microregimens   268

17.3 Clustering Multilevel Systems   269
    17.3.1 A two-level statistical model   270
    17.3.2 Estimating parameters by the EM algorithm   270
17.4 Extracting Dietary Patterns from the Nutritional
    Data   271
References   273

**18 Neural Networks: An Application for Predicting
Smear Negative Pulmonary Tuberculosis**   **275**
A. M. Santos, B. B. Pereira, J. M. Seixas,
F. C. Q. Mello, and A. L. Kritski

18.1 Introduction   276
18.2 Materials and Methods   277
    18.2.1 Data set   277
    18.2.2 Neural network design   278
    18.2.3 Data selection for network design   279
18.3 Relevance of Explanatory Variables   283
18.4 Results   283
18.5 Conclusions   284
References 285

**19 Assessing Drug Resistance in HIV Infection Using
Viral Load Using Segmented Regression**   **289**
H. Liang, W.-Y. Tan, and X. Xiong

19.1 Introduction   289
19.2 The Model   292
    19.2.1 The likelihood function   294
    19.2.2 The prior distribution   294
    19.2.3 The posterior distributions   295
19.3 The Gibbs Sampling Procedure   297
19.4 Analysis of the ACTG 315 Data   298
19.5 Conclusion and Dicussion   301
References 303

**20 Assessment of Treatment Effects on HIV Pathogenesis
Under Treatment By State Space Models**   **305**
W.-Y. Tan, P. Zhang, X. Xiong, and P. Flynn

20.1 Introduction   305
20.2 A Stochastic Model for HIV Pathogenesis Under
    Treatment   306
    20.2.1 Stochastic differential equations of
        state variables   307
    20.2.2 The probability distribution of state
        variables   308

20.3 A State Space Model for HIV Pathogenesis Under
    Antiretroviral Drugs   309
20.4 Estimation of Unknown Parameters and State
    Variables   310
20.5 An Illustrative Example   311
20.6 Conclusions and Discussion   314
References   317

PART VI: SAFETY AND EFFICACY ASSESSMENT

21 Safety Assessment Versus Efficacy Assessment   **323**
M. A. Foulkes

21.1 Introduction   323
21.2 Design Issues   324
    21.2.1 Outcomes   324
    21.2.2 Power   325
    21.2.3 Population   326
    21.2.4 Comparison   326
21.3 Analytic Issues   326
    21.3.1 Compliance   326
    21.3.2 Missing data   327
    21.3.3 Confounding   327
    21.3.4 Bias   328
    21.3.5 Misclassification   328
    21.3.6 Multiplicity   328
21.4 Analytic Approaches   329
21.5 Inferences   330
21.6 Conclusions   330
References   332

**22 Cancer Clinical Trials with Efficacy and Toxicity
Endpoints: A Simulation Study to Compare
Two Nonparametric Methods**   **335**
A. Letierce and P. Tubert-Bitter

22.1 Introduction   336
22.2 Setting   337
22.3 Method for the Simulation Study   340
22.4 Results   342
22.5 Conclusion   346
References   347

**23 Safety Assessment in Pilot Studies When
Zero Events Are Observed**   **349**
R. E. Carter and R. F. Woolson

23.1 Introduction   349
23.2 Clinical Setting   350
23.3 Notation   351
23.4 Binomial Setting   351
23.5 Geometric Setting   352
23.6 Bayesian Credible Interval   354
23.7 Clinical Setting: Revisited   356
23.8 Summary   357
References   357

PART VII: CLINICAL DESIGNS

**24 An Assessment of Up-and-Down Designs and
Associated Estimators in Phase I Trials**   **361**
H. K. T. Ng, S. G. Mohanty, and N. Balakrishnan

24.1 Introduction   361
24.2 Notation and Designs   362
    24.2.1 The biased coin design (BCD)   363
    24.2.2 The k-in-a-row rule (KROW)   364
    24.2.3 The Narayana rule (NAR)   364
    24.2.4 Continual reassessment method (CRM)   364
24.3 Estimation of Maximum Tolerated Dose   365
24.4 Simulation Setting   367
24.5 Comparison of Estimators   368
24.6 Comparison of Designs   369
References   385

**25 Design of Multicentre Clinical Trials with
Random Enrolment**   **387**
V. V. Anisimov and V. V. Fedorov

25.1 Introduction   387
25.2 Recruitment Time Analysis   389
25.3 Analysis of Variance of the Estimated ECRT   393
25.4 Inflation of the Variance Due to Random
    Enrolment   395
25.5 Solution of the Optimization Problem   396
25.6 Conclusions   398
Appendix   398
References   400

**26 Statistical Methods for Combining Clinical Trial
Phases II and III** **401**
N. Stallard and S. Todd

26.1 Introduction   401
26.2 Background   402
    26.2.1 The clinical evaluation programme for
        new drugs   402
    26.2.2 Combining clinical trial phases II and III   403
    26.2.3 Background to sequential clinical trials   404
26.3 Methods for Combining Phases II and III   407
    26.3.1 Two-stage methods   408
    26.3.2 A multistage group-sequential method   408
    26.3.3 A multistage adaptive design method   409
    26.3.4 Example—a multistage trial comparing
        three doses of a new drug for the
        treatment of Alzheimer's disease   410
26.4 Discussion and Future Directions   413
References   415

**27 SCPRT: A Sequential Procedure That Gives
Another Reason to Stop Clinical Trials Early** **419**
X. Xiong, M. Tan, and J. Boyett

27.1 Introduction   420
27.2 The SCPRT Procedure   421
    27.2.1 Controlling the boundary   423
    27.2.2 Boundaries in terms of P-values   423
27.3 An Example   424
27.4 SCPRT with Unknown Variance   426
27.5 Clinical Trials with Survival Data   428
27.6 Conclusion   432
References   432

PART VIII: MODELS FOR THE ENVIRONMENT

28 Seasonality Assessment for Biosurveillance Systems **437**
E. N. Naumova and I. B. MacNeill

28.1 Introduction   438
    28.1.1 Conceptual framework for seasonality
        assessment   438
28.2 δ-Method in Application to a Seasonality Model   440
    28.2.1 Single-variable case   440
    28.2.2 Two-variables case   441

    28.2.3 Application to a seasonality model   442
    28.2.4 Potential model extension   443
    28.2.5 Additional considerations   444
28.3 Application to Temperature and Infection
     Incidence Analysis   446
28.4 Conclusion   449
References   450

**29 Comparison of Three Convolution Prior Spatial
   Models for Cancer Incidence   451**
*E.-A. Sauleau, M. Musio, A. Etienne,
and A. Buemi*

29.1 Introduction   451
29.2 Materials and Methods   453
    29.2.1 ICAR model   455
    29.2.2 Distance model based on the exponential
           function   455
    29.2.3 Two-dimensional P-splines model   456
    29.2.4 Implementation of the models   456
29.3 Results   456
29.4 Discussion   459
References   463

**30 Longitudinal Analysis of Short-Term Bronchiolitis
   Air Pollution Association Using Semiparametric
   Models   467**
S. Willems, C. Segala, M. Maidenberg, and M. Mesbah

30.1 Introduction   467
30.2 Data   469
    30.2.1 Sanitary data   469
    30.2.2 Environmental data   469
30.3 Methods   470
    30.3.1 Generalized additive models   470
    30.3.2 Air pollution time series studies strategy   471
    30.3.3 Criticism about the use of standard statistical
           software to fit GAM to epidemiological time
           series data   474
30.4 Results   475
    30.4.1 Series of number of hospital consultations:
           Results with S-Plus   475
    30.4.2 Series of number of hospital consultations:
           Results with R   482
    30.4.3 SAS results   483

30.5 Discussion   484
References   486

PART IX: GENOMIC ANALYSIS

31 Are There Correlated Genomic Substitutions?   **491**
M. Karnoub, P. K. Sen, and F. Seillier-Moiseiwitsch

31.1 Introduction   491
31.2 The Probabilistic Model   492
31.3 Parameter Estimation   496
31.4 New Test Statistic   497
31.5 Power Studies   500
31.6 Numerical Studies   501
31.7 Data Analysis   504
31.8 Discussion   507
Appendix 31.1   509
Appendix 31.2   510
References   513

PART X: ANIMAL HEALTH

**32 Swiss Federal Veterinary Office Risk
Assessments: Advantages and Limitations
of the Qualitative Method**   **519**
R. Hauser, E. Breidenbach, and K. D. C. Stärk

32.1 Introduction   520
32.2 Health Risks from Consumption of Milk and
    Dairy Products: An Example of a Qualitative
    Risk Assessment   521
    32.2.1 Risk profile   521
    32.2.2 Hazard identification   521
    32.2.3 Risk network   522
    32.2.4 Risk estimation   523
    32.2.5 Recommendations for random sample planning
        and risk managers   524
32.3 Advantages and Disadvantages of Qualitative
    Risk Assessment   525
32.4 Statistics' Part in Qualitative Risk Assessment   526
References   526

**33 Qualitative Risk Analysis in Animal Health:
A Methodological Example**   **527**
B. Dufour and F. Moutou

33.1 Introduction   528
33.2 Global Presentation of the Method   528
33.3 Qualitative Appreciation of the Probability of
     Each Event   530
33.4 Qualitative Risk Appreciation   531
33.5 Qualitative Appreciation Examples   532
33.6 Discussion   534
References   536

Index   **539**

Preface

Statistical methods have become an increasingly important and integral part of research in health sciences. For this reason, we organized an *International Conference on Statistics in Health Sciences* during June 23–25, 2004, at Université de Nantes, Nantes, France. This conference, with the participation of over 200 researchers from numerous countries, was very successful in bringing together experts working on statistical methodology and applications into several different aspects and problems in health sciences.

This volume comprises a selection of papers that were presented at the conference. All the articles presented here have been peer reviewed and carefully organized into 33 chapters. For the convenience of the readers, the volume has been divided into the following parts:

- PROGNOSTIC STUDIES AND GENERAL EPIDEMIOLOGY
- PHARMACOVIGILANCE
- QUALITY OF LIFE
- SURVIVAL ANALYSIS
- CLUSTERING
- SAFETY AND EFFICACY ASSESSMENT
- CLINICAL DESIGNS
- MODELS FOR THE ENVIRONMENT
- GENOMIC ANALYSIS
- ANIMAL HEALTH

As is evident, these cover a wide range of topics pertaining to statistical methods in health sciences.

Our sincere thanks go to all the authors who have contributed to this volume, and for their cooperation, patience, and support throughout the course of the preparation of the volume. We are also indebted to the referees for helping us in the evaluation of the manuscripts and in improving the quality of this publication.

Special thanks are due to Mrs. Debbie Iscoe for the excellent typesetting of the entire volume, and to Mr. Thomas Grasso (Editor, Birhäuser, Boston) and Ms. Regina Gorenshteyn (Assistant Editor, Birkhäuser, Boston) for their encouragement and help.

Jean-Louis Auget
Université de Nantes
Nantes, France

N. Balakrishnan
McMaster University
Hamilton, Canada

Mounir Mesbah
Université de Pierre et Marie Curie
Paris, France

Geert Molenberghs
Hasselt University
Diepenbeek, Belgium

Contributors

Abrams, Keith R. Centre for Biostatistics and Genetic Epidemiology, 22-28 Department of Health Sciences, University of Leicester Princess Road West, Leicester, UK
kra1@le.ac.uk

Altman, Douglas G. Cancer Research UK Medical Statistics Group Centre for Statistics in Medicine, Wolfson College Oxford OX2 6UD, UK
doug.altman@cancer.org.uk.

Anisimov, Vladimir V. Research Statistics Unit, GlaxoSmithKline NFSP-South, Third Avenue, Harlow Essex CM19 5AW, UK
Vladimir.V.Anisimov@gsk.com

Arnau, A. Clinical Epidemiology and Research Department, Vic General Hospital, 08500 Vic, Spain
aarnau@hgv.es

Balakrishnan, N. Department of Mathematics and Statistics, McMaster University, Hamilton, Ontario, Canada L8S 4K1
bala@univmail.cis.mcmaster.ca

Begaud, B. Université Victor Segalen, 146 rue Léo Saignat, 33076 Bordeaus Cedex, France
bernard.begaud@pharmaco.u-bordeaux2.fr

Bordes, L. Université de Technologie de Compiègne, LMAC Royallieu, BP 525, 60205 Compiègne, France
Laurent.Bordes@utc.fr

Boyett, James St. Jude Children's Research Hospital, Memphis, TN 38105-2794, USA
jim.boyett@stjude.org

Breidenbach, E. Federal Veterinary Office Department of Monitoring, P.O. Box CH-3003, Bern, Switzerland
Eric.Breidenbach@bvet.admin.ch

Breuils, C. Lab. de Math. Nicolas Oresme, Université de Caen, BP 5186, 14032 Caen Cedex, France
christelle.breuils@maths.unicaen.fr

Buemi, Antoine Cancer Registry of Haut-Rhin, Mulhouse, France
buemia@ch-mulhouse.fr

Calle, M. L. Systems Biology Department, Universitat de Vic, 13, Laura St., E-08500 Vic, Spain
malu.calle@uvic.es

Carter, Rickey E. Department of Biostatistics, Bioinformatics and Epidemiology, Medical University of South Carolina, Charleston, SC 29425, USA
carterre@musc.edu

Challa, Tariku Center for Statistics, Hasselt University, Agoralaan - building D, 3590 Diepenbeek, Belgium
tariku_c@yahoo.com

Christensen, Karl Bang National Institute of Occupational Health, Lerso Parkallé 105, 2100 Copenhagen, Denmark
kbc@ami.dk

Ciampi, Antonio Department of Epidemiology and Biostatistics, McGill University, Montreal, Quebec, Canada, H2T 2T4
antonio.ciampi@mcgill.ca

Cypser, James W. Institute for Behavioural Genetics, University of Colorado at Boulder, Boulder, CO 80309-0447, USA

Czene, Kamila Department of Medical Epidemiology and Biostatistics, Karolinska Institute, Stockholm, Sweden

Deheuvels, Paul Université Pierre et Marie Curie, Laboratoire de Statistique Théorique et Appliquée, Boîte 158, Bureau 8A25, 175 rue du Chevaleret, 75013 Paris, France
pd@ccr.jussieu.fr

Derzko, Gérard Sanofi-Aventis, 371 rue du Pr Joseph Blayac, 34184 Montpellier Cedex 4, France
gerard.derzko@sanofi-aventis.com

Dufour, Barbara UP Maladies contagieuses, École Nationale Vétérinaire d'Alfort, 7 Avenue du Général-de-Gaulle, 94704 Maisons-Alfort Cedex, France
bdufour@vet-alfort.fr

Etienne, Arnaud Cancer Registry of Haut-Rhin, Mulhouse, France
  `arno.etienne@free.fr`

Federov, Valerii V. Research Statistics Unit, GlaxoSmithKline, 1250 S. Collegeville Rd., Collegeville, PA 19426-0989, USA
  `Valeri.V.Fedorov@gsk.com`

Flynn, Pat Department of Biostatistics, St. Jude Children's Research Hospital, Memphis, TN 38105-2794, USA

Foulkes, Mary A. U.S. Food Drug Administration Center for Biologics Evaluation and Research, Office of Biostatistics and Epidemiology, 1401 Rockville Pike, HFM-210, Rockville, MD 20852, USA
  `foulkes@cber.fda.gov`

Fourrier, A. Université Victor Segalen, 146 rue Léo Saignat, 33076 Bordeaux Cedex, France
  `annie.fourrier@pharmaco.u-bordeaux2.fr`

Gerville-Réache, L. Mathematical Statistics and Its Applications, BP 26, University Victor Segalen Bordeaux 2, 33076 Bordeaux, France
  `leo.gerville@u-bordeaux2.fr`

Harris, Adrian L. Cancer Research UK Oncology Unit, Churchill Hospital, Oxford, UK

Hauser, R. Swiss Federal Veterinary Office (SFVO), Monitoring Schwarzenburgstrasse 161, CH-3003 Bern, Switzerland
  `ruth.hauser@bvet.admin.ch`

Holländer, N. Institute of Medical Biometry and Medical Informatics, Freiburg, Stefan-Meier Str. 26, 79104 Freiburg, Germany
  `noh@imbi.uni-freiburg.de`

Johnson, Thomas E. Institute for Behavioural Genetics, University of Colorado at Boulder, Boulder, CO 80309, USA

Karnoub, M. Population Genetics, GlaxoSmithKline, 5 Moore Drive, Box 13398, Research Triangle Park, NC 27709, USA
  `mac31876@glaxowellcome.com`

Klar, Neil Cancer Care Ontario, Ontario, Canada

Kritski, A. L. Faculty of Medicine and Tuberculosis, Research Unit-IDT-Federal, University of Rio de Janeiro, Rio de Janeiro, Brazil

Lachenbruch, Peter A. FDA/CBER/OBE, 1401 Rockville Pike HFM-215, Rochville, MD 20852, USA
lachenbruch@cber.fda.gov

Lambert, Paul C. Centre for Biostatistics and Genetic Epidemiology, Department of Health Sciences, University of Leicester, 22-28 Princess Road West, Leicester, UK
pl4@le.ac.uk

Lechevallier, Yves Institut National de Recherche en Informatique et en Automatique, Rocquencourt 78153, Le Chesnay Cedex, France
Yves.Lechevallier@inria.fr

Leiva, A. Clinical Epidemiology and Research Department, Vic General Hospital, 08500 Vic, Spain
arfons74@hotmail.com

Letierce, Alexia Unité de Recherche Clinique Paris Sud, Hôpital Bicêtre, 78 rue de Gé'eral Leclerc, 94807 Le Kremlin-Bicêtre Cedex, France
alexia.letierce@bct.aphp.fr

Liang, Hua Department of Biostatistics and Computational Biology, University of Rochester, Rochester, NY 14642, USA
hliang@bst.rochester.edu

Lichtenstein, Paul Department of Medical Epidemiology and Biostatistics, Karolinska Institute, Stockholm, Sweden

Lipshultz, Steven Department of Pediatrics, University of Miami School of Medicine, Miami, FL 33136, USA

Lipsitz, Stuart Department of Biostatistics, Bioinformatics and Epidemiology, Medical University of South Carolina, Charleston, SC 29425, USA

MacNeill, Ian B. Department of Statistical and Actuarial Sciences, University of Western Ontario, London, Ontario, Canada N6G 1S3
macneill@uwo.ca

Maidenberg, Manuel Association Respirer, 57 rue de la Convention, 75015 Paris, France
Manuel.maidenberg@wanadoo.fr

McHenry, M. Brent Department of Biostatistics, Bioinformatics and Epidemiology, Medical University of South Carolina, Charleston, SC 29425, USA

Mello, F. C. Q. Universidade Federal de Rio de Janeiro, TB Unit-HUCFF/ UFRJ, Rio de Janiero, Brazil

Mesbah, Mounir Université Pierre et Marie Curie, Laboratoire de Statistique Théorique et Appliquée, Bote 158, Bureau 8A25, 175 rue du Chevaleret, 75013 Paris, France
mesbah@ccr.jussieu.fr

Mohanty, S. G. Department of Mathematics and Statistics, McMaster University, Hamilton, Ontario, Canada L8S 4K1
mohanty@mcmaster.ca

Moutou, François Unité d'Epidémiologie, AFSSA LERPAZ, BP 67, 94703 Maisons-Alfort Cedex, France
f.moutou@afssa.fr

Musio, Monica Department of Mathematics and Informatics, Cagliari University, Cagliari, Italy
mmusio@unica.it

Natarajan, Sundar The Department of Medicine, New York University School of Medicine and the VA New York Harbor Healthcare System, New York, NY 10010, USA
sundar.natarajan@med.nyu.edu

Naumova, Elena N. Department of Family Medicine and Community Health, Tufts University School of Medicine, Boston, MA 02111, USA
elena.naumova@tufts.edu

Ng, H. K. T. Department of Statistical Science, Southern Methodist University, Dallas, TX 75275-0332, USA
ngh@mail.smu.edu

Nikulin, M. Mathematical Statistics and Its Applications, BP 26, University Victor Segalen Bordeaux 2, 33076 Bordeaux, France
nikou@sm.u-bordeaux2.fr

Orazio, S. Mathematical Statistics and Its Applications, BP 26, University Victor Segalen Bordeaux 2, 33076 Bordeaux, France

Pastorino, Ugo European Institute of Oncology, Milano, Italy

Pereira, B. B. Post Graduate School of Engineering, Federal University of Rio de Janeiro and Faculty of Medicine and Tuberculosis Research Unit, University of Rio de Janeiro, Rio de Janeiro, Brazil
basilio@nesc.ufrj.br

Pezzella, Francesco   Cancer Research UK Pathology Unit, John Radcliffe Hospital, Oxford, UK

Riley, Richard D.   Centre for Biostatistics and Genetic Epidemiology, 22-28 Department of Health Sciences, University of Leicester, Princess Road West, Leicester, UK
rdr3@le.ac.uk

Roura, P.   Clinical epidemiology and Research Department, Hospital General de Vic 1, Francesc Pla St E., 08500 Vic, Spain
proura@hgv.es

Roux, E.   INSERM U642 (LTSI) Université Rennes 1 Campus Beaulieu, Bât 22, 35042 Rennes, France
rouxemmanuel@free.fr

Santos, A. M.   Department of Mathematics, Federal University of Maranhão, Maranhão, Brazil amirandas@terra.com.br

Sauerbrei, W.   Institute of Medical Biometry, University Hospital Freiburg, Stefan-Meier-Str. 26, 79104 Freiburg, Germany
wfs@imbi.uni-freiburg.de

Sauleau, Erik-A.   Registre des Cancers du Haut-Rhin, 9 rue du Dr Mangeney, BP 1370, 68070 Mulhouse, France
sauleauea@ch-mulhouse.fr

Sébille, Véronique   Faculté de Pharmacie Lab de Biomathématique-Biostatistique, 1 rue Gaston Veil, 44035 Nantes Cedex 01, France
veronique.sebille@univ-nantes.fr

Segala, Claire   SEPIA-Santé, 18 bis, rue du Calvaire, F-56310 Merland, France
sepia@sepia-sante.com

Seixas, J. M.   Signal Processing Laboratory, Federal University of Rio de Janeiro, Rio de Janeiro, Brazil

Seillier-Moiseiwitsch, F.   Department of Biostatistics, Bioinformatics and Biomathematics, Georgetown University Medical Center, Washington, DC 20057-1484, USA
seillier@georgetown.edu

Semenchenko, Ganna V.   Max Planck Institute for Demographic Research, Konrad Zuse Str. 1, 18057 Rostock, Germany
semenchenko@demogr.mpg.de

Sen, P. K. Department of Biostatistics, University of North Carolina, Chapel Hill, NC 27599-7420, USA
pksen@bios.unc.edu

Stallard, Nigel Warwick Medical School, The University of Warwick, Coventry CV4 7AL, UK
n.stallard@warwick.ac.uk

Stärk, K. D. C. Swiss Federal Veterinary Office, Department of Monitoring, P.O. Box CH-3003, Bern, Switzerland
katharina.staerk@bvet.admin.ch

Sun, Jianguo Department of Statistics, University of Missouri, Columbia, MI 65211, USA
tsun@stat.missouri.edu

Sutton, Alex J. Centre for Biostatistics and Genetic Epidemiology, 22-28 Department of Health Sciences, University of Leicester, Princess Road West, Leicester, UK
ajs22@le.ac.uk

Tan, Ming Greenbaum Cancer Center, University of Maryland, Baltimore, MD 21201, USA
ming.tan@umm.edu

Tan, Wai-Yuan Department of Mathematical Sciences, University of Memphis, Memphis, TN 38152, USA
waitan@memphis.edu

Thiessard, F. Université Victor Segalen, 146 rue Léo Saignat, 33076 Bordeaux Cedex, France
Frantz.Thiessard@isped.u-bordeaux2.fr

Todd, Susan Medical and Pharmaceutical Statistics Research Unit, The University of Reading, UK, P.O. Box 240, Earley Gate, Reading RG6 6FN, UK
s.c.todd@reading.ac.uk

Trivella, Marialena Cancer Research, UK Medical Statistics Group Centre for Statistics in Medicine, Wolfson College, Oxford OX2 6UD, UK

Tubert-Bitter, Pascale INSERM Unit 780, Unité de Recherche en Epidémiologie et Biostatistiques, 16 avenue Paul Vaillant Couturier, 94807 Villejuif Cedex, France
tubert@vjf.inserm.fr

Wienke, Andreas Institute of Medical Epidemiology, Biostatistics and Informatics, Martin-Luther-University Halle-Wittenberg, Halle, Germany
andreas.wienke@medizin.uni-halle.de

Willems, Sylvie Unité de neuropsychologie Faculté de Psychologie et de Sciences de l'Education, Université de Liège, B33 B-4000 Liège, Belgium
swillems@ulg.ac.be

Wittes, Janet Statistics Collaborative, 1625 Massachusetts Ave. NW, Suite 600, Washington, DC 20036, USA
janet@statcollab.com

Woolson, Robert F. Department of Biostatistics, Bioinformatics and Epidemiology Medical, University of South Carolina, Charleston, SC 29425, USA
woolson@musc.edu

Xiong, Xiaoping Department of Biostatistics, St. Jude Children's Research Hospital, Memphis, TN 38105-2794, USA
xiaoping.xiong@stjude.org

Yáñez, A. Clinical Epidemiology and Research Department, VIC General Hospital, 08500 Vic, Spain
ayanez@hgv.es

Yashin, Anatoli I. Demographic Studies, Duke University, Durham, NC 27708-0408, USA
Yashin@cds.duke.edu

Zhang, P. Department of Mathematical Sciences, University of Memphis, Memphis, TN 38152, USA

Zhu, Chao Department of Statistics, University of Missouri, Columbia, MI 65211, USA

List of Tables

Table 1.1   Problems encountered with data sets in PILC study   **10**

Table 2.1   Estimated hazard ratios (HR), AIC, and BIC in Cox models: Results from the univariate Cox model (no adjustment), the full model and a selected model obtained by backward elimination with $\alpha = 0.05$ (BE(0.05)) assuming (A) a (log-)linear relationship for continuous covariates and (B) categorising continuous covariates as predefined in the first analysis of the GBSG-2 study   **26**

Table 2.2   Selected prognostic markers, AIC, and BIC for different model selection strategies. Included markers marked by dots   **27**

Table 2.3   Estimated hazard ratios (HR) for prognostic subgroups derived in the GBSG-2 study by using the selected Cox model with categorised covariates (COX) and a modification of the simple tree displayed in Figure 2.2B (CART*). Validation of the HRs in the Freiburg-DNA study   **32**

Table 2.4   Summary of important issues for the analysis of single prognostic marker studies   **34**

Table 4.1   Posterior probability that the event rate is less than π as a function of various prior distributions   **72**

Table 5.1   Fuzzy characterization of the variables   **82**

Table 5.2   Average and standard deviation (in brackets), over the 1000 simulated datasets, of the prior parameters of Du-Mouchel's model, estimated by means of maximum likelihood   **88**

Table 6.1   Predictors of the number of absence spells. Results from Poisson regression with random person effects   **102**

Table 6.2   Results from Poisson regression with random person ef-   **103**
             fects including (i) the observed raw sum score, (ii) esti-
             mated values for each person, or (iii) latent covariate (cf.
             (6.6)) as predictors. All analyses are adjusted for effect
             of gender, age, and job group
Table 6.3   Predictors of the number of absence spells. Effect of the   **104**
             latent covariate skill discretion on job group level

Table 7.1   Type I error probability for the sequential probability ra-   **117**
             tio test (SPRT) and the triangular test (TT) (nominal
             $\alpha = \beta = 0.05$). Data are $\hat{\alpha}$ (standard errors)
Table 7.2   Power for the sequential probability ratio test (SPRT)   **117**
             and the triangular test (TT) (nominal $\alpha = \beta = 0.05$).
             Data are $1 - \hat{\beta}$ (standard errors)
Table 7.3   Average sample number (ASN) and 90th percentile (P90)   **118**
             of the number of patients required to reach a conclusion
             under H_0 for the sequential probability ratio test (SPRT)
             and the triangular test (TT) (nominal $\alpha = \beta = 0.05$)
Table 7.4   Average sample number (ASN) and 90th percentile (P90)   **118**
             of the number of patients required to reach a conclusion
             under H_1 for the sequential probability ratio test (SPRT)
             and the triangular test (TT) (nominal $\alpha = \beta = 0.05$)
Table 7.5   Type I error probability for the sequential probability ra-   **119**
             tio test (SPRT) and the triangular test (TT) for different
             amounts of items with one overlapping category (nominal
             $\alpha = \beta = 0.05$). Overlap is the proportion of overlapping
             category. Data are $\hat{\alpha}$ (standard errors)
Table 7.6   Power for the sequential probability ratio test (SPRT)   **119**
             and the triangular test (TT) for different amounts of
             items with one overlapping category (nominal $\alpha = \beta =
             0.05$). Overlap is the proportion of overlapping category.
             Data are $1 - \hat{\beta}$ (standard errors)
Table 7.7   Average sample number (ASN) and 90th percentile (P90)   **120**
             of the number of patients required to reach a conclusion
             under H_0 for the sequential probability ratio test (SPRT)
             and the triangular test (TT) for different amounts of
             items with one overlapping category (nominal $\alpha = \beta =
             0.05$). Overlap is the proportion of overlapping category.
             Data are ASN/P90

Table 7.8   Average sample number (ASN) and 90th percentile (P90)   **120**
of the number of patients required to reach a conclusion
under H_1 for the sequential probability ratio test (SPRT)
and the triangular test (TT) for different amounts of
items with one overlapping category (nominal $\alpha = \beta =$
0.05). Overlap is the proportion of overlapping category.
Data are ASN/P90

Table 9.1 (4×3) table from answers to the two health status ques-   **140**
tions from the parent questionnaire from the childhood
leukemia study

Table 9.2 (4×5) table from answers to the two health status ques-   **141**
tions from the 2002 United States National General Social
Survey (GSS)

Table 9.3 (2×2) table of cell counts at cutpoints j and k **143**

Table 9.4 (2×2) table of probabilities at cutpoints j and k **143**

Table 9.5   Table of six Kappa coefficients at all cutpoints using the   **145**
childhood leukemia study. Estimates and 95% confidence
intervals obtained from SAS Proc Freq

Table 9.6 (2×2) table corresponding to $\hat{\kappa}_{22} = 0.463$ in Table 9.5   **145**

Table 9.7   Table of 12 Kappa coefficients at all cutpoints using the   **146**
2002 United States National General Social Survey. Es-
timates and 95% confidence intervals obtained from SAS
Proc Freq

Table 9.8 (2×2) table corresponding to $\hat{\kappa}_{23} = 0.858$ in Table 9.7   **146**

Table 10.1   Correlated gamma frailty model applied to breast cancer   **158**
data

Table 10.2   Correlated gamma frailty model with observed covariates   **159**

Table 10.3   Correlated gamma frailty model without and with a cure   **162**
fraction

Table 11.1   Risk coefficient estimates for model 11.1   **173**

Table 12.1   Lifespan characteristics in the groups of nematodes   **187**
Caenorhabditis elegans subjected to heat shock of different duration

Table 12.2   Parameter estimates of the semiparametric model of het-   **189**
erogeneous mortality for groups of nematodes *Caenorhab-
ditis elegans* subjected to heat shock of different duration

Table 14.1 N_d behavior for various values of d ($\beta_0 = 1$, censorship   **214**
              rate: 48%)
Table 14.2 $N_{0.5}$ with respect to β_0 **215**

Table 16.1   Model comparison for Pima Indians data   **255**
Table 16.2   Test set classification error   **256**
Table 16.3   Proportion of time the hard tree test set classification   **256**
              error (E_H) is greater than the soft node test set classifi-
              cation error (E_S)

Table 17.1   French center sample   **264**
Table 17.2   Proportion of the six regimens: overall and by center   **273**

Table 18.1   Composition of the training and testing sets selected   **283**
Table 18.2   Efficiencies of classification   **284**

Table 19.1   Estimates of the parameters of four subjects   **300**

Table 20.1   The observed numbers of HIV RNA virus load of an HIV-   **313**
              infected patient
Table 20.2   The history of drug treatment   **314**
Table 20.3   The estimate of parameters   **315**

Table 21.1   Differences that affect the assessments of safety and effi-   **331**
              cacy throughout product/intervention development

Table 22.1   Type I error rate estimates for $n = 50$ and $n = 100$ **343**
              patients in each group, for the association parameter $\alpha =$
              2 and $\alpha = 5$, obtained from 1000 simulations. *LR* and
              ST refer to the MULTIN tests for the likelihood ratio
              ordering and the stochastic ordering
Table 22.2   Power estimates for the one-sided comparison of treat-   **344**
              ment A versus treatment B, with $n = 50$ patients in each
              group, based on 1000 simulations. See Table 22.1 for the
              column names
Table 22.3   Power estimates for the one-sided comparison of treat-   **345**
              ment A versus treatment B, with $n = 100$ patients in
              each group, based on 1000 simulations. See Table 22.1
              for the column names

Table 24.1   Bias and MSE of the estimators under biased-coin design   **372**
              with $N = 15$

Table 24.2   Bias and MSE of the estimators under biased-coin design **373**
with $N = 25$

Table 24.3   Bias and MSE of the estimators under biased-coin design **374**
with $N = 35$

Table 24.4   Bias and MSE of the estimators under biased-coin design **375**
with $N = 50$

Table 24.5   T-Bias and T-MSE of the estimators under biased-coin **376**
design with $N = 15$

Table 24.6   T-Bias and T-MSE of the estimators under biased-coin **377**
design with $N = 25$

Table 24.7   T-Bias and T-MSE of the estimators under biased-coin **378**
design with $N = 35$

Table 24.8   T-Bias and T-MSE of the estimators under biased-coin **379**
design with $N = 50$

Table 24.9   Ratio of MSE for ISLOG to biased coin design **380**

Table 24.10   Ratio of T-MSE for ISLOG to biased coin design **380**

Table 24.11   Ratio of MSE for MMLE to biased coin design **381**

Table 24.12   Ratio of T-MSE for MMLE to biased coin design **381**

Table 24.13   Ratio of TE to biased coin design **382**

Table 24.14   Ratio of TOX to biased coin design **382**

Table 26.1   Critical values for the Stallard and Todd (2003) and **411**
Bauer and Kieser (1999) designs for the galantamine trial

Table 26.2   Observed test statistics for the galantamine trial **412**

Table 27.1   Boundary coefficient a for given K and ρ **422**

Table 27.2   OC for the adaptive SCPRT with unknown variance **428**

Table 28.1   Characteristics of seasonal curves for ambient tempera- **448**
ture and *Salmonella* cases

Table 29.1   Estimation of parameters for the three models **458**

Table 30.1   Summary of the introduction of the different pollutants **480**

Table 30.2   Summary of the test comparing the model including a **480**
linear term and the one with a LOESS function

Table 30.3   Summary of the estimates of the final models **482**

Table 30.4   Summary of the estimates of the final models **483**

Table 31.1   Contingency table summarizing the observed characters   **493**
              (either amino acids or nucleotides) at two generic posi-
              tions

Table 31.2   Percentages of statistics falling above given percentiles of   **502**
              the χ^2-distribution with 4 degrees of freedom. * indi-
              cates that an entry is farther than 2 S.D.s away from the
              expected percentage

Table 31.3   Percentages of statistics falling above given percentile of   **503**
              the χ^2-distribution with 9 degrees of freedom. * indi-
              cates that an entry is farther than 2 S.D.s away from the
              expected percentage

Table 31.4   Results of analysis with new statistic and other ap-   **504**
              proaches. Q denotes the proposed statistic. Entries are
              left blank when the test statistic does not reach the 0.99
              significance level. * indicates that the test statistic falls
              above the 99.5 percentile, ** above the 99.9 percentile,
              and *** outside the support of the reference distribution

Table 31.5   Data for positions 12 and 18   **507**
Table 31.6   Data for positions 14 and 19   **508**

Table 32.1   Expert opinion: Factors with negative effects, probability   **523**
              of occurrence, and consequences for the end product

Table 32.2   Probability of contamination above threshold limits   **525**

Table 33.1   Results of the combination of the different qualitative ap-   **533**
              preciations used in the qualitative risk analysis (Nu =
              Null, N = Negligible, L = Low, M = Moderate, and H =
              High)

Table 33.2   Global and reduced risk appreciation following the conta-   **535**
              mination route by *Coxiella burnetii* from small domestic
              ruminants [Anonymous (2004)]

List of Figures

Figure 2.1   Different risk functions for the effect of age obtained in   **24**
              the GBSG-2 study: categorised risk function (solid line),
              linear risk function (dashed line), and fractional polyno-
              mial (dotted line)

Figure 2.2   Classification and regression trees obtained for the   **29**
              GBSG-2 study: (A) no P-value correction and all cut-
              points allowed (no prespecification) and (B) with P-value
              correction and prespecification of cutpoints

Figure 2.3   Kaplan–Meier estimates of event-free survival probabil-   **31**
              ities for the prognostic subgroups derived from a Cox
              model with categorised covariates (COX) and the simple
              tree displaced in Figure 2.2B (CART)

Figure 3.1   Forest plot for the $MYCN$ overall survival (OS) meta-   **43**
              analysis from the neuroblastoma review including the 45
              studies that allowed the $\log_e$(hazard ratio) and its stan-
              dard error to be estimated [Riley $et\ al.$ (2004a)]. N.B.
              There were 107 other studies which provided $MYCN$ re-
              sults or IPD in relation to prognosis but not in sufficient
              detail to allow the $\log_e$(hazard ratio) and its standard er-
              ror to be obtained; hence, the meta-analysis pooled haz-
              ard ratio result below must be treated with caution, as it
              is not possible to include much of the overall evidence in
              the evidence synthesis

Figure 3.2   Types of prognostic marker studies, as suggested by Alt-   **44**
              man and Lyman (1998)

Figure 3.3   Funnel plot of the overall survival $\log_e$(hazard ratio) es-   **47**
              timates for $MYCN$ with Begg's pseudo 95% confidence
              limits [Begg and Mazumdar (1994)]

Figure 3.4   Key areas where improved research and better statisti-   **50**
              cal practice are needed within primary prognostic marker
              studies

Figure 3.5   Summary of the main problems preventing clinically use-   **53**
                ful meta-analysis of summary statistics extracted from
                published prognostic marker studies

Figure 3.6   Summary of the main potential benefits of having individ-   **53**
                ual patient data (IPD) for a meta-analysis of prognostic
                marker studies

Figure 4.1   Power of the sentinel event test as a function of R, the   **69**
                ratio of the mean time between events under the null and
                alternative hypotheses

Figure 5.1   Drug life cycle   **79**
Figure 5.2   Trapezoidal membership function of a fuzzy subset F of   **81**
                the variable V, and fuzzy membership value for an ob-
                served value x
Figure 5.3   Fuzzy rule base for the reporting probability determina-   **83**
                tion. In each cell of the table are given the conclusions
                associated with a serious event (upper part of the cell)
                and to a mild event (lower part of the cell). VH is for
                'Very high,' H for 'High,' M for 'Medium,' L for 'Low,'
                and VL for 'Very low'
Figure 5.4   Principle of the fuzzy reasoning implementation and val-   **84**
                ues used for defuzzification
Figure 5.5   Sequential data generation process for one (drug i, event **85**
                j) couple
Figure 5.6   Reporting probabilities (a) and cumulative number of re-   **87**
                ports (b), (c), and (d)

Figure 6.1   Overview of the relation between variables in the regres-   **99**
                sion model

Figure 7.1   Stopping boundaries based on the triangular test (TT)   **116**
                for $\alpha = \beta = 0.05$ with an effect size (ES) of 0.5

Figure 11.1   Mean profile of functional status   **169**
Figure 11.2   Mean profile of nutritional status   **170**
Figure 11.3   Multistate model with two intermediate events to de-   **171**
                scribe all possible paths from admission to death
Figure 11.4   Multistate model with one intermediate event to describe   **172**
                all possible paths from admission to death
Figure 11.5   Predicted residual survival curves for patients two months **175**
                after admission

Figure 11.6   Predicted residual survival curves for patients four   **176**
               months after admission
Figure 11.7   Probability of death during the next six months as a func-   **177**
               tion of the time t from admission

Figure 12.1   Dependence of survival function for the experimental   **185**
               group on changes in the baseline hazard
Figure 12.2   Dependence of survival function for the experimental   **186**
               group on changes in the frailty distribution
Figure 12.3   (a) Estimated baseline hazard for the control group of   **189**
               nematodes compared to the estimates of observed hazard
               and (b) empirical and modeled conditional survival func-
               tions for experimental groups of worms (survival func-
               tion for the control group is approximated by gamma–
               Gompertz model with parameters $\alpha = 4.4\text{e-}4$ (3e-4; 5e-4),
               $\beta = 0.42$ (0.4; 0.43), $\sigma^2 = 0.83$ (0.81; 0.85))

Figure 15.1   Estimated standard deviations with $b = 1$ **231**
Figure 15.2   Estimated standard deviations with $b = 2$ **232**
Figure 15.3   Estimated survival function and 95% confidence bands   **233**

Figure 16.1   ANN and prediction models   **242**
Figure 16.2   Linear predictor   **244**
Figure 16.3   Additive predictor   **246**
Figure 16.4   Prediction tree and its associated ANN   **247**
Figure 16.5   Alternative architecture: hierarchy of experts   **249**
Figure 16.6   Example of soft tree   **251**
Figure 16.7   Soft tree for Pima Indians data   **254**
Figure 16.8   Hard tree for Pima Indians data   **255**
Figure 16.9   Hard tree for car mileage data   **257**
Figure 16.10   Soft tree for car mileage data   **258**
Figure 16.11   Extended soft tree   **258**

Figure 17.1   Initialization of PCA   **267**
Figure 17.2   Kohonen map   **267**
Figure 17.3   Relation between center and regimens   **269**
Figure 17.4   The six regimens by Zoom Stars   **272**

Figure 18.1   Example of cross-validation for $k = 10$ **280**
Figure 18.2   Relevance for data description using 12 variables   **285**

Figure 19.1   Viral load data for ACTG 315 study   **291**

Figure 19.2   Illustrative plot of three segments used to explore viral   **293**
               load trajectory
Figure 19.3   Diagnostic plots. Left panel: the number of MCMC iter-   **299**
               ations and posterior means; right panel: the densities of
               the posterior means
Figure 19.4   The estimated population mean curve obtained by using   **300**
               ACTG 315 data and Bayesian approach. The observed
               values are indicated by plus
Figure 19.5   Profiles of four arbitrarily selected patients for ACTG 315 **301**
               data. The dotted and solid lines are estimated individual
               and population curves. The observed values are indicated
               by the circle signs

Figure 20.1   Plots showing the estimated numbers of infectious and   **312**
               noninfectious virus, and productively HIV-infected CD4
               T cells per ml of blood

Figure 22.1   The five sets of points (X, Y) on the $Q \times Q$ square. Points   **339**
               $\mathbf{a}(X, Y)$, $\mathbf{a}'(X', Y)$, and $\mathbf{a}''(X, Y')$ illustrate the DISCR
               method. They satisfy $X' > X$ and $Y' < Y$

Figure 23.1   Upper limit of the $100(1 - \alpha)\%$ one-sided confidence in- **353**
               terval for the true underlying adverse event rate, π, for
               increasing sample sizes when zero events of interests are
               observed
Figure 23.2   Comparisons of upper limit of a 90% Bayesian credible   **355**
               interval for values of a and b

Figure 24.1   Dose–response curves with parameters $a = -6.0$, $b = 1.0$ **383**
Figure 24.2   Dose–response curves with parameters $a = -4.5$, $b = 0.5$ **383**
Figure 24.3   Dose–response curves with parameters $a = -3.0$, $b = 0.5$ **384**
Figure 24.4   Dose–response curves with parameters $a = -6.0$, $b = 0.5$ **384**
Figure 24.5   Dose–response curves with parameters $a = -1.5$, $b = 0.25$ **385**

Figure 25.1   Comparison of recruitment times. $n = 160, N = 20$.   **393**
               Competitive time: **1** – fixed rates with $\lambda = 2$; **2** – gamma
               rates, $\mathbf{E}[\lambda] = 2, \mathbf{Var}[\lambda] = 0.5$. Balanced time: **3** – fixed
               rates with $\lambda = 2$; **4** – gamma rates, $\mathbf{E}[\lambda] = 2, \mathbf{Var}[\lambda] = 0.5$

Figure 26.1   Group-sequential stopping boundary and sample paths   **412**
               for the galantamine trial with efficient score, Z, plotted
               against observed Fisher's information, V

Figure 27.1   Sequential test statistic S_t simulated under H_0: $\mu_x - \mu_y = 0$ **425**

Figure 27.2   Sequential test statistic S_t simulated under H_a: $\mu_x - \mu_y = 0.3$ **426**

Figure 27.3   Clinical trial with historical control: survival curves at different looks   **431**

Figure 28.1   Characteristics of seasonality: Graphical depiction and definition for daily time series of exposure (ambient temperature) and outcome (disease incidence) variables   **439**

Figure 28.2   Seasonal curve for ambient temperature in temperate climate of Massachusetts, USA. Solid line is the fitted mean-value function   **445**

Figure 28.3   Seasonal curve for *Salmonella* cases in Massachusetts, USA. Solid line is the fitted mean-value function   **446**

Figure 28.4   Temporal pattern in daily *Salmonella* cases (Z-axis) with respect to ambient temperature values in C° (Y-axis) over time (X-axis)   **447**

Figure 29.1   Standardized incidence ratios for lung cancer by geographical unit   **460**

Figure 29.2   Mapping of spatial effects for lung cancer (exponential of the values)   **461**

Figure 30.1   Daily number of hospital consultations for bronchiolitis   **476**

Figure 30.2   Autocorrelations of the daily number of hospital consultations for bronciolitis   **476**

Figure 30.3   Residuals of model (30.14)   **478**

Figure 30.4   Partial autocorrelation of the residuals after introduction of the time   **478**

Figure 30.5   LOESS function corresponding to the time   **479**

Figure 30.6   LOESS function for the minimal temperature   **479**

Figure 30.7   Comparison between LOESS function and linear term for $pm10A5$ **481**

Figure 32.1   The four elements of risk analysis. [Source: OIE, Terrestrial Animal Health Code (2003)]   **520**

Figure 32.2   Risk network, origin, and identification of hazards in dairy product manufacture   **522**

Figure 32.3   Qualitative assessment of hard cheese. The probability of contamination   **524**

Figure 32.4   Qualitative assessment of yoghurt and curdled milk. The   **524**
                probability of contamination
Figure 33.1   The components of risk estimation   **529**
Figure 33.2   Presentation of the global chart of the analysis. [From   **530**
                OIE (2001)]

Advances in Statistical Methods
for the Health Sciences

PART I

PROGNOSTIC STUDIES AND GENERAL EPIDEMIOLOGY

1

Systematic Review of Multiple Studies of Prognosis: The Feasibility of Obtaining Individual Patient Data

Douglas G. Altman,[1] **Marialena Trivella,**[1] **Francesco Pezzella,**[2] **Adrian L. Harris,**[3] **and Ugo Pastorino**[4]

[1]*Cancer Research UK/NHS Centre for Statistics in Medicine, Oxford, UK*
[2]*Cancer Research UK Pathology Unit, John Radcliffe Hospital, Oxford, UK*
[3]*Cancer Research UK Oncology Unit, Churchill Hospital, Oxford, UK*
[4]*Istituto Nazionale Tumori, Milan, Italy*

Abstract: Studies of prognosis have received rather little attention by those carrying out systematic reviews. Such reviews are increasingly being attempted but the poor quality of published 'primary' studies leads to serious difficulties. Thus there have been calls for such reviews to be based on individual patient data (IPD) but such studies are as yet rare.

We consider the advantages of IPD for reviews of prognostic variables and describe in detail a systematic review of microvessel density counts as a prognostic variable for patients with non-small cell lung cancer. We show that such a study is feasible, but note that it may not be cost-effective to attempt to obtain all relevant data.

Keywords and phrases: Prognostic markers, systematic review, meta-analysis, individual patient data

1.1 Introduction

Prognostic studies include clinical studies of variables predictive of future events as well as epidemiological studies of aetiological risk factors. While they often explore several factors simultaneously, many studies examine the prognostic importance of a single specified variable, such as a tumour marker. Such studies are the focus of this paper.

The number of published prognostic studies continues to grow, but unfortunately additional studies have often led to more confusion than clarification [Simon and Altman (1994)]. As multiple similar studies accumulate, it becomes increasingly important to identify and evaluate all of the relevant work in order to develop a more reliable overall assessment [Altman and Lyman (1998)]. As with other types of research, all the relevant evidence is best assessed in a systematic review; see Altman (2001) for a systematic identification and structured appraisal of multiple research studies of the same topic. (Such studies are often called meta-analyses, but we prefer to reserve that term for the statistical synthesis of the results of several studies, as discussed below.)

Systematic reviews help both to clarify scientific findings and identify gaps in the literature. At their best, they may also contribute to policy making and adoption of new clinical practices. Compared with randomised controlled trials (RCTs) and epidemiological studies of risk factors, studies of prognosis have received rather little attention by those carrying out systematic reviews. Such studies are increasingly being attempted. Although our main emphasis in this chapter will be on studies of tumour markers, reviews of prognostic studies are also seen in other medical fields and in other types of research including epidemiological studies; see Kuijpers *et al.* (2004), Brocklehurst and French (1998), Ebell, White, and Weismantel (2000), Ray (1998), Sauerbrei, Blettner, and Royston (2001), and Kosmas, Tatsioni, and Ioannidis (2004).

When there are several published studies for a single marker, they frequently yield conflicting results. Broadly speaking, the inconsistent findings may be due to variation in some or all of patient characteristics, laboratory methods, and methodological quality (including data analysis), as well as chance variation. It is important to consider carefully the details of each study as misleading results from individual studies may distort the results of any subsequent meta-analyses. Unfortunately, the generally poor standards of reporting in published articles seriously impedes efforts to make sense of the literature [Riley *et al.* (2003)].

The key steps of a systematic review are: (1) define a clear and concise question, (2) define explicit inclusion and exclusion criteria, (3) identify potentially relevant studies (using a defined search strategy), (4) select eligible studies, (5) appraise methodological quality using standardised criteria, (6) extract information about methods of each study and its results, (7) analyse and present results of all the studies (including, if appropriate, a statistical synthesis using meta-analysis and investigation of possible reasons for heterogeneous results across studies), and (8) interpret the combined results; see Selvin *et al.* (2004).

The specific features of prognostic investigations are such that, however desirable it might be, applying these general principles is not straightforward. Particular concerns include the inability to extract adequate information about the details of how the study was done, inconsistent methods of data analysis (especially relating to cutpoints and adjustment for other variables), inadequate reporting of the results of the study (linked to the specific issues for summarising survival data), and the likelihood of publication bias. This last point should not be underestimated; increasingly systematic reviews are showing a relation between sample size and observed effect, strongly suggestive of publication bias.

Such an effect has been strongly suggested, for example, in recent reviews of thymidylate synthase expression in colorectal cancer [see Popat, Matakidou, and Houlston (2004)] and glycosylated haemoglobin and cardiovascular disease in diabetes mellitus [see Selvin *et al.* (2004)]. As Simon (2001) wrote: ". . . the literature is probably cluttered with false-positive studies that would not have been submitted or published if the results had come out differently." The consequence is that published studies will tend to overestimate the prognostic value of tumour markers.

The difficulties of carrying out a systematic review using published data have been widely recognised; see Altman and Lyman (1998), Altman (2001), Riley *et al.* (2006), Williamson *et al.* (2002), and Parmar, Torri, and Stewart (1998). Such problems seriously undermine the key goal of a systematic review to provide reliable evidence. It is not unusual for systematic reviewers to conclude that a set of prognostic studies was either too diverse or too poor to allow a meaningful meta-analysis. Several authors have noted that reviews of published studies are of limited value and that instead reviewers should attempt to acquire the individual patient data from each study; see Altman and Lyman (1998), Altman (2001), Riley *et al.* (2006), Piedbois and Buyse (2004), and Blettner *et al.* (1999).

The vast majority of systematic reviews are based on published studies, primarily because of the relative ease with which they can be done (even though it is not that easy) [Piedbois and Buyse (2004)]. The alternative of obtaining the individual patient data (IPD) from multiple studies [Clarke and Stewart (2000), Stewart and Clarke (1995), and Oxman, Clarke, and Stewart (1995)] is in principle far more valuable but also potentially problematic.

We believe that there have been very few IPD systematic reviews of prognostic marker studies. Here we consider the issues that arise when carrying out an IPD systematic review, based on our experience of carrying out such a study in patients with lung cancer. Although it was clear that the IPD approach was desirable, we aimed to assess whether such a study was feasible.

1.2 Systematic Review Based on Individual Patient Data

The broad reasons in favour of IPD reviews together with the principal benefits over reviews based on published studies are summarised by Riley *et al.* (2006). Key advantages include being able to analyse the data in a consistent manner and reducing (if not eliminating) the effect of publication bias. Noteworthy disadvantages are the considerable resources needed to carry out such a review and difficulties encountered in obtaining the data sets, particularly if they were created a long time ago.

The general idea of an IPD systematic review is that the raw data for each individual are obtained directly from the researchers/data owners irrespective of whether a particular study has been published. These data are checked and validated, and ideally are brought up to date (i.e., if extended follow up information is available). The data are (re-)analysed centrally by the review group using consistent statistical methods, including meta-analysis if appropriate.

IPD meta-analyses have most famously been carried out by the Early Breast Cancer Trialists Collaborative Group (1998) when evaluating the impact of therapies for early breast cancer. Although the IPD approach has been used increasingly for reviewing results of RCTs, even here such studies remain in a small minority because of the resources needed. By contrast, there seem to have been very few attempts to carry out IPD reviews on prognostic studies; see Look *et al.* (2002).

For IPD reviews of trials, rather than simply asking each group to provide their data, a recommended approach is to establish a multicentre collaborative framework; see Stewart and Clarke (1995). Such a partnership, including group authorship of the resulting article(s), is more likely to lead to obtaining the raw data from as many relevant studies as possible.

We note the importance of investing adequate time at the outset in carefully planning the IPD systematic review, including producing a detailed study protocol. Among key issues to be decided are developing strategies to identify studies, specifying study inclusion criteria, drawing up a careful list of variables to be requested, developing a simple and flexible data collection procedure, and prespecifying methods of statistical analysis.

1.3 A Case Study: Microvessel Density in Non-Small Cell Lung Cancer

The Prognosis in Lung Cancer (PILC) project was setup as an international cooperative group aiming to clarify the area of prognostic factors in lung cancer. In the first instance, it was decided to examine microvessel density counts (MVD) (a measure of angiogenesis) as a potential prognostic factor in non-small cell lung cancer (NSCLC); see Trivella *et al.* (2006).

A pilot study was first carried out to identify published studies. Online searches of Medline and CancerLit databases and a trawl of the references included in identified publications initially revealed 23 eligible studies investigating MVD as a prognostic factor in NSCLC. The key words used for the search were: lung cancer, lung carcinomas, angiogenesis, neovascularisation, and microvessel.

As well as meeting some clinical criteria, studies were required to have used the median or mean MVD as a cutpoint to define patients with high or low vascularisation, and to have reported overall survival (%) after at least five years of follow-up. Studies that reported results on partially overlapping sets of data were excluded.

Despite these rather loose criteria only 9 out of the 23 papers (39%) provided suitable data for inclusion in a meta-analysis. In total, data relating to 1573 patients were analysed; 691 classified as high and 882 as low MVD. The Mantel–Haenszel method was used to perform a meta-analysis of the relative risk (RR) from each study. The pooled overall estimate of risk showed a lower risk of death at five years (RR 0.77, 99% CI 0.68 to 0.88; $P < 0.001$) for patients with lower MVD. However, there was highly significant heterogeneity (variability between estimates) among the 9 studies.

The PILC steering committee comprised an oncologist, a surgeon, a pathologist, and two statisticians, one of whom worked full time on the project. The committee provided general advice on the project as well as detailed clinical and pathological expertise. A key objective was to explore the feasibility and practical difficulties of doing individual patient data (IPD) systematic reviews in studies of prognosis. In this chapter, we thus focus on the logistic issues as they provide the greatest challenges and take the majority of the total time of such a project. The findings of the analysis will be presented elsewhere.

In the following sections, we discuss general issues and then describe how we dealt with these issues in PILC.

1.3.1 Identifying studies (data sets) and obtaining the data

For systematic reviews based on published data, it is generally the aim to include as many studies as possible. For IPD systematic reviews, it is natural to adopt the same philosophy. However, identifying all relevant studies and obtaining the data can be very time-consuming, especially if efforts are made to obtain unpublished data, so that the goal of including data from all relevant studies may often be impossible to achieve.

The natural first step is to carry out a careful search of electronic databases for relevant studies. It is advisable not to rely only on PubMed; other databases may be fruitful. Strategies for searching for prognostic studies have been described by McKibbon *et al.* (1995). However, in the present context, searching needs to be more comprehensive than just searching for published results as the aim here is to identify groups who might have relevant data. Thus, for example, it would be useful also to identify published studies of the comparison of assays or methods of measuring the marker of interest in patients with the disease of interest.

Emphasis should be placed on also trying to identify and include as many unpublished studies as possible, to try to reduce the impact of publication bias. Finding unpublished studies is not easy. An unpublished prognostic 'study' may be merely a set of data sitting on a computer, possibly with little documentation. Indeed, their existence may well be nearly forgotten.

Unpublished studies can be identified through a variety of strategies including asking personal contacts, advertising the project on the Internet, on email lists, or at conferences, and writing to appropriate departments. It is particularly relevant to ask groups who are known to have relevant data if they know of other groups with similar data.

Once potential collaborators have been identified, the reviewers should provide a detailed protocol of the study as well as any relevant and/or helpful information that may persuade them to participate and offer their data. They should also be made aware of future authorship arrangements and be assured that their data contribution will be used in a responsible and confidential manner.

Even after groups have agreed to collaborate, there may be some delay in acquiring all the data. It pays to be persistent and polite and when possible to send regular reminders to those who have failed to respond by the requested deadline. An easy-to-use reply form might also increase the response rate. The multinational approach to such a study may also introduce language difficulties. It is important to establish good relationships and effective ways of communication with each potential collaborator from a very early stage. Occasional newsletters may be helpful, reporting on the overall progress of the project.

The few previous IPD studies of prognostic factors seem to have begun with a collaborative network already in place; see Look *et al.* (2002). For PILC, however, there was no existing group. We believed that relatively few groups worldwide had studied microvessel density counts in non-small lung cancer, so our intention was to identify all such studies done anywhere and try to obtain individual patient data from as many research centres as possible, regardless of whether the studies had been published. Careful searching of the published literature combined with a network of personal contacts revealed a number of research groups around the world working on lung cancer. Also, the project was presented at an international conference abroad. A speculative letter was drawn up presenting a draft proposal of the project and inviting research groups to collaborate as well as asking the recipients to forward the letter to anyone they thought appropriate.

Of the 38 groups initially contacted, 28 (73%) replied positively, but one group could not participate due to lack of resources. There was no response from the remaining 10 centres (some of which may not have been reliably identified). The 28 groups that were willing to participate were sent a second letter requesting their data; 18 (67%) of the centres had appropriate data. Ultimately, 17 centres were able to supply the required data within the (very flexible) deadline, giving data for about 3200 patients. To safeguard the project against possible accusations of irresponsible use of data and to ensure that collaborators felt at ease with the way their data would be treated, at least one investigator in each group was asked to sign a consent form.

1.3.2   Checking the data

Obtaining individual patient data from each collaborating group opens a new phase of the study. It is essential also to gain a full understanding about how each study was carried out, including details of methods of measurement and coding of key variables. These simple steps mask several common difficulties, so that checking all the data sets can be a very slow process.

Even the simplest data checking procedures may reveal inconsistencies that would otherwise have gone undetected. For example, a patient coded as alive in one field might by mistake have a date of death entered elsewhere in the data set and thus they could be misanalysed in a survival analysis. When data are conflicting, it is necessary to seek a resolution from the data owner.

To facilitate data checking in PILC, a 'Data Characteristics Form' was sent to each group requesting information on a series of key questions regarding data collection procedures, criteria for inclusion of patients, and details of the laboratory methods used for obtaining the data. The information gathered proved invaluable for checking and validating the data, and provided an understanding of the structure of each data set. As was expected, however, the standardisation process was far from straightforward. Table 1.1 lists some of the most profound problems encountered. For data sets that were compiled a long time ago, it will be hard (at best) to resolve questions about the data, such as contradictory fields or invalid codes.

Direct communication with the data owners means that it is possible to resolve errors and misunderstandings concerning the collection, coding, and storage of the data. In fact, this is one of the greatest advantages of IPD meta-analysis over systematic review of only published studies. Also, older data sets might have been in the meantime updated, so the corrected/updated data can be used.

A detailed journal was kept of PILC's daily activity. This exercise, although time consuming, proved invaluable given the complex process of checking multiple data sets over a long period. A key part of the cleaning and preparation of each dataset was the implementation of standardised coding of variables common to all PILC data sets, without which sensible analysis would have been impossible. Particular issues arose in relation to the MVD measurements, as outlined in the next section.

After data checking, an 'Individual Profile' for each data set was prepared based on information extracted from the Data Characteristics Forms and included simple descriptive and basic statistical analysis. These profiles were sent

Table 1.1: Problems encountered with data sets in PILC study

During visual inspection and basic checking of the data sets

- In a few data sets, for some patients the disease-free survival time was larger than the total survival.

- In one data set, the sex of the patient was not available and had to be determined from the patient's first name.

- Very often, the survival time had been calculated manually and many inaccuracies were observed.

- The variable for cancer stage was calculated wrongly on a number of records.

- Numerous live patients had a date of death recorded.

- While dealing with numerical errors, it was discovered that some records in question should not have been included in the database in the first place. The most common reason was that the patient had not undergone surgery but only had a biopsy performed.

- Dead patients were coded as "alive" because the cause of death was not related to the lung cancer.

- On one occasion whilst enquiring about a numerical mistake, the data owner discovered that his data were 'randomised;' in a sorting attempt in Excel, only half the columns were sorted.

- Different centres use the numbers '0' and '9' in different ways. For instance, in some data sets '0' MVD means it is missing whereas in others it means that no vessels were identified in the slide.

From the individual profiles

- The data distributions were different from what the researchers expected, indicating errors in the data.

- The shapes of the summary Kaplan–Meier curves prompted researchers to recheck their data and correct errors.

---

back to the centres to ensure that all the information had been correctly understood and interpreted. As a consequence, some further details were amended.

1.3.3 MVD measurements

Particular issues arose in the PILC study relating to the MVD measurements. Ideally all the studies would have used identical or at least similar laboratory methods, as even minor differences could affect the quantification. In the event when all data sets used immunohistochemistry for angiogenesis quantification, two main approaches were used and we discovered considerable variability in their implementation. The *Chalkley* method uses an eyepiece with 25 random points and the pathologist attempts to match as many of the points as possible with the vessels on the slide, counting only the matched vessels. The *all vessels* method requires the pathologist to count all visible stained vessels. For both methods, areas showing a concentration of vessels are chosen to be measured, known as 'hotspots.' In brief, all vessels is a density method whereas Chalkley produces an area estimate.

In addition to there being two counting methods, there was considerable variation in the methods of preparation of the slides (three staining agents) in the decision about where to do the counting (choice of 'hotspots'), the numbers of readings, the numbers of observers, and in the microscope magnification used. Furthermore, some recorded the mean of several counts whereas others recorded the maximum.

Perhaps not surprisingly, therefore, we found that the all vessels counts varied considerably across studies, both in terms of the average count and the shape of the distribution. The Chalkley measurements were rather more consistent across studies.

Fortunately, three studies had used both methods enabling us to make a direct comparison. Analysis of these data sets showed rather poor agreement. As a result, it was decided that all subsequent data analyses would be performed separately for Chalkley and all vessels data. Three other data sets were also used to develop an empirical correction to convert data recorded as maximum counts to give estimated mean counts.

With individual patient data and accompanying details of study methodology, we were able to get far more detailed information than would have been possible in a review of only published studies.

To illustrate the value of collecting IPD, 14/17 data sets needed data corrections, some of them major. We were able to remove duplicates as several studies had been done on overlapping patient groups. Three of the 17 data sets had not previously been published, and for 6 of the remaining 14 we obtained extended follow-up compared to the data that had been used for the published analyses.

1.3.4   Meta-analysis

There are several important advantages of IPD when conducting a meta-analysis. All of these were implemented in the PILC study. Thus we were able to carry out a Cox proportional hazards regression analysis for each data set, keeping the MVD measurements as continuous and also adjusting for the same covariates (stage of cancer and age) in each case. The resulting log hazard ratios for MVD count and standard errors were combined using random effects meta-analysis to get an overall assessment of the prognostic value of MVD counts. All analyses were performed separately for Chalkley and all vessels MVD counts.

In addition, we were able to explore subgroups in a consistent way; in particular, we examined the prognostic value of MVD within groups defined by stage of cancer. The results of all the analyses are presented elsewhere; see Trivella *et al.* (2006).

1.4   Discussion

Prognostic studies are mainly retrospective observational studies. Individually they are generally too small, and too poorly designed and analysed to provide reliable evidence. As a consequence of the poor quality of research, prognostic markers may remain under investigation for many years after initial studies without any resolution of the uncertainty. An obvious way forward is to carry out a systematic review and meta-analysis to identify and synthesise the available relevant information.

Carrying out such studies is more of a challenge than for randomised trials, however. Published reports of prognostic studies are often lacking in methodological reporting, use poorly chosen statistical techniques, and often fail to report the numerical results that are necessary for inclusion in meta-analysis. There is to date no accepted set of guidelines on how to assess the quality of such studies. In addition, as noted earlier, there are serious concerns about the impact of publication bias, such that publication is more likely among studies showing that a marker has a statistically significant association with prognosis.

Meta-analysis based on published information may thus be difficult or impossible; see Altman and Lyman (1998) and Riley *et al.* (2006). Although such meta-analyses may sometimes be useful, especially when the study characteristics do not vary too much and only the best studies are included, the findings will rarely be convincing. Some, if not all, of these obstacles may be overcome by obtaining IPD. For example, the widespread use of dichotomisation of continuous variables reduces power and offers a breeding ground for publication bias when multiple cutpoints are explored; see Altman *et al.* (1994). The availability of IPD avoids bias by enabling the original measurements to be used.

The IPD approach is perhaps especially useful for studies with time-to-event data (for example, prognostic studies) inasmuch as such data are generally not well summarised in publications; see Riley *et al.* (2003). Indeed, those systematic reviews and meta-analyses of RCTs that have been performed using IPD have largely assessed time-to-event outcomes.

1.4.1 Systematic review of prognostic studies using individual patient data

Systematic reviews (with meta-analysis) of individual patient data have mainly been of randomised trials. Consequently, publications with advice on how to conduct and analyse such studies have concentrated on experiences from RCTs; see Clarke and Stewart (2000) and Stewart and Clarke (1995).

The PILC project was the first known concerted collaborative effort to obtain IPD for a prognostic marker from as many centres as possible, with the view to put them through meta-analysis. The few previous similar efforts have been largely restricted to acquiring data from a limited number of centres, perhaps as an existing collaborative group; see Look *et al.* (2002).

For the PILC project, individual patient data were collected from all contributing centres, and unpublished data were sought and included. Methods were devised to obtain much more detailed information about study methods than appeared in publications. The data were carefully checked and standardised, and in addition to analysing the data as continuous, a uniform cut-off point was adopted. Moreover, all analyses were performed separately for the single most contributory factor of variation, the method of MVD counting. The reliability of MVD measurement techniques, the choice of cut-off points, and the number of patients and events in each study were major contributing factors to study quality. Finally, random-effects meta-analysis was employed to synthesize the available data.

Although just a single case study, many of the lessons learnt from PILC will apply broadly to IPD studies of prognosis in cancer and indeed in other medical areas. Our experiences accord with what has been written by others about IPD studies, and may be summarised as follows

1. Obtaining and combining raw data from prognostic studies is a long, expensive, and rather laborious process, although it offers clear compensation in avoiding methodological pitfalls.

2. Identifying unpublished data is difficult and time-consuming.

3. Individual studies are likely to be heterogeneous in terms of measurement methods (e.g., assays) used.

4. Reported results and publications from participating groups are usually lacking in detail and laboratory and statistical methods lack consistency.

5. Data checking and standardisation should be given particular attention and are inevitably time-consuming.

6. Standardising patient inclusion/exclusion criteria is possible and should be done.

7. Many data sets will benefit from corrected data and extended follow-up.

8. Detailed record keeping is of primary importance.

9. Appropriateness of analyses can be ensured, including maintaining key data as continuous and applying consistent adjustment for covariates.

10. Variation in the methods of measuring ostensibly the same variable are a serious impediment to clear conclusions – consensus methods should be developed.

The main advantages of collecting IPD in systematic reviews of prognostic studies are the inclusion of extended follow-up for studies that were published; inclusion of unpublished studies with reduced risk of publication bias; ability to check the data; standardised data analysis, including correct analysis of continuous variables; analysis based on time-to-event for each patient; and ability to analyse patient subgroups.

IPD meta-analysis is thus clearly desirable. We have shown that it is feasible, but it may not be cost-effective as implemented here. As one of the key factors is the number of data sets, an obvious option to consider is to restrict the study to a smaller number of centres with the larger data sets, and perhaps also to seek only those studies using consistent laboratory methods. Of course, if not all studies are sought, then the selection of data sets should be made independently of the study's findings. In the future, it may be possible to carry out such studies using high-quality samples stored in tissue banks.

1.4.2   The need for higher-quality prognostic studies

It is encouraging that systematic reviews have expanded into the area of prognosis despite the practical difficulties; see Altman (2001). The approach is the best available in attempting to efficiently utilise published information. However, the quality of a systematic review reflects the quality of the primary studies, and there is ample evidence that primary studies are often poorly reported and poorly conducted; see Riley *et al.* (2003, 2006) and Sauerbrei (2005). In time, we may hope that reporting guidelines for primary prognostic studies may lead to better quality published information; see McShane, Altman, and Sauerbrei (2005).

Individual patient data undoubtedly provide the best quality of information for any systematic review. The great disadvantage is that it is tremendously time-consuming – the whole process can take several years. Also, we note that it cannot overcome either deficiencies of individual studies or heterogeneity of methodological approaches, although such issues will become much clearer in an IPD systematic review. Consideration needs to be given to valid strategies for IPD systematic reviews on subsets of studies, perhaps defined by sample size or methodological features.

Systematic reviews of prognostic studies, whether based on the literature or on IPD, will generally fail to yield a very clear answer. They will, however, be able to draw attention to the paucity of good-quality evidence and pave the way for higher-quality future research, as in the following example.

> From this analysis it becomes evident that further retrospective investigations will not contribute to the solution of the problem and thus are obsolete. There is an obvious need for standardization of the assay procedure and the assessment of the specimens as well as for the initiation of a prospective multicenter trial to provide definite answers. [Schmitz-Dräger *et al.* (2000)]

Acknowledgements. This project was supported by a project grant from Imperial Cancer Research Fund (now Cancer Research UK).

We thank the collaborators in all of the PILC centres for providing their data and answering many questions about their studies: E. Brambilla, CHU Albert Michallon, Grenoble, France; A. Cariello, Ospedale Santa Maria delle Croci, Ravenna, Italy; G. Cox, St James' Hospital, Dublin, Ireland; C. Dazzi, Ospedale Santa Maria delle Croci, Ravenna, Italy; G. Fontanini, University of Pisa, Pisa, Italy; K. Gatter, John Radcliffe Hospital, Oxford, UK; G. Giaccone, Vrije Universiteit Medical Center, Amsterdam, The Netherlands; A. Giatromanolaki, Democritus University of Thrace, Alexandroupolis, Greece; D. Harpole, Duke University Medical Center, Durham, NC, USA; M. Koukourakis, Democritus University of Thrace, Alexandroupolis, Greece; J. Mattern, German Cancer Research Center, Heidelberg, Germany; M.-B. Moore, Duke University Medical Center, Durham, NC, USA; A. Nicholson, Royal Brompton Hospital, London, UK; K. O'Byrne, St James' Hospital, Dublin, Ireland; B. Offersen, Aarhus University Hospital, Aarhus, Denmark; P. Pääkkö, University of Oulu, Oulu, Finland; F. Pasini, University of Verona, Azienda Ospedaliera di Verona, Verona, Italy; G. Pelosi, University of Milan School of Medicine, European Institute of Oncology, Milan, Italy ; N. Pendleton, University of Manchester, Hope Hospital, Manchester, UK; S. Pilotti, Istituto Nazionale Tumori, Milano, Italy; A. Schor, The Dental School, University of Dundee, Dundee, UK; J. Sikora, National Institute of Tuberculosis, Warsaw, Poland; M. Volm, German Cancer Research Center, Heidelberg, Germany; and Y. Yamazaki, Hokkaido University School of Medicine, Kitaku, Sapporo, Japan.

References

1. Altman, D. G. (2001). Systematic reviews of evaluations of prognostic variables, *British Medical Journal*, **323**, 224–228.

2. Altman, D. G., Lausen, B., Sauerbrei, W., and Schumacher, M. (1994). Dangers of using "optimal" cutpoints in the evaluation of prognostic factors, *Journal of the National Cancer Institute*, **86**, 829–835.

3. Altman, D. G., and Lyman, G. H. (1998). Methodological challenges in the evaluation of prognostic factors in breast cancer, *Breast Cancer Research Treatment*, **52**, 289–303.

4. Blettner, M., Sauerbrei, W., Schlehofer, B., Scheuchenpflug, T., and Friedenreich, C. (1999). Traditional reviews, meta-analyses and pooled analyses in epidemiology, *International Journal of Epidemiology*, **28**, 1–9.

5. Brocklehurst, P., and French, R. (1998). The association between maternal HIV infection and perinatal outcome: A systematic review of the literature and meta-analysis, *British Journal of Obstetrics and Gynaecology*, **105**, 836–848.

6. Clarke, M. J., and Stewart, L. A. (2000). Obtaining individual patient data from randomised controlled trials, In *Systematic Reviews in Health Care: Meta-analysis in Context* (Eds., M. Egger, G. Davey Smith, and D. G. Altman), pp. 109–121, BMJ Books, London.

7. Early Breast Cancer Trialists' Collaborative Group (1998). Tamoxifen for early breast cancer: An overview of the randomised trials, *Lancet*, **351**, 1451–1467.

8. Ebell, M. H., White, L. L., and Weismantel, D. (2000). A systematic review of troponin T and I values as a prognostic tool for patients with chest pain, *The Journal of Family Practice*, **49**, 746–753.

9. Egger, M., and Davey Smith, G. (2004). Principles of and procedures for systematic reviews, In *Systematic Reviews in Health Care. Meta-analysis in Context* (Eds., M. Egger, G. Davey Smith and D. G. Altman), pp. 23–42, BMJ Books, London.

10. Kosmas, I. P., Tatsioni, A., and Ioannidis, J. P. (2004). Association of C677T polymorphism in the methylenetetrahydrofolate reductase gene with hypertension in pregnancy and pre-eclampsia: A meta-analysis, *Journal of Hypertension*, **22**, 1655–1662.

11. Kuijpers, T., van der Windt, D. A., van der Heijden, G. J., and Bouter, L. M. (2004). Systematic review of prognostic cohort studies on shoulder disorders, *Pain*, **109**, 420–431.

12. Look, M. P., van Putten W. L., Duffy, M. J., Harbeck, N., Christensen, I. J., Thomassen, C., Kates, R., Spyratos, F., Ferno, M., Eppenberger-Castori, S., Sweep, C. G., Ulm, K., Peyrat, J. P., Martin, P. M., Magdelenat, H., Brunner, N., Duggan, C., Lisboa, B. W., Bendahl, P. O., Quillien, V., Daver, A., Ricolleau, G., Meijer-van Gelder, M. E., Manders, P., Fiets, W. E., Blankenstein, M. A., Boret, P., Romain, S., Daxenbichler, G., Windbichler, G., Cufer, T., Borstnar, S., Kueng, W., Beex, L. V., Klijn, J. G., O'Higgins, N., Eppenberger, U., Janicke, F., Schmitt, M., and Foekens, J. A. (2002). Pooled analysis of prognostic impact of urokinase-type plasminogen activator and its inhibitor PAI-1 in 8377 breast cancer patients, *Journal of the National Cancer Institute*, **94**, 116–128.

13. McKibbon, K. A., Walker-Dilks, C., Haynes, R.B., and Wilczynski, N. (1995). Beyond ACP Journal Club: How to harness MEDLINE for prognosis problems, *ACP Journal Club*, **123**. A12–A14.

14. McShane, L. M., Altman, D. G., Sauerbrei, W., Taube, S. E., Gion, M., Clark, G. M. for the Statistics Subcommittee of the NCI/EORTC Working Group on Cancer Diagnostics (2005). Reporting recommendations for tumor marker prognostic studies (REMARK), *Journal of the National Cancer Institute*, **97**, 1180–1184.

15. Oxman, A. D., Clarke, M. J., and Stewart, L. A. (1995). From science to practice. Meta-analyses using individual patient data are needed, *Journal of the American Medical Association*, **274**, 845–846.

16. Parmar, M. K., Torri, V., and Stewart, L. (1998). Extracting summary statistics to perform meta-analyses of the published literature for survival endpoints, *Statistics in Medicine*, **17**, 2815–2834.

17. Piedbois, P., and Buyse, M. (2004). Meta-analyses based on abstracted data: A step in the right direction, but only a first step, *Journal of the National Clinical Oncology*, **22**, 3839–3841.

18. Popat, S., Matakidou, A., and Houlston, R. S. (2004). Thymidylate synthase expression and prognosis in colorectal cancer: A systematic review and meta-analysis, *Journal of Clinical Oncology*, **22**, 529–536.

19. Ray, J. G. (1998) Meta-analysis of hyperhomocysteinemia as a risk factor for venous thromboembolic disease, *Archives of Internal Medicine*, **158**, 2101–2106.

20. Riley, R. D., Abrams, K. R., Sutton, A. J., Lambert, P. C., Jones, D. R., Heney, D., and Burchill, S. A. (2003). Reporting of prognostic markers: Current problems and development of guidelines for evidence-based practice in the future, *British Journal of Cancer*, **88**, 1191–1198.

21. Riley, R. D., Abrams, K. R., Lambert, P. C., Sutton, A. J., and Altman, D. G. (2006). Where next for evidence synthesis of prognostic marker studies? Improving the quality and reporting of primary studies to facilitate clinically relevant evidence-based results, *in this volume*.

22. Sauerbrei, W. (2005). Prognostic factors. Confusion caused by bad quality design, analysis and reporting of many studies, *Advances in Otorhinolaryngology*, **62**, 184–200.

23. Sauerbrei, W., Blettner, M., and Royston, P. (2001). On alcohol consumption and all-case mortality, *Journal of Clinical Epidemiology*, **54**, 537–540.

24. Schmitz-Dräger, B. J., Goebell, P. J., Ebert, T., and Fradet, Y. (2000). p53 immunohistochemistry as a prognostic marker in bladder cancer. Playground for urology scientists? *European Urology*, **38**, 691–699.

25. Selvin, E., Marinopoulos, S., Berkenblit, G., Rami, T., Brancati, F. L., Powe, N. R., and Golden, S. H. (2004). Meta-analysis: Glycosylated hemoglobin and cardiovascular disease in diabetes mellitus, *Annals of Internal Medicine*, **141**, 421–431.

26. Simon, R. (2001). Evaluating prognostic factor studies, In *Prognostic Factors in Cancer* (Eds., M. K. Gospodarowicz, D. E. Henson, R. V. P. Hutter, B. O'Sullivan, L. H. Sobin, and C. Wittekind), pp. 49–56, Wiley-Liss, New York.

27. Simon, R., and Altman, D. G. (1994). Statistical aspects of prognostic factor studies in oncology, *British Journal of Cancer*, **69**, 979–985.

28. Stewart, L. A., and Clarke, M. J. (1995). Practical methodology of meta-analyses (overviews) using updated individual patient data. Cochrane Working Group, *Statistics in Medicine*, **14**, 2057–2079.

29. Trivella, M. H., Altman, D. G., Pezzella, F., Pastorino, U., and Harris, A. L. (2006). Angiogenesis as a prognostic factor in non-small cell lung carcinoma. A meta-analysis using individual patient data, *Submitted for publication*.

30. Williamson, P. R., Smith, C. T., Hutton, J. L., and Marson, A. G. (2002). Aggregate data meta-analysis with time-to-event outcomes, *Statistics in Medicine*, **21**, 3337–3351.

2

On Statistical Approaches for the Multivariable
Analysis of Prognostic Marker Studies

N. Holländer and W. Sauerbrei

Institute of Medical Biometry and Medical Informatics, Freiburg, Germany

Abstract: Various statistical methods to analyse prognostic marker studies are available and are used in practice. Issues of multivariable model building will be discussed in the framework of regression models and classification and regression trees (CART). It is shown that the choice of one specific statistical method has a strong influence on the results and, therefore, on the interpretation of a prognostic marker. Within regression models we compare the full model with models obtained by backward variable selection considering also transformations of continuous covariates. We discuss problems caused by the uncritical application of CART and outline advantages of small and simple trees. Furthermore, we show how to form risk groups with different prognoses and we illustrate the necessity to validate results in an independent study. Data of two breast cancer studies are used for illustration.

Keywords and phrases: Prognostic markers, model building, regression, trees, validation

---

2.1 Introduction

The identification and assessment of prognostic markers (also termed as prognostic factors) is an important task in clinical research. Studies on prognostic markers attempt to determine a prediction of the course of disease for groups of patients defined by the values of prognostic markers. In contrast to therapeutic studies, however, where statistical principles and methods are well developed and generally accepted, this is not the case for the evaluation of prognostic markers. Deficiencies in design [see Riley *et al.* (2006)] and analysis of prognostic marker studies (e.g., no proper multivariable analysis) explain to some

19

extent why prognostic markers are discussed controversially. In addition to issues such as small sample size, publication bias, and inappropriate reporting
[see Riley *et al.* (2003)], differences of statistical methods used to analyse single studies are an important reason hindering a sensible summary assessment
of a prognostic marker. Many prognostic markers or prognostic classification
schemes do not survive a rigorous validation in new data [see Sauerbrei *et al.*
(1997)]. Consequently, prognostic markers derived from these studies are often
not accepted for general use [see Wyatt and Altman (1995) and Boracchi and
Biganzoli (2003)].

In this chapter, we show for a specific example that the choice of the statistical method and various specific assumptions have a strong influence on the
results and, therefore, on the interpretation of prognostic markers. Focusing
on the statistical analysis of prognostic markers in oncology, we discuss issues
of model building in the framework of regression models and of classification
and regression trees. Within regression models, we compare the full model
with models selected by backward elimination procedures and consider also different assumptions with respect to the functional form of continuous markers.
Applying CART, we discuss problems caused by an uncritical application of
tree-building approaches and outline advantages of small and simple trees. For
illustration, we use the data of two studies in patients with node-positive breast
cancer (Section 2.2). The statistical methods are described in Section 2.3. Results obtained in the larger of the two breast cancer studies are given in Section
2.4. In Section 2.5, we show how to classify, based on a selected regression
model or tree, the patient population into risk groups with different prognoses.
Using the data of a second smaller breast cancer study, we demonstrate the
necessity of an independent validation of the results.

2.2 Examples: Two Prognostic Studies in
Breast Cancer

We consider the data of two studies of patients with node-positive breast
cancer. The first, a clinical trial [GBSG-2 study, $n = 686$ patients, 299 events
for event-free survival (EFS)] is used to identify prognostic markers and to
investigate the influence of different model-building strategies. This dataset
was used previously for prognostic modelling [for example, by Sauerbrei
and Royston (1999) and Schumacher *et al.*   (2006)] and is available at
http://www.blackwellpublishers.com/rss/.   The data of the second, smaller
Freiburg-DNA study ($n = 139$ patients, 76 events for EFS) are exclusively
used to validate the results obtained in the GBSG-2 study. Prognostic markers evaluated in both studies were patient's age, menopausal status, tumour

size, estrogen, and progesterone receptor, tumour grade, and number of involved lymph nodes. More details with references are given in Schumacher *et al.* (2006).

2.3   Statistical Methods

There are several statistical methods to analyse prognostic marker studies. In this chapter, we consider regression models and classification and regression trees.

2.3.1   Regression models

For survival data, a standard tool to analyse multiple prognostic markers simultaneously is the Cox proportional hazards regression model. If we denote the prognostic markers under consideration by $X_1, X_2, \ldots, X_p$, then the model is given by

$$\lambda(t|X_1, X_2, \ldots, X_p) = \lambda_0(t) \exp(\beta_1 X_1 + \beta_2 X_2 + \cdots + \beta_p X_p), \qquad (2.1)$$

where $\lambda(t \mid \cdot) = \lim_{h \to 0} (1/h) Pr(t \leq T < t + h \mid T \geq t, \cdot)$ denotes the hazard function of the event-free or overall survival time random variable T and $\lambda_0(t)$ is an unspecified baseline hazard. The assumption of a (log-)linear effect of a continuous prognostic marker X_j (e.g., tumour size) is one of the standard assumptions in the Cox regression model; here, $\exp(\beta_j)$ represents the increase or decrease in risk if X_j is increased by one unit. If X_j is binary (e.g., menopausal status), then $\exp(\beta_j)$ is simply the hazard ratio (HR) of category 1 (e.g., postmenopausal) to the reference category ($X_j = 0$, e.g., premenopausal).

Continuous markers

Due to this easy interpretation, continuous prognostic markers are often categorised into two or more subgroups. Doing so, in formula (2.1) the corresponding prognostic marker is replaced by dummy variables for the different categories (e.g., two dummies for three categories). Then the hazard ratio is estimated with respect to one reference category. For more details, see standard textbooks by Marubini and Valsecchi (1995) and Therneau and Grambsch (2000). However, the categorisation of a continuous prognostic marker has several disadvantages such as loss of information [see Royston, Altman, and Sauerbrei (2006)]. On the other hand the assumption of a (log-)linear relationship may be wrong. As an alternative, Royston and Altman (1994) proposed the fractional polynomial (FP) approach which provides more flexibility by allowing non-linear relationships of continuous covariates while preserving simplicity of the final model to an acceptable degree.

Variable selection

An important aspect in the analysis of prognostic marker studies is the selection of markers with influence on the outcome. To select relevant covariates in the framework of regression models, variable selection methods such as stepwise methods or selection based on an information criterion (e.g., Akaike's AIC) are commonly applied [see Weissberg (2005)].

In this chapter, we apply backward elimination (BE) using different nominal significance levels and compare the results to the full model. We will use the common significance level $\alpha = 0.05$ [BE(0.05)], BE with significance level $\alpha = 0.157$ [BE(0.157)], which corresponds asymptotically to AIC if selection of one variable is considered, and $\alpha = 0.01$ [BE(0.01)] leading to a more stringent selection of markers. Combining the selection of a FP transformation for continuous covariates with selection of variables by backward elimination, Sauerbrei and Royston (1999) and Sauerbrei *et al.* (1999) have extended the FP-approach to a model-building strategy, which is referred to as the *multivariable fractional polynomial* (MFP) approach. This MFP approach also allows the incorporation of basic medical knowledge, that is, the increase or decrease in risk must be monotonic. Software is generally available [see Sauerbrei *et al.* (2006)].

To assess the selected models, we use the Akaike Information Criterion (AIC) and the Bayesian Information Criterion (BIC). The latter depends on sample size and puts more penalty on each covariate in the selected model than the AIC. A smaller value of AIC and BIC, respectively, corresponds to a better model.

2.3.2   Classification and regression trees (CART)

Hierarchical trees are a popular approach for nonparametric modelling of the relationship of several potential prognostic markers and a response variable. Briefly, the idea of classification and regression trees (CART) is to construct subgroups that are internally as homogeneous as possible with respect to the outcome (here, EFS) and externally as separated as possible. Thus, CART leads directly to prognostic subgroups defined by the selected prognostic markers. This is achieved by a recursive tree-building algorithm. Although the principles of the approach have been available for a long time, the monograph of Breiman *et al.* (1984) is often considered as the important "starting point" of tree-based methods. Here we will use CART as a synonym for these approaches. The original version of CART has been modified in various directions, but here we concentrate on the application to survival data. The log-rank test is used to split the data recursively into subgroups. As a stopping rule for the tree-building process, we use $p_{stop} = 0.05$ as an upper bound of the minimal p value and $n_{min} = 20$ as minimum number of patients in a subgroup. Furthermore, we restricted the possible splits to the range between the 10% and 90% quantiles of the empirical distribution of each continuous marker. Within this range, all splits are considered as potential cutpoints and CART selects the cutpoint corresponding to the minimum p-value p_{min} of the log-rank test that is used for the comparison of the resulting two subgroups. More details with references are given in Schumacher *et al.* (2006).

Because of the well-known problem resulting from multiple testing, it is obvious that the selection of the minimum p-value cannot lead to correct results of the log-rank test. To account for this problem, we used a P-value correction of Lausen and Schumacher (1992).

2.3.3   Formation of risk groups

Quite often, the aim is to develop a prognostic classification scheme. The final subgroups obtained in a regression tree are well suited for this task. Depending on the number of final nodes and their separation, some combination of these subgroups to a prognostic subgroup might be indicated, especially if the prognosis is comparable. For more complex trees systematic approaches to prune and amalgamate nodes have been proposed [see Breiman *et al.* (1984)]. For smaller trees, medical knowledge and subjective preferences can be incorporated to define a prognostic classification scheme [see Sauerbrei *et al.* (1997)].

For the regression approaches considered in Section 2.3, prognostic subgroups can be formed by dividing the distribution of the prognostic index $\hat{\beta}_1 X_1 + \hat{\beta}_2 X_2 + \cdots + \hat{\beta}_p X_p$ into quartiles.

2.4   Results in the GBSG-2 Study

In this section, we apply the different statistical methods to the data of the GBSG-2 study. Some results will be used to form risk groups in Section 2.5.

2.4.1   Regression models – standard applications

In regression models for the GBSG-2 data, all analyses were adjusted for hormonal treatment.

Table 2.1 shows results of univariate Cox models as well as the results of the full model and the model selected by BE(0.05). For continuous covariates, we use both approaches, assuming either a linear effect (A) or using cutpoints to categorise the variables (B). Cutpoints were chosen independently from the data as predefined in the original analysis of the GBSG-2 study; for more details, see Schumacher *et al.* (2006). Results are given in terms of estimated hazard ratios (HRs). HRs should be given with confidence intervals, but we have omitted them for brevity. With BE(0.05), we select with both approaches a model containing the three markers: tumour grade, number of involved lymph nodes, and progesterone receptor. Using AIC and BIC for model assessment, the two models with categorised covariates fit better than the corresponding models based on the assumption of a linear effect of continuous covariates. For both approaches, the model selected by BE(0.05) would be preferred to the corresponding full model due to smaller values of AIC and BIC.

BE(0.01) yields the same model as BE(0.05) when a linear effect is assumed, whereas only two markers (number of lymph nodes, progesterone receptor) were selected with BE(0.01) for categorised data (Table 2.2). Applying BE(0.157) in the latter situation, age and menopausal status were included in the selected model, but both markers were eliminated when assuming a linear effect. However, tumour size is now included. Assessing models by BIC, the smallest model would be preferred due to the large penalty term for additional markers; the smallest AIC value was obtained with BE(0.05) for categorised covariates. However, in spite of the better fit, the categorisation can always be criticised because of some degree of arbitrariness and subjectivity concerning the number of cutpoints, the specific cutpoints chosen, and a loss of information [see Royston, Altman, and Sauerbrei (2006)].

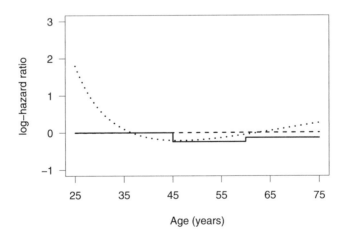

Figure 2.1: Different risk functions for the effect of age obtained in the GBSG-2 study: categorised risk function (solid line), linear risk function (dashed line), and fractional polynomial (dotted line)

2.4.2 Regression models – the MFP-approach

Applying the MFP-approach to the GBSG-2 data with significance level $\alpha =$ 0.05, the following markers were selected: number of positive lymph nodes, tumour grade, progesterone receptor, and age, for the latter two a FP transformation was chosen. This model yields an AIC value of 3072.22 corresponding to an improvement of the log-likelihood of 8.7 as compared to the model selected by BE(0.05) with categorised covariates (Table 2.2). For more details, see Table 4 in Sauerbrei and Royston (1999). With the MFP-approach, a highly significant nonlinear effect of age was detected (likelihood ratio test for age gives $P < 0.001$) with a strong increase in risk for younger patients. Corresponding to the results in Table 2.1, we illustrate in Figure 2.1 that there is hardly any prognostic effect of age if we assume linearity or after categorising age into the subgroups based on the predefined cutpoints.

The analysis of the GBSG-2 study has shown that the final regression model may strongly depend on the underlying model-building strategy and that standard assumptions such as linearity for continuous covariates may not correspond to the data.

2.4.3 Summary assessment – implication of the modelling strategy

As shown in Figure 2.1, we observed hardly any effect of age when assuming linearity or when categorising age using the prespecified cutpoints. However, using a single cutpoint of 40 years the resulting HR (95% confidence interval) comparing patients > 40 years, with patients ≤ 40 years in a multivariable regression model is 0.624 (0.424,0.918) indicating, in contrast to scenario B (Table 2.1), a larger and significant age effect. This simple example demonstrates that the choice of a specific cutpoint can strongly influence the estimated HR in one single study. This also affects the pooled estimate if such a study is included in a meta-analysis.

Furthermore, in meta-analyses based on published data, adjusted estimates of a specific prognostic marker are often not available for several studies [see Riley *et al.* (2006)]. It is not uncommon to calculate a pooled estimate of the HR from all data available, which means that estimated effects from unadjusted analyses and adjusted analyses are averaged. To illustrate differences between results from adjusted and unadjusted analyses, we have included univariate analyses for the GBSG-2 data (see Table 2.1). For some variables, unadjusted HRs are much larger giving a very optimistic view on the prognostic value of the corresponding marker. In our example, this is more apparent for the model with the categorised risk markers. For example, the unadjusted estimated HR for tumour grades 2 and 3 are 2.369 and 3.056, respectively, as compared to patients with grade 1 tumours. However, adjusting for the other prognostic

Table 2.1: Estimated hazard ratios (HR), AIC, and BIC in Cox models. Results from the univariate Cox model (no adjustment), the full model and a selected model obtained by backward elimination with $\alpha = 0.05$ (BE(0.05)) assuming (A) a (log-)linear relationship for continuous covariates and (B) categorising continuous covariates as predefined in the first analysis of the GBSG-2 study

Marker	A: Continuous, Linear Effect†			Categorisation	B: Categorised Markers		
	Univariate HR#	Full Model HR#	BE(0.05) HR#		Univariate HR#	Full Model HR#	BE(0.05) HR#
Age (years)	1.000	0.991	—	≤ 45	1	1	—
				$46 - 60$	0.790	0.672	—
				> 60	0.901	0.687	—
Menopausal status	1.166	1.310†	—	Pre	1	1	—
				Post	1.166	1.307	—
Tumour size (mm)	1.015**	1.008*	—	≤ 20	1**	1	—
				$21 - 30$	1.354	1.240	—
				> 30	1.751	1.316	—
Tumour grade	1.534**	1.321**	1.340	1	1**	1	1
				2	2.369	1.723	1.709
				3	3.056	1.746	1.777
No. of lymph nodes	1.059**	1.051**	1.057	$1 - 3$	1**	1**	1
				$4 - 9$	2.153	1.976	2.071
				≥ 10	3.975	3.513	3.662
Progesterone receptor (fmol/ml)	0.997**	0.998**	0.998	< 20	1**	1**	1
				≥ 20	0.464	0.545	0.536
Estrogen receptor (fmol/ml)	0.999	1.000	—	< 20	1	1	—
				≥ 20	0.663	0.994	—
$\text{AIC} = -2\log L + 2p$	-	3120.2	3117.9		-	3087.2	3083.6
$\text{BIC} = -2\log L + \log(\tilde{n})p$	-	3146.1	3129.0		-	3128.1	3102.1

p Number of covariates in the model, $\tilde{n}$ denotes effective sample size $\tilde{n} = 299$.

† Except for menopausal status, which is binary; grade coded 1,2,3.

HR given without confidence intervals for better illustration only.

*, ** Likelihood ratio test significant at significance level * $\alpha = 0.05$ and ** $\alpha = 0.01$.

Table 2.2: Selected prognostic markers, AIC, and BIC for different model selection strategies. Included markers marked by dots

Marker	A: Continuous, Linear Effect				B: Categorised Markers			
	Full Model	BE(0.157)	BE(0.05)	BE(0.01)	Full Model	BE(0.157)	BE(0.05)	BE(0.01)
Age	•				•			
Menopausal status	•				•	•		
Tumour size	•	•			•	•		
Tumour grade	•	•	•	•	•	•	•	
No. of lymph nodes	•	•	•	•	•	•		
Progesterone receptor	•	•	•	•	•	•	•	•
Estrogen receptor	•				•		•	•
$\text{AIC} = -2\log L + 2p$	3120.2	3116.6	3117.9	3117.9	3087.2	3084.5	3083.6	3085.1
$\text{BIC} = -2\log L + \log(\tilde{n})p$	3146.1	3131.4	3129.0	3129.0	3128.1	3114.1	3102.1	3096.2

p Number of covariates in the model, $\tilde{n}$ denotes effective sample size $\tilde{n} = 299$.

markers in the full model, the corresponding estimated HRs reduced to 1.723 and 1.746, respectively. In a chapter in this volume Riley *et al.* (2006) illustrate a possible influence of this issue on the result of a meta-analysis by calculating pooled estimates for adjusted and unadjusted effects of a prognostic marker (*MYCN*) for neuroblastoma [see Riley *et al.* (2006)]. As in our analysis, for a single study the estimated HRs from the unadjusted analysis were larger. Consequently, a meta-analysis mixing unadjusted and adjusted risk estimates from the primary studies produces pooled estimates whose interpretation is very difficult.

2.4.4   Application of classification and regression trees

Using the CART procedure with our choice of specific parameters for the analysis of the GBSG-2 data, we obtained the large complex tree displayed on the left side of Figure 2.2. We start with the whole group of 686 patients (the 'root') with 299 observed events corresponding to an event rate of 43.6%. The marker with the smallest minimum p-value is 'number of involved lymph nodes' (in Figure 2.2 denoted as NODES), and the whole group is split at an estimated cutpoint of 9 positive nodes yielding subgroups of 585 patients with less than or equal to 9 positive lymph nodes (event rate 38.8%) and a subgroup of 103 patients with more than 9 positive nodes (event rate 70.9%). Repeating this procedure in the latter smaller subgroup, progesterone receptor (PROGREZ) with cutpoint 23 fmol leads to the smallest minimum p-value and the 103 patients are subdivided into subgroups of 60 and 43 patients, respectively. In these two subgroups, no further splits are possible because of the p_{stop} criterion. In the group of 585 patients with maximally 9 positive lymph nodes, again NODES appeared to be the strongest marker with a cutpoint of 3 positive nodes. In this left part of the tree, the resulting subgroups are then subdivided by PRO-GREZ; further subdivisions are based on the markers tumour size (TUSIZE), age (AGE), and/or estrogen receptor (ESTREZ). Finally, the tree-building algorithm leads to 12 final subgroups, which are illustrated by the boxes in Figure 2.2.

This uncritical application of CART has several disadvantages. (i) For continuous markers, the cutpoint is selected from a large set of possible splits. Because of the well-known problem resulting from multiple testing, it is obvious that the selection of the minimum p-value cannot lead to correct results of the log-rank test. Ignoring this problem, continuous variables are likely to be chosen for data splitting, even if they have hardly any prognostic effect. Furthermore, the tree-building algorithm produces too many splits and ends up with too many final subgroups. However, this problem can be reduced by using a corrected p-value p_{cor} instead of the minimum p-value [see Lausen and Schumacher (1992)]. Additionally, it is questionable whether all selected cutpoints are sensible. In the subgroup of the 103 patients with more than 9 positive

A   **B**

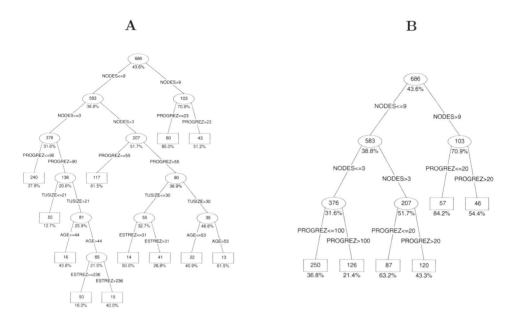

Figure 2.2: Classification and regression trees obtained for the GBSG-2 study: (A) no *p*-value correction and all cutpoints allowed (no prespecification) and (B) with *p*-value correction and prespecification of cutpoints

nodes, for example, we obtained for the progesterone receptor a cutpoint of 23 fmol. The same value would be obtained when using a corrected instead of the minimum *p*-value. However, the choice of 23 fmol is somewhat arbitrary and may not be reproducible or comparable to cutpoints obtained in other studies. In medical studies, cutpoints of 5, 10, or 20 fmol/ml are often used to classify into receptor-positive and receptor-negative patients. Thus, another useful restriction to be implemented in the tree-building process may be the definition of a set of predefined possible cutpoints. For the progesterone and estrogen receptors we chose 5, 10, 20, 100, and 300 fmol as possible splits. Defining also prespecified cutpoints for age and tumour size and using corrected *p*-values of the log-rank test, we obtained the small tree displayed on the right side of Figure 2.2. NODES with a cutpoint of 9 positive lymph nodes is again used to split the complete population. The corrected *p*-value is still highly significant ($p_{\text{cor}} < 0.0001$) indicating the strong prognostic effect of this marker. Further splits are based on NODES with cutpoint 3 and on PROGREZ. In contrast to the first complex tree, we obtained a simple small tree, which is based on the two important prognostic markers only, with 6 final subgroups. Generally, the interpretation of such simple trees is easier and the chance that results are reproducible is much higher as compared to that from large complex trees.

2.5   Formation and Validation of Risk Groups

Using the small tree (Figure 2.2B) we form four prognostic subgroups out of the six final subgroups:

  I: NODES $\leq$ 3 and PROGREZ > 100.
 II: NODES $\leq$ 3 and PROGREZ $\leq$ 100 or 4 $\leq$ NODES $\leq$ 9 and PROGREZ > 20.
III: 4 $\leq$ NODES $\leq$ 9 and PROGREZ $\leq$ 20 or NODES > 9 and PROGREZ > 20.
 IV: NODES > 9 and PROGREZ $\leq$ 20.

The Kaplan–Meier estimates of the event-free survival curves for subgroups I–IV, which are given in Figure 2.3 under the heading 'CART,' show a good separation between the selected prognostic subgroups.

Kaplan–Meier estimates of EFS for the prognostic subgroups derived from the prognostic index of the Cox regression model selected by BE(0.05) with categorised variables are displayed in Figure 2.3 as 'COX.' Again, we obtained a clear separation between prognostic subgroups.

Although both approaches use the same two strong prognostic markers the resulting prognostic subgroups need not necessarily contain the same patients. The group with the worst prognosis obtained by COX, for instance, contains 180 patients, whereas subgroup IV of CART contains only 57 patients. Furthermore, it should be taken into account that we estimated the difference between prognostic subgroups with the same data that we used for model building. As a consequence, the differences between risk groups are most likely overestimated and results have to be validated in an independent study.

Validation

We attempt to validate the two prognostic classification schemes with the data of the Freiburg-DNA study that covers the same patient population and prognostic markers as the GBSG-2 study. Despite the good agreement, which could not be taken for granted in practice, CART is not directly applicable, because only progesterone and estrogen receptor status (positive: > 20 fmol and negative: $\leq$ 20 fmol) are recorded in the Freiburg-DNA study. Therefore, we modify CART by replacing the value 100 for PROGREZ by 20. We replace subgroups I and II by new subgroups I* and II*; the modified classification approach is referred to as CART*. Except for the adaption for PROGREZ, no further modifications were necessary. However, this good agreement between studies is an exception rather than a rule.

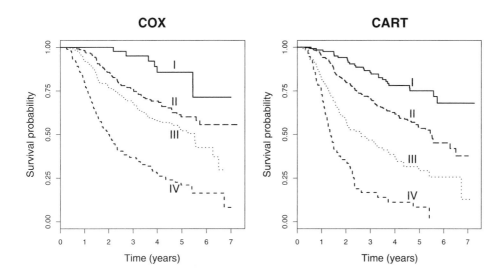

Figure 2.3: Kaplan–Meier estimates of event-free survival probabilities for the prognostic subgroups derived from a Cox model with categorised covariates (COX) and the simple tree displaced in Figure 2.2B (CART)

Table 2.3 shows the estimated hazard ratios with 95% confidence intervals for the prognostic groups derived from the two classification schemes. The HRs were estimated by using dummy variables defining the risk groups and by taking the group with the best prognosis as reference. To obtain prognostic subgroups in the Freiburg-DNA study, the definitions and categorisation derived in the GBSG-2 study are used. The results show that there is some shrinkage in the HRs when estimated in the Freiburg DNA study. For several reasons, such as the baseline category in COX includes only 7.6% of patients in contrast to 35.4% in the baseline category of CART, a comparison of the amount of shrinkage is difficult. It seems to be that shrinkage is more pronounced in the CART* classification scheme (reduction by 47% in the high-risk group) as compared with COX (reduction by 28% in the high-risk group).

To sum up, the assessment of prognostic classification schemes should not be performed in the same data set that is used for model building and formation of risk groups. If no validation data are available, data-splitting as cross-validation or bootstrap resampling methods could be applied to obtain different data sets for model building and assessment of results.

Table 2.3: Estimated hazard ratios (HR) for prognostic subgroups derived in the GBSG-2 study by using the selected Cox model with categorised covariates (COX) and a modification of the simple tree displayed in Figure 2.2B (CART*). Validation of the HRs in the Freiburg-DNA study

	GBSG-2 study			Freiburg-DNA study[†]		
	HR (95% CI)	n	(percent)	HR (95% CI)	n	(percent)
COX						
I	1	52	(7.6)	1	33	(23.7)
II	2.68 (1.23, 5.83)	218	(31.8)	1.78 (0.73, 4.31)	26	(18.7)
III	3.95 (1.83, 8.51)	236	(34.4)	3.52 (1.65, 7.30)	58	(41.7)
IV	9.92 (4.62,21.29)	180	(26.2)	7.13 (2.56,17.18)	14	(10.7)
CART*						
I*	1	243	(35.4)	1	50	(36.0)
II*	1.82 (1.34, 2.47)	253	(36.9)	1.99 (1.05, 3.75)	38	(27.3)
III	3.48 (2.51, 4.82)	133	(19.4)	3.19 (1.70, 5.97)	33	(23.7)
IV	8.20 (5.52,11.98)	57	(8.3)	4.34 (1.85,10.15)	11	(7.9)

[†] Complete case analysis, observations with missing values deleted.

2.6   Discussion

In this chapter, we presented several statistical methods which are used to analyse prognostic marker studies. It was shown that results can strongly depend on the modelling approach. We demonstrated that a so-called *final* multivariable regression model is often the result of a more or less extensive model-building process which may involve the categorisation and/or transformation of markers as well as the selection of variables in an automatic or subjective manner. Several assumptions are always required. Investigating prognostic markers by means of classification and regression trees, corrected p-values should be applied to overcome problems caused by multiple testing in continuous markers. Furthermore, the prespecification of cutpoints and the definition of sensible stopping rules are important to provide interpretable trees.

Considering only 7 potential prognostic markers in our example, we have shown that standard assumptions of the Cox model may be violated and that a careful multivariable modelling is needed to select relevant markers and to assess their effect. Obviously, these problems increase with an increasing number of potential prognostic markers. Even before the first results of gene expression studies were published, the effect of more than 200 potential prognostic markers in breast cancer were controversially discussed, and by 2001 about 1000 papers have been published on this issue. Considering only several variables, the 'full' model is often not sensible, although its use is postulated in theoretical papers or some textbooks [e.g., Harrell (2001)]. One important reason is that the full model avoids data-dependent modelling providing unbiased parameter estimates and meaningful confidence intervals. On the negative side, it has to be stressed that the choice of variables in the full model is rather unclear. Generally, a large number of different variables are recorded in a clinical trial and also in a clinical cancer registry. Which of these variables belong to the full model? The 'pro' to avoid data-dependent modelling leads to the 'con' that the full model includes some variables with a negligible effect [see Sauerbrei (1999)] and usually assumes linear effects for continuous covariates. However, this assumption may not agree with the dose–response relationship in the data. Investigating possible nonlinearity with the MFP approach, this was most obvious for age in our example. Model building by selection of variables and functional forms for continuous variables may cause bias of estimates in the *final* multivariable regression model. Therefore, the model-building process should be taken into account when judging the results of a prognostic study; in practice, it is usually neglected. Simplicity should be an important aim of model building [see Sauerbrei (1999)]. This also helps with issues such as stability and reproducibility of the selected model or tree. Bootstrap resampling methods may be used to investigate stability of regression models [see Royston and Sauerbrei (2003)] and to correct for bias caused by model building [see Schumacher, Holländer, and Sauerbrei (1997) and Holländer, Sauerbrei, and Schumacher (2004)]. Procedures to combine variable selection with shrinkage have been proposed [see Breiman (1995) and Tibshirani (1997)]. To improve the predictive ability of trees, stabilising methods based on resampling, such as bagging have been proposed [see Breiman (2001) and Hothorn *et al.* (2004)]. Furthermore, to assess their usefulness, prognostic models should be validated in independent data [see Simon and Altman (1994) and Altman and Royston (2000)]. Using the classification scheme developed in the GBSG-2 study to form prognostic subgroups in the validation study, we observed some shrinkage with respect to the separation of the resulting subgroups.

In addition to the statistical approaches described in this chapter, there are many other modelling approaches available and more statistical issues to consider for the analysis of a single study. To handle these issues, authors have specific preferences but general recommendations are currently not available [see Schumacher *et al.* (2006), Concato, Feinstein, and Holford (1993), Harrell, Lee, and Mark (1996), Pajak *et al.* (2000), McShane and Simon (2001), and Biganzoli, Borachi, and Marubini (2003)]. A variety of methods is used in real studies; conflicting results concerning the prognostic relevance of single markers may be caused by the choice and/or the (inadequate) application of a specific statistical method. In Table 2.4, we have summarised important issues concerning the analysis of single studies. In addition to the topics discussed here, we have also listed a few points requiring more attention in future studies.

Table 2.4: Summary of important issues for the analysis of single prognostic marker studies

---

1. **Treatment of Study Population**
- Ideally patients without any systemic adjuvant therapy, but unrealistic in many diseases
- Standardisation or randomisation of treatment preferable; adjustment for treatment in the analysis

2. **Model-Building Process**
- Multivariable model required to assess the effect of a marker
- Many approaches available; no general agreement concerning preferable strategies
- Our preference is regression models; other approaches can give complementary information

2a. **Regression Models**
- Problems caused by categorisation of continuous covariates
- Standard assumption of a (log-)linear effect of continuous markers may be wrong
- Variable selection methods sensible to select relevant markers; complexity of the "final" regression model depends on nominal significance level
- Different variable selection strategies may result in different "final" regression models

2b. **Trees**
- Uncritical application of trees can lead to large, unstable, and uninterpretable trees
- p-value correction and prespecification of cutpoints for continuous variables

2c. **Other Approaches**
- Many methods available, none without problems

3. **Formation of Risk Groups**
- Different model-building strategies may result in different risk groups
- Avoid too-small risk groups

4. **Validation of Results**
- Overestimation of effects caused by data-dependent modelling
- Validation of prognostic relevance of markers and models in independent validation study

5. **Issues Requiring More Attention in Future Studies**
- Stability investigation of selected models
- Combining variable selection with shrinkage
- Differentiation between studies developing a prediction model from studies with main interest in one specific marker

---

In general, the evaluation of a prognostic marker requires a summary assessment from several studies. For individual studies, it is generally accepted that a multivariable analysis is required. Consequently, a pooled estimate from several studies should be based on adjusted estimates from individual studies. Ideally all studies use the same variables for adjustment. This may be possible with individual patient data (IPD) and simple models containing a small number of 'important' markers only. For new markers, it is more promising that research groups start cooperation when designing new studies with the aim of a prospectively planned pooled analysis, a concept sometimes used in epidemiological research [see Blettner *et al.* (1999)]. With the current situation of trying to summarise poorly published estimates based on different ways of analysis, a reliable assessment of the prognostic value of a marker is nearly impossible. Many important problems illustrating the difficulties of performing a pooled analysis using published studies and the feasibility of obtaining IPD are addressed in two chapters in this volume by Riley *et al.* (2006) and Altman *et al.* (2006).

References

1. Altman, D. G., and Royston, P. (2000). What do we mean by validating a prognostic model? *Statistics in Medicine*, **19**, 453–473.

2. Altman, D. G., Trivella, M., Pezzella, F., Harris, A. L., and Pastorino, U. (2006). Systematic review of multiple studies of prognosis: The feasibility of obtaining individual patient data, *in this volume*.

3. Biganzoli, E., Borachi, P., and Marubini, E. (2003). Biostatistics and tumour marker studies in breast cancer: Design, analysis and interpretation issues, *The International Journal of Biological Markers*, **18**, 40–48.

4. Blettner, M., Sauerbrei, W., Schlehofer, B., Scheuchenpflug, T., and Friedenreich, C. (1999). Traditional reviews, meta-analyses and pooled analyses in epidemiology, *International Journal of Epidemiology*, **28**, 1–9.

5. Boracchi, P., and Biganzoli, E. (2003). Markers of prognosis and response to treatment: Ready for clinical use in oncology? A biostatistician's viewpoint, *The International Journal of Biological Markers*, **18**, 65–69.

6. Breiman, L. (1995). Better subset regression using the nonnegative Garotte, *Technometrics*, **37**, 373–384.

7. Breiman, L. (2001). Random forests, *Machine Learning*, **45**, 5–32.

8. Breiman, L., Friedman, J. H., Olsen, R. J., and Stone, C. J. (1984). *Classification and Regression Trees*, Wadsworth, Monterey, California.

9. Concato, J., Feinstein, A. R., and Holford, T. R. (1993). The risk of determining risk with multivariable models, *Annals of Internal Medicine*, **118**, 201–210.

10. Harrell, F. E., Jr. (2001). *Regression Modelling Strategies: With Applications to Linear Models, Logistic Regression, and Survival Analysis*, Springer-Verlag, New York.

11. Harrell, F. E., Lee, K. L., and Mark, D. B. (1996). Multivariable prognostic models: Issues in developing models, evaluating assumptions and accuracy, and measuring and reducing errors, *Statistics in Medicine*, **15**, 361–387.

12. Holländer, N., Sauerbrei, W., and Schumacher, M. (2004). Confidence intervals for the effect of a prognostic factor after selection of an 'optimal' cutpoint, *Statistics in Medicine*, **23**, 1701–1713.

13. Hothorn, T., Lausen, B., Benner, A., and Radespiel-Tröger, M. (2004). Bagging survival trees, *Statistics in Medicine*, **23**, 77–91.

14. Lausen, B., and Schumacher, M. (1992). Maximally selected rank statistics, *Biometrics*, **48**, 73–85.

15. Marubini, E., and Valsecchi, M. G. (1995). *Analysing Survival Data from Clinical Trials and Observational Studies*, John Wiley & Sons, New York.

16. McShane, L. M., and Simon, R. (2001). Statistical methods for the analysis of prognostic factor studies, In *Prognostic Factors in Cancer* (Eds., M. K. Gospodarowicz, D. E. Henson, R. V. P. Hutter, *et al.*), 2nd ed., John Wiley & Sons, Lisbon.

17. Pajak, T. F., Clark, G. M., Sargent, D. J., McShane, L. M., and Hammond, M. E. H. (2000). Statistical issues in tumour marker studies, *Archives of Pathology and Laboratory Medicine*, **124**, 1011–1015.

18. Riley, R. D., Abrams, K. R., Lambert, P. C., Sutton, A. J., and Altman, D. G. (2006). Where next for evidence synthesis of prognostic marker studies? Improving the quality and reporting of primary studies to facilitate clinically evidence-based results, *in this volume*.

19. Riley, R. D., Abrams, K. R., Sutton, A. J., Lambert, P. C., Jones, D. R., Heney, D., and Burchill, S. A. (2003). Reporting of prognostic markers: Current problems and development of guidelines for evidence-based practice in the future, *British Journal of Cancer*, **88**, 1191–1198.

20. Royston, P., and Altman, D. G. (1994). Regression using fractional polynomials of continuous covariates: parsimonious parametric modelling (with discussion), *Applied Statistics*, **43**, 429–467.

21. Royston, P., Altman, D. G., and Sauerbrei, W. (2006). Dichotomizing continuous predictors in multiple regression: A bad idea, *Statistics in Medicine*, **25**, 127–141.

22. Royston, P., and Sauerbrei, W. (2003). Stability of multivariable fractional polynomial models with selection of variables and transformations: A bootstrap investigation, *Statistics in Medicine*, **22**, 639–659.

23. Sauerbrei, W. (1999). The use of resampling methods to simplify regression models in medical statistics, *Applied Statistics*, **48**, 313–329.

24. Sauerbrei, W., Hübner, K., Schmoor, C., and Schumacher, M. (1997). Validation of existing and development of new prognostic classification schemes in node negative breast cancer, *Breast Cancer Research and Treatment*, **42**, 149–163.

25. Sauerbrei, W., Meier-Hirmer, C., Benner, A., and Royston, P. (2006). Multivariable regression model building by using fractional polynomials: description of SAS, STATA and R programs, *Computational Statistics & Date Analysis*, **50**, 3464–3485.

26. Sauerbrei, W., and Royston, P. (1999). Building multivariable prognostic and diagnostic models: Transformation of the predictors by using fractional polynomials, *Journal of the Royal Statistical Society, Series A*, **162**, 71–94.

27. Sauerbrei, W., Royston, P., Bojar, H., Schmoor, C., and Schumacher, M. (1999). Modelling the effects of standard prognostic factors in node-positive breast cancer, *British Journal of Cancer*, **79**, 1752–1760.

28. Schumacher, M., Holländer, N., and Sauerbrei, W. (1997). Resampling and cross-validation techniques: A tool to reduce bias caused by model building? *Statistics in Medicine*, **16**, 2813–2827.

29. Schumacher, M., Holländer, N., Schwarzer, G., and Sauerbrei, W. (2006). Prognostic factor studies, In *Handbook of Statistics in Clinical Oncology* (Eds., J. Crowley and D. P. Ankerst), 2nd ed., pp. 307–351, CRC, Boca Raton, Florida.

30. Simon, R., and Altman, D. G. (1994). Statistical aspects of prognostic factor studies in oncology. *British Journal of Cancer*, **69**, 979–985.

31. Therneau, T. M., and Grambsch, P. M. (2000). *Modeling Survival Data: Extending the Cox Model*, Springer-Verlag, New York.

32. Tibshirani, R. (1997). The lasso method for variable selection in the Cox model, *Statistics in Medicine*, **16**, 385–395.

33. Weissberg, S. (2005). *Applied Linear Regression*, Third ed., John Wiley & Sons, New York.

34. Wyatt, J. C., and Altman, D. (1995). Prognostic models: Clinically useful or quickly forgotten? Commentary, *British Medical Journal*, **311**, 1539–1541.

3

Where Next for Evidence Synthesis of Prognostic Marker Studies? Improving the Quality and Reporting of Primary Studies to Facilitate Clinically Relevant Evidence-Based Results

Richard D. Riley,[1] **Keith R. Abrams,**[1] **Paul C. Lambert,**[1] **Alex J. Sutton,**[1] **and Douglas G. Altman**[2]

[1] *University of Leicester, Princess Road West, Leicester, UK*
[2] *Wolfson College, Oxford, UK*

Abstract: Prognostic markers can help to identify patients with different risks of specific outcomes, facilitate treatment choice, and aid patient counselling. Unfortunately, within any given disease area, the wealth of conflicting and heterogeneous evidence makes it difficult for the clinician to ascertain the overall evidence about specific markers and how to use them in practice. The application of formal methods (e.g., a systematic review and meta-analysis) of obtaining and synthesising evidence is therefore greatly needed in the prognostic marker field. However, in this chapter we illustrate and discuss the reasons why currently poor standards of design, clinical relevance, and reporting in primary studies limit statistically reliable and clinically relevant evidence-based results for prognostic markers. These problems add to those issues for the statistical analysis in primary studies that are discussed in another chapter in this volume. To help overcome the problems we highlight guidelines for conducting and reporting primary prognostic research, and we particularly discuss why the availability of individual patient data would help realise the evidence-based use of prognostic markers in clinical practice.

Keywords and phrases: Meta-analysis, prognosis, predictive marker, individual patient data, systematic review

3.1 Introduction and Aims

3.1.1 Prognostic markers and prognostic marker studies

Prognostic markers (also called prognostic factors or prognostic variables) are important clinical tools as they help to identify patients with different risks of specific outcomes (e.g., recurrence of disease) and can thereby facilitate the most appropriate treatment strategies and aid patient counselling. They can include simple measures such as age, sex, stage of disease, or size of tumour, but also more complex factors such as abnormal levels of proteins or catecholamines, and unusual genetic mutations. In oncology, hundreds of prognostic marker studies are published each year [see Riley *et al.* (2003b)] with assessments made about the association of one or more markers with *overall survival* (i.e., whether patients were alive or dead at the end of the study) and *disease-free survival* (i.e., whether patients were alive or had either died or suffered a recurrence of disease by the end of the study). However, prognostic marker studies are common in many other research fields, such as heart disease [Hemingway and Marmot (1999)] and dementia [Mitchell *et al.* (2004)], and are also used in relation to many other outcomes such as surgical complications [Carpeggiana *et al.* (2004)] and arthritis [Deodhar *et al.* (2003)].

3.1.2 The need for formal evidence syntheses of prognostic marker studies

Unfortunately, within any given disease area, the results across different primary prognostic marker studies are often inconsistent and contradictory [Simon and Altman (1994)]. Across studies, many different markers are assessed in relation to heterogeneous subpopulations, treatments, and outcomes. Furthermore, many studies have small numbers of patients and therefore a low statistical power of detecting treatment or survival benefits arising out of using prognostic markers. This wealth of conflicting and heterogeneous evidence makes it difficult for clinicians to ascertain the overall evidence about specific markers and, even for those known to be important, how to use them in practice (e.g., to which patients, using which cut-off levels, and applying which treatment regimen). Clinicians thus need help in establishing evidence-based results and guidelines about prognostic markers. The application of formal methods of obtaining and synthesising evidence is therefore greatly needed in the prognostic marker field, otherwise there will continue to be large uncertainty and subjective, perhaps inappropriate, use of prognostic markers in practice.

Since about 1990, there has been a growing movement toward evidence-based clinical practice and the formation of evidence-based clinical and public health policies. The most commonly applied evidence synthesis method is a *systematic review*, which is a transparent framework for the collection, critical appraisal, and synthesis of the current evidence from published and (if possible) unpublished studies [Egger, Davey Smith, and Altman (2001)]. If appropriate, a *meta-analysis* can be performed at the end of a systematic review, which is a statistical approach that combines the quantitative evidence from all the individual studies (or the subset of better quality studies) to produce overall evidence-based results [Egger, Davey Smith, and Altman (2001)]. In order to facilitate a meta-analysis approach, it is common for a summary statistic (e.g., hazard ratio) of interest to be chosen and extracted, where possible, from each published (and unpublished) study. Alongside the estimate of the summary statistic chosen, one also requires a measure of the uncertainty about the estimate obtained [e.g., standard error of the $\log_e$(hazard ratio)], so that the meta-analysis can give relatively more weight to those estimates with small uncertainty and, conversely, relatively smaller weight to those estimates with large uncertainty. A systematic review with meta-analysis is an ideal approach for a formal evidence synthesis of prognostic marker studies. However, we have recently demonstrated that a reliable and clinically useful systematic review and meta-analysis will often not be feasible in this field, especially if one seeks to extract and synthesise summary statistics from published articles [Riley *et al.* (2003a)]. One major problem is that the primary studies to be synthesised are poorly reported, in terms of both statistical information (e.g., solely *p*-values are often presented instead of a hazard ratio and confidence interval) and clinical information (e.g., treatment used and age of patients is often not reported). This problem restricts the extraction of summary statistics and makes it difficult to perform reliable meta-analyses that determine the clinical importance of each marker studied based on the overall evidence [Altman (2001) and Altman and Lyman (1998)].

3.1.3 Aims of this chapter

Chapter 2 in this volume by Holländer and Sauerbrei (2006) highlights issues associated with an appropriate statistical analysis within primary prognostic studies. It is shown that different analysis strategies can give different results concerning the effect of a factor. However, good research and appropriate statistical practice is required throughout the whole study, not just at the analysis stage, and so the first aim for this chapter is to highlight further areas where improvements are needed within primary research of prognostic markers. Our second aim is to emphasise why there is a need, alongside improvements in the primary studies, for individual patient data (IPD) to be commonly made available from each study to help those performing meta-analysis; the practicalities of actually realising the IPD approach are assessed by Altman *et al.* (2006), Chapter 1 in this volume.

3.2   Difficulties of an Evidence Synthesis of Prognostic Marker Studies

3.2.1   Poor and heterogeneous reporting

We recently performed a large-scale systematic review of prognostic tumour markers in neuroblastoma and used it as an empirical investigation of the feasibility of producing evidence-based results of prognostic marker studies from the published literature [Riley *et al.* (2003a)]. The review identified 260 prognostic studies and in these there were 575 different reports where levels of one of 13 different tumour markers were related to overall survival (OS) or disease-free survival (DFS) by summary statistics or IPD. From each of these reports an estimate of the $\log_e$(hazard ratio) and its variance were sought, but only 204 (35.5%) of the reports enabled both these statistics to be obtained. Furthermore, the $\log_e$(hazard ratio) and its variance were both directly provided on only three occasions in the 575 reports (0.005%); the other 201 estimates required either indirect estimation methods (160 estimates), as suggested by Parmar *et al.* (1998), or used the IPD provided in the published articles to calculate the estimates directly using Cox regression (41 estimates). IPD was sometimes presented within the published literature because many studies had a small sample size due to the rarity of neuroblastoma disease, however, in general the availability of IPD from cancer studies is not common [Altman *et al.* (2006)].

In the neuroblastoma review, we used the estimates extracted to perform meta-analyses for each of the 13 markers considered, for each of OS and DFS where possible [Riley *et al.* (2004a)]. For example, the OS meta-analysis result for *MYCN*, the most commonly studied prognostic marker in neuroblastoma (152 studies in total presented OS results or IPD for *MYCN*), is shown in Figure 3.1 and it suggests that high levels of *MYCN* are strongly associated with an increased risk of death. However, the reliability and clinical interpretability of this meta-analysis result is clearly limited because: (i) 107 studies (70.4 %) could not be included in the evidence synthesis because the *MYCN* results or IPD relating to prognosis were not provided in sufficient detail to allow the $\log_e$(hazard ratio) and its standard error to be estimated for OS; and (ii) the results across studies were heterogeneous in clinical factors assessed, such as stage of disease and age of patients, and in the cut-off level used to dichotomise the data (Figure 3.1). In particular, the multitude of missing summary statistics in (i) makes one concerned that the set of available summary statistics does not actually reflect the truth. There is a strong potential for the OS (and similarly

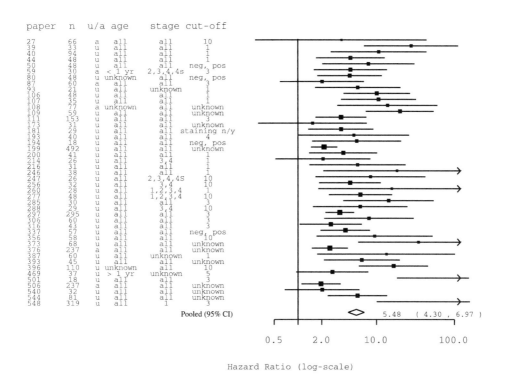

paper	n	u/a	age	stage	cut-off
27	66	a	all	all	10
39	33	u	all	all	1
40	94	u	all	all	1
44	48	u	all	all	1
50	48	u	all	all	neg, pos
59	30	a	< 1 yr	2,3,4,4s	3
80	48	u	unknown	all	neg, pos
87	60	a	all	all	3
93	21	u	all	unknown	3
106	48	u	all	all	1
107	35	u	all	all	1
108	77	a	unknown	all	unknown
109	59	u	all	all	unknown
111	153	u	all	all	3
173	31	u	all	all	unknown
181	29	u	all	all	staining n/y
193	40	u	all	all	4
194	18	u	all	all	neg, pos
199	492	u	all	all	unknown
200	41	u	all	all	1
214	26	u	all	3,4	1
216	31	u	all	all	1
246	38	u	all	all	1
247	26	u	all	2,3,4,4S	10
256	32	u	all	3,4	10
260	28	u	all	1,2,3,4	1
277	48	u	all	1,2,3,4	10
285	30	u	all	all	3
288	29	u	all	3,4	10
297	295	u	all	all	3
306	60	u	all	all	3
316	43	u	all	all	3
337	57	u	all	all	neg, pos
355	58	u	all	all	10
375	68	u	all	all	unknown
376	237	a	all	all	unknown
387	60	u	all	unknown	1
393	45	u	all	all	unknown
396	110	u	unknown	all	10
469	37	u	> 1 yr	unknown	5
501	18	u	all	all	3
506	237	a	all	all	unknown
540	32	u	all	all	unknown
544	81	u	all	all	unknown
548	319	u	all	1	3

Pooled (95% CI)   5.48 (4.30 , 6.97)

0.5   2.0   10.0   100.0

Hazard Ratio (log-scale)

paper = study id number, n = number of patients, u/a = unadjusted or adjusted hazard ratio; stage = stage of disease; all stages = all of stages 1,2,3,4,and 4s were represented by the n patients, all ages = ages < 1 year and > 1 year were represented by the n patients, and cut-off = cut-off level used to dichotomise *MYCN* into 'low-risk' and 'high-risk' levels.

Figure 3.1: Forest plot for the *MYCN* overall survival (OS) meta-analysis from the neuroblastoma review including the 45 studies that allowed the $\log_e$(hazard ratio) and its standard error to be estimated [Riley *et al.* (2004a)]. N.B. There were 107 other studies which provided *MYCN* results or IPD in relation to prognosis but not in sufficient detail to allow the $\log_e$(hazard ratio) and its standard error to be obtained; hence, the meta-analysis pooled hazard ratio result below must be treated with caution, as it is not possible to include much of the overall evidence in the evidence synthesis

the DFS) meta-analysis result to be biased if some of the missing summary statistics were not missing at random, perhaps because of publication bias or other related dissemination biases (see Section 3.2.5) [Riley *et al.* (2004b)].

The key reporting problems (such as no hazard ratio or confidence interval) that prevented us from obtaining 64.5% of the evidence base in the neuroblastoma review are presented elsewhere, with guidelines also made for improved reporting in the future [Riley *et al.* (2003a)]. To complement this work, we will now discuss some of the other underlying reasons why primary prognostic studies often severely limit a clinically useful meta-analysis of the overall evidence.

3.2.2   Poor study design and problems clarifying study purpose

Altman and Lyman (1998) present suitable criteria that those initiating a primary prognostic study should consider, and they suggest that every effort should be made to limit potential biases and to emulate the design standards of a clinical trial. They propose three main study types for assessing specific markers (Figure 3.2), based on Simon and Altman (1994). Although Phases I to III have not yet been universally accepted, at the very least they provide an important starting point for prognostic marker research, particularly as currently many published primary studies are not properly designed. For example, often no justification is made for the sample size used, or whether the

---

1. **Phase I:** exploratory studies (hypothesis generating) which seek an association between a prognostic marker and characteristics of disease thought to have prognostic importance.
2. **Phase II:** exploratory studies attempting to use values of a prognostic marker to
   (a) discriminate between patients at high and low risk of disease progression or death; or to
   (b) indicate which subsets of patients are likely to benefit from therapy.
3. **Phase III:** confirmatory studies of a priori hypotheses attempting to use values of a prognostic marker to
   (a) discriminate between patients at high and low risk of disease progression or death; or to
   (b) indicate which subsets of patients are likely to benefit from therapy.

Figure 3.2: Types of prognostic marker studies, as suggested by Altman and Lyman (1998)

markers, subpopulations, and outcomes assessed were determined prior to the study beginning [Simon and Altman (1994)]; furthermore, the characteristics of patients assessed in a study may often not be described and thus one may have little idea of who the samples of patients selected are. Such problems make one concerned that the reasons regarding how and what results are published from a study may be subject to bias, which limits their reliability for clinical practice (see Section 3.2.5). The further problem for evidence synthesis is that, due to poor reporting of information across the large majority of studies [Riley *et al.* (2003a)], it is generally very difficult to differentiate those studies which were properly designed from those studies that were poorly designed.

A related problem is distinguishing those primary studies that were originally initiated for the same purpose [Altman and Lyman (1998)]. The majority of prognostic marker studies have the purpose to establish the association between a single putative marker of interest to some outcome (e.g., OS or DFS), and these were the predominant studies included in the neuroblastoma review introduced previously [Riley *et al.* (2004a)]. However, there are also some studies that do not have this primary purpose (e.g., studies to develop or validate a classification rule [Sauerbrei *et al.* (1997)]), yet still report summary statistics or IPD relating markers to outcome as secondary results. Some meta-analysts may deem that, other things being equal, only those studies that were specifically designed for the purposes of evaluating one or more markers should be included in the meta-analysis (i.e., those where prognostic marker results were the primary endpoint) [Egger *et al.* (2003)]. Unfortunately, as the original study aims are rarely specified in a published article, it is often hard to ascertain whether prognostic results were a primary or secondary objective. Indeed, a study may have started off with prognostic results as a secondary aim but then, perhaps after witnessing the results obtained, may have switched the primary focus of the published study to the prognostic markers.

3.2.3 Little indication of how to implement markers in clinical practice

Prognostic markers that can be specifically used to predict the response to therapy or treatment are called *predictive markers* (or predictive factors or predictive variables). For example, estrogen receptor and progesterone receptors are predictive markers used to select those breast cancer patients most likely to respond to hormone therapy [Duffy (2005)]. If the results from prognostic studies are to be most directly relevant to clinical practice, then as well as being properly designed (see Section 3.2.2), they must also take into account the treatment or therapeutic strategy involved in order to identify specific predictive markers [Windeler (2000)]. Such *predictive studies* relate to the Phase II(b) and III(b) studies in Figure 3.2 and they should ideally be integrated within an RCT, where the predictive ability of the marker can be assessed in relation to the treatment groups assessed. Unfortunately, there are few high-quality Phase II(b) and III(b) studies, and even when they are published it is often difficult to identify them from most other prognostic studies due to the type of study (e.g., exploratory – Phase I, confirmatory – Phase III) and the treatment received by patients not being reported. It is highly likely that the majority of prognostic studies in the published literature are actually Phase I or II because, as seen in the neuroblastoma review [Riley *et al.* (2003a)], they often contain small numbers of patients and report a large number of results for a variety of possible markers, and therefore do not seem to be focused on making confirmatory conclusions for a few markers in relation to specific treatments. Thus, even if a marker appears to have prognostic value, it will be very difficult to utilise it in clinical practice when there is a lack of identifiable, high-quality studies that relate its results to specific treatments. This problem will clearly also limit a clinically relevant evidence synthesis.

3.2.4   Small sample sizes

Small sample sizes is a particular problem for rare diseases, such as neuroblastoma or other childhood cancers, and leads to individual studies having low statistical power. It also leads to a greater number of similar, but ultimately slightly different, studies of the same prognostic markers as each research group reports the results for their own small sample. This in turn leads to heterogeneity and inconsistency in how and what results were reported, especially regarding the adjustment factors used, the characteristics of patients included, and the cut-off levels used to dichotomise the continuous markers into "high-risk" and "low-risk" levels (Figure 3.1). All these problems ultimately limit meta-analysis conclusions. For example, in the neuroblastoma review, if the hazard ratio was not reported we used indirect estimation methods to obtain an approximate value for the unavailable hazard ratios where possible [Parmar, Torri, and Stewart (1998)]. Such indirect methods more closely estimate the true values when the sample size is large, however, in the neuroblastoma review only 196 of 318 reports for which indirect estimation was required included more than 25 patients. Multiple studies with small sample sizes also cause the problem of overlapping sets of patients across different studies. Although prospective studies are the ideal ones [Altman and Lyman (1998)], most prognostic studies are retrospective, using information that has already been collected from stored samples (e.g., in a tumour bank), and so there is a large potential for different studies to report results for many of the same patients. However, it is practically very difficult to elicit those published studies that use the same or overlapping sets of patients, and this again weakens meta-analysis [Riley *et al.* (2003b)].

3.2.5   Publication bias, selective within-study reporting, and selective analyses

For prognostic marker studies, there is likely to be the common problem of publication bias, where results that do not generate formal statistically significant or clinically valuable findings may not be published. Other related dissemination bias problems may also exist. For example, within-study selective reporting may occur and in particular nonstatistically significant or negative results may not be reported in as much detail as significant or positive results, thus making the extraction of desired summary statistics for meta-analysis more difficult (e.g., '$p > 0.05$' is often presented) [Hahn, Williamson, and Hutton (2002)]. This may often be a consequence of a reluctance of journals or researchers to report negative findings in detail. Other forms of dissemination bias may include outcome reporting bias, subgroup reporting bias, and language bias [Egger, Dickersin, and Davey Smith (2001)]. In the meta-analysis of OS estimates for *MYCN* from the neuroblastoma review, there was a strong suggestion that dissemination bias may be affecting the results. For instance, consider a plot of all the $\log_e$(hazard ratio) estimates for OS against their standard error (Figure 3.3). The assumption is that this plot should form a funnel shape if dissemination bias is not present, as estimates from smaller studies will be more widely spread about the mean effect due to larger standard errors [Sterne, Egger, and Davey Smith (2001) and Duval and Tweedie (2000)]. However, the plot is not indicative of a very funnel-like shape, and asymmetry is apparent, with a gap in the bottom right of the plot (Figure 3.3). Furthermore, two statistical tests indicated that dissemination bias was likely to exist assuming that this was the main cause of funnel

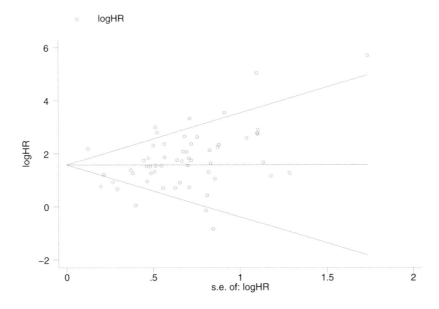

Figure 3.3: Funnel plot of the overall survival $\log_e$(hazard ratio) estimates for *MYCN* with Begg's pseudo 95% confidence limits [Begg and Mazumdar (1994)]

plot asymmetry ($p < 0.001$) [Egger *et al.* (1997) and Begg and Mazumdar (1994)]. It appears that some studies with less positive results than those obtained were missing from the meta-analysis, and this suggests that the true underlying pooled $\log_e$(hazard ratio) for OS is likely to be somewhat smaller than the estimated pooled value of 1.70 (equivalent to a hazard ratio of 5.48) [Riley *et al.* (2004b)].

It is important to note many problems of dissemination bias may also be introduced during a prognostic study and not just at the final reporting stage. For example, the type of statistical analysis used has an influence on the result which then may influence the dissemination bias [Holländer and Sauerbrei (2006)]. The choice of cut-off level used to dichotomise the marker, and thus define a low-risk and a high-risk group of patients, may also be specifically chosen to optimise the difference between groups and produce a result with the maximum statistical or clinical significance possible [Altman *et al.* (1994)]. The difficulty for meta-analysis is again distinguishing those properly conducted studies from those where biased choices of cut-off levels, analyses, and samples were used. Excluding studies with a small number of patients from the evidence synthesis may help alleviate the potential problem of bias, as these studies are likely to be of poorest quality. However, this issue relates to currently unanswered questions facing meta-analysts about which studies should generally be included in a meta-analysis [Egger *et al.* (2003)].

3.2.6   Lack of appreciation or validation of previous findings

Evidence-based reviews are facilitated when new primary studies specifically build on the results of previous studies, thus forming a collective drive toward answering questions of real clinical importance. For example, when a primary study assesses the potential of a new marker, it should do so in relation to those other markers previously identified as important and currently used in clinical practice. However, in reality many studies only report unadjusted results, and the adjusted results that are presented across studies are often highly inconsistent in the set of adjustment factors used [Riley *et al.* (2003a)]. For example, of the 17 adjusted hazard ratio estimates for OS and DFS that were obtained for *MYCN* from the neuroblastoma review, only 2 were adjusted for exactly the same set of factors, and both these were from the same article.

It would appear that a lack of collaboration across research groups combined with poorly designed studies (see Section 3.2.2) is causing there to be many similar but slightly different prognostic studies, with many not building on previous findings. Indeed, there may be a deliberate ploy to make a new primary study slightly different from those previously published in order to increase the opportunity for 'new' findings. Validation of previous findings is considered less important, and such studies may have a smaller chance of publication. Unfortunately, this leads to substantial clinical and methodological heterogeneity across studies. For example, the pooled *MYCN* meta-analysis result for OS was based on 45 hazard ratios, of which 6 were adjusted and 39 were unadjusted, and these related to at least 7 different cut-off levels, 3 different age groups, and 5 different stage groups (Figure 3.1). Other factors such as treatment received and how the marker was measured are likely to add further heterogeneity problems. This heterogeneity makes it very difficult for clinicians to interpret or use the *MYCN* pooled OS result in practice; for instance, which cut-off level should they use, which patients and treatments should *MYCN* be used for, and how should *MYCN* be used alongside other prognostic markers? The meta-analysis cannot provide answers to such questions.

To help try to make the meta-analysis results clearer, it may often be possible to perform separate meta-analysis for different subgroups of estimates. In Figure 3.1, we have pooled the 45 unadjusted and adjusted hazard ratios together in one analysis to obtain a pooled HR of 5.48 (95% CI: 4.30 to 6.97). Alternatively, if we just combine the 39 unadjusted results, then a pooled HR of 6.032 (95% CI: 4.640 to 7.842) is obtained; similarly, if we just combine the 6 adjusted results, then a pooled HR of 2.886 (95% CI: 1.823 to 4.569) is obtained. The fact that the unadjusted pooled result is substantially larger than the adjusted pooled result emphasises the difficulty in interpreting one overall meta-analysis that synthesises both types of estimates together [Holländer and Sauerbrei (2005)]. Furthermore, even the interpretation of the separate unadjusted and adjusted subgroup meta-analyses is practically impossible due to the additional heterogeneity in, amongst many other factors, treatment received, age of patients, and the cut-off level used across studies. Indeed, it was impossible to synthesise even two different *MYCN* unadjusted estimates that reflected patients and studies with similar features. The heterogeneity affecting the *MYCN* OS dataset therefore demonstrates that even subgroup meta-analyses may not easily allow clinically relevant evidence-based prognostic marker results.

3.3 What Improvements Are Needed in Primary Prognostic Marker Studies?

Given the discussion in Section 3.2, there are perhaps four main areas where improvements in primary prognostic marker studies are needed: study design, clinical relevance, statistica analysis, and study reporting. The key aspects of how each of these areas needs to improve are summarised in Figure 3.4, and these are based on four previous publications [Riley *et al.* (2003a), Altman and Lyman (1998), Holländer and Sauerbrei (2006), and Windeler (2000)]. Improvements in each of these four areas would not only improve the clinical relevance and validity of the primary studies themselves, but would also greatly facilitate evidence-based reviews in this field as discussed in Section 3.2.

- **Study design** – see Altman and Lyman (1998). Improvements need to arise through greater consideration of, amongst other things:
  – Study type (e.g., Phase I, II or III).
  – Study purpose (e.g., what is the primary objective?).
  – Sample size (e.g., what is the desired power to detect meaningful differences in outcome).
  – Inclusion/exclusion criteria.
  – Prior hypotheses and the prior specification of which markers and outcomes are to be considered (e.g., in a study protocol).
- **Clinical relevance** – see Windeler(2000). Primary studies need to produce more clinically useful results by, amongst other things:
  – Collaborating across research groups to achieve larger sample sizes and consistency in method of measuring the marker, cut-off levels, adjustment factors, and outcomes assessed.
  – Building on the results of previous studies, and assessing new markers in relation to those markers and treatments currently used in practice.
  – Being high-quality, large-scale Phase III studies and relating assessments to specific treatment strategies so that predictive markers can be identified for clinical practice.
- **Statistical analysis** – see Holländer and Sauerbrei (2006). The statistical analysis in primary studies should consider:
  – Multivariable analyses that adjust for standard factors.
  – Whether a Cox regression model is appropriate.
  – The analysis and reporting of continuous markers on their original scale (rather than using a cut-off level).
  – Analyses in subgroups only if there is strong justification and if sample size is sufficient.
  – Whether the main assumptions of the model are plausible.
  – The use of sensitivity analyses for important issues.
  – The potential issue of overoptimism when the same data are used for model development, estimation of parameters, and also model assessment.
- **Study reporting** - see Riley *et al.* (2003a). Improved reporting of prognostic marker studies is greatly needed with regard to, amongst other things:
  – Reporting the results of all markers and outcomes considered, not just those statistically significant (to reduce the threat of publication bias and within-study selective reporting).
  – Reporting an effect estimate (e.g., hazard ratio) with confidence interval, rather than solely a p-value.
  – Reporting marker results adjusted for other prognostic factors and treatments of recognised and accepted clinical importance.
  – Making individual patient data available for those performing evidence synthesis.

Figure 3.4: Key areas where improved research and better statistical practice are needed within primary prognostic marker studies

To help achieve improvements in study design, we strongly recommend those researchers initiating and carrying out prognostic studies refer to the study design criteria proposed by Altman and Lyman (1998). In particular, those involved in primary studies should decide from the outset whether their study is to be a Phase I, Phase II, or Phase III study (Figure 3.2), and then clearly state this in the eventual published article. Indeed, there needs to be a general move away from Phase I or II studies toward a greater number of large, protocol-driven (preferably prospective), high-quality Phase III studies. Furthermore, in order to identify predictive markers, there is also a need to directly relate marker assessments to a specific treatment regimen (i.e., more Phase III(b) studies are required). Such a move will inevitably require research groups to collaborate wherever possible to achieve greater sample sizes; for example, Look *et al.* (2002) have successfully initiated a multicentre study of prognostic markers within the breast cancer field. To help achieve improvements in the analysis and reporting of results in published studies, we refer to Chapter 2 by Holländer and Sauerbrei (2006) in this volume and to those reporting guidelines provided by Riley *et al.* (2003a). In particular, all markers assessed (and not just those statistically significant) should be reported, because this would help to reduce publication and other related biases, as would the reporting of prespecified hypotheses within a clear and readily available study protocol [Altman and Lyman (1998)]. We also recommend that continuous markers should not be dichotomised because, amongst other reasons, this approach discards potentially important quantitative information and considerably reduces the power to detect a real association between the marker and outcome [Altman *et al.* (1994)]. We encourage researchers to analyse and report results (e.g., hazard ratio estimates) of continuous markers on their original continuous scale [Altman *et al.* (1994)]. Furthermore, the most appropriate analysis of continuous prognostic markers may require nonlinear modelling techniques, as highlighted by Sauerbrei *et al.* (1999).

3.4 Evidence Synthesis Using Individual Patient Data Rather than Summary Statistics

Meta-analysis of survival studies using summary statistics extracted from the published literature can be beneficial [Tudur *et al.* (2001)], and improved reporting of literature-based results is therefore clearly important [Riley *et al.* (2003a)]. However, even if all studies are well-designed and clinically important Phase III studies, there is increasing evidence that unless IPD is also made available from these studies, a clinically useful evidence-based review and meta-analysis may still be limited because of the differing study characteristics, statistical analyses, and reporting standards used [Riley *et al.* (2003a) and Holländer and Sauerbrei (2006)]. The main problems limiting meta-analysis of summary statistics from the published literature are shown in Figure 3.5, and improved reporting of summary statistics in primary studies is likely to reduce rather than remove these problems [Riley *et al.* (2003a)]. For example, even if reporting standards improve, it is highly likely that for some studies not all the summary statistics and outcomes desired would be available, and it is perhaps inevitable that there will always be some heterogeneity across studies in cut-off levels, markers assessed, and adjustment factors used. The main potential advantages for an IPD evidence synthesis of prognostic marker studies are shown in Figure 3.6. For example, IPD including exact marker levels would allow data to be reanalysed where cut-off levels, and adjustment factors were not consistent [Holländer and Sauerbrei (2006)], and would allow continuous marker results where originally a cut-off level was used. Furthermore, it may increase the opportunity to evaluate combinations of markers, which may produce more specific and accurate prognostic assessments than the individual markers themselves. Furthermore, Lambert *et al.* (2002) have shown that IPD is generally required when investigating patient characteristics as effect modifiers in a meta-analysis.

We acknowledge that having IPD from every primary study may still not necessarily solve all the problems for meta-analysis of prognostic studies [Stewart and Tierney (2002)]. In particular, not all the information required to calculate the desired estimates will always be available in the IPD; for example, if time of disease recurrence had not been recorded, it would not be possible to assess DFS, and if continuous marker levels are presented as dichotomised, then one could not choose a consistent cut-off level across studies. Publication bias may also affect which IPD is available across studies, and indeed what is exactly reported in the IPD itself. For example, information about some outcomes or patients may be deliberately omitted if they produce less interesting or contradictory findings. The availability of IPD will also not overcome the problems of poor study design or that the study does not consider clinically relevant issues, and there is little benefit of obtaining IPD from previous studies of poor quality. Obtaining IPD is also likely to be more costly and time-consuming than extracting literature-based results [Altman *et al.* (2006) and Stewart and Tierney (2002)] and there is the potential for the IPD available to simply relate to those studies which were the best reported in the first place. Of course, even when prioritising the IPD approach, the meta-analyst will in practice end up with a mixture of estimates obtained from IPD and estimates obtained from summary statistics; hence, novel meta-analysis methods which take these different sources into account are also needed [Steyerberg *et al.* (2000)]. The practical feasibility of actually initiating, obtaining, and synthesising IPD is considered in further detail Chapter 1 by Altman *et al.* (2006) in this volume.

- Missing and poorly reported outcomes and summary statistics across studies, possibly due to within-study selective reporting
- The threat of publication bias, and other related dissemination biases
- Direct estimates (e.g., of the hazard ratio) for some studies, only indirect estimates for others
- Heterogeneous choice and use of adjustment factors across studies
- Heterogeneous and biased choice of cut-off levels across studies
- Other heterogeneity across studies in type of statistical analysis used, method of measuring the markers, treatment the patients received, and stage of disease
- Possibly overlapping sets of patients across studies
- Difficulty in assessing whether patient characteristics are effect modifiers across studies
- Difficulty in assessing the benefits of a prognostic marker over time and in relation to time-dependent covariates such as treatment received and stage of disease

Figure 3.5: Summary of the main problems preventing clinically useful meta-analysis of summary statistics extracted from published prognostic marker studies

Availability of IPD from the primary studies has the potential to allow one to:
- Obtain estimates for those missing or poorly reported outcomes and summary statistics across studies; it may thus reduce the problem of selective within-study reporting
- Obtain more direct estimates (e.g., of the hazard ratio) where previously only indirect estimates were available
- Standardise strategy of statistical analysis across studies
- Produce more adjusted estimates where previously only unadjusted estimates were available
- Use a (small) consistent set of adjustment factors across studies
- Use a consistent cut-off level across studies, or produce continuous marker results where originally a cut-off level was used (or vice versa)
- Assess the benefits of using combinations of markers
- Assess specific subgroups of patients across studies (e.g., premenopausal, stage 4 disease), and assess whether patient-level characteristics (such as age and treatment) are effect modifiers across studies
- Identify those studies which contain the same or overlapping sets of patients
- Assess model assumptions in each study, such as proportional hazards
- Assess markers over time and in relation to time-dependent covariates such as treatment received and stage of disease

Figure 3.6: Summary of the main potential benefits of having individual patient data (IPD) for a meta-analysis of prognostic marker studies

3.5   Discussion

In this paper we have identified several areas of primary prognostic marker studies that need to be improved in order to allow more clinically relevant results from both the individual studies themselves and also from evidence-based reviews in this field. It is clearly important that the design, clinical relevance, and reporting of studies are all collectively improved, and this follows on from the message in another chapter in this volume [Holländer and Sauerbrei (2006)] that there is a need to improve and partly standardise the statistical analysis in primary studies. It only takes one of these four areas to be poor for the usefulness of the individual study to be limited. For example, no improvements in study reporting can overcome poor study design or that the study did not consider those questions of clinical relevance. Guidelines for the design [Altman and Lyman (1998)], purpose [Altman and Lyman (1998)], analysis [Holländer and Sauerbrei (2006)], and reporting [Riley et al. (2003a)] of prognostic marker studies are clearly very important, and indeed new reporting guidelines have just been considered by McShane et al. (2005). However, there is little evidence to suggest that solely publishing such guidelines will cause the changes in practice required. Perhaps the most pivotal role in ensuring the guidelines are adhered to is held by the editors of and reviewers for clinical journals. Editors can be considered as the 'gate-keepers' to publication, and they can therefore enforce standards that an article must meet if it is to be considered for publication. Indeed, some editors ensure certain standards are met at an early stage through the prospective registration of trials with their journal (e.g., *The Lancet*). However, it may be more difficult to take this approach with prognostic marker studies as there is usually no intervention as such and many aspects have already been performed before the study is initiated (e.g., tumour samples already taken and stored in a tumour bank).

We have also discussed in this paper the importance of IPD for evidence synthesis of prognostic marker studies, and highlighted how this has substantial benefits over the literature-based approach. Authors of primary studies are encouraged to make their IPD available for those performing meta-analysis. Other steps toward clinically useful evidence-based results are also needed. For instance, the initiation of tumour banks may help as these store patient tumour samples in a central repository and allow retrospective analyses [Kerr (2003)]. This set-up allows new potentially important prognostic markers to be retrospectively analysed in comparison to the set of markers previously found to be important. Hence, if IPD were also stored for each study, a patient's tumour sample could be reassessed and the information for the new marker placed alongside the other marker details already available in the IPD. The UKCCSG have initiated such an approach for storing tumour samples of childhood cancers [Mott, Mann, and Stiller (1997)].

The need for IPD combined with the need for new studies that are properly designed and appropriately targeted suggests that evidence synthesis of prognostic marker studies may be best achieved through prospectively planned pooled analyses [Blettner *et al.* (1999)]. To achieve this, collaborative groups are required to work toward a number of high quality primary studies with the collective, long-term aim of pooling together the IPD from each study to formulate evidence-based results. In this situation, the primary studies themselves could be developed with a prospective meta-analysis in mind, so that it would be pre-specified which clinical questions to address in the studies and one could achieve consistency in design, markers assessed, marker measurement, treatments received, patients included, outcomes recorded, and method of analysis amongst other pertinent factors. It would also allow authors of primary studies to know right from the beginning that their IPD would be needed, which should, one would hope, make them more amenable to recording and maintaining high-quality IPD that they are also willing to make available at the end of their study. Prospectively planned pooled analyses are already used in epidemiological research [Blettner *et al.* (1999)], and their initiation within the prognostic marker field is something we strongly recommend.

Acknowledgements. Richard Riley is funded by the Department of Health NCCRCD as a Post-doctoral Research Scientist in Evidence Synthesis.

References

1. Altman, D. G. (2001). Systematic reviews of evaluations of prognostic variables, *BMJ*, **323**, 224–228.

2. Altman, D. G., Lausen, B., Sauerbrei, W., and Schumacher, M. (1994). Dangers of using "optimal" cutpoints in the evaluation of prognostic factors, *Journal of the National Cancer Institute*, **86**, 829–835.

3. Altman, D. G., and Lyman, G. H. (1998). Methodological challenges in the evaluation of prognostic factors in breast cancer, *Breast Cancer Research and Treatment*, **52**, 289–303.

4. Altman, D. G., Trivella, M., Pezzella, F., Harris, A. L., and Pastorino, U. (2006). Systematic review of multiple studies of prognosis: The feasibility of obtaining individual patient data, *In this volume*.

5. Begg, C. B., and Mazumdar, M. (1994). Operating characteristics of a rank correlation test for publication bias, *Biometrics*, **50**, 1088–1101.

6. Blettner, M., Sauerbrei, W., Schlehofer, B., Scheuchenpflug, T., and Friedenreich, C. (1999). Traditional reviews, meta-analyses and pooled analyses in epidemiology, *International Journal of Epidemiology*, **28**, 1-9.

7. Carpeggiani, C., L'Abbate, A., Landi, P. *et al.* (2004). Early assessment of heart rate variability is predictive of in-hospital death and major complications after acute myocardial infarction, *International Journal of Cardiolology*, **96**, 361–368.

8. Deodhar, A. A., Brabyn, J., Pande, I., Scott, D. L., and Woolf, A. D. (2003). Hand bone densitometry in rheumatoid arthritis, a five year longitudinal study: An outcome measure and a prognostic marker, *Annals of the Rheumatic Disease*, **62**, 767–770.

9. Duffy, M. J. (2005). Predictive markers in breast and other cancers: A review, *Clinical Chemistry*, **51**, 494–503.

10. Duval, S., and Tweedie, R. (2000). Trim and fill: A simple funnel-plot-based method of testing and adjusting for publication bias in meta-analysis, *Biometrics*, **56**, 455–463.

11. Egger, M., Davey Smith, G., Schneider, M., and Minder, C. (1997). Bias in meta-analysis detected by a simple, graphical test, *BMJ*, **315**, 629–634.

12. Egger, M., Davey Smith, G., and Altman, D. G. (2001). *Systematic Reviews in Health Care: Meta-Analysis in Context*, BMJ, London.

13. Egger, M., Dickersin, K., and Davey Smith, G. (2001). Problems and limitations in conducting systematic reviews, In *Systematic Reviews in Health Care: Meta-analysis in Context* (Eds., M. Egger, G. Davey Smith, and D. G. Altman), pp. 43–68, BMJ, London.

14. Egger, M., Juni, P., Bartlett, C., Holenstein, F., and Sterne, J. (2003). How important are comprehensive literature searches and the assessment of trial quality in systematic reviews? Empirical study, *Health Technology Assessment*, **7**, 1–76.

15. Hahn, S., Williamson, P. R., and Hutton, J. L. (2002). Investigation of within-study selective reporting in clinical research: Follow-up of applications submitted to a local research ethics committee, *Journal of Evaluation in Clinical Practice*, **8**, 353–359.

16. Hemingway, H., and Marmot, M. (1999). Evidence based cardiology: Psychosocial factors in the aetiology and prognosis of coronary heart disease. Systematic review of prospective cohort studies, *BMJ*, **318**, 1460-1467.

17. Holländer, N., and Sauerbrei, W. (2006). On statistical approaches for the multivariable analysis of prognostic factor studies, *in this volume*.

18. Kerr, C. (2003). UK launch "virtual" tumour bank to improve treatment research, *Lancet Oncology*, **4**, 264.

19. Lambert, P. C., Sutton, A. J., Abrams, K. R., and Jones, D. R. (2002). A comparison of summary patient-level covariates in meta-regression with individual patient data meta-analysis, *Journal of Clinical Epidemiology*, **55**, 86–94.

20. Look, M. P., van Putten, W. L., Duffy, M. J. *et al.* (2002). Pooled analysis of prognostic impact of urokinase-type plasminogen activator and its inhibitor PAI-1 in 8377 breast cancer patients, *Journal of the National Cancer Institute*, **94**, 116–128.

21. McShane, L. M., Altman, D. G., Sauerbrei, W., Taube, S. E., Gion, M., and Clark, G. M. (2005). REporting recommendations for tumor MARKer prognostic studies (REMARK), *European Journal of Cancer*, **41**, 1690–1696.

22. Mitchell, S. L., Kiely, D. K., Hamel, M. B., Park, P. S., Morris, J. N., and Fries, B. E. (2004). Estimating prognosis for nursing home residents with advanced dementia, *Journal of the American Medical Association*, **291**, 2734–2740.

23. Mott, M. G., Mann, J. R., and Stiller, C. A. (1997). The United Kingdom children's cancer study group–the first 20 years of growth and development, *European Journal Cancer*, **33**, 1448–1452.

24. Parmar, M. K., Torri, V., and Stewart, L. (1998). Extracting summary statistics to perform meta-analyses of the published literature for survival endpoints, *Statistics in Medicine*, **17**, 2815–2834.

25. Riley, R. D., Abrams, K. R., Sutton, A. J. *et al.* (2003a). Reporting of prognostic markers: Current problems and development of guidelines for evidence-based practice in the future, *British Journal of Cancer*, **88**, 1191–1198.

26. Riley, R. D., Burchill, S. A., Abrams, K. R. *et al.* (2003b). A systematic review and evaluation of the use of tumour markers in paediatric oncology: Ewing's sarcoma and neuroblastoma, *Health Technology Assessment*, **7**, 1–162.

27. Riley, R. D., Heney, D., Jones, D. R. *et al.* (2004a). A systematic review of molecular and biological tumor markers in neuroblastoma, *Clinical Cancer Research*, **10**, 4–12.

28. Riley, R. D., Sutton, A. J., Abrams, K. R., and Lambert, P. C. (2004b). Sensitivity analyses allowed more appropriate and reliable meta-analysis conclusions for multiple outcomes when missing data was present, *Journal of Clinical Epidemiology*, **57**, 911–924.

29. Sauerbrei, W., Hubner, K., Schmoor, C., and Schumacher, M. (1997). Validation of existing and development of new prognostic classification schemes in node negative breast cancer, *German Breast Cancer Study Group, Breast Cancer Res. Treat.*, **42**, 149–163.

30. Sauerbrei, W., Royston, P., Bojar, H., Schmoor, C., and Schumacher, M. (1999). Modelling the effects of standard prognostic factors in node-positive breast cancer. German Breast Cancer Study Group (GBSG), *British Journal of Cancer*, **79**, 1752–1760.

31. Simon, R., and Altman, D. G. (1994). Statistical aspects of prognostic factor studies in oncology, *British Journal of Cancer*, **69**, 979–985.

32. Sterne, J. A., Egger, M., and Davey Smith, G. (2001). Systematic reviews in health care: Investigating and dealing with publication and other biases in meta-analysis, *BMJ*, **323**, 101–105.

33. Stewart, L. A., and Tierney, J. F. (2002). To IPD or not to IPD? Advantages and disadvantages of systematic reviews using individual patient data, *Evaluation and Health Professions*, **25**, 76–97.

34. Steyerberg, E. W., Eijkemans, M. J., Van Houwelingen, J. C., Lee, K. L., and Habbema, J. D. (2000). Prognostic models based on literature and individual patient data in logistic regression analysis, *Statistics in Medicine*, **19**, 141–160.

35. Tudur, C., Williamson, P. R., Kahan, S., and Best, L. Y. (2001). The value of the aggregated data approach to meta-analysis with time-to-event outcomes, *Journal of the Royal Statistical Society, Series A*, **164**, 357–370.

36. Windeler, J. (2000). Prognosis - What does the clinician associate with this notion? *Statistics in Medicine*, **19**, 425–430.

PART II
Pharmacovigilance

4

Sentinel Event Methods for Monitoring Unanticipated Adverse Events

Peter A. Lachenbruch and Janet Wittes

U.S. Food and Drug Administration, Rockville, MD, USA
Statistical Collaborative, Washington, DC, USA

Abstract: We propose an approach to monitoring unanticipated adverse events in a clinical trial. For a specific type of event, the methods allow the first occurrence, the first few occurrences, or an elevated rate to trigger a formal monitoring plan to identify whether that event occurs more frequently in the treated than in the control arm. The methods can apply either to rare events or to common events not expected to occur at an elevated rate in the treated group. We offer some simple models, emphasizing that, by the very nature of its rarity, a rare event is quite difficult to monitor.

Keywords and phrases: Safety, data monitoring, sentinel events, group sequential plans, time to event analyses, progressive censoring

4.1 Introduction

A clinical trial studying a new product, or a new use for an already approved product, aims to assess the product's safety and efficacy. Available statistical methods allow rigorous assessment of efficacy: one specifies null and alternative hypotheses along with an appropriate statistical test. At the end of the trial, one applies the test to the data and ends with a conclusion regarding efficacy. Trials with a Data Safety Monitoring Board (DSMB) that observes the data over time might adopt a group-sequential interim monitoring plan that allows early stopping to declare efficacy with preservation of the Type 1 error rate. Such procedures are well known [see, e.g., Jennison and Turnbull (2000)].

Monitoring safety poses more difficult problems. Although some trials explicitly aim to determine whether a product is safe, the primary aim of most trials is to show efficacy, with safety a byproduct of the design. We generally assess efficacy with a single prespecified primary endpoint. For safety, by

61

contrast, multiplicity abounds and important safety issues may not be clearly defined before the clinical trial begins. Strict safety stopping rules may not apply because a DSMB may wish more flexibility in its decision-making for safety than for efficacy. We note that the FDA has adopted the term Data Monitoring Committee (DMC); however, we use DSMB to emphasize the "safety" aspect of the function of these boards. Many different types of events can occur; at the end of the trial, identifying which, if any, the product under study causes is daunting both statistically and medically. Even more difficult is the dilemma for a DSMB observing the data over time: a DSMB that stops a trial early for an observed excess of events may be reacting to chance phenomena; failure to stop may put subjects in the trial at unnecessary risk. This paper proposes sentinel event approaches, both classical and Bayesian, for a DSMB to use in monitoring the safety of a product during a clinical trial. We consider here confirmatory (Phase 3) controlled or uncontrolled trials; see FDA Guidance for Clinical Trial Sponsors (2006). Uncontrolled Phase 3 trials, although not common in most situations, are sometimes used to study orphan diseases or medical devices.

We start with three examples (Section 4.2) to provide the context for the methods. We then present a brief description of usual approaches, both formal and informal, for monitoring specific adverse events (Section 4.3). We propose to use the first recognition of an unanticipated adverse event as a sentinel alerting the DSMB to monitor the trial for this event. Not all such first recognitions would lead to such monitoring; only those deemed sufficiently worrisome would qualify. After the sentinel event, we apply statistical procedures that control the Type 1 error rate. This chapter presents some examples of the approach. For specific cases, the DSMB should devise a method appropriate to the situation, accounting for such items as the stage of recruitment, the planned follow-up time, and, of course, the nature of the study and of the sentinel event.

For monitoring in response to a few sentinel events, or a single one (Section 4.4), we present methods for trials with a fixed follow-up time for each subject where all events occur in the treated group (Section 4.4.1) and for trials with a common closeout time, that is, follow-up censored on a fixed calendar date where events occur in both the treated and control group (Section 4.4.2).

For large trials with many events, we propose using the first recognition that the rate of a particular event is higher in the treated arm; this type of sentinel event is really a sentinel rate (Section 4.5).

We end with a simple Bayesian model (Section 4.6) applied to one of the examples and some concluding remarks (Section 4.7).

4.2 Examples

This section presents three examples. The first shows when a single rare, unanticipated adverse event could serve as a sentinel for further monitoring. In the second, the sentinel is a small number of unanticipated events of a specific type. The third case provides an example where an increased rate of an adverse event could trigger further formal monitoring.

Example 4.2.1 (A single sentinel event.) A death occurred early in the course of a clinical trial of a childhood vaccine. The trial was so small that any death was unexpected. Consequently, the death caused serious concern for the DSMB; members wanted to be confident that the death did not indicate an unanticipated problem with the vaccine.

Example 4.2.2 (A small number of events comprising the sentinel.) In a clinical trial randomizing subjects to either a new or a control vaccine, three subjects in about 900 in the new vaccine group and one of 300 in the control vaccine group experienced a specific serious adverse event. The p-value for the difference in these rates is 0.6. The FDA was consulted about the findings and was worried not about the difference between the two rates, but about the overall event rate itself, because the anticipated serious adverse event rate had been roughly 1 in 10,000, substantially lower than the observed rate of $1/300$.

Example 4.2.3 (A sentinel event rate.) The Women's Health Initiative (WHI) was composed of four trials. Here we discuss the PERT trial (Progesterone–Estrogen Replacement Therapy), the component that studied the hypothesis that postmenopausal treatment with estrogen and progesterone reduces the rate of myocardial infarction. This trial, designed to last 12 years, had many endpoints and several major hypotheses. The investigators and the DSMB published their monitoring plan for safety and efficacy [Freedman *et al.* (1996)]. The investigators anticipated that estrogens would reduce the rate of myocardial infarction, hip fracture, and colorectal cancer, but increase the rate of invasive breast cancer, pulmonary embolism, and endometrial cancer. Stroke was a "monitored" endpoint, that is, one that the DSMB was to look at carefully over the course of the trial, but no a priori hypothesis was established concerning the direction of the effect.

Early in the trial, the DSMB noted a higher incidence of stroke and pulmonary embolism, and a lower rate of breast cancer in the PERT group. Quite surprisingly and contrary to the primary hypothesis of the study, the PERT group also had an early higher incidence of myocardial infarction than the placebo group. The trends for pulmonary embolism, stroke, and myocardial infarction continued throughout the trial, and the breast cancer rates became higher in the PERT than in the placebo group.

The DSMB of the WHI recommended stopping the PERT trial early because interim results showed:

- An excess of invasive breast cancer on the treated arm. This excess exceeded the prespecified boundary for harm for breast cancer.

- A myocardial infarction rate in the treated arm substantially higher than in the placebo arm. The monitoring plan for the WHI included an O'Brien–Fleming bound for benefit on myocardial infarction. Because the plan had no a priori bound for harm, the observed excess did not cross any prespecified monitoring boundary.

- Accounting for both positive and negative effects on seven monitored endpoints, an adverse effect of treatment that was consistent with the prespecified boundary for overall harm.

The National Heart, Lung, and Blood Institute, the sponsor of the trial, stopped the PERT trial soon after the DSMBs recommendation [Writing Group for the Womens Health Initiative Investigators (2002)].

Monitoring the PERT trial was complicated by the fact that the WHI included an estrogen-alone (ERT) trial, which studied women who had a hysterectomy prior to randomization. Early in the course of the study, the DSMB had observed more myocardial infarctions in both hormone-treated groups (ERT and PERT) than in their respective placebo groups. In response to these observations, the DSMB requested periodic updates on the overall event rates and based the decision to continue the study on its best judgment at each meeting. The DSMB could have regarded the excess rate of myocardial infarction as a sentinel rate.

4.3 Usual Approaches to Monitoring Safety

Many adverse events that occur during the course of a trial are expected. Some may be due to the disease itself. Others may be caused by the product under study, by comorbidities, or by drug interactions. For studies of drugs or biologicals, sometimes a particular class of product may be known to cause specific adverse events. Early phase studies should have already elucidated the mechanism of action of the drug and its pharmacokinetics, so that common adverse events attributable to the drug should have already been identified. In Phase 3 trials of diseases that are not life-threatening, serious adverse events will usually occur only rarely. In life-threatening disease, adverse experiences that reflect the process of the disease are common, but their rates are expected to be similar in the treated and control groups. Of particular concern are unanticipated serious or life-threatening events that arise during the course of the trial.

Standard statistical guidelines can specify methods for monitoring anticipated adverse events. When prior experience provides a background rate, a formal statistical monitoring plan can detect rates in excess of expectation. For example, many injected vaccines cause injection site reactions, such as soreness or redness. Similarly, bleeding is common in trials of antithrombotic agents. If historical data provide an expected event rate, the investigators can design a monitoring plan to identify an unacceptably high rate. Although it is generally preferable to assess safety by comparing the event rates by treatment group, sometimes it is also useful to compare the rates within a trial to the rates expected from historical data. A DSMB should know if the rates in the trial in both the treatment and control arms are meaningfully above expectation. As we show below, for very rare events, a few occurrences in the treated group and none in the control can lead to concern.

For unanticipated events, a DSMB risks reacting to a falsely "discovered" endpoint [Jennison and Turnbull (2000) and Mehrotra and Heyse (2004)], for the event may have occurred in the treatment arm purely by chance. Therefore, DSMBs typically wish to dampen a rush to judgment about the product or intervention. In prevention trials among healthy volunteers or in trials of diseases or conditions not usually accompanied by many types of serious adverse events (e.g., relief of minor headache pain), one analysis might compare the total number of adverse events to a standard rate known from historical data (a hurdle) or to the comparator (a placebo or active control). The observation that the patients in the test group had more adverse events than expected or more than those in the comparator might be disconcerting.

Trials in diseases with many associated adverse events (e.g., Type 2 diabetes) may compare only the aggregate of all serious adverse events to those that lead to hospitalization or are life-threatening. For diseases in which many serious adverse events occur over a short time period (e.g., sepsis), such an approach will generally not be useful, for nearly all patients will experience serious adverse events. Instead, focusing on particular serious adverse events will likely increase the specificity of the comparison.

A DSMB that encounters a worrisome excess of adverse events in a Phase 3 clinical trial typically responds by monitoring that event more frequently or spending more time discussing it. Sometimes, the DSMB waits until the difference between the number of events in the treated and control group hits some nominal level of significance. The statisticians often complain that such an approach is biased, because it includes the event that led to the monitoring, nonrigorous, because it does not preserve the Type 1 error rate, and is woefully lacking in power. We have rarely seen a DSMB institute a formal plan for subsequent monitoring of that event.

4.4   Methods for Sentinel Events

Without sufficient data, as in the case of rare events, a plausible statistical model, coupled with reasonable sensitivity analyses, may enlighten the DSMB's interpretation of the observations. In this section, we present a number of procedures as examples of our approach. The procedures share some simple features. First, they identify a sentinel event. Next, they establish a statistical method for monitoring subsequent occurrences of that event. The method must exclude any occurrence of the sentinel event that led to the monitoring. Furthermore, the method should have reasonably high power. It should be statistically unbiased, but its Type 1 error rate may be set at a one-sided level higher than the conventional 0.025.

For individual events, we may consider (a) the number of nonevents until the kth event or (b) the time until the next (or kth) event. For groups of patients in whom the sentinel "event" is an unexpectedly high rate, we can use (c) the event rate in the future patients.

Various statistical models suggest themselves: for individual events the negative binomial model or a binomial sequential probability ratio test is natural for problem (a) whereas the exponential or gamma distribution is appropriate for problem (b). Normal models lend themselves to problem (c).

The remainder of this section deals with two specific examples of the approach. In the first example (Section 4.4.1), all subjects have the same follow-up time and all events occur in the treated group (or the monitoring is based only on the treated group). The second example (Section 4.4.2) provides an approach when the follow-up times differ and we are comparing the occurrences of the event in the treated group to a historical rate or to the control group.

4.4.1   Constant follow-up time

When all subjects in the trial have the same follow-up time, one can define a sentinel event that triggers a monitoring activity but is not itself included in the monitoring. An example of such a trigger is the occurrence of a single rare event following administration of the product, where "rare" might be defined as an event that would be expected to occur in less than $1/1500$ administrations. An important question is whether only patients randomized after this subject should contribute to the monitoring set. If the DSMB uses the exponential distribution to model the distribution of time to event, the exponential distribution's lack of memory allows inclusion of early patients. To keep the statistical analysis simple, we consider the time to such presumably rare events to be exponentially distributed and then monitor the time to the *next* event (or next k events). Our first example, the single death in a trial of a childhood vaccine, provides a case of this type. Here we consider the case in which all events occur in the treated group.

For trials with a single administration of a drug (or a short-term treatment period), we might count the number of nonevents (i.e., the number of administrations of the drug not followed by an adverse event) until the kth event occurs, where k is small. The relevant time is the time from randomization. Thus, the DSMB might consider events within a specific number of days, T, after administration. The analysis applies only to the people who have had an event or who have had at least T days of follow-up. In such a case, the traditional significance level of 0.05 seems too stringent. Instead, a safety monitor or DSMB might decide that a probability below 0.1 or 0.2 should lead to more frequent monitoring or to a pause in the trial for further reflection.

A second statistical model might consider the time until the kth event. Assuming a short period of enrollment, an exponential distribution for time to event yields a gamma distribution for the time to the kth event. In some cases, only adverse events that occur within T days after the end of therapy are plausibly considered. Such a model would lead to a progressively censored sample. Of course, the distribution of time to event should be examined carefully, for a cluster of events that occur soon after T may in fact be related to therapy.

To increase power, we might wish to estimate the mean time to an event. For the exponential distribution, this estimated mean time $\hat{\mu} = \{\sum t_i + [N - n] \times T\}/n = V/n$, where N is the number of subjects in the treated group, n the number with an event, and $2V/\mu$ has a $\chi^2(2n)$ distribution. In situations where μ is expected to be large, say 1500 days, an estimate of 500 days would be troubling.

Consider a design with moderately high power at μ_0/R, $(R < 1)$, where R is the ratio of the mean time to event under the hypothesis of "no safety concern." For example, if $\mu_0 = 1500$ and $T = 30$, we might want to test for $R = 3$ at 80% power and use $k = 2$ (i.e., the distribution of total time to the second event after the sentinel event). Note we count each person's time from the administration of the product, not from the start of the study. One might use $k = 2$ if the event were quite serious and one did not wish to wait long to determine risk. The critical region would be

$$2[(t_1 + t_2) + 30(N - 2)]/1500 \leq 0.711,$$

where N is the number of people enrolled after the person with the sentinel event. For each person with an event, we calculate the time from administration of the product until the event.

For example, suppose after the sentinel event, two new events occur immediately upon administration of the vaccine. That is, both events occur at $t = 0$.

In this situation, being within the critical region would require that $N < 20$. Consider, for example, a vaccine study where subjects are recruited over time, perhaps a short time. In order to conclude that the event represents a safety concern, this second event after the sentinel event must occur before the 20th person enrolled after the person with the sentinel event receives the vaccine. If the second event did not occur until $N = 30$, then $V = (t_1 + t_2) + 30(N - 2) > 840$, $\chi^2 \geq 1680/1500 = 1.12$, and we could not conclude that there was a safety concern.

The power of this procedure, namely, the probability that $2V/\mu < 0.711$ when $= 500$, is low:

$$P\left(\frac{2V}{1500} \leq 0.711 | \mu = 500\right) = P(\chi_4^2 \leq 2.133) = 0.29.$$

Achieving high power requires either more than two events or specifying a more extreme difference. For example, a mean time to the event of 5000 days and $R = 10.1$ would give power:

$$P\left(\frac{2V}{5000} \leq 0.711 | \mu = 500\right) = P(\chi_4^2 \leq 7.11) = 0.87.$$

This model could reliably detect a large difference from expected mean time to event with only two events in the treated group and none in the control.

Note that this approach rejects for small, not large, values of V creating a trap for the unwary statistician because most χ^2 tests reject for large values of the test statistic.

The following curves, see Figure 4.1, show the power of this test for various ratios of mean time to event under the null and the alternative hypothesis when $(= 0.05$ and $0.10)$. Here, n is the number of events and $2n$ the number of degrees of freedom. If the ratio R is very high, or the number of events monitored is large, this method yields adequate power. For as few as four events, this method can detect a ratio of at least five with a power of 0.80.

4.4.2 Censoring at a fixed calendar time

We use a type I censoring model if censoring occurs at a fixed calendar time, rather than after a fixed exposure period. The maximum likelihood estimate of μ is

$$\hat{\mu} = \frac{\sum t_i + \sum T_j}{n},$$

where t_j are the event times and T_j are the times of censored observations. Using the observed information, we find

$$z = \frac{\hat{\mu} - \mu}{\sqrt{\frac{\hat{\mu}^2}{k}}} = \sqrt{k}\frac{\hat{\mu} - \mu}{\hat{\mu}} .$$

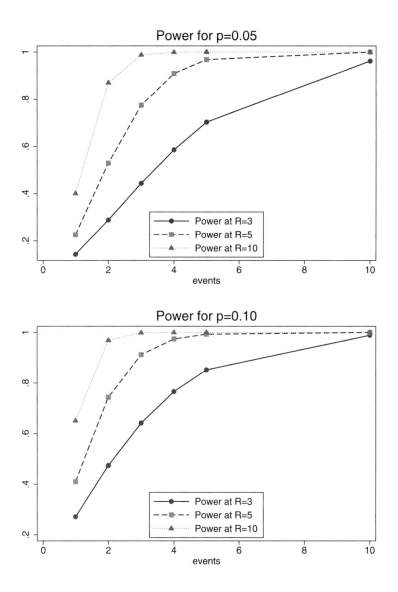

Figure 4.1: Power of the sentinel event test as a function of R, the ratio of the mean time between events under the null and alternative hypotheses

Because this estimate of μ lacks nice distributional properties, the statistic z requires large samples for the normal approximation to hold; bootstrapping would give approximately valid tests.

We can adapt this model to compare two arms of a study. Because $2V/\mu$ is distributed χ^2 with $2n$ d.f., the quantity

$$F = (V_T/n_T)/(V_C/n_C)$$

has an F distribution with $2n_T$ and $2n_C$ d.f., where V_T and V_C are the total exposure times for the treatment and control arms, and n_T and n_C are the numbers on each arm. (If the allocation to the two arms is not 1:1, the expected mean number of events will differ in proportion to the allocation. For example, if $n_T = 3n_C$, we would expect V_T to be approximately $3V_C$ when the rates do not differ.)

Generally, tests based on F distributions will have low power unless the means μ_T and μ_C differ considerably or the number of events is moderately large. Even a tenfold difference in means will be difficult to detect with a total of four events in both arms.

Revisiting our second example in Section 4.3, suppose the DSMB had wanted be sure that the adverse event rate was below $1/2000 = 0.0005$. In this case, the 95% two-tail confidence intervals are (0.0007 to 0.0097) if we observe three events per 900 and (0.0008 to 0.0184) if we observe one per 300. Both of these intervals exclude the 0.0005 target. Each participant received one immunization and was observed for 21 days. Four events occurred at about 10 days after vaccination. Thus, $\sum t_i = 40$ so $V = 40 + (21 \times 896) = 18,856$. The maximum likelihood estimate, $\hat{\mu} = 18,856/4 = 4714$ days to event, is substantially greater than 2000. The expected rate was $1/10,000$ implying that the median number of days to event would be about 6930. This calculation suggests that μ is somewhat smaller than the expected 10,000 days but perhaps not small enough to be of concern. Pooling both vaccine and control groups, the test for an overall mean of 6930 days to event is $\chi^2 = 2 \times 18,856/6930 = 5.44$ ($p < 0.71$), insufficient evidence to reject a mean of 10,000 days to event for this vaccine.

Recall that $n_T = 900$ and $n_C = 300$, so the two sample test,

$$\begin{aligned} F_{6,2} &= [(30 + 21 \times 897)/900]/[(10 + 21 \times 299)/300] \\ &= [18,846/900]/[6289/300] = 0.998 \end{aligned}$$

gives $p < 0.58$, which provides no statistical evidence of a difference between the vaccines on the control and new vaccine arms.

The FDA, when informed of the adverse events, became concerned even though the rates were the same in the treated and control groups. Because of the prior experience with vaccines for this disease, a high rate would have caused concern even if the control had been a placebo. The medical severity of the events was sufficient to cause the trial to pause.

4.5 Methods for Sentinel Event Rates

Consider now a large trial with many adverse events. Suppose a DSMB observes an elevated event rate of a specific adverse event. The first observation of such a rate would correspond to the sentinel "event." In such a case, the DSMB could initiate a monitoring scheme (perhaps a group sequential plan) and modify or halt the trial when the adverse event rate exceeded a given level. Once again, the monitoring scheme would apply only to subjects randomized after the observation of the sentinel event (the high event rate, in this case). For a single elevated rate, the result follows directly from the earlier material. A monitoring scheme might examine outcomes among every 100 patients. Monitoring multiple events for safety may require statistical adjustment to protect against overzealous stopping; the chance of exceeding any one endpoint is greater than the chance of exceeding a single specified endpoint. Suppose, for example, in a study of several thousand people, the DSMB met for the first time after 200 people in each of the treated and control groups had been randomized and imagine that six strokes, five in the treated group and one in control, had been reported. The exact two-sided p-value for a five-to-one split is 0.21; the exact one-sided p-value is 0.11. Thus, the event, although worrisome, does not reach conventional levels of significance even if we disregard multiple looks. Nonetheless, a 5:1 split in a very serious adverse event would worry a DSMB. It might then institute an α-spending function approach to apply to the next patients randomized. It might choose to spend α linearly [i.e., $\alpha(t) = \alpha t$] or, perhaps, quadratically. An O'Brien–Fleming boundary is often too stringent at early times, when it is important to stop administering a bad drug, or at least to inform the investigators and participants of a newly discovered risk. The bounds would apply only to the newly randomized participants so that a new stroke that occurred to the first cohort of 400 participants would not count in the formal monitoring. This approach—defining a boundary during the course of the study—allows the DSMB to use data from the study to generate hypotheses and then subsequent data to test them.

The DSMB for the WHI could have instituted such a plan when it first noted excess rates of stroke and myocardial infarction in the treated arm.

Table 4.1: Posterior probability that the event rate is less than π as a function of various prior distributions: 3 events; 897 nonevents

	Prior Distribution			Posterior Probability Rate $< \pi$ π			
a	*b*	*Mean*	*s.d.*	*0.0005*	*0.001*	*0.005*	*0.01*
1	1	0.5	0.289	0.0109	0.0628	0.8271	0.9939
0.1	19.9	0.005	0.015	0.0093	0.0572	0.8234	0.9940
1	999	0.001	0.001	0.0712	0.2960	0.9959	1.000
10	9990	0.001	0.0003	0.0041	0.3002	1	1
10	19990	0.0005	0.00016	0.2523	0.9742	1	1

4.6 Bayesian Models

When we can view adverse events in a clinical trial as arising from a binomial distribution, a Bayesian analysis with a beta prior distribution offers a different approach to the problem of monitoring safety in response to sentinel events. We provide examples of five arbitrarily chosen beta priors to illustrate the impact of the prior on the posterior. Assume the parameter p, the adverse event rate, has a beta distribution with parameters a and b. Recall that the mean and variance of the beta(a, b) prior are $a/(a + b)$ and $ab/[(a + b)^2(a + b + 1)]$, respectively. Returning to our second example, a trial of 900 patients with three events would have a beta posterior distribution with parameters $a + 3$ and $b + 897$. The pair of parameters $(a, b) = (1, 1)$, which produces a rather flat prior, requires strong evidence from the data to demonstrate a low posterior event rate.

The prior ($a = b = 1$) gives very little assurance that the adverse event rate is 0.0005 or less. No case in Table 4.1, even when the prior has a very low mean, gives a posterior probability above 0.9 that the adverse event rate is below 0.0005. The above analysis shows that the data at hand provide little evidence that the adverse event rate is below 0.001.

In summary, for the second example, with 900 observations, neither a classical nor a Bayesian approach provides sufficient statistical evidence to declare the adverse event rate is below 0.001.

4.7 Summary

The statistical issues posed by monitoring for safety differ considerably from the issues posed by monitoring for efficacy. In the latter case, prior hypotheses govern the design of the study and the consequent data monitoring boundaries. For safety monitoring, however, the hypotheses are often data-driven. We suggest that a DSMB can react to an observed worrisome adverse event by establishing monitoring procedures in response to a sentinel event.

We have discussed some practical issues in implementing this process. First, we have concentrated on phase 3 studies, however, investigators will study potentially high-risk products (e.g., gene therapy) in phase 1 and 2 studies. Although these are typically smaller, often single-arm, studies, the ideas regarding sentinel events can be useful for them as well. In particular, the methods that assess whether a safety standard has been exceeded are relevant. We can apply this same approach to phase 4 single arm studies. In these cases, information about specific safety events may be available so the sentinel event has already occurred and we can establish a monitoring plan.

The level of evidence needed to raise a concern is relevant to both the size (the type I error rate) and the power we select in assessing safety. We used $k = 2$ events for our vaccine example with progressive censoring. The first event occurred soon after the study started, making our level of concern high. Choosing k in other situations will depend on the severity of the event as well as our prior experience. A sentinel event that occurs after a few participants have been exposed may lead us to believe the event rate is higher than anticipated and so we base our power calculations on that higher rate. For example, if the first event occurs on the 10th patient where $T = 30$ days, then the estimated mean time to event is $(t + 30 \times 9)/1 = 270 + t < 300$ days, but if it occurs after the 1000th patient the estimated number of days is $(t + 999 \times 30)/1 = 29,970 + t$. In the first case, we might choose a small value of k because of a concern that the mean time to event is much shorter than expected, whereas for the second we might choose a substantially larger k because the mean is consistent with our prior experience.

A DSMB or safety monitor should not be bound by purely statistical considerations. It may recommend termination of a study when no statistical difference in safety can be shown because of the medical implications of an adverse event. The statistical criteria should be an adjunct to the DSMB's judgment, not a governor of it. If possible, we suggest the DSMB examine the safety analyses at the same time as the efficacy analyses; however, if the efficacy analyses are spaced widely, such a schedule will not provide satisfactory assurance for safety.

Statistical stringency is often less crucial for safety than for efficacy analyses. We believe that the traditional significance level of 0.05 is often too stringent. Instead, a safety monitor or DSMB might decide that a probability below 0.1 or 0.2 should lead to more frequent monitoring or to a pause in the trial for further reflection and analysis.

To recapitulate, efficacy endpoints are frequently assessed by group sequential tests. Because safety endpoints are usually not known at the start of the trial, formal testing procedures cannot be in place from the onset. Instituting a formal testing procedure that includes the event bringing the problem to attention compromises the size of the statistical test. We suggest starting a formal monitoring procedure on the basis of a sentinel event. We suggest adopting a definition of "event" as broad as necessary for the purposes of the monitoring.

Acknowledgements. We thank Susan Ellenberg and Mary Foulkes for thoughtful comments on the manuscript. George Gentile provided useful information on some vaccine issues.

References

1. Benjamini, Y., and Hochberg, Y. (1955). Controlling the false discovery rate: A new and powerful approach to multiple testing, *Journal of the Royal Statistical Society, Series B*, **57**, 1289–1300.

2. FDA Guidance for Clinical Trial Sponsors (2006). On the establishment and operation of clinical trial data monitoring committees.

3. Freedman, L., Anderson, G., Kipnis, V., Prentice, R., Wang, C. Y., Rossouw, J., Wittes, J., and DeMets, D. (1996). Approaches to monitoring the results of long-term disease prevention trials: Examples from the Womens Health Initiative, *Controlled Clinical Trials*, **17**, 509–525.

4. Jennison, C., and Turnbull, B. (2000). *Group Sequential Methods with Applications to Clinical Trials*, Chapman & Hall/CRC, Boca Raton, Florida.

5. Mehrotra, D. V., and Heyse, J. F. (2004). Use of the false discovery rate for evaluating clinical safety data, *Statistical Methods in Medical Research*, **13**, 227–238.

6. National Institutes of Health (1998). NIH policy for data and safety monitoring, Available at: http://grants.nih.gov/grants/guide.

7. Writing Group for the Womens Health Initiative Investigators (2002). Risks and benefits of estrogen plus progestin in healthy postmenopausal women, *Journal of the American Medical Association*, **288**, 321–333.

5

Spontaneous Reporting System Modelling for the Evaluation of Automatic Signal Generation Methods in Pharmacovigilance

E. Roux,[1] **F. Thiessard,**[2] **A. Fourrier,**[3] **B. Bégaud,**[3] **and P. Tubert-Bitter**[4]

[1] *INSERM U642, Rennes, France*
[2] *Université Victor Segalen, Bordeaux, France*
[3] *INSERM U657, Université Victor Segalen, Bordeaux, France*
[4] *INSERM U 780, Villejuif, France*

Abstract: Pharmacovigilance aims at detecting adverse effects of marketed drugs. It is generally based on a Spontaneous Reporting System (SRS) that consists of the spontaneous reporting, by health professionals, of events that are supposed to be adverse effects of marketed drugs. SRS supply huge databases, the human-based exploitation of which cannot be exhaustive. Automated signal generation methods have been proposed in the literature but no consensus exists concerning their efficiency and applicability due to the difficulties in evaluating the methods on real data.

The objective is to propose SRS modelling in order to simulate realistic data sets that would permit completion of the methods' evaluation and comparison. In fact, as the status of the drug–event relationships is known in the simulated data sets, generated signals can be labelled as "true" or "false."

The spontaneous reporting is viewed as a Poisson process depending on: the drug's exposure frequency, the delay from the drug's launch, the adverse events' background incidence and seriousness, and the reporting probability. This reporting probability, quantitatively unknown, is derived from the qualitative knowledge found in the literature and expressed by experts. This knowledge is represented and exploited by means of a set of fuzzy rules.

Then, we show that the SRS modelling permits to evaluate the automatic signal generation methods proposed within pharmacovigilance and contribute to generate a consensus on drugs' postmarketing surveillance strategies.

Keywords and phrases: Adverse drug reaction reporting systems, modelling, fuzzy system, computer simulation, data mining, validation studies

5.1   Introduction

Clinical trials are efficient for identifying the most frequent adverse effects of a
drug prior to marketing. However, for obvious reasons, the effects of rare occurrences cannot be detected. Such effects can be specific to a population subgroup
and/or can have a latency longer than the trial duration. The identification of
such effects is the scope of pharmacovigilance, whose role includes the postmarketing surveillance of adverse effects based on the spontaneous reporting by
the medical community of adverse events suspected to be related to a medication. The Spontaneous Reporting System (SRS) supplies huge databases with a
continuous flow. For example, in 1997, 35,000 new reports were added quarterly
to the Uppsala Monitoring Centre (UMC) database that gathers the reports of
47 countries of the World Health Organization (WHO) Collaborating Program
for International Drug Monitoring [Bate *et al.* (1998)]. DuMouchel (1999) mentioned that the Food and Drug Administration (FDA) database contained 1.2
million different reports. On 1 January 2000, the Netherlands Pharmacovigilance Foundation LAREB contained 26,555 reports concerning 17,330 different
drug–event combinations [Van Puijenbroek *et al.* (2002)]. At the end of 2001,
the French pharmacovigilance database contained about 200,000 reports referring to about 185,000 different drug–event couples [Thiessard *et al.* (2003)].
Such massive databases preclude human-based exploration. In such a context,
pharmacovigilance would benefit from an automatic signal generation method
that would exploit all the available information.

A good evaluation of the suspicious character of a drug–event couple of the
database would be to determine to what extent the observed number of reports
referring to this couple exceeds the expected number of reports, assuming the
independence between exposure to the drug and the adverse event. Such a
direct assessment is not permitted by the SRS. Spontaneous Reporting Systems
are based on the subjective appreciation of the medical community and do not
provide an exhaustive reporting of the adverse effects. At first the adverse event
has to be diagnosed and next, it has to be judged new and serious enough to be
reported [Tubert-Bitter *et al.* (1998)]. It is impossible to know the proportion
of adverse events that is reported. Moreover, the reported events are supposed
to be causally related to the prescribed drugs but the simultaneous presence
of an adverse event and of a drug can be coincidental. In other words, not
all the adverse effects are reported (and the proportion of reported events is
unknown), and the adverse events reported are not all adverse drug reactions.
Moreover, the background incidence of the events in the whole population and
the number of patients exposed to the drugs are unknown. This prevents reliable
computation of an expected number of reports for drug–event couples.

A solution proposed in the literature is to use Data Mining (DM) methods that only exploit the intrinsic information of the database in order to estimate, for a given couple, the expected number of reports by means of the data related to all the other drugs and events. DM methods act as automatic hypotheses generators that pharmacovigilance experts then have to confirm or invalidate. All the methods use an association measure that evaluates to what extent drugs and events are statistically related. Decision on the status of the drug–event relations can then be made according to a threshold. It is also possible to rank the drug–event couples from the most to the least suspicious according to the values of the measure [DuMouchel (1999)]. Methods essentially differ from one to the other by the association measure they use. A large variety of measures has been proposed: the Proportional Reporting Ratio (PRR) [Evans, Waller, and Davis (2001)], the Reporting Odds Ratio (ROR) [Van Puijenbroek *et al.* (2002), Rothman, Lanes, and Sacks (2004), Egberts, Meyboom, and Van Puijenbroek (2002), Van Puijenbroek, Diemont, and Van Grootheest (2003) and Waller *et al.* (2004)], the Yule's Q [Van Puijenbroek *et al.* (2002)], the Sequential Probability Ratio Test (SPRT) [Evans (2003)], the statistics based on Poisson or Chi-square distributions [Van Puijenbroek *et al.* (2002)], the Information Component [Bate *et al.* (1998), Van Puijenbroek *et al.* (2002), and Gould (2003)], and the Empirical Bayes Method [DuMouchel (1999) and Gould (2003)]. The former ones are very simple and intuitive disproportionality measures and the two last ones are more complicated Bayesian measures, demanding more statistical and computational skills.

Due to the fact that the events' Relative Risk (RR), the background incidence of the events, and the number of patients exposed to the drugs are unknown, the signals generated by the DM methods cannot be labelled as 'true' or 'false.' This prevents us from absolutely evaluating the methods' performances in identifying suspicious drug–event couples. So no consensus exists concerning the DM method(s) to be used and routine application of such methods in pharmacovigilance is still limited. Van Puijenbroek *et al.* (2002) circumvented this difficulty by comparing methods' results with the results of one of them, considered as the reference one. In this way, methods can be compared in a relative manner. However, it is necessary to approach the absolute performances of the methods in order to draw conclusions about their efficiency. Moreover, it would be interesting to study the sensitivity of the methods' results according to the drug and/or event characteristics.

The objective of this paper is to propose a SRS modelling in order to simulate realistic data. The evaluation of the DM methods could then be completed, as the status of the drug–event relationships and the drug and event characteristics as well are known in the simulated dataset. It is important to obtain data as realistic as possible in order to be able to derive knowledge of the efficiency of DM methods with real data.

The chapter is organized as follows: the SRS modelling is described in the first section. The model takes into account the qualitative knowledge expressed by pharmacovigilance experts and found in the literature, by means of a fuzzy representation of knowledge and a fuzzy inference system. Then, the Application section proposes a set of simulation parameter values that aims at obtaining realistic situations within the French pharmacovigilance context. The empirical Bayes method [DuMouchel (1999)] is then described. Generated data are described and results relative to the data mining method are presented in the Results section. The data mining method evaluation is not the main issue tackled by this paper. It is only presented as an illustration of what information can be derived from simulations.

5.2   Methods

5.2.1   Spontaneous reporting system modelling

In the present study, a pharmacovigilance database is simply viewed as a two-entry table: one entry for the events and the other for the drugs. The cell corresponding to the (drug i, event j) couple contains the cumulated reports number N_{ij}, associated with this couple, that is, the total number of reports concerning this couple since the launch of the drug.

The probability distribution of the numbers of reports n_{ij}, during a given period Δ_t, is assumed to be Poisson with a mean report number δ_{ij} [Tubert (1993) and Tubert *et al.* (1992)]:

$$\delta_{ij} = RR_{ij} I_j T_i p_{ij}, \tag{5.1}$$

where RR_{ij} is the drug–event relative risk of a (drug i, event j) combination. When $RR_{ij} > 1$, the drug exposure increases the probability of event; however, some drug–event associations may still be coincidental. Note that the objective of a signal generation method is to identify the couples (drug i, event j) with $RR_{ij} > 1$ – such an identification is a 'true signal' – while keeping low the proportion of 'false signals' corresponding to the couples with $RR_{ij} = 1$. I_j is the background incidence of the event j and T_i the exposure frequency, that is, the number of patients exposed to the drug i during the given period Δ_t. Assuming that the probability of observing the event without the exposure to the drug is comparable to the probability to observe the event in the whole population, that is, the background incidence of the event, the product $RR_{ij} \cdot I_j \cdot T_i$ represents the expected number of events j associated with the drug i during Δ_t.

As seen in the Introduction section, cases are not systematically reported. So a reporting probability, p_{ij}, completes the Spontaneous Reporting System modelling. No particular constraint is imposed on the definition of I_j in the present version of the SRS modelling. We now describe in detail the other parameters of the model.

5.2.2 Exposure to the drug (T_i)

The exposure to the drug, T_i, is time dependent and is defined, in our study, by the drug life cycle characterised by the five periods: 'Launch,' 'Growth,' 'Maturity,' 'Decline,' and 'End of life' (see Figure 5.1). In the present paper, the only parameter required for defining the whole cycle is the maximal exposure, T_{imax}, corresponding to the exposure during the Maturity phase. T_i is supposed to reach $T_{imax}/10$ at the end of the Launch period, to reach its maximal value after the Growth period, and to decline exponentially after the Maturity phase, so that at ten years, $T_i = T_{imax}/2$. The bounds of the cycle phases and the exposure values associated with these bounds can be adapted to different situations and can be different from one drug to another. However, by fixing some values, we choose to limit the number of parameter values that have to be defined for simulation.

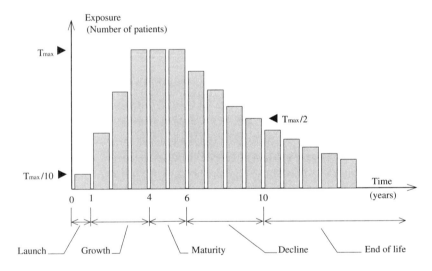

Figure 5.1: Drug life cycle

5.2.3 Events' relative risk (RR_{ij})

A proportion of coincidental drug–event associations that will give 'false' reports (i.e., with $RR_{ij} = 1$) is defined. The remaining couples, with $RR_{ij} > 1$, are associated with 'true' reports and are supposed to generate a signal. The same proportions of couples with $RR_{ij} = 1$ and $RR_{ij} > 1$ are imposed on each data subset having the same value for T_i, I_j, event seriousness and delay since the drug's launch. For each subset, the RR_{ij} values are randomly attributed to the drug–event couples. The set of $RR_{ij} > 1$ is assumed to be exponentially distributed so that $\{RR_{ij} > 1\} \subset [RR_{\min}, RR_{\max}]$, with $RR_{\min} > 1$.

5.2.4 Reporting probability (p_{ij})

The submodel concerning the static and dynamic characteristics of the reporting probability is the most original point of the present paper. In Tubert (1993), a learning model already attempts to reproduce the changes, over time, of the reporting probability magnitude for a given drug–event couple. However, the two major differences with the model of the present paper are: the fact that in Tubert (1993), the probability of detecting and reporting the event can only improve with time, and the fact that the learning model is a mathematical expression with parameters, the values of which can be quite difficult to determine and interpret for pharmacovigilance experts. In fact, the pharmacovigilance experts have only general and/or qualitative knowledge of p_{ij}. In order to obtain realistic simulated data, this qualitative knowledge has to be exploited and has to be easily updated if a change occurs in it. Fuzzy set theory and fuzzy logic permit us to represent such knowledge and to exploit it to perform humanlike deductive reasoning. So we propose to derive a set of fuzzy rules from the literature and pharmacovigilance experts' advice. These fuzzy rules represent three basic intuitions of the experts concerning reporting probability, that have been confirmed by quantitative analysis of real data [Tubert-Bitter *et al.* (1998)]: (1) the more serious the event is, and the more reported it is; (2) the more unknown the causal relationship between a drug and an event is, the more reported the event is; (3) the more recent the drug is, the more reported the event is. These rules are imposed to distinguish serious and mild events, to characterise the delay since the drug launch, and the knowledge of the causal relationship between a drug and an event. We simply consider the seriousness of an event as a binary variable with two modalities: serious and mild. We assume that the more a drug–event couple is reported, the more the medical community suspects the causal relationship between the drug and the event and considers it as known. So the knowledge the medical community has on a given drug–event association is assumed to be characterised by the cumulative number of reports, for the considered drug–event couple, since the launch date of the drug.

Fuzzy coding

The delay from the drug launch, the cumulative number of reports, and the reporting probability are characterized by fuzzy subsets as presented in Figure 5.2. The delay since the drug launch is coded according to the five modalities that characterize the drug life cycle presented in Figure 5.1, that is, 'Launch,' 'Growth,' 'Maturity,' 'Decline,' and 'End of life.' The fuzzy subsets corresponding to these modalities are defined by the values in Table 5.1. The cumulative number of reports is partitioned into three fuzzy modalities: 'Low,' 'Medium,' and 'High,' corresponding to the intervals [0,5], [0,20], and [5, +∞], respectively. Three modalities correspond to an intuitive partitioning of the variable's domain and do not demand the definition of an unmanageable number of rules. Eventually the reporting probability is coded with five modalities: 'Very low,' 'Low,' 'Medium,' 'High,' and 'Very high,' corresponding to the intervals [0,0.0125], [0,0.025], [0.0125,0.05], [0.025,0.1], and [0.05,0.1], respectively. Note that the reporting probability is assumed to be at most equal to 0.1, according to the literature; see Tubert *et al.* (1992) and Weber (1986). The five modalities of the reporting probability permit us to define enough rules in order to represent the whole available knowledge. They especially permit a better representation of the gradual knowledge previously cited and expressed as 'The more [. . .] is, the higher the reporting probability is.'

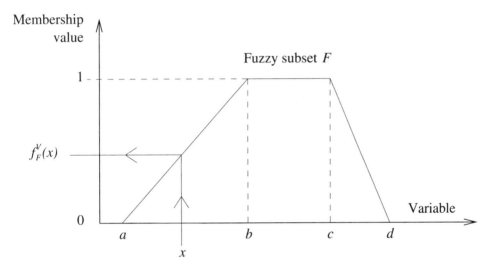

Figure 5.2: Trapezoidal membership function of a fuzzy subset F of the variable V, and fuzzy membership value for an observed value x

The membership value of an observed value x of a variable V, for the fuzzy subset F, is, due to the trapezoidal shape of the membership functions (or triangular when $b = c$, see Figure 5.2):

$$f_F^V(x) = \max\left(\min\left(\frac{x-a}{b-a}, 1, \frac{d-x}{d-c}\right), 0\right). \qquad (5.2)$$

For example, a drug–event couple that has been reported ten times belongs to the modality 'Medium' with a membership value equal to 2/3 and to the modality 'High' with a membership value equal to 1/3.

Table 5.1: Fuzzy characterization of the variables

Variable	Fuzzy Subset	a	b	c	d
Cumulative	Low	0	0	0	5
reports number	Medium	0	5	5	20
	High	5	20	$+\infty$	$+\infty$
Delay since	Launch	0	0	0	1
drug launch	Growth	0	1	1	4
(years)	Maturity	1	4	6	10
	Decline	6	10	10	50
	End of life	10	50	$+\infty$	$+\infty$
Reporting	Very low	0	0	0	0.0125
probability	Low	0	0.0125	0.0125	0.025
	Medium	0.0125	0.025	0.025	0.05
	High	0.025	0.05	0.05	0.1
	Very High	0.05	0.1	0.1	0.1

Fuzzy rules definition

Given the three basic rules previously stated and the coding of the variables, the rule base presented in Figure 5.3 is defined. The fuzzy conclusions associated with the cells of the table (Figure 5.3) are chosen to represent the gradual knowledge of the type 'the more [...] is, the higher the reporting probability is.' The exceptions are the rules associated to the fuzzy subset 'Launch,' for which the reporting probability is 'Very high' (or 'High' for mild events) whatever the cumulative number of reports is. This is justified by the fact that during the 'Launch' period, the potential causal relationship between the drug and an observed event is a priori unknown. Another exception is the increase of the reporting probability when moving up from the 'Launch' to the 'Growth' period and while keeping with a 'Low' cumulative number of reports. This increase of the reporting probability is supposed to model, before the 'maturity' period of the drug, a learning phase during which the medical community and pharmacovigilance experts are more focused on the new drug–event couples, before the true status of the drug–event relationships is known; see Tubert (1993).

Rules activation

The fuzzy implication and the generalised modus ponens operator are the *minimum (min)* operator [Bouchon-Meunier and Marsala (2003)]. For instance, consider the rule (R) *'IF the event is mild AND IF the cumulative number*

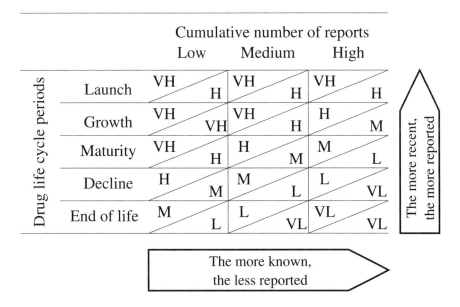

Figure 5.3: Fuzzy rule base for the reporting probability determination. In each cell of the table are given the conclusions associated with a serious event (upper part of the cell) and to a mild event (lower part of the cell). VH is for 'Very high,' H for 'High,' M for 'Medium,' L for 'Low' and VL for 'Very low'

of reports is Low AND IF the delay since the drug launch corresponds to the Launch period, THEN the reporting probability is High.' Now consider, for a given drug–event couple, the observations N_{obs} and D_{obs} for the total number of reports and the delay since the drug launch, respectively. N_{obs} and D_{obs} are 'fuzzified' according to Eq. (5.2); that is, the membership values $f_{Low}^N(N_{obs})$ and $f_{Launch}^{delay}(D_{obs})$ are computed. Then the rule (R) is fired; that is, the fuzzy conclusion $C_R(N_{obs}, D_{obs})$ is computed as follows

$$C_R(N_{obs}, D_{obs})$$
$$= \min_{x \in [0.025, 0.1]} \left(f_{High}^{pij}(x), \min \left(f_{Low}^N(N_{obs}), f_{Launch}^{delay}(D_{obs}) \right) \right). \quad (5.3)$$

The principle for obtaining the fuzzy conclusion is also presented graphically in Figure 5.4. Note that several rules can lead to the same conclusion. So these fuzzy conclusions are aggregated with the maximum operator.

At this stage, the conclusion is still fuzzy and cannot be exploited directly by Eq. (5.1). It has to be "defuzzified." This operation is realised by the Height Method (HM) [Eklund, Kallin, and Riissanen (2000)], using the following expression

$$p_{ij} = \frac{\sum_{k=1}^K \mu_k \times p_k}{\sum_{k=1}^K \mu_k},$$

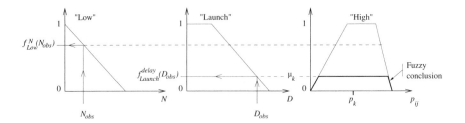

Figure 5.4: Principle of the fuzzy reasoning implementation and values used for defuzzification

where K is the number of fuzzy subsets characterizing p_{ij}, that is, five in the present model (cf. Table 5.1). p_k is the mean of the maxima of the membership function associated with the kth fuzzy subset of p_{ij} and μ_k is the minimum of the membership values of the conditions of the rule [cf. Eq. (5.3) and Figure 5.4].

This defuzzification method does not requires defining the membership functions for all the values of p_{ij} but only determining the intervals of the fuzzy subset that correspond to the maxima of the membership functions. Such a defuzzification method is simple and fast. Moreover, it permits us to reach the extreme values of p_{ij} (i.e., 0 and 0.1), unlike the centre of gravity method, for example.

5.2.5 Data generation process

The model of the SRS described above can be used to generate simulated data associated with virtual drugs and events. Given a set of parameter values chosen for simulation, data are generated sequentially with respect to the procedure described in Figure 5.5. A total duration of the reporting process, corresponding to the maximal delay since the drug launch we want to consider, must be defined. The period Δ_t between two successive generations has to be chosen too. As a new drug can be launched during the generation process, it is possible to have, at the same time, drugs with different delays since launch.

5.3 Application

5.3.1 Values of the model parameters

In the present study, ten years of the Spontaneous Reporting System were simulated, with a generation period of six months. We considered 150 virtual drugs and 100 virtual adverse events. The maximal exposures to the drugs over the ten-year period, $T_{i\ max}$, were three million, 300,000 and 30,000, each value being

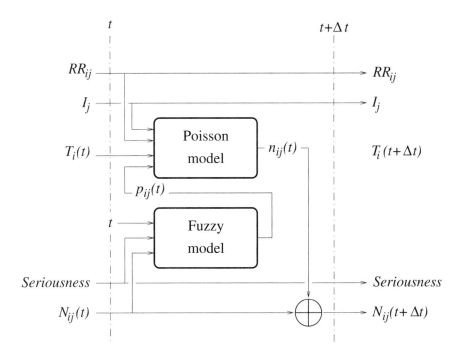

Figure 5.5: Sequential data generation process for one (drug i, event j) couple

associated with one third of the drugs. For each maximal exposure value, five drugs were launched each year during the ten year reporting process, leading to ten different delays since launch, from one to ten years. Background incidences of adverse events, I_j, were 1/50,000 and 1/10,000, each associated with one half of the events. For each value of background incidence, half of the events were considered as serious and the remaining ones as mild. This repartition corresponds approximately to the one in the French pharmacovigilance database, where 46% of the events are labelled serious [Thiessard *et al.* (2003)]. Ten percent of the drug–event couples were associated with a relative risk, RR_{ij}, in the interval [1.2, 10]. The remaining couples (90%) had a relative risk equal to 1. In fact, the results provided by DuMouchel's method [DuMouchel (1999)] on the FDA database (this method is described in the next section) tend to show that about 1/10 of dependent drug–event couples are present in the database, even if DuMouchel himself does not go so far concerning the interpretation of his results. In our simulated datasets, this repartition was imposed to each data subset having the same value for $T_{i\ max}$, I_j, event seriousness, and delay since the drug launch. Simulations have been performed with the R language and environment.

5.3.2 Application of the empirical Bayes method

In order to illustrate the kind of information we can derive from the simulated data, we apply the empirical Bayes method proposed by DuMouchel (1999). In this method, the distribution of the number of reports is assumed to be Poisson, with an expectation μ_{ij} for the (drug i, event j) couple. Then DuMouchel considers the rate

$$\lambda_{ij} = \frac{\mu_{ij}}{\frac{n_{i.} \cdot n_{.j}}{N}},$$

where $n_{i.}$ and $n_{.j}$ are the total report numbers for the drug i and for the event j, respectively. N is the total report number in the database and $(n_{i.}n_{.j})/N$ is the expected report number for the (drug i, event j) couple, assuming the independence between the rows and the columns in the dataset. Large values – larger than 1 – of λ_{ij} indicate that the couple (i, j) is more reported than expected. Then a prior mixture of two gamma distributions is assumed for λ_{ij}:

$$\lambda_{ij} \overset{a\ priori}{\sim} P \cdot \Gamma_1(\alpha_1, \beta_1) + (1 - P) \cdot \Gamma_2(\alpha_2, \beta_2),$$

where P is the weight of the component $\Gamma_1(\alpha_1, \beta_1)$ in the mixture. A prior distribution with five parameters is quite flexible to model the data. The 'empirical' character of the method comes from the estimation of the prior distribution parameters $\theta = \{P, \alpha_1, \beta_1, \alpha_2, \beta_2\}$, by means of maximum likelihood estimation from the data. The posterior distribution is a mixture of two gamma distributions too. It is then possible to obtain the exact posterior mean of λ_{ij}, denoted EBAM_{ij}. DuMouchel proposes using this value [in fact, DuMouchel uses the geometric mean derived from $\log_2(\lambda_{ij})$] to rank the drug–event couples. The proper objective of the present study is not the method description and evaluation but the SRS modelling. We refer to the following articles for a more detailed description of the method [see Bate *et al.* (1998), DuMouchel (1999), and Gould (2003)].

5.4 Results

One thousand data sets have been generated. Figure 5.6 shows the reporting probability and the cumulative number of reports in three different cases and as a function of the time. On average, 10,502 (standard deviation, SD = 35) drug–event combinations have been reported at least once. Two thousand (SD = 37) drug-event couples have been reported only once, 1181 (SD = 29) twice, 770 (SD = 25) three times, and 6551 (SD = 23) at least four times. These numbers correspond to 19.0%, 11.3%, 7.3%, and 62.4% of the reported couples, respectively. The average maximal report number for a drug–event couple was

537 (SD = 19). The average number of 'true associations,' that is, the number of couples whose relative risk exceeds one, was 1182 (SD = 10) and corresponds to 11.3% of the reported couples.

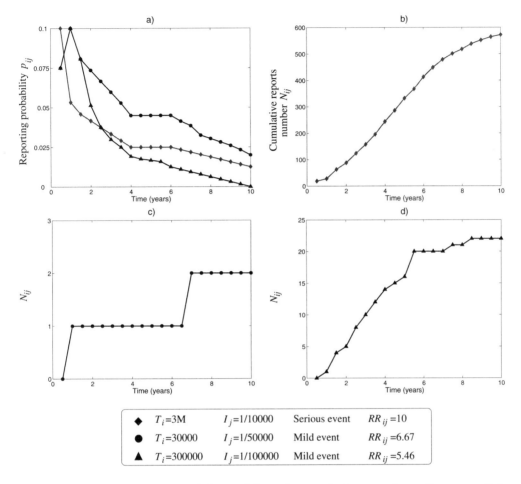

Figure 5.6: Reporting probabilities (a) and cumulative number of reports (b), (c), and (d)

For each of the generated data sets, DuMouchel's method has been applied. Table 5.2 shows the prior parameters of the mixture model, obtained by means of maximum likelihood estimation. These results can be interpreted as follows. A proportion of $P = 0.096$ (9.6%) of the drug–event combinations is associated with λ_{ij} values that stem from a gamma distribution with a mean superior to one ($\alpha_1/\beta_1 = 2.8$). The remaining couples ($1 - P = 0.904$) are associated with values of λ_{ij} that stem from a gamma distribution with a mean of 0.86 (< 1). So $P = 0.096$ can be compared to the 11.3% of the drug–event couples with $RR_{ij} > 1$, that is, the proportion of the drug–event combinations that have to be identified by a signal generation method.

Table 5.2: Average and standard deviation (in brackets), over the 1000 simulated datasets, of the prior parameters of DuMouchel's model, estimated by means of maximum likelihood

θ					1st Mixture Component		2nd Mixture Component	
					Mean	Variance	Mean	Variance
α_1	β_1	α_2	β_2	P	$\frac{\alpha_1}{\beta_1}$	$\frac{\alpha_1}{(\beta_1)^2}$	$\frac{\alpha_2}{\beta_2}$	$\frac{\alpha_2}{(\beta_2)^2}$
5.188	1.820	146.687	171.098	0.0964	2.847	1.571	0.858	0.006
(0.466)	(0.134)	(59.028)	(69.711)	(0.0038)	(0.065)	(0.096)	(0.004)	(0.002)

The knowledge of the 'true' status of the drug–event associations, in terms of relative risk, allows us to label the signals generated by the data mining methods as 'true' or 'false.' As DuMouchel proposes to rank the drug-event couples by means of the values of the empirical Bayes measure of association, without defining a threshold, it seems appropriate to evaluate the method by means of the percentage of the false positive signals among a predefined number of the most highly ranked couples. For 100, 200, and 500 of the most highly ranked drug–event combinations, the empirical Bayes method provides 0.0%, 0.3%, and 4.0% of false positive signals, respectively. If a threshold is proposed to generate signals, then method performances can be studied in terms of sensitivity, specificity, and the like.

5.5   Discussion

The aim of this paper is to obtain realistic simulated data sets in order to evaluate data mining methods, and not to reproduce the reporting process associated with a real drug–event combination. Consequently, we discuss model validity at the data set scale. However, the difficulties encountered for the data mining method evaluation prevent us from easily validating the SRS modelling too. Nevertheless, qualitative validation can be performed. In fact, the changes of the reporting probability follow the expected ones, described in the literature and by experts (Figure 5.6). In Figure 5.6 we notice the increase of the probability during the first year after the drug launch, corresponding to the 'learning phase,' except for frequent drug–event associations with serious events that are supposed to be known very quickly and whose reporting probabilities remain high in the long term.

The estimation of the prior parameters of the mixture model of DuMouchel (Table 5.2) shows that the prior probability associated with the mixture component with a mean exceeding one and the prior expectations of the two models' components (0.0964, 2.847, and 0.858, respectively), are of the same order as the ones found by DuMouchel with real data (0.0969, 3.509, and 0.7699, respectively).

An effort should be made to make the distributions of the marginal numbers (i.e., $n_{i.}$ and $n_{.j}$) comparable to the real ones for a size-comparable subset of the real pharmacovigilance database. Firstly, these numbers are exploited by the data mining methods to determine the expected numbers of reports. Secondly, to study the distributions of these numbers is, to our knowledge, the only manner to quantitatively evaluate the SRS model. In the present paper, the repartition of the numbers of the drug–event couples according to the report numbers seems to be realistic even if the very low numbers of reports are less represented in the simulated data sets than in the real ones. In fact, in the Dutch database used by Van Puijenbroek *et al.* (2002), the proportions of combinations with one, two, three, and four or more reports were 68,4%, 14.2%, 6.2%, and 11.2%, respectively. On the other hand, the FDA database used by DuMouchel (1999) contained 35.5% of drug–event couples with one report. So the features of real databases vary from one country to another and, when performing stratification of the databases according to sex, age, and so on, from one stratum to another. This creates the need to go further into the quantitative evaluation of the model of secondary importance. However, the influence of the values of each model parameter on the methods' results should be further investigated in order to contextualize the methods' performances and to study the robustness of the results.

Some SRS features have not been taken into account in the previously described model. The most important one is the drug interactions, that is, the fact that some events can be caused by the simultaneous exposure to two or more drugs and not by the drugs taken alone. DuMouchel proposes a method to identify the associations between an event and more than one drug by means of the 'all-two-factor' model [DuMouchel and Pregibon (2001)]. In order to evaluate such a method, it seems necessary to model drugs' interactions in the simulated data sets.

5.6   Conclusion

This paper proposes a model of the SRS that permits us to generate realistic data and to perform the quantitative evaluation of the data mining methods proposed for pharmacovigilance. Although the quantitative validation of the model needs further investigations that are difficult to realize, the qualitative knowledge exploited by the model, especially in order to determine realistic values for the reporting probability, is accepted by pharmacovigilance experts. Fuzzy set theory and fuzzy logic are not only interesting for modelling qualitative knowledge but also to actualise this knowledge by pharmacovigilance experts themselves. They contribute to make the model adjustable and intelligible for the experts and to make the simulated data interpretable. So Spontaneous Reporting System modelling participates in knowledge discovery on the SRS itself and is of particular interest for pharmacovigilance experts. By attempting to reproduce the reporting process of a specific drug–event couple of the real database, for which exposure to the drug over the time and the event's incidence and seriousness are known, it would be possible to approximate the unobservable features of the couple, and especially the event relative risk. SRS modelling permits not only the evaluation of data mining methods but also the support of pharmacovigilance experts in defining and testing surveillance strategies. Surveillance strategies of databases are sequential and much information can be derived from the evolution of the report numbers over time [Bate *et al.* (1998) and Gould (2003)]. As the data generation process in the present study is sequential, the evaluation of surveillance strategies including time consideration is straightforward.

Acknowledgements. This work has been carried out at the Biostatistics and Epidemiology Unit (U 472) of the French Institute of Health and Medical Research (INSERM). It has been supported by the INSERM within the engineers hosting program.

References

1. Bate, A., Lindquist, M., Edwards, I. R., Olsson, S., Orre, R., Lansner, A., and De Freitas, R. M. (1998). A Bayesian neural network method for adverse drug reaction signal generation, *European Journal of Clinical Pharmacology*, **54**, 315–321.

2. Bouchon-Meunier, B., and Marsala, C. (2003). Méthodes de raisonnement, In *Logique floue, principes, aide à la décision*, Hermès Science, London, England.

3. DuMouchel, W. (1999). Bayesian data mining in large frequency tables, with an application to the FDA spontaneous reporting system, *The American Statistician*, **53**, 177–190.

4. DuMouchel, W., and Pregibon, D. (2001). Empirical Bayes screening for multi-item associations, In *Proceedings of 7th ACM SIGKDD Inter-*

national Conference on Knowledge Discovery and Data Mining (KDD 2001), San Francisco, California, USA.

5. Egberts, A. C. G., Meyboom, R. H. B., and Van Puijenbroek, E. P. (2002). Use of measure of disproportionality in pharmacovigilance – three Dutch examples, *Drug Safety*, **25**, 453–458.

6. Eklund, P., Kallin, L., and Riissanen, T. (2000). Fuzzy systems, *Report*, pp. 27–32, Umeå University.

7. Evans, S. (2003). Sequential probability ratio tests applied to public health problems, *Controlled Clinical Trials*, **24**, 67S.

8. Evans, S. J., Waller, P. C., and Davis, S. (2001). Use of proportional reporting ratios (PRRs) for signal generation from spontaneous adverse drug reaction reports, *Pharmacoepidemiology and Drug Safety*, **10**, 483–486.

9. Gould, A. L. (2003). Practical pharmacovigilance analysis strategies, *Pharmacoepidemiology and Drug Safety*, **12**, 559–574.

10. Rothman, K. J., Lanes, S., and Sacks, S. T. (2004). The reporting odds ratio and its advantages over the proportional reporting ratio, *Pharmacoepidemiology and Drug Safety*, **13**, 519–523.

11. Thiessard, F., Miremont-Salame, G., Fourrier, A., Haramburu, F., Auriche, P., Kreft-Jais, C., Tubert-Bitter, P., Roux, E., and Bégaud, B. (2003). Description of the French pharmacovigilance system: Reports from 1985 to 2001, In *Proceedings of 19th International Conference on Pharmacoepidemiology and 1st International Conference on Therapeutic Risk Management*, pp. 22–24, Philadelphia, Pennsylvania, USA.

12. Tubert, P. (1993). Modelling in pharmacovigilance, In *Methodological Approaches in Pharmacoepidemiology* (Eds., ARME-P). pp. 151–156, Elsevier Science Publishers B.V., Amsterdam, The Netherlands.

13. Tubert, P., Bégaud, B., Péré, J.-C., Haramburu, F., and Lellouch, J. (1992). Power and weakness of spontaneous reporting: A probabilistic approach, *Journal of Clinical Epidemiology*, **45**, 283–286.

14. Tubert-Bitter, P., Haramburu, F., Bégaud, B., Chaslerie, A., Abraham, E., and Hagry, C. (1998). Spontaneous reporting of adverse drug reactions: Who reports and what? *Pharmacoepidemiology and Drug Safety*, **7**, 323–329.

15. Van Puijenbroek, E. P., Bate, A., Leufkens, H., Lindquist, M., Orre, R. and Egberts, A. C. G. (2002). A comparaison of measures of disproportionality for signal detection in spontaneous reporting systems for adverse drug reaction, *Pharmacoepidemiology and Drug Safety*, **11**, 3–10.

16. Van Puijenbroek, E. P., Diemont, W. L. and Van Grootheest, K. (2003). Application of quantitative signal detection in the Dutch spontaneous reporting system for adverse drug reactions, *Drug Safety*, **26**, 293–301.

17. Waller, P., Van Puijenbroek, E., Egberts, A. and Evans, S. (2004). The reporting odds ratio versus the proportional reporting ratio: 'deuce', *Pharmacoepidemiology and Drug Safety*, **13**, 525–526.

18. Weber, J. C. P. (1986). Mathematical models in adverse drug reaction assessment, In *Iatrogenic Diseases* (Eds., P. F. Arcy, and J. P. Griffin), Oxford University Press, London, England.

PART III
QUALITY OF LIFE

6

Latent Covariates in Generalized Linear Models: A Rasch Model Approach

Karl Bang Christensen

National Institute of Occupational Health, Denmark
University of Copenhagen, Copenhagen, Denmark

Abstract: Study of multivariate data in situations where a variable of interest is unobservable (latent) and only measured indirectly is widely applied. Item response models are powerful tools for measurement and have been extended to incorporate latent structure. The (log-linear) Rasch model is a simple item response model where tests of fit and item parameter estimation can take place without assumptions about the distribution of the latent variable. Inclusion of a latent variable as predictor in standard regression models such as logistic or Poisson regression models is discussed, and a study of the relation between psychosocial work environment and absence from work is used to illustrate and motivate the results.

Keywords and phrases: Rasch models, latent regression, generalized linear models, measurement error, random effects

6.1 Introduction

In many applied research situations, many of the variables of interest are unobservable (latent) and are only measured indirectly using indicators. The rationale behind the construction of a psychometric scale using item response theory [van der Linden and Hambleton (1997)] is to provide a translation of manifest variables (item responses) to an underlying latent variable with values on the real line, that is, translation from a discrete scale to an interval scale. Inference about the latent variable should thus not uncritically be based directly on observed item responses or the observed raw sum score.

This is important when considering a latent covariate, indirectly measured using categorical items, because a standard approach would be to include the sum of the observed item responses (the raw sum score) in a regression model, thus ignoring the measurement error. The literature on measurement error models is large, but deals mostly with linear measurement error models. Measurement error models have been applied in different research areas to model errors-in-variables problems, incorporating error in the response as well as in the covariates.

This chapter provides a view on Rasch models within a GLM context. A very general description of this can be found in De Boeck and Wilson (2004) with focus on modelling latent variables as outcome in regression models, using observed item responses. Here it is examined how a latent covariate can be included in a generalized linear model when the latent covariate is measured using either a Rasch model [Rasch (1960) and Fischer and Molenaar (1995)] or a more general log-linear Rasch model [Kelderman (1984,1992)]. Section 6.2 describes an extension of generalized linear models with subject-level random effects and shows how a linear regression model with a latent variable as outcome (a latent regression model) can be formulated as a generalized linear mixed model. The interpretation of regression parameters in the presence of random effects is discussed in Section 6.3. The results are motivated by an occupational health example where observed covariates (gender, age, and education) and a latent covariate (skill discretion) is included in a Poisson regression analysis of absence rates (Section 6.5).

6.2   Generalized Linear Mixed Models

Generalized linear models [Nelder and Wedderburn (1972) and McCullagh and Nelder (1989)] are a class of regression models that includes normal, logistic, and Poisson regression models.

Consider a sample of subjects $j = 1, \ldots, N$ and let $y_1, \ldots, y_N$ denote the observed values of the outcome variable. It is assumed that the distribution of y_j is a one-parameter exponential family:

$$p(y_j | \eta_j) = \exp(y_j \eta_j - b(y_j, \eta_j) + c(y_j)) \qquad (j = 1, \ldots, N), \qquad (6.1)$$

where $\eta_1, \ldots, \eta_N$ are parameters called linear predictors and the bs and cs are constants. Let X_j denote the vector of observed covariates for the jth subject (the jth row in the design matrix). Exponential families such as (6.1) are the basis of generalized linear models by assuming the linear structure

$$\eta_j = X_j \beta \qquad (j = 1, \ldots, N). \qquad (6.2)$$

The distribution of the ys is determined by the Xs and the βs. These will often be of interest because they have a straightforward interpretation (for example, as difference in means in normal regression model parameters and as the log of odds-ratios in logistic regression models). For Poisson and logistic regression models the predictor can be extended with residual variation; that is,

$$\eta_j = X_j\beta + \epsilon_j, \qquad \epsilon_j \sim N(0, \sigma^2) \qquad (j = 1, \ldots, N) \qquad (6.3)$$

The result is a simple generalized linear mixed model (the term simple is used to indicate that only subject-level random effects are introduced). The residual ϵ_j can be interpreted as over dispersion, for example, from unobserved covariates.

Let $\theta_1, \ldots, \theta_N$ denote the values of the latent covariate of interest. In what follows, it is assumed that the latent covariate is measured using a Rasch model [Rasch (1960) and Fischer and Molenaar (1995)] or a log-linear Rasch model [Kelderman (1984)] with known item parameters. Whether such a model fits the data should of course be examined carefully, and the approaches discussed in what follows have little merit if a (log-linear) Rasch model does not fit the data.

6.2.1   Latent regression models

When the values $\theta_1, \ldots, \theta_N$ of the latent covariate have been measured using a (log-linear) Rasch model where the item parameters are known, the distribution of the raw scores $t_1, \ldots, t_N$ comes from a one-parameter exponential family [Christensen *et al.* (2004)], and the generalized linear mixed model given by the structure

$$\theta_j = Z_j\delta + \xi_j \qquad \xi_j \sim N(0, \omega^2) \qquad (j = 1, \ldots, N) \qquad (6.4)$$

is called a latent regression model. Since the pioneering work of Andersen and Madsen (1977), models of this kind have been discussed by many authors for dichotomous Rasch models [Zwinderman (1991), Hoijtink (1995), Kamata (2001), and Maier (2001)], polytomous Rasch models [Anderson (1994), Zwinderman (1997), and Christensen *et al.* (2004)], and more general dichotomous item response theory models [Janssen *et al.* (2000) and Fox and Glas (2001)].

Latent regression models are a powerful tool for comparing groups with respect to the value of a latent variable. Inference based on the observed raw scores $t_1, \ldots, t_N$ has been shown to yield invalid results [Embretson (1996)] and statistics based on estimated values $\hat{\theta}_1, \ldots, \hat{\theta}_N$ for each person can yield biased results [Hoijtink and Boomsma (1996)].

It should be noted that, although there is no mathematical difference in the way the variables θ and η are used in the regression models, they are in fact fundamentally different. In the latent regression model, θ is the variable of interest and the use of the observed raw sum score t is a technical detail. In the regression model for the observed outcome, the outcome variable y is the variable of interest and the introduction of the predictor η is a technical detail.

6.3   Interpretation of Parameters

The inclusion of random effects changes the interpretation of the parameters β because the predictor η is a stochastic variable. Interpretation of regression parameters in the presence of random effects has been discussed for logistic regression models by Larsen *et al.* (2000), and for latent regression models by Christensen *et al.* (2004) focusing on the advantages of reporting of the random effect as the median of the absolute difference.

Here Poisson regression models with subject-level random effects (the regression models used in the example in Section 6.5) are considered. In a Poisson regression model, (6.1) is $p(y_j|\eta_j) = \exp(y_j\eta_j - \exp(\eta_j) - \log(y_j!))$, and the parameter β_1, say, in (6.2) can be interpreted as the logarithm of the rate ratio between two groups of subjects.

In the presence of random effects, for example, (6.3), differences between subjects on the link scale are stochastic variables. For two randomly chosen subjects who have the same value of all fixed effects covariates (i.e., $X_{j_1} = X_{j_2}$), the median is

$$\mathrm{med}(|\eta_{j_1} - \eta_{j_2}|) = \sqrt{2\sigma^2\mathrm{med}(\chi_1^2)} \simeq 0.954 \cdot \sigma \qquad (6.5)$$

because $\eta_{j_1} - \eta_{j_2}$ is normally distributed with mean zero and variance $2\sigma^2$. The median (6.5) is a measure of heterogeneity on the same scale as the contrasts. In the example in Section 6.5, where the number of absence days is studied using a Poisson regression model, (6.5) is the logarithm of the ratio between the largest and smallest number of absence days for two randomly chosen subjects in the same group (i.e., with the same value of the covariates).

6.4   Generalized Linear Models with a Latent Covariate

Assuming for all $j = 1, \ldots, N$ that y_j and t_j are conditionally independent given η_j and θ_j, the joint distribution of (y_j, t_j) is a two-dimensional exponential family, and the model described in the following is the result of imposing a simpler structure on the variables (θ_j, η_j), for $j = 1, \ldots, N$ and including residual correlation.

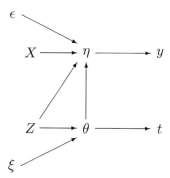

Figure 6.1: Overview of the relation between variables in the regression model

   This section describes a one-dimensional regression model for the observed outcome variable y using the raw sum score t and the known item parameters to model the relation between η and θ. The interpretation of the parameters is discussed and a two-stage estimation algorithm is proposed.

6.4.1   Model

The latent covariate θ can be included in a regression model for the observed outcomes by inserting the θs in (6.3), that is, by imposing the structure

$$
\begin{pmatrix} \eta_j \\ \theta_j \end{pmatrix} = \begin{pmatrix} X_j\beta + \gamma\theta_j + \epsilon_j \\ Z_j\delta + \xi_j \end{pmatrix} \quad \begin{pmatrix} \epsilon_j \\ \xi_j \end{pmatrix} \sim N(0,\Sigma) \quad \Sigma = \begin{pmatrix} \sigma^2 & 0 \\ 0 & \omega^2 \end{pmatrix} \quad (6.6)
$$

for $j = 1,\ldots,N$. This extension is a very simple structural equation model [Bollen (1989)] formulated for the variables (η,θ); an example of the structural relationship between variables imposed by this model is shown in Figure 6.1.
   The standard approach would be to include the observed raw sum scores in (6.3), that is, $\eta_j = X_j\beta + t_j\gamma + \epsilon_j$, $\epsilon_j \sim N(0,\sigma^2)$ for $j = 1,\ldots,N$, thereby indirectly postulating a relation between the responses y_j and values θ_j of the latent covariate. Because the raw sum score is not on an interval scale, another model is required and a better approach would be to include estimated values, $\eta_j = X_j\beta + \gamma\hat{\theta}_j + \epsilon_j$, $\epsilon \sim N(0,\sigma^2)$ for $j = 1,\ldots,N$, but two subjects with the same raw sum score do not have exactly the same value of the latent covariate, and this approach will ignore estimation error. The model (6.6) on the other hand takes variation into account by using θ as a random effect.

6.4.2   Interpretation of parameters

For two subjects j_1 and j_2, mean values can be compared using the difference

$$
\eta_{j_1} - \eta_{j_2} = (X_{j_1} - X_{j_2})\beta + \gamma(\theta_{j_1} - \theta_{j_2}) + (\epsilon_{j_1} - \epsilon_{j_2}) \qquad (6.7)
$$

on the η-scale. If the random effects (ϵ_{j_1} and ϵ_{j_2}) are disregarded, the parameters β and γ are differences on this scale: β_1, say, is the difference between subjects for whom $X_{1j_1} = X_{1j_2} + 1$ and $X_{ij_1} = X_{ij_2}$, for $i \neq 1$ and $\theta_{j_1} = \theta_{j_2}$, and γ is the difference between subjects for whom $\theta_{j_1} = \theta_{j_2} + 1$, and $X_{j_1} = X_{j_2}$.

When the random effects are included, the difference (6.7) is a stochastic variable, and this changes the interpretation of the parameters β and γ. The difference between subjects for whom $X_{1j_1} = X_{1j_2} + 1$ and $X_{ij_1} = X_{ij_2}$, for $i \neq 1$ and $\theta_{j_1} = \theta_{j_2}$ is normally distributed with mean β_1 and variance $2\sigma^2$. The difference between subjects for whom $\theta_{j_1} = \theta_{j_2} + 1$, and $X_{j_1} = X_{j_2}$ is normally distributed with mean γ and variance $2\sigma^2$.

When a linear structure is imposed on the latent covariate, θ_j can be replaced by $X_j\delta + \xi_j$ in (6.7) yielding

$$\eta_{j_1} - \eta_{j_2} = (X_{j_1} - X_{j_2})\beta + (X_{j_1} - X_{j_2})\gamma\delta + \gamma(\xi_{j_1} - \xi_{j_2}) + (\epsilon_{j_1} - \epsilon_{j_2})$$

$$(6.8)$$

and the difference between subjects for whom $X_{1j_1} = X_{1j_2} + 1$ and $X_{ij_1} = X_{ij_2}$, for $i \neq 1$ and $X_{j_1} = X_{j_2}$ is normally distributed with mean β_1 and variance $2\gamma^2\omega^2 + 2\sigma^2$. If $X_{1j_1} = X_{1j_2} + 1$, $X_{1j_1} = X_{1j_2} + 1$ and $X_{ij_1} = X_{ij_2}$, $X_{ij_1} = X_{ij_2}$, for $i \neq 1$ the mean of the difference is $\beta_1 + \gamma\delta_1$. This has special implications when a covariate influences both η and θ: the effect on the outcome y is divided into a direct effect, and a indirect (or mediated) effect through the effect on the latent covariate θ (cf. Figure 6.1).

6.4.3 Parameter estimation

The joint probabilities specified by (6.6) are

$$\Pr(y_j, t_j) = \int \int p(y_j | X_j\beta + \gamma(X_j\delta + \xi_j) + \epsilon_j)$$
$$\times q(t_j | X_j\delta + \xi_j)\phi_{\omega^2}(\xi_j)\phi_{\sigma^2}(\epsilon_j)$$

$$(6.9)$$

where ϕ_{ω^2} is the density function of the normal distribution with mean zero and variance ω^2. This yields the log-likelihood function

$$l(\beta, \gamma, \delta, \sigma^2, \omega^2) = \sum_{j=1}^{N} \log(\Pr(y_j, t_j)).$$

$$(6.10)$$

This log-likelihood function can be maximized using PROC NLMIXED in SAS. This procedure uses an adaptive Gaussian quadrature, found to be one of the best methods in a comparison of several different integrated likelihood approximations [Pinheiro and Bates (1995)].

Realistic starting values for the parameters β, δ, and γ will decrease computing time greatly and these could be obtained by (i) numerical solution of the fixed effects model (given by $\eta = X\beta + \gamma\theta$ and $\theta = X\delta$); (ii) solving the score equations

$$U(\beta, \delta, \gamma) = \sum_{j=1}^{N} X_j(y_j - E(y_j|X_j\beta + X_j\gamma\delta)) + \sum_{j=1}^{N} X_j(t_j - E(t_j|X_j\delta)) = 0,$$

because this leads to consistent estimates even though the correlation structure is ignored [Liang and Zeger (1986)]; or (iii) by using the following adaptation of the Iterative Weighted Least Squares (IWLS) algorithm [see Nelder and Wedderburn (1972) and McCullagh and Nelder (1989)]. Estimates of the parameters $\hat{\beta}$, $\hat{\delta}$, and $\hat{\gamma}$ yield a vector $\hat{\theta} = X\hat{\delta}$ of predicted θ-values and thereby also a vector $\hat{\eta} = X\hat{\beta} + \hat{\gamma}\hat{\theta}$ of predicted η-values. Because the mean and variance in one-parameter exponential families are uniquely determined by the parameter predictors η and θ this yields estimates of the mean vectors and variance–covariance matrices for y and t. Starting values for the parameters β, γ, and δ can be obtained by iteratively solving the equations

$$(X|\theta)'V(y)^{-1}(X|\theta) \begin{pmatrix} \beta \\ \gamma \end{pmatrix} = (X|\theta)V(y)^{-1}y^*$$
$$X'V(t)^{-1}X\delta = X'V(y)^{-1}t^*,$$

where $y^* = (y - E(y))V(y)^{-1}$ and $t^* = (t - E(t))V(t)^{-1}$ are updated in each step. This algorithm is very fast and works in many situations, but will not always converge when the fixed effects model is not identified.

6.5   Example

In 1997, the Danish National Institute of Occupational Health conducted a study of the psychosocial work environment in a random sample of 4000 people from a general population between 20 and 60 years (response rate = 62%). The data collection yielded responses from a total of 1858 people who were employed. In this example, the subsample of people employed in offices, trade, and industry, who had complete item responses, are considered (504 employees in all: 268 office workers, 99 trade workers, and 137 workers in industry). The research question concerns how differences in sickness absence rates can be attributed to the observed covariates: gender, age, job group, and education [no education, skilled, vocational education (three years), higher education] and to the latent covariate skill discretion.

Let Y_j denote the number of sickness absence spells for person j. Table 6.1 shows estimated parameters from a Poisson regression model with random person effects ($\eta_j = X_j\beta + \epsilon_j$).

Table 6.1: Predictors of the number of absence spells. Results from Poisson regression with random person effects

	Estimate	95% CI	p
Gender (being a woman)	0.247	(0.008, 0.487)	0.043
Age (10 years)	−0.134	(−0.229,−0.038)	0.006
Trade workers	0	—	—
Office workers	0.202	(−0.083, 0.487)	0.164
$\hat{\sigma}$	0.645	(0.530, 0.759)	—

The number of sickness absence spells is seen to differ among job groups, industry workers having 41% more sickness absence spells than trade workers [$\exp(0.347) = 1.41$] and it is also apparent that there is substantial variation between persons. The median (6.5) is $0.954 \cdot 0.645 = 0.615$ and thus the ratio between largest and smallest number of absence days for two randomly chosen subjects with the same value of the covariates is $\exp(0.618) = 1.850$.

6.5.1   Latent covariate

Three items were used to measure skill discretion (Does your job require you to take the initiative? Do you have the possibility of learning new things through your work? Can you use your skills or expertise in your work? Responses: To a large extent, To some extent, Somewhat, Not very much, To a very small extent). The answer categories were scored $0, 1, 2, 3, 4$, and total scores t_j taking values $0, 1, \ldots, 12$ were computed. The Rasch model was found to fit adequately to the data and based on this model a value $\hat{\theta}_j$ of the latent covariate can be estimated for each person.

Three Poisson regression models are compared introducing skill discretion in the model by: (i) including the raw scores $\eta_j = X_j\beta + \gamma_{(i)}t_j + \epsilon_j$, (ii) including estimated values for each person $\eta_j = X_j\beta + \gamma_{(ii)}\hat{\theta}_j + \epsilon_j$, or (iii) by the model (6.6)

$$\eta_j = X_j\beta + \gamma_{(iii)}\theta_j + \epsilon_j$$
$$\theta_j = \delta_0 + \xi_j.$$

The estimated effects $\hat{\gamma}_{(i)}, \hat{\gamma}_{(ii)}, \hat{\gamma}_{(iii)}$ of skill discretion on the number of sickness absence spells in these three models are shown in Table 6.2

The model (6.6) discloses a substantial reduction and is the only model to disclose a significant effect. The parameters $\gamma_{(ii)}$ and $\hat{\gamma}_{(iii)}$ are immediately comparable because they are on the same scale.

Table 6.2: Results from Poisson regression with random person effects including (i) the observed raw sum score, (ii) estimated values for each person, or (iii) latent covariate (cf. (6.6)) as predictors. All analyses are adjusted for effect of gender, age, and job group

	Estimate	95% CI	p
$\gamma_{(i)}$	-0.051	$(-0.106, 0.004)$	0.064
$\gamma_{(ii)}$	-0.087	$(-0.187, 0.013)$	0.088
$\gamma_{(iii)}$	-0.213	$(-0.423, -0.003)$	0.046

The parameter γ quantifies the effect of a one-point increase on the latent scale, cf. (6.7), the proposed model estimates that this effect is a reduction of absence rates by 19.2% ($\exp(-0.213) = 0.808$), whereas the predicted effect based on estimated θ_js is a reduction by 8.3%, presumably because the measurement error inherent in the estimates is not taken into account.

6.5.2 Job group level effect of the latent covariate

Next, a more general model incorporating job group levels of skill discretion is considered

$$\eta_j = X_j\beta + \gamma_{(iii)}\theta_j + \epsilon_j$$
$$\theta_j = Z_j\delta + \xi_j.$$

This structural equation model [Bollen (1989)] for the variables θ, η yields a better description of the distribution of the latent variable in the population, and a latent regression model that fits better [Christensen and Kreiner (2004)]. The estimated parameters are shown in Table 6.3.

In this model, the difference between office workers and trade workers is

$$\eta_{office} - \eta_{trade} = \beta_{office} + \gamma\delta_{office} = 0.183 + 0.135 \cdot 0.206$$
$$= 0.183 + 0.028 = 0.211;$$

this difference is of the same magnitude as the one in Table 6.1, but the effect on sickness absence is divided into a direct effect, and a indirect (or mediated) effect through the effect on the latent covariate: $0.028/0.211 = 13.3\%$ of this job group difference is explained by differences in skill discretion.

Table 6.3: Predictors of the number of absence spells. Effect of the latent covariate skill discretion on job group level

Parameter	Estimate	S.E.
β_{woman}	0.205	0.122
β_{age}	−0.140	0.048
β_{trade}	0	—
β_{office}	0.183	0.145
$\beta_{industry}$	0.315	0.166
γ	−0.135	0.063
δ_{trade}	0	—
δ_{office}	−0.206	0.156
$\delta_{industry}$	−0.144	0.175
σ	0.629	—
ω	1.044	—

6.6 Discussion

A simple approach to including a latent variable indirectly measured through item responses in a generalized linear model was discussed here. Many other latent variable models have been proposed; see, for example, Muthén (1984, 1989), Rabe-Hesketh, Skrondal, and Pickles (2004), Skrondal and Rabe-Hesketh (2003), and Fox and Glas (2001, 2002). A special feature of the approach used here is that the separation between measurement models and structural models inherent in the Rasch model is used by inserting known item parameters in the distribution of the raw sum score. This distribution then comes from a one-parameter exponential family and (6.4) yields a generalized linear mixed model. This situation is approximated when consistent conditional maximum likelihood estimates of item parameters are used. The consequences of this two-stage estimation procedure have been studied: the procedure yields consistent estimates of regression parameters, but standard errors are too small, and this problem is constant over sample sizes but gets smaller if the number of items is increased, that is, with increased measurement precision [Christensen *et al.* (2004)].

Because this approach is based on the distribution of the total score and not the distribution of single item responses, the framework is easily expanded to measurement using log-linear Rasch models [Kelderman (1984) and Christensen *et al.* (2004)]. Complex relationships between variables (e.g., local dependence structures) can thus be included [Kreiner and Christensen (2002, 2004)]. The use of generalized linear models allows for standard interpretation (e.g., the rate ratios in the example). When consistent conditional maximum likelihood estimates of item parameters are inserted, the distribution of the raw sum score t is a one-parameter exponential family and a model including both latent variables and Poisson distributed variables is straightforward.

Most applications of random effect models require specialized standalone software, e.g., HLM [Raudenbush *et al.* (2000), MLwiN [Goldstein *et al.* (1998)] and Mplus [Muthén and Muthén (1998)], an exception being `gllamm` [Rabe-Hesketh, Pickles, and Skrondal (2001)] implemented in Stata. The approaches discussed here are implemented in SAS [Christensen and Bjorner (2003)].

References

1. Andersen, E. B. (1994). Latent regression analysis, *Research Report 106*, Department of Statistics, University of Copenhagen, Denmark.

2. Andersen, E. B., and Madsen, M. (1977). Estimating the parameters of the latent population distribution, *Psychometrika*, **42**, 357–374.

3. Bollen, K. A. (1989). *Structural Equations with Latent Variables*, John Wiley & Sons, New York.

4. Christensen, K. B., and Bjorner, J. B. (2003). SAS macros for Rasch based latent variable modelling, *Technical Report 03/13*, Department of Biostatistics, University of Copenhagen, Denmark
   http://pubhealth.ku.dk/bs/publikationer.

5. Christensen, K. B., Bjorner, J. B., Kreiner, S., and Petersen, J. H. (2004). Latent regression in loglinear Rasch models, *Communications in Statistics —Theory and Methods*, **33**, 1295–1313.

6. Christensen, K. B., and Kreiner, S. (2004). Testing the fit of latent regression models, *Communications in Statistics—Theory and Methods*, **33**, 1341–1356.

7. De Boeck, P., and Wilson, M. (2004). *Explanatory Item Response Models. A Generalized Linear and Nonlinear Approach*, Springer-Verlag, New York.

8. Embretson, S. E. (1996). Item response theory models and spurious interaction effects in factorial ANOVA designs, *Applied Psychological Measurement*, **20**, 201–212.

9. Fischer, G. H., and Molenaar, I. W. (1995). *Rasch Models—Foundations, Recent Developments, and Applications*, Springer-Verlag, New York.

10. Fox, J. P., and Glas, C. A. W. (2001). Bayesian estimation of a multilevel IRT model using Gibbs sampling, *Psychometrika*, **66**, 271–288.

11. Fox, J. P., and Glas, C. A. W. (2002). *Modeling Measurement Error in a Structural Multilevel Model*, pp. 245–269, Lawrence Erlbaum, Hillsdale, NJ.

12. Fox, J. P., and Glas, C. A. W. (2003). Bayesian modeling of measurement error in predictor variables using item response theory, *Psychometrika*, **68**, 169–191.

13. Goldstein, H., Rasbash, J., Plewis, I., Draper, D., Browne, W., Yang, M., Woodhouse, G., and Healy, M. (1998). *A User's Guide to mlwin*, Multilevel Models Project, Institute of Education, University of London, England.

14. Hoijtink, H. (1995). Linear and repeated measures models for the Person parameters, In *Rasch Models—Foundations, Recent Developments, and Applications* (Eds., G. H. Fischer, and I. W. Molenaar), pp. 203–214, Springer-Verlag, New York.

15. Hoijtink, H., and Boomsma, A. (1996). Statistical inference based on latent ability estimates, *Psychometrika*, **61**, 313–330.

16. Janssen, R., Tuerlinckx, F., Meulders, M., and De Boeck, P. (2000). A hierarchial IRT model for criterion-referenced measurement, *Journal of Educational and Behavioral Statistics*, **25**, 285–306.

17. Kamata, A. (2001). Item analysis by the hierarchial generalized linear model, *Journal of Educational Measurement*, **38**, 79–93.

18. Kelderman, H. (1984). Loglinear Rasch model tests, *Psychometrika*, **49**, 223–245.

19. Kelderman, H. (1992). Computing maximum likelihood estimates of loglinear models from marginal sums with special attention to loglinear item response theory, *Psychometrika*, **57**, 437–450.

20. Kreiner, S., and Christensen, K. B. (2002). *Graphical Rasch Models*, pp. 187–203, Kluwer Academic, Dordrecht, The Netherlands.

21. Kreiner, S., and Christensen, K. B. (2004). Analysis of local dependence and multidimensionality in graphical loglinear rasch models, *Communications in Statistics—Theory and Methods*, **33**, 1239–1276.

22. Larsen, K., Petersen, J. H., Budtz-Jørgensen, H., and Endahl, L. (2000). Interpreting parameters in the logistic regression model with random effects, *Biometrics*, **56**, 909–914.

23. Liang K. Y., and Zeger, S. (1986). Longitudinal data analysis using generalized linear models, *Biometrika*, **73**, 13–22.

24. Maier, K. S. (2001). A Rasch hierarchial measurement model, *Journal of Educational and Behavioral Statistics*, **26**, 307–330.

25. McCullagh, P., and Nelder, J. A. (1989). *Generalized Linear Models*, Second edition, Chapman and Hall, London, England.

26. Muthén, B. (1984). A general structural equation model with dichotomous, ordered categorical, and continous latent variable indicators, *Psychometrika*, **49**, 115–132.

27. Muthén, B. (1989). Latent variable modeling in heterogenous populations, *Psychometrika*, **54**, 557–585.

28. Muthén, L. K., and Muthén, B. (1998). *Mplus: The Comprehensive Modelling Program for Applied Researchers, Users Manual*, Muthén & Muthén, Los Angeles.

29. Nelder, J. A., and Wedderburn, R. W. M. (1972). Generalized linear models, *Journal of the Royal Statistical Society, Series A*, **135**, 370–384.

30. Pinheiro, J. C., and Bates, D. M. (1995). Approximations to the log-likelihood function in the nonlinear mixed-effects model, *Journal of Computational and Graphical Statistics*, **4**, 12–35.

31. Rabe-Hesketh, S., Pickles, A., and Skrondal, A. (2001). Gllamm manual, *Technical Report 2001/01*, Department of Biostatistics and Computing, Institute of Psychiatry, King's College, London, http://www.iop.kcl.ac.uk/IoP/Departments/ BioComp/programs/gllamm.html.

32. Rabe-Hesketh, S., Skrondal, A., and Pickles, A. (2004). Generalised multilevel structural equation modelling, *Psychometrika*, **69**, 183–206.

33. Rasch, G. (1960). *Probabilistic Models for Some Intelligence and Attainment Tests*, Danish National Institute for Educational Research, Copenhagen, Denmark; Expanded edition, University of Chicago Press, Chicago, 1980.

34. Raudenbush, S. W., Bryk, A. S., Cheong, Y. F., and Congdon, Jr., R. T. (2000). *HLM 5. Hierarchical Linear and Nonlinear Modeling*, Scientific Software International, Inc., Lincolnwood, IL.

35. Skrondal, A., and Rabe-Hesketh, S. (2003). Multilevel logistic regression for polytomous data and rankings, *Psychometrika*, **68**, 267–287.

36. van der Linden, W. J., and Hambleton, R. K. (Eds.) (1997). *Handbook of Modern Item Response Theory*, Springer-Verlag, New York.

37. Zwinderman, A. H. (1991). A generalized Rasch model for manifest predictors, *Psychometrika*, **56**, 589–600.

38. Zwinderman, A. H. (1997). Response models with manifest predictors, In *Handbook of Modern Item Response Theory* (Eds., W. J. van der Linden, and R. K. Hambelton), pp. 245–258, Springer-Verlag, New York.

7

Sequential Analysis of Quality of Life Measurements with the Mixed Partial Credit Model

Véronique Sébille,[1] **Tariku Challa,**[2] **and Mounir Mesbah**[3]

[1] *Université de Nantes, Nantes, France*
[2] *Limburgs Universitair Centrum, Diepenbeek, Belgium*
[3] *Université Pierre et Marie Curie Paris VI, Paris, France*

Abstract: Early stopping of clinical trials either in the case of beneficial or deleterious effect of treatment on quality of life (QoL) is an important issue. QoL is usually evaluated using self-assessment questionnaires and responses to the items are combined into scores assumed to be normally distributed (which is rarely the case). An alternative is to use item response theory (IRT) models such as the partial credit model (PCM) for polytomous items which takes into account the categorical nature of the items.

Sequential analysis and mixed partial credit models were combined in the context of phase II noncomparative trials. The statistical properties of the sequential probability ratio test (SPRT) and of the triangular test (TT) were compared using mixed PCM and traditional average scores methods (ASM) by means of simulations.

The type I error of the sequential tests was correctly maintained for both methods, the mixed PCM being more conservative than the ASM. Although remaining a bit underpowered, the mixed PCM displayed higher power than the ASM for both sequential tests. Both methods allowed substantial reductions in average sample numbers as compared with fixed sample designs. Overlapping of item category particularly affected the ASM by inflating the type I error and power. The use of IRT models in sequential analysis of QoL endpoints is promising and should provide a more powerful method to detect therapeutic effects than the traditional ASM.

Keywords and phrases: Quality of life, item response theory, partial credit model, mixed models, sequential tests, clinical trials

7.1   Introduction

Many clinical trials attempt to measure health-related quality of life (QoL) which refers to 'the extent to which one's usual or expected physical, emotional and social well-being are affected by a medical condition or its treatment' [Cella and Bonomi (1995) and Fairclough (2002)]. QoL endpoints, reflecting the patient's perception of his or her well-being and satisfaction with therapy, are important health outcomes to consider. However, each domain of health can have several components (e.g., symptoms, ability to function, disability) and translating these various domains of health into quantitative values to measure quality of life is a complex task, drawing from the field of psychometrics, biostatistics, and clinical decision theory. In clinical trials in which specific therapeutic interventions are being studied, QoL is usually evaluated using self-assessment questionnaires that consist of a set of questions called items, which are often polytomous and frequently combined to give scores for scales or subscales. The common practice is to work on average scores that are generally assumed to be normally distributed. However, these average scores are rarely normally distributed and usually do not satisfy a number of basic measurement properties including sufficiency, unidimensionality, or reliability. Moreover, these scores are often used as a reduction of a larger amount of data without introducing clearly the mechanism of such reduction in the likelihood.

Item response theory (IRT), which was first mostly developed in educational testing, takes into account the multiplicity and categorical nature of the items by introducing an underlying response model [Fisher and Molenaar (1995)] relating those items to a latent parameter having the nice property to be interpreted as the true individual QoL. In this framework, the probability of response of a patient on an item depends upon two different parameters: the 'ability level' of the person (which reflects his or her current QoL) and the 'difficulty' of the item (which reflects somehow the capacity of that specific item in discriminating between good and bad QoL).

QoL endpoints are often studied in noncomparative phase II trials, which are commonly designed to evaluate therapeutic efficacy as well as further investigation of the side-effects and potential risks associated with therapy. Early stopping of clinical trials either in the case of beneficial or deleterious effect of the treatment on QoL is an important matter [Cannistra (2004)]. Several early termination procedures, allowing for repeated statistical analyses on accumulating data and for stopping a trial as soon as the information is sufficient to conclude, have been developed over the last few decades [Jennison and Turnbull (1999) and Whitehead (1997)]. Although sequential methodology is often used in clinical trials, IRT modelling, as a tool for scientific measurement, is not quite well established in the clinical trial framework despite a number of advantages offered by IRT to analyse clinical trial data [Holman *et al.* (2003a)]. Moreover, it has been suggested that IRT modelling offers a more accurate measurement of health status and thus should be more powerful to detect treatment effects [McHorney *et al.* (1997) and Kosinski *et al.* (2003)]. Hence, IRT modelling could be an interesting alternative to traditional sequential analysis of QoL endpoints based only on average scores. In fact, the benefit of combining sequential analysis and IRT methodologies using mixed Rasch models for binary items has already been studied [Sébille and Mesbah (2006)] and seems very promising. However, because QoL is much more often assessed in clinical trials using scales with polytomous items, our previous work was extended to mixed partial credit modelling for polytomous items in the context of phase II noncomparative trials. We performed sequential analysis of QoL endpoints (obtained from the observed data) using mixed partial credit models and we compared the use of such IRT modelling methods with the traditional use of average scores methods.

7.2 Methods

7.2.1 The partial credit model

The partial credit model is an IRT model that allows for the analysis of responses to ordinal items [Masters (1982)]. The model considers one parameter (called the item difficulty parameter) per positive response to each item. Let the ordinal categories be represented by scores $0, 1, \ldots, m$. Under the partial credit model, the probability that the ith patient with health status (QoL) level θ_i will respond (X_{ij}) in category k rather than any other category on item j, given the item difficulty parameters vector $\beta_j = (\beta_{j0}, \beta_{j1}, \ldots, \beta_{jm})$, where $\beta_{j0} = 0$ is given by:

$$P(X_{ij} = k/\theta_i, \beta_j) = f\left(X_{ij}/\theta_i; \beta_j\right) = \frac{\exp\left(\sum_{l=0}^{k}(\theta_i - \beta_{jl})\right)}{\sum_{c=0}^{m}\exp\left(\sum_{l=0}^{c}(\theta_i - \beta_{jl})\right)}.$$

Where $k = 0, 1, 2, \ldots, m$, and m is the number of categories minus one, $j = 1, 2, \ldots, J$, and J is the number of items in the questionnaire, $i = 1, 2, \ldots, N$, and N is the number of patients.

The parameter β_{jl} can be thought of as an item step difficulty to respond in category l rather than in category $l - 1$. That is, β_{jl} is the health status, as measured by the latent trait, one would require to expect a 50–50 chance of responding in category l rather than in category $l - 1$. The item difficulty parameter values can take any order and the possible reverse order of these thresholds leads to the phenomenon of overlapping. For well-constructed items, the thresholds are ordered. This implies that some grouping of categories might be required in the case of overlapping.

7.2.2 Estimation of the parameters

Several methods are available for estimating the parameters (the θs and βs) in the partial credit model [Hamon and Mesbah (2002)] including: joint maximum likelihood (JML), conditional maximum likelihood (CML), and marginal maximum likelihood (MML). The MML is used when the partial credit model is interpreted as a mixed model with θ as a random effect having distribution $h(\theta, \zeta)$ with unknown parameters ζ. The distribution h is often assumed to belong to some family distribution (often Gaussian) and its parameters are jointly estimated with the item parameters. The MML estimators for the item parameters are asymptotically efficient [Thissen (1982)]. Furthermore, because MML does not presume existence of a sufficient statistic (unlike other methods), it is applicable to virtually any type of IRT model.

7.2.3 Sequential analysis

The ethical desirability of terminating a trial that shows an early therapeutic advantage or disadvantage is the primary motivation for the use of sequential analysis. In a sequential trial the decision to stop admission to the trial depends on the nature of the evidence accumulated thus far. In this section we shall discuss the methodological aspect of sequential analysis performed either under the partial credit mixed model or under the average scores approach on QoL data.

7.2.4 The Z and V statistics

Two sample statistics play an important role in the investigation of a parameter of interest, say φ, and are fundamental to sequential trials [Whitehead (1997)]. One is a cumulative measure of the advantage of a therapy and is called the efficient score (Z) and the other indicates the amount of information about φ contained in Z and is called Fisher information (V). Both can be calculated at any stage of a clinical trial; V will increase as the trial progresses. The form of the efficient score Z for a parameter of interest and of Fisher information V can be derived from an appropriate likelihood function.

The model being used to describe the behaviour of the data is assumed to be known, apart from the value of the parameter of interest and the other parameters ϕ are treated as nuisances and in particular the likelihood of φ and ϕ based on the data will be known. The maximum likelihood estimates of the nuisance parameters at a given value of φ are used in order to derive the Z and V statistics that are needed for sequential analysis. The log-likelihood will be denoted by $l(\varphi, \phi)$ and the maximum likelihood estimate of ϕ at a given value of φ by $\hat{\phi}(\varphi)$. The consistency of $\hat{\phi}(\varphi)$ implies that in large samples $l(\varphi, \hat{\phi}(\varphi))$ will provide a good approximation to $l(\varphi, \phi)$ with the advantage that it depends only on φ. This property guarantees that an expansion in the power of φ can be made. From the Taylor expansion of $l(\varphi, \hat{\phi}(\varphi))$ about $(0, \hat{\phi}(0))$ it can be shown that

$$Z = l_\varphi(0, \hat{\phi}(0))$$

$$V = -l_{\varphi\varphi}(0, \hat{\phi}(0)) + \left\{ l_{\varphi\phi}(0, \hat{\phi}(0)) \right\}' \left\{ l_{\phi\phi}(0, \hat{\phi}(0)) \right\}^{-1} l_{\varphi\phi}(0, \hat{\phi}(0))),$$

where the subscripts indicate the derivatives of the log-likelihood with respect to φ, ϕ, or both φ and ϕ. For small φ and large samples, Z is assumed to have a normal distribution with mean φV and variance V. More details on the theoretical background of the two statistics can be found in well-known references [Whitehead (1997) and Jennison and Turnbull (1999)].

7.2.5 Traditional sequential analysis

In the traditional framework of sequential analysis [Wald (1947), Whitehead (1997), and Jennison and Turnbull (1999)], θ_i is assumed to be observed (not to be a latent value) and the observed score S_i is used as a 'surrogate' of the true latent trait θ_i. This leads to the classical framework of sequential analysis. For N patients, a normal distribution of the observed scores is assumed: $S_1, S_2, \ldots, S_N \sim N(\mu, \sigma)$. Let μ_0 be the mean score before treatment, the hypotheses of interest after receiving treatment can be expressed as: H_0: $\mu = \mu_0$ versus H_1: $\mu > \mu_0$. Let $\varphi = (\mu - \mu_0)/\sigma$; the above hypotheses can be rewritten as H_0: $\varphi = 0$ versus H_1: $\varphi > 0$. The statistics Z and V depending on the observed scores S, say $Z(S)$ and $V(S)$, can then be derived as previously described using the log-likelihood of φ and σ based on the N observations. More details can be found elsewhere [Whitehead (1997)].

7.2.6 Sequential analysis based on partial credit measurements

We shall now focus on the latent case, that is, the case where θ_i is unobserved. Thus, the likelihood will be different, because the likelihood is traditionally a function of the observations, not of the unobserved variables.

The derivation of the Z and V statistics using the partial credit model is less straightforward. The response of a patient X_{ij} $(i = 1, \ldots, N)$ to each item j $(j = 1, \ldots, J)$ depends, under the partial credit model, on two parameters: the latent trait θ_i and the item difficulty parameters $\beta_j = (\beta_{j0}, \beta_{j1}, \ldots, \beta_{jm})$. We assumed a normal distribution $g(\theta_i)$ for the latent trait θ_i with mean μ and variance σ^2, and the item difficulty parameters β_j to be known. The hypotheses of interest can be written as H_0: $\mu = \mu_0$ versus H_1: $\mu > \mu_0$.

$$\text{Let } f\left(X_{ij}/\theta_i; \beta_j\right) = \frac{\exp(\sum\limits_{l=0}^{k}(\theta_i - \beta_{jl}))}{\sum\limits_{c=0}^{m} \exp(\sum\limits_{l=0}^{c}(\theta_i - \beta_{jl}))}.$$

The joint distribution of the responses, X_i, of the ith subject with latent trait θ_i, assuming local independence of the items, is given by

$$f(X_i, \theta_i) = \prod_{j=1}^{J} f(X_{ij}/\theta_i)\, g(\theta_i).$$

Thus, the marginal contribution of the ith subject to the likelihood is

$$f(X_i, .) = \int \prod_{j=1}^{J} f(X_{ij}/\theta_i)\, g(\theta_i)\, d\theta_i.$$

Therefore, the likelihood, assuming patients are independent, is given by

$$L(\theta_1, \theta_2, \ldots, \theta_N; \mu, \sigma\,(\mu)) = \prod_{i=1}^{N} \int \prod_{j=1}^{J} f(X_{ij}/\theta_i)\, g(\theta_i)\, d\theta_i.$$

Substituting the actual distributions of f and g under the partial credit model, we obtain the following likelihood.

$$L\left(\theta_1, \theta_2, \ldots, \theta_N, \mu, \sigma\,(\mu)\right)$$
$$= \prod_{i=1}^{N} \int \prod_{j=1}^{J} \left\{ \frac{\exp(\sum\limits_{l=0}^{k}(\theta_i - \beta_{jl}))}{\sum\limits_{c=0}^{m} \exp(\sum\limits_{l=0}^{c}(\theta_i - \beta_{jl}))} * \frac{\exp(-\frac{1}{2}\left(\frac{\theta_i - \mu}{\sigma}\right)^2)}{\sigma\sqrt{2\pi}}\, d\theta_i \right\}.$$

Once we have the likelihood, the procedure for finding the Z and the V statistics can be used. This time, the statistics Z and V will depend on X, the responses to the items, which contain all the information on the items and will be denoted $Z(X)$ and $V(X)$. Estimation of $Z(X)$ and $V(X)$ was done by maximising the marginal likelihood, obtained from integrating out the random effects. Numerical integration methods had to be used because it was not possible to provide an analytical solution. We used the well-known adaptive Gauss–Hermite quadrature to obtain numerical approximations [Pinheiro and Bates (1995)].

7.2.7 The sequential probability ratio test and the triangular test

The statistics Z and V were denoted $Z(S)$ and $V(S)$ in the case of traditional sequential analysis based on sufficient scores and $Z(X)$ and $V(X)$ in the case of a joint sequential and partial credit analysis based directly on observed items. However, for ease of the general presentation of the tests we shall use the notations Z and V here. The sequential probability ratio test (SPRT) and the triangular test (TT) use a sequential plan defined by two perpendicular axes, the horizontal axis corresponds to Fisher's information V, and the vertical axis corresponds to the efficient score Z which represents the benefit as compared with H_0. The TT appears in Figure 7.1. For a one-sided test, the boundaries of the test delineate a continuation region (situated between these lines), from the regions of nonrejection of H_0 (situated beneath the bottom line) and of rejection of H_0 (situated above the top line). The boundaries depend on the statistical hypotheses (values of the expected treatment benefit, α and β) and on the number of subjects included between two analyses. They can be adapted at each analysis when this number varies from one analysis to the other, using the 'Christmas tree' correction [Siegmund (1979)]. The expressions of the boundaries for one-sided tests [Sébille and Bellissant (2001)] are given in the appendix. At each analysis, the values of the two statistics Z and V are computed and Z is plotted against V, thus forming a sample path as the trial goes on. The trial is continued as long as the sample path remains in the continuation region. A conclusion is reached as soon as the sample path crosses one of the boundaries of the test: nonrejection of H_0 if the sample path crosses the lower boundary, and rejection of H_0 if it crosses the upper boundary.

7.2.8 Simulation design

We simulated 1000 noncomparative clinical trials with patient's item responses generated according to a partial credit model. The latent trait θ_i was assumed to follow a normal distribution with mean μ and variance $\sigma^2 = 1$ and the trial we considered involved the comparison of the two hypotheses: H_0: $\mu = \mu_0 = 0$ against H_1: $\mu > 0$. We considered a QoL questionnaire with ten items and four ordinal categories. The items were first assumed to be well constructed, meaning that there was no overlapping in the categories of the items and hence the thresholds (item difficulty parameters) of the items were ordered. We sampled the item difficulty parameters from a uniform distribution ranging from -3 to 3 in an increasing order according to the categories. The statistical properties of the SPRT and of the TT were studied in the setting of one-sided noncomparative trials. We studied the type I error (α), power ($1-\beta$), average sample number (ASN), and 90th percentile (P90) of the number of patients required to reach a conclusion using simulations. The sequential tests

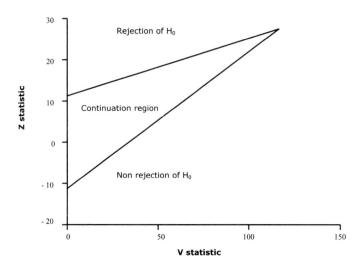

Figure 7.1: Stopping boundaries based on the triangular test (TT) for $\alpha = \beta = 0.05$ with an effect size (ES) of 0.5

were compared with the traditional method using the SPRT or TT based on the averages of patient's scores. We investigated different expected effect sizes $[(\mu - \mu_0)/\sigma = \mu$, ranging from 0.4 to 0.6], sequential analyses were performed every 20 included patients with working significance level 0.05, and power 0.95.

We also investigated the impact of overlapping category items on the properties of the sequential tests using either the partial credit model or the average scores approach. Items with overlapping categories usually require removal or collapsing of categories in order to improve the validity of the scale. We considered the case of none, 20%, 30%, 40%, and 50% of items with one overlapping at the third category and sequential analyses were performed using the same design as before with an effect size of 0.5.

7.3 Results

Table 7.1 summarises the type I error rate of the SPRT and TT for different values of the effect size using either the partial credit model or the average scores method. The significance levels achieved by the SPRT and TT were found to be lower than the working significance level, both under the partial credit model and the average scores approach. In particular, the SPRT under the partial credit model for all effect sizes was found to have lower type I error probability than the average scores method and hence appeared to be more conservative. Moreover, the type I error seemed to decrease as the effect size increased for both SPRT and TT, especially under the partial credit model.

Table 7.1: Type I error probability for the sequential probability ratio test (SPRT) and the triangular test (TT) (nominal $\alpha = \beta = 0.05$). Data are $\widehat{\alpha}$ (standard errors)

Effect Size	Partial Credit Model		Average Scores Method	
	SPRT	TT	SPRT	TT
0.4	0.026 (0.005)	0.035 (0.006)	0.039 (0.006)	0.038 (0.006)
0.5	0.014 (0.004)	0.030 (0.005)	0.038 (0.006)	0.043 (0.006)
0.6	0.008 (0.003)	0.023 (0.005)	0.033 (0.006)	0.043 (0.006)

Table 7.2 shows the power achieved by the SPRT and TT for different values of the effect size using either the partial credit model or the average scores method. The power remained more accurate under the partial credit model as compared with the average scores approach, especially for the SPRT.

Table 7.2: Power for the sequential probability ratio test (SPRT) and the triangular test (TT) (nominal $\alpha = \beta = 0.05$). Data are $1 - \widehat{\beta}$ (standard errors)

Effect Size	Partial Credit Model		Average Scores Method	
	SPRT	TT	SPRT	TT
0.4	0.941 (0.007)	0.928 (0.008)	0.920 (0.009)	0.917 (0.009)
0.5	0.922 (0.008)	0.905 (0.009)	0.909 (0.009)	0.897 (0.010)
0.6	0.935 (0.008)	0.881 (0.010)	0.926 (0.008)	0.905 (0.009)

Table 7.3 summarises the ASN and P90 of the number of patients required to reach a conclusion under H_0 for the SPRT and TT for different values of the effect size using either the partial credit model or the average scores method. We also computed for comparison purposes the approximate number of patients required by a single-stage design (SSD) using IRT modelling from the results published in a recent paper [Holman *et al.* (2003a)]. As expected, the ASN and P90 all decreased as the expected effect sizes increased whatever the method used. The ASN and P90 under H_0 were always much smaller for both methods based either on the average scores approach or the partial credit model than for the SSD for whatever values of effect size considered. The decreases in the ASN were a bit larger for the average scores method as compared with the partial credit model: -70% and -66% on average, respectively.

Table 7.3: Average sample number (ASN) and 90th percentile (P90) of the number of patients required to reach a conclusion under H_0 for the sequential probability ratio test (SPRT) and the triangular test (TT) (nominal $\alpha = \beta = 0.05$)

Effect Size	SSD – IRT*	Partial Credit Model		Average Scores Method	
		SPRT	TT	SPRT	TT
0.4	125	46.3/80	47.9/80	37.9/80	41.1 /60
0.5	100	33.6 60	33.3/60	27.8/40	28.0 /40
0.6	80	26.7/40	25.8/40	24.0/40	23.1 /40

*Approximate number of subjects required in a single-stage design (SSD) using IRT modelling. Data are ASN/P90.

Tables 7.4 summarises the ASN and P90 of the number of patients required to reach a conclusion under H_1 for the SPRT and TT for different values of the effect size using either the partial credit model or the average scores method. The approximate number of patients required by a single-stage design using IRT modelling was also computed. The same kind of behaviour was observed for both methods with a reduction in sample size for the average scores method and the partial credit model as compared with the SSD of -67% and -58% on average, respectively, the ASN being a bit larger under H_1 as compared with what was observed under H_0.

Table 7.4: Average sample number (ASN) and 90th percentile (P90) of the number of patients required to reach a conclusion under H_1 for the sequential probability ratio test (SPRT) and the triangular test (TT) (nominal $\alpha = \beta = 0.05$)

Effect Size	SSD – IRT*	Partial Credit Model		Average Scores Method	
		SPRT	TT	SPRT	TT
0.4	125	58.1/100	56.0/80	44.1/80	46.5 /80
0.5	100	42.2/80	39.5/60	32.5/60	32.3 /40
0.6	80	36.8/60	30.0/40	26.4/40	24.5 /40

*Approximate number of subjects required in a single-stage design (SSD) using IRT modelling. Data are ASN/P90.

Table 7.5 shows the type I error rate of the SPRT and TT for different amounts of items with one overlapping category in the scale using either the partial credit model or the average scores method. The type I error probabilities of both sequential procedures under the partial credit model appeared to be unaffected by the amount of items with one overlapping category and were always lower than the working significance level (0.05). In contrast, under the average scores method, the type I error probabilities of both sequential procedures increased as more items with one overlapping category appeared in the scale.

Table 7.5: Type I error probability for the sequential probability ratio test (SPRT) and the triangular test (TT) for different amounts of items with one overlapping category (nominal $\alpha = \beta = 0.05$). Overlap is the proportion of overlapping category. Data are $\hat{\alpha}$ (standard errors)

Overlap	Partial Credit Model		Average Scores Method	
	SPRT	TT	SPRT	TT
0	0.014 (0.004)	0.030 (0.005)	0.038 (0.006)	0.043 (0.006)
20	0.010 (0.003)	0.028 (0.005)	0.062 (0.008)	0.052 (0.007)
30	0.013 (0.004)	0.036 (0.006)	0.101 (0.010)	0.108 (0.010)
40	0.012 (0.003)	0.025 (0.005)	0.116 (0.010)	0.141 (0.011)
50	0.012 (0.003)	0.028 (0.005)	0.167 (0.012)	0.172 (0.012)

Table 7.6 shows the power achieved by the SPRT and TT for different amounts of items with one overlapping category in the scale using either the partial credit model or the average scores method. The power achieved by the SPRT and TT under the partial credit model appeared to be unaffected by the amount of items with one overlapping category, the TT being more underpowered, however, than the SPRT. In contrast, under the average scores method, the power achieved by the sequential procedures increased as more items with one overlapping category appeared in the scale.

Table 7.6: Power for the sequential probability ratio test (SPRT) and the triangular test (TT) for different amounts of items with one overlapping category (nominal $\alpha = \beta = 0.05$). Overlap is the proportion of overlapping category. Data are $1 - \hat{\beta}$ (standard errors)

Overlap	Partial Credit Model		Average Scores Method	
	SPRT	TT	SPRT	TT
0	0.922 (0.008)	0.905 (0.009)	0.909 (0.009)	0.897 (0.010)
20	0.931 (0.008)	0.898 (0.010)	0.941 (0.007)	0.936 (0.008)
30	0.917 (0.009)	0.892 (0.010)	0.964 (0.006)	0.964 (0.006)
40	0.929 (0.008)	0.892 (0.010)	0.972 (0.005)	0.971 (0.005)
50	0.931 (0.008)	0.903 (0.009)	0.982 (0.004)	0.978 (0.005)

Tables 7.7 and 7.8 summarise the ASN and P90 of the number of patients required to reach a conclusion under H_0 and H_1 for the SPRT and TT for different amounts of items with one overlapping category in the scale using either the partial credit model or the average scores method. The ASN and P90 of the number of patients required to reach a conclusion for the SPRT and TT under the partial credit model appeared to be unaffected by the amount of the item with one overlapping category. Furthermore, the influence of the item category overlapping was only slight when using the average scores approach; the ASN appeared to increase or decrease as more items with one overlapping category were used under H_0 and H_1, respectively.

Table 7.7: Average sample number (ASN) and 90th percentile (P90) of the number of patients required to reach a conclusion under H_0 for the sequential probability ratio test (SPRT) and the triangular test (TT) for different amounts of items with one overlapping category (nominal $\alpha = \beta = 0.05$). Overlap is the proportion of overlapping category. Data are ASN/P90

Overlap	Partial Credit Model		Average Scores Method	
	SPRT	TT	SPRT	TT
0	33.6/60	33.3/60	27.8/40	28.0/40
20	32.7/60	32.3/60	29.5/60	29.9/40
30	32.8/60	32.1/60	31.9/60	30.9/40
40	33.2/60	33.0/60	35.2/60	33.4/60
50	32.8/60	32.6/60	35.7/60	33.8/60

Table 7.8: Average sample number (ASN) and 90th percentile (P90) of the number of patients required to reach a conclusion under H_1 for the sequential probability ratio test (SPRT) and the triangular test (TT) for different amounts of items with one overlapping category (nominal $\alpha = \beta = 0.05$). Overlap is the proportion of overlapping category. Data are ASN/P90

Overlap	Partial Credit Model		Average Scores Method	
	SPRT	TT	SPRT	TT
0	42.2/80	39.5/60	32.5/60	32.3/40
20	44.3/80	40.0/60	31.1/60	31.4/40
30	41.5/80	36.4/60	27.4/40	28.5/40
40	45.6/80	40.2/60	28.2/40	29.5/40
50	44.5/80	39.8/60	26.4/40	28.2/40

7.4 Discussion

We evaluated the benefit of combining sequential analysis and IRT methodologies in the context of phase II noncomparative clinical trials using QoL endpoints. We studied and compared the statistical properties of the SPRT and of the TT using either a mixed partial credit model or the traditional average scores method. Simulation studies showed that: (i) the type I error α was correctly maintained but seemed to be lower for the mixed partial credit model as compared with the average scores method; (ii) both methods seemed to be a bit underpowered, especially the average scores method, the power being higher when using the mixed partial credit model; (iii) as expected using sequential analysis, both methods allowed substantial reductions in ASNs as compared with the SSD; and (iv) overlapping of item category particularly affected the average score method by inflating the type I error and power.

The observed difference between the mixed partial credit model and the average scores method with respect to the statistical properties of the sequential procedures might be partly explained by the plausibility of the distributional assumption of the Z and V statistics. From the results of normality assessment (Kolmogorov–Smirnov test) under H_0, the normality assumption for the Z statistic was found to hold more often under the mixed partial credit model as compared with the traditional average scores method. Moreover, the estimation of Z was always lower when it was performed using the mixed partial credit model ($\hat{Z}(X)$) as compared with the average scores method ($\hat{Z}(S)$, $p < 0.01$, for all cases), which might explain why partial credit modelling methods seemed to be more conservative than the average scores method in terms of significance level. Furthermore, the variance of $\hat{Z}$ was always lower when the estimation was performed using the Partial Credit modelling method as compared with the average scores method suggesting that the estimator of Z using mixed partial credit modelling might be more efficient.

Several limitations to our study are worth being mentioned. The items considered were assumed studied and the difficulty parameters were assumed known before designing the sequential analysis. The motivation for this assumption was the existence of calibrated item banks from which items for a specific study can be obtained [Holman *et al.* (2003b)]. A two-stage [Andersen (1977)] estimation embedded in the sequential analysis can be performed by first estimating the item difficulty parameters from the data and then estimating the Z and V statistics. However, because often few patients are involved in phase II trials, the data might be insufficient to satisfactorily estimate the item difficulty parameters and hence will make this approach difficult and further work is needed.

The impact of item overlapping which might often occur in practice seemed to be quite important for the average scores method as compared with mixed partial credit modelling and further investigations (different amounts of overlapping in scales including different numbers of items) are needed. Moreover, evaluating the impact on the statistical properties of the sequential tests of the amount of missing data (often encountered in practice) and missing data mechanisms (missing completely at random, missing at random, non ignorable missing data) and studying the statistical properties of other group sequential methods could also be investigated such as spending functions [Lan and De Mets (1983)], and Bayesian sequential methods [Grossman *et al.* (1994)], for instance. Finally, these combined methodologies (IRT modelling and sequential procedures) are currently being developed in the context of comparative clinical trials (phase III trials) which frequently include QoL endpoint assessments when comparing one therapeutic strategy against another (work in progress).

7.5   Conclusion

Item response theory usually provides more accurate assessment of health status as compared with summation methods [McHorney *et al.* (1997) and Kosinski *et al.* (2003)]. Sequential analysis taking into account the specific nature of QoL data seems to give more accurate results with respect to the statistical properties of the sequential procedures and might provide a more powerful method to detect therapeutic effects than the traditional summation method.

The use of IRT methods in the context of sequential analysis of QoL endpoints is promising and combining both methods to evaluate the effect of different therapeutic strategies on QoL endpoints is appropriate and correct both from the measurement point of view and from the plausibility of response distributional assumption.

Appendix

Stopping boundaries for the one-sided SPRT and TT

The stopping boundaries, allowing us to detect an effect size (ES) with working significance level α and power $1 - \beta$ (with $\beta = \alpha$), are:

$Z = -a + bV$ (lower boundary) and $Z = a + bV$ (upper boundary) for the one-sided SPRT,

$Z = -a + 3cV$ (lower boundary) and $Z = a + cV$ (upper boundary) for the one-sided TT,

with $a = a' - 0.583\sqrt{I}$, $b = \frac{1}{2} \cdot ES$, $c = \frac{1}{4} \cdot ES$, and $I = V_i - V_{i-1}$ where V_i is the information available at inspection i ($V_0 = 0$) for both tests, and $a' = (1/ES)\log[(1-\alpha)/\alpha]$ for the one-sided SPRT, and $a' = (2/ES)\log(1/2\alpha)$ for the one-sided TT.

The correction $0.583\sqrt{I}$ is used to adjust for the discrete monitoring of the data [Siegmund (1979)]. When $\beta \neq \alpha$, a corrected value of the effect size ES must be used to compute the equations of the boundaries. In this case, the boundaries of the tests are computed from an exact formula.

References

1. Andersen, E. B. (1977). Estimating the parameters of the latent population distribution, *Psychometrika*, **42**, 357–374.

2. Cannistra, S. A. (2004). The ethics of early stopping rules: Who is protecting whom? *Journal of Clinical Oncology*, **22**, 1542–1545.

3. Cella, D. F., and Bonomi, A. E. (1995). Measuring quality of life: 1995 update, *Oncology*, **9**, 47–60.

4. Fairclough, D. L. (2002). *Design and Analysis of Quality of Life Studies in Clinical Trial*, Chapman and Hall/CRC, Boca Raton, Florida.

5. Fisher, G. H., and Molenaar, I. W. (1995). *Rasch Models, Foundations, Recent Developments, and Applications*, Springer-Verlag, New York.

6. Grossman, J., Parmar, M. K., Spiegelhalter, D. J., and Freedman, L. S. (1994). A unified method for monitoring and analysing controlled trials, *Statistics in Medicine*, **13**, 1815–1826.

7. Hamon, A., and Mesbah, M. (2002). Questionnaire reliability under the Rasch model, In *Statistical Methods for Quality of Life Studies: Design, Measurements and Analysis* (Eds., M. Mesbah, B. F.Cole, and M. L. T. Lee), Kluwer, Amsterdam, The Netherlands.

8. Holman, R., Glas, C. A., and de Haan, R. J. (2003a). Power analysis in randomized clinical trials based on item response theory, *Controlled Clinical Trials*, **24**, 390–410.

9. Holman, R., Lindeboom, R., Glas, C. A. W., Vermeulen M., and de Haan, R. J. (2003b). Constructing an item bank using item response theory: The AMC linear disability score project, *Health Services Outcome Research Methods*, **4**, 19–33.

10. Jennison, C., and Turnbull, B. W. (1999). *Group Sequential Methods with Applications to Clinical Trials*, Chapman and Hall/CRC, Boca Raton, Florida.

11. Kosinski, M., Bjorner, J. B., Ware, J. E. Jr, Batenhorst, A., and Cady R. K. (2003). The responsiveness of headache impact scales scored using 'classical' and 'modern' psychometric methods: A re-analysis of three clinical trials, *Quality of Life Research*, **12**, 903-912.

12. Lan, K. K. G., and De Mets, D. L. (1983). Discrete sequential boundaries for clinical trials, *Biometrika*, **70**, 659–663.

13. Masters, G. N. (1982). A Rasch model for partial credit scoring, *Psychometrika*, **47**, 149–174.

14. McHorney, C. A., Haley, S. M., and Ware, J.E. Jr. (1997). Evaluation of the MOS SF-36 Physical Functioning Scale (PF-10): II. Comparison of relative precision using Likert and Rasch scoring methods, *Journal of Clinical Epidemiology*, **50**, 451–461.

15. Pinheiro, J. C., and Bates, D. M. (1995). Approximations to the log-likelihood function in the nonlinear mixed-effects model, *Journal of Computational and Graphical Statistics*, **4**, 12–35.

16. Sébille, V., and Bellissant, E. (2001). Comparison of the two-sided single triangular test to the double triangular test, *Controlled Clinical Trials*, **22**, 503–514.

17. Sébille, V., and Mesbah, M. (2006). Sequential Analysis of Quality of Life Rasch Measurements, In *Probability, Statistics and Modelling in Public Health*, (Eds., M. Nikulin, D. Commenges, and C. Huber) Springer-Verlag, New York.

18. Siegmund, D. (1979). Corrected diffusion approximations in certain random walk problems, *Advances in Applied Probability*, **11**, 701–719.

19. Thissen, D. (1982). Marginal maximum likelihood estimation for the one-parameter logistic model, *Psychometrika*, **47**, 175–186.

20. Wald, A. (1947). *Sequential Analysis*, John Wiley & Sons, New York.

21. Whitehead, J. (1997). *The Design and Analysis of Sequential Clinical Trials*, Second edition, John Wiley & Sons, Chichester, U.K.

8

A Parametric Degradation Model Used in Reliability, Survival Analysis, and Quality of Life

M. Nikulin, L. Gerville-Réache, and S. Orazio
Université Victor Segalen Bordeaux 2, Bordeaux, France

Abstract: A parametric degradation model based on the Wiener process is studied. The best unbiased estimators are constructed for the parameters of this model.

Keywords and phrases: Accelerated life, conjoint model, degradation process, failure time, longevity, MVUE, nuisance parameter, path model, reliability, quality of life, soft failure, survival analysis, traumatic failure, unbiased estimator

8.1 Introduction

Degradation and failure time data in reliability, bioreliability, biology, and medical statistics are usually used to estimate the survival or the intensity functions. Degradation data are obtained when quantities characterizing degradation of individuals during a course of disease are measured. It is the information used in addition to censored failure time data. This paper deals with the modeling and simultaneous analysis of failure time data and degradation. Traditional failure time analysis methods for estimating component reliability record only the time to failure (for units that fail) or the running time (for units that do not fail). In life testing of highly reliable components, there will be few or no failures, making reliability assessment difficult. Degradation data can, particularly in applications in which few or no failures are expected, provide considerably more reliability information than would be available from traditional censored failure time data.

Linear degradation models were used by Suzuki, Maki, and Yokogawa (1993) to model the increase in a resistance measurement over time and by Tseng, Hamada, and Chiao (1994) for modeling lumen output from fluorescent light bulbs over time. Nelson (1990) and Meeker and Escobar (1998) described many different applications and models for accelerated degradation and described Arrhenius analysis for data involving a destructive testing. Lu and Meeker (1993) use the convex degradation model for the growth rate of fatigue cracks. Concave degradation models are used by Carey and Koenig (1991) and Meeker and Luvalle (1995) to describe degradation of components in electronic circuits. A few years later, Meeker and Escobar (1998) proposed using the so-called path models. This approach is very interesting and it often gives good results. See also, Lawless (2003), Bagdonavičius and Nikulin (2001, 2002, 2004), and Duchesne (2004). More examples can be found in Meeker and Escobar (1998). The next important step in the development of degradation models was done by Doksum and Hoyland (1992), Singpurwalla (1995), and Whitemore (1995) when they proposed the model based on the Wiener process; see also Doksum and Normand (1995, 1996), Kahle and Wendt (2005), and Lehmann (2004). Later, Wendt and Kahle (2004), Singpurwalla (1997), Singpurwalla and Youngren (1998), Bagdonavičius and Nikulin (2002), and Harlamov (2004) studied models based on Gamma, Levy and other processes. Influence of covariates on degradation is also modelled by Bagdonavičius and Nikulin (2001, 2002) to estimate reliability when the environment is dynamic. Couallier (2004) compared the parametric and semiparametric estimates in the model described by Bagdonavičius and Nikulin (2001). The semiparametric analysis of several new degradation and failure time regression models without and with covariates is described by Bagdonavičius et al. (2002a,b), Bagdonavičius and Nikulin (2002), and Bagdonavičius, Haghighi, and Nikulin (2005). Levuliene (2002) considered semiparametric estimates and goodness-of-fit tests for tire wear analysis. Barberger-Gateau et al. (2004) proposed the so-called conjoint accelerated degradation model to analyze the impact of dementia and sex on disablement in the elderly, to verify that a hierarchical relationship exists between the concepts of activities daily living, instrumental activities of daily living and mobility, and to use this model to study the evolution of disability; see also Barberger-Gateau et al. (2006). For more about the applications of degradation and accelerated life models in biology, demography, medicine, biophysics, and sports, one may refer to Antonov et al. (2004), Bellamy (1995), Bohm et al. (2005), Ellis et al. (2005), Gail et al. (2005), Guyatt et al. (1985), Felson et al. (1998, 1987), Stucki and Simon (2005), and Younger et al. (2005).

We shall consider here a simple parametric degradation model for which we can describe a good estimation procedure in the sense that we shall construct the best estimators for the parameters of the considered model.

8.2   Degradation Process

To describe the degradation, we shall use a simple degradation model based on a diffusion degradation process $X(t)$, whose parameters can be estimated using its values in the moments $t_1, t_2, \ldots, t_n$.

We call a failure of an individual natural or soft if the degradation process attains a critical level.

Other failures (death, for example, one of them) are called *traumatic*. Traumatic failures may be of various modes; see, for example, Bagdonavičius, Haghighi, and Nikulin (2005). It is interesting to consider models when the intensities of traumatic failures of different modes depend on degradation. As a rule, these intensities are increasing functions of degradation process $X(t)$.

Using the degradation process, we can also consider a continuous time multi-state *illness–death* model in terms of a semi-Markovian process, when competing risk between a disease, described in terms of degradation process, and the death are assumed.

Here we consider the estimation problem for the parameters of a simple degradation process $X(t)$, which is of interest in applications in biomedical research, such as sports medicine and public health.

Suppose we observe on the set $\mathcal{T} = \{t_1, t_2, \ldots, t_n\} \subset [0, T]$ a random process

$$X(t) = \exp\{a(\theta; t)\} \exp\left\{ \sigma W(t) - \frac{\sigma^2 t}{2} \right\}, \qquad (8.1)$$

where $W(t)$ is the standard Wiener process on $[0, \infty)$. Here, the unknown function $a(\theta; t)$ to be estimated belongs to the given parametric set $\mathcal{L}$ and unknown $\sigma > 0$ is the nuisance parameter. Clearly,

$$\mathbf{E} \, X(t) = \exp\{a(\theta, t)\}.$$

We have to estimate the function $a(\cdot, \cdot)$ based on observations $X(t), t \in \mathcal{T}$. It is convenient to deal with another process

$$Z(t) = \ln X(t) = a(\theta; t) - \frac{\sigma^2 t}{2} + \sigma W(t).$$

We set

$$Z_*(t) = \ln X(t) + \frac{\sigma^2 t}{2} = a(\theta; t) + \sigma W(t) = Z(t) + \frac{\sigma^2 t}{2}.$$

We suppose that the set $\mathcal{L}$ is a linear set

$$\mathcal{L} = sp\{\varphi_0, \varphi_1, \ldots, \varphi_m\},$$

where the system $\{\varphi_0, \varphi_1, \ldots, \varphi_m\}$ is a basis of $\mathcal{L}$.

We assume that

$$\varphi_0(t) = ct \qquad (8.2)$$

for some appropriately chosen constant c. Thus,

$$a(\theta;t) = \sum_{j=0}^{m} \theta_j \varphi_j(t), \qquad \text{where } \theta = (\theta_0, \theta_1, \dots, \theta_m).$$

It is clear that we are free in the selection of the basis $\{\varphi_0, \varphi_1, \dots, \varphi_m\}$.

8.3 Estimation Problem

To begin, suppose that σ is known and we have to estimate the unknown parameter θ from the observations $Z_*(t), t \in \mathcal{T}$. As the risk function we take the quadratic function

$$R(\hat{a}, a) = \mathbf{E} \sum_{k=1}^{n} (\hat{a}(t_j) - a(t_j))^2. \qquad (8.3)$$

We construct a convenient linear unbiased estimator $\hat{a}$ for a. We assume that $\hat{a} \in \mathcal{L}$,

$$\hat{a}(\theta;t) = \sum_{j=0}^{m} \hat{\theta}_j \varphi_j(t).$$

Denote by $\mathbb{R}$ the space of functions defined on $\mathcal{T}$ with the inner product

$$(\varphi, \psi) = \sum_{j=1}^{n} \varphi(t_j)\psi(t_j),$$

and the norm

$$\|\varphi\| = \sqrt{(\varphi, \varphi)}.$$

We also consider another Hilbert structure on $\mathbb{R}$ which is defined by the relations

$$(\varphi, \psi)_W = \sum_{i,j=1}^{n} \varphi(t_i)\psi(t_j) t_i \wedge t_j,$$

$$\|\varphi\|_W = \sqrt{(\varphi, \varphi)_W}.$$

It is easy to see that

$$(\varphi, \psi)_W = \mathbf{E}\left\{ \sum_{j=1}^{n} \varphi(t_j)W(t_j) \sum_{i=1}^{n} \varphi(t_i)W(t_i) \right\}$$

and

$$||\varphi||_W^2 = \mathbf{E} \left(\sum_{j=1}^{n} \varphi(t_j) W(t_j) \right)^2 .$$

We suppose that the system $\{\varphi_0, \ldots, \varphi_m\}$ is an orthonormal basis of $\mathcal{L}$ in the space $\mathbb{R}$ with inner product $(\cdot, \cdot)$:

$$(\varphi_k, \varphi_r) = \delta_{kr}.$$

We obtain from (8.3)

$$R(\hat{a}, a) = \mathbf{E} \sum_{j=0}^{m} \left(\hat{\theta}_k - \theta_k \right)^2 .$$

8.4 Linear MVUE for a

We now want to construct the best linear unbiased estimator $\hat{\theta}_k$ for θ_k for all $k = 0, 1, \ldots, m$; see, for example, Voinov and Nikulin (1993). It is clear that

$$\hat{\theta}_k = \sum_{j=1}^{n} \psi_k(t_j) Z_*(t_j), \tag{8.4}$$

where the function ψ_k satisfies the relation

$$(\psi_k, \varphi_r) = \delta_{kr}. \tag{8.5}$$

In this case,

$$\mathbf{E} \left(\hat{\theta}_k - \theta_k \right)^2 = \sigma^2 \mathbf{E} \left(\sum_{j=1}^{n} \psi_k(t_j) W(t_j) \right)^2 = \sigma^2 ||\psi_k||_W. \tag{8.6}$$

So we have to minimize (8.6) under the condition (8.5).

8.5   Solution of the Optimization Problem

Denote by $\mathcal{L}^\perp$ the orthogonal complement to $\mathcal{L}$ in the space $\mathbb{R}$ with the inner product $(\cdot, \cdot)$. It is easy to see that

$$\psi_k = \varphi_k - \varphi^k$$

for an element $\varphi^k \in \mathcal{L}^\perp$. So it follows from (8.4) that the element φ^k is defined by

$$\|\varphi_k - \varphi^k\|_W = \inf_{\varphi \in \mathcal{L}^\perp} \|\varphi_k - \varphi\|_W.$$

Thus, we have

$$\varphi^k = P_W\left(\mathcal{L}^\perp\right) \varphi_k.$$

Here we denote by $P_W\left(\mathcal{L}^\perp\right)$ the orthoprojector in the space $\mathbb{R}$ with the inner product $(\cdot, \cdot)_W$ onto the subspace $\mathcal{L}^\perp$. It is clear that if the system

$$\{\xi_1, \ldots, \xi_d\}, \qquad d = n - m - 1,$$

is an orthonormal basis of $\mathcal{L}^\perp$ in the space $\mathbb{R}$ with the inner product $(\cdot, \cdot)_W$; then for any $\varphi \in \mathbb{R}$

$$P_W\left(\mathcal{L}^\perp\right) \varphi = \sum_{j=1}^{d} (\varphi, \xi_j)\, \xi_j,$$

So,

$$\varphi^k = P_W\left(\mathcal{L}^\perp\right) \varphi_k = \sum_{j=1}^{d} (\varphi_k, \xi_j)\, \xi_j.$$

8.6   Estimation of σ^2 and θ_0

Suppose we construct estimators $\hat{\theta}_1, \ldots, \hat{\theta}_m$. It follows from (8.3) and (8.5) that for $k \neq 0$ the estimator

$$\hat{\theta}_k = (Z_*, \psi_k) = (Z, \psi_k)$$

does not depend on σ.

Actually, σ is unknown. To estimate it, we consider the random variables

$$Y_j = (Z, \xi_j) = \sigma\,(W, \xi_j), \qquad j = 1, \ldots, d.$$

It is clear that
$$\mathbf{E}\, Y_i = 0, \quad \mathbf{E}\, Y_i Y_j = \sigma\, (\xi_i, \xi_j)_W = \sigma \delta_{ij}.$$

$Y_1, \ldots, Y_d$ is the sequence of i.i.d. random variables and $Y_j \in N(0, \sigma^2)$; so we may take as estimator for σ^2

$$\hat{\sigma}^2 = \frac{1}{d-1} \sum_{j=1}^{d} \left(Y_j - \overline{Y}\right)^2, \qquad \overline{Y} = \frac{1}{d} \sum_{j=1}^{d} Y_j$$

and take as estimator for θ_0 the statistic

$$\hat{\theta}_0 = (Z, \psi_0) + \frac{\hat{\sigma}^2 c}{2}, \qquad \text{where } c \text{ is as defined in (8.2).}$$

It is clear that

$$\hat{\theta}_0 = \theta_0 + \frac{c}{2} \left(\hat{\sigma}^2 - \sigma^2\right).$$

Now let $X_j(t), j = 1, \ldots, N$ be independent copies of the process $X(t), t \in T$:

$$X_j(t) = \exp\{a(\theta; t)\} \exp \left\{\sigma W_j(t) - \frac{\sigma^2 t}{2}\right\}.$$

We denote by $\hat{\sigma}_j^2$ the unbiased estimator for σ^2 that is constructed on the process X_j:

$$\hat{\sigma}_j^2 = \frac{1}{d-1} \sum_{k=1}^{d} (\ln X_j, \xi_k)^2 - \left(\frac{1}{d} \sum_{k=1}^{d} (\ln X_j, \xi_k)\right)^2.$$

We consider a new estimator for σ^2 as

$$\hat{\sigma}^2 = \frac{1}{N} \sum_{k=1}^{N} \hat{\sigma}_k^2.$$

In the same way, we consider estimators

$$\hat{\theta}_k = \frac{1}{N} \sum_{k=1}^{N} \hat{\theta}_k^j \qquad (k = 1, \ldots, m),$$

where we denote by $\hat{\theta}_k^j$ the best unbiased estimator for θ_k, based on the process X_j. Thus,

$$\hat{\theta}_k = \theta_k + \frac{1}{N} \sum_{k=1}^{N} U_k^j.$$

Here, for $k = 0, \ldots, m$, we denote

$$U_k^j = \frac{\sigma}{N} \sum_{k=1}^{N} (W_j, \psi_k).$$

The estimator $\hat{\theta}_0$ is defined by the relation

$$\hat{\theta}_0 = \frac{1}{N} \sum_{k=1}^{N} \hat{\theta}_0^j,$$

where

$$\hat{\theta}_0^j = \frac{1}{N} \sum_{k=1}^{N} (\ln X_j, \psi_0) + \frac{\hat{\sigma}^2 c}{2}.$$

So

$$\hat{\theta}_0^j = \theta_0 + \frac{c}{2} (\hat{\sigma}^2 - \sigma^2) + \frac{1}{N} \sum_{k=1}^{N} U_0^j.$$

Suppose $N \to \infty$, $n \to \infty$. It is then clear that in this case

$$\sqrt{N} \left(\hat{\theta}_N - \theta \right) \to N(0, \Sigma).$$

Here $\hat{\theta}_N = \left(\hat{\theta}_0, \ldots, \hat{\theta}_m \right)$, $\theta = (\theta_0, \ldots, \theta_m)$, and Σ is the covariance matrix of Gaussian vector $\left(U_0^j, \ldots, U_m^j \right)$, which does not depend on j.

Acknowledgements. The authors wish to thank V. Solev, V. Bagdonavičius, and V. Couallier for valuable comments and suggestions.

References

1. Antonov, V., Huber, C., Nikulin, M., and Polischook, V. (2004). *Longevity, Aging and Degradation Models*, Politechique University, Saint Petersburg.

2. Bagdonavičius, V., Bikelis, A., Kazakevicius, A., and Nikulin, M. (2002a). Non-parametric estimation from simultaneous degradation and failure data, *Comptes Rendus, Academie des Sciences de Paris*, **335**, 183–188.

3. Bagdonavičius V., Bikelis, A., Kazakevicius, V., and Nikulin, M. (2002b). Estimation from simultanuous degradation and failure time data, In *Mathematical Statistic and Its Applications*, 29 pp, Université Victor Segalen Bordeaux 2, France.

4. Bagdonavičius V., Haghighi, F., and Nikulin M. (2005). Statistical analysis of general degradation path model and failure time data with multiple failure modes, *Communications in Statistics—Theory and Methods*, **34**, 1643–1662.

5. Bagdonavičius, V., and Nikulin, M. (2001). Estimation in degradation models with explanatory variables, *Lifetime Data Analysis*, **7**, 85–103.

6. Bagdonavičius V., and Nikulin M. (2002). *Accelerated Life Models: Modeling and Statistical Analysis*, Chapman & Hall, Boca Raton, Florida.

7. Bagdonavičius, V., and Nikulin, M. (2004). Semiparametric analysis of degradation and failure time data with covariate, In *Parametric and Semiparametric Models with Applications to Reliability, Survival Analysis, and Quality of Life* (Eds., M. Nikulin, N. Balakrishnan, M. Mesbah, and N. Limnios), pp. 41–65, Birkhaüser, Boston.

8. Barberger-Gateau P., Zdorova-Cheminade, O., Nikulin, M., and Bagdonavičius, V. (2004). The conjoint accelerated degradation model and statisticsal analysis of the impact of dementia and sex on the disablement in the elderly for survival and longitudinal data measured with noise, Preprint 0104, IFR *Santé Publique*, Université Victor Segalen Bordeaux 2, Bordeaux, France.

9. Barberger-Gateau, P., Bagdonavičius, V., Nikulin, M., and Zodorova-Cheminade, O. (2006). The impact of dementia and sex on disablement in the elderly, In *Probability, Statistics, and Modelling in Public Health*, (Eds., M. Nikulin, D. Commenges, and C. Huber), pp. 37–52, Springer-Verlag, New York.

10. Bellamy, N. (1995). *WOMAC Ostheoarthritis Index: A User's Guide*, London, Ontario, Canada.

11. Bohm, B. B., Aigner, T., Roy, B., Brodie, T. A., Blobel, C. P., and Burkhardt, H. (2005). Homeostatic effects of the metalloproteinase disintegrin ADAM15 in degenerative cartilage remodeling, *Arthritis & Rheumatism*, **52**, 1100–1109.

12. Carey, M., and Koenig, R. (1991). Reliability assessment based on accelerated degradation: A case study, *IEEE Transactions on Reliability*, **40**, 499–506.

13. Couallier, V. (2004). Comparison of parametric and semi-parametric in joint models with covariables and traumatic censoring, In *Parametric and Semiparametric Models with Applications to Reliability, Survival Analysis, and Quality of Life* (Eds., M. Nikulin, N. Balakrishnan, M. Mesbah, and N. Limnios), pp. 81–99, Birkhaüser, Boston.

14. Doksum, K. A., and Hoyland, A. (1992). Models for variable-stress accelerated life testing experiment based on Wiener processes and the inverse Gaussian distribution, *Technometrics*, **34**, 74–82.

15. Doksum, K. A., and Normand, S.-L. T. (1995). Gaussian models for degradation processes - Part I: Methods for the analysis of biomarker data, *Lifetime Data Analysis*, **1**, 131–144.

16. Doksum K. A., and Normand S.-L. T. (1996). Models for degradation processes and event times based on Gaussian processes, In *Lifetime Data: Models in Reliability and Survival Analysis*, pp. 85–91, Kluwer, Dordrecht, The Netherlands.

17. Duchesne, T. (2004). Regression models for lifetime given the usage history, In *Abstracts of MMR'2004*, Santa Fe, California.

18. Ellis, W. C., Mahlooji, M., and Matis, J. H. (2005). Models for estimating parameters of neutral detergent fiber digestion by ruminal microorganism, *Journal of Animal Science*, **83**, 1591–1601.

19. Felson, D., Couropmitree, N., Chaisson, C, Hannan, M, Zhang, Y., Mc Alindon, T., La Valley, M., Levy, D., and Myers R. (1998). Evidence for a mendelin gene in a segregation analysis of generalized radiographic osteoarthrisis, *Arthritis & Rheumatism*, **41**, 1064–1071.

20. Felson, D., Naimark, A., Anderson, J., Kazis, L., Castelli, W., and Meenan, R. (1987). The prevalence of knee osteoarthrisis in the elderly. The Framingham Osteoarthrisis Study, *Arthritis & Rheumatism*, **30**, 914–918.

21. Gail, D., Nancy, E., Robert, L., Michael, G., Matthew, B., and Stephen, C. (2000). Effectiveness of manual physical therapy and exercise in osteoarthritis of the knee, *Annals of Internal Medecine*, **132**, 173–181.

22. Guyatt, G., Sullivan, M., Thompson, P., Fallen, E., Pugsley, S., and Taylor D. (1985). The 6-minute walk: A new measure of exercise capacity in patients with chronic heart failure, *Canadian Medical Association Journal*, **132**, 919–923.

23. Harlamov, B. (2004). Inverse gamma-process as a model of wear, In *Longevity, Aging and Degradation Models in Reliability, Health, Medicine and Biology*, volume 2 (Eds., V. Antonov, C. Huber, M. Nikulin, and V. Politschook), pp. 180–190, St. Petersburg State Politechnical University, Saint Petersburg, Russia.

24. Kahle, W., and Wendt, H. (2005). Statistical analysis of some parametric degradation models, In *Probability, Statistics and Modelling in Public Health* (Eds. M. Nikulin, D. Commenges and C. Huber), pp. 266–279, Springer-Verlag, New York.

25. Lawless, J. (2003). *Statistical Models and Methods for Lifetime Data*, Second edition, John Wiley & Sons, Hoboken, New Jersey.

26. Lehmann, A. (2004). On a degradation-failure models for repairable items, In *Parametric and Semiparametric Models with Applications to Reliability, Survival Analysis, and Quality of Life* (Eds., M. Nikulin, N. Balakrishnan, M. Mesbah and N. Limnios), pp. 65–80, Birkhaüser, Boston.

27. Levuliene, R. (2002). Semiparametric estimates and goodness-of-fit tests for tire wear and failure time data, *Nonlinear Analysis: Modelling and Control*, **7**, 61–95.

28. Lu, C., and Meeker, W.(1993). Using degradation measures to estimate a time-to-failure distribution, *Technometrics*, **35**, 161–174.

29. Meeker, W., and Escobar, L. (1998). *Statistical Methods for Reliability Data*, John Wiley & Sons, New York.

30. Meeker, W., Escobar, L., and Lu, C. (1998). Accelerated degradation tests: Modeling and analysis, *Technometrics*, **40**, 89–99.

31. Meeker, W., and Luvalle, M. (1995). An accelerated life test model based on reliability kinetics, *Technometrics*, **37**, 133–146.

32. Nelson, W. (1990). *Accelerated Testing: Statistical Models, Test Plans, and Data Analysis*, John Wiley & Sons, New York.

33. Sandmark, H., and Vingard, E. (1999). Sport and risk for severe osteoartrosis of the knee, *Scandinavian Journal of Medicine & Science in Sports*, **9** 279–284.

34. Singpurwalla, N. (1995). Survival in dynamic environnements, *Statistical Science*, **1**, 86–103.

35. Singpurwalla, N. (1997). Gamma processes and their generalizations: An overview, In *Engineering Probabilistic Design and Maintenance for Flood Protection* (Eds., R. Cook, M. Mendel, and H. Vrijling), pp. 67–73, Kluwer, Dordrecht, The Netherlands.

36. Singpurwalla, N., and Youngren, M. (1998). Multivariate distributions induced by dynamic environments, *Scandinavian Journal of Statistics*, **20**, 251–261.

37. Stucki, J. W., and Simon, H. U. (2005). *Journal of Theoretical Biology*, **4**, 123–131.

38. Suzuki, K., Maki, K., and Yokogawa, K. (1993). An analysis of degradation data of a carbon film and properties of the estimators, In *Statistical Sciences and Data Analysis* (Eds., K. Matusita, M. L. Puri, and T. Hayakawa), VSP, Utrecht, The Netherlands.

39. Tseng, S., Hamada, M., and Chiao, H. (1994). Using degradation data from a fractional experiment to improve fluorescent lamp reliability, *Research Report RR-94-05*, University of Waterloo, Waterloo, Canada.

40. Voinov, V., and Nikulin, M. (1993). *Unbiased Estimators and Their Applications, Volume 1: Univariate Case*, Kluwer, Dordrecht, The Netherlands.

41. Wendt, H., and Kahle, W. (2004). On parametric estimation for a position-dependent marking of a doubly stochastic Poisson process, In *Parametric and Semiparametric Models with Applications to Reliability, Survival Analysis, and Quality of Life* (Eds. M. Nikulin, N. Balakrishnan, M. Mesbah, and N. Limnios), pp. 473–486, Birkhaüser, Boston.

42. Whitmore, G. A. (1995). Estimating degradation by a Wiener diffusion process subject to measurement error, *Lifetime Data Analysis*, **1**, 307–319.

43. Whitmore, G. A., Crowder, M. I., and Lawless, J. F. (1998). Failure inference from a marker process based on bivariate model, *Lifetime Data Analysis*, **4**, 229–251.

44. Whitmore, G. A., and Schenkelberg, F. (1997). Modelling accelerated degradation data using Wiener diffusion with a time scale transformation, *Lifetime Data Analysis*, **3**, 27–45.

45. Younger, J. M., Fan, C. T., Chen, L., Rosser, M. F., Patterson, C., and Cyr, D. M. (2005). Cystic fibrosis transmembrane conductance as a model substrate to study endoplasmic reticulum protein quality control in mammalian cells, *Methods in Molecular Biology*, **301**, 293–303.

9

Agreement Between Two Ratings with Different Ordinal Scales

Sundar Natarajan,[1] **M. Brent McHenry,**[2] **Stuart Lipsitz,**[2]
Neil Klar,[3] **and Steven Lipshultz**[4]

[1] *New York University School of Medicine and the VA New York Harbor
Healthcare System, New York, NY, USA*
[2] *Medical University of South Carolina, Charleston, SC, USA*
[3] *Cancer Care Ontario, ON, Canada*
[4] *University of Miami School of Medicine, Miami, FL, USA*

Abstract: Agreement studies, where several observers may be rating the same
subject for some characteristic measured on an ordinal scale, provide important
information. The weighted Kappa coefficient is a popular measure of agreement
for ordinal ratings. However, in some studies, the raters use scales with different
numbers of categories. For example, a patient quality of life questionnaire may
ask 'How do you feel today?' with possible answers ranging from 1 (worst) to
7 (best). At the same visit, the doctor reports his impression of the patient's
health status as very poor, poor, fair, good, or very good. The weighted Kappa
coefficient is not applicable here because the two scales have a different number
of categories. In this paper, we discuss Kappa coefficients to measure agreement
between such ratings. In particular, with R categories of one rating, and C
categories of another, by dichotomizing the two ratings at all possible cutpoints,
there are $(R-1)(C-1)$ possible (2×2) tables. For each of these (2×2) tables, we
estimate the Kappa coefficient for dichotomous ratings. The largest estimated
Kappa coefficients suggest the cutpoints for the two ratings where agreement
is the highest and where categories can be combined for further analysis.

Keywords and phrases: Measure of agreement, Kappa coefficient, ordinal
data

9.1 Introduction

Studies of agreement are common in medical research [Kraemer *et al.* (2002)].
For example, in order to evaluate a child's health in a study of childhood asthma,
both parents may be asked to rate the child's symptoms. In order to assess
the reliability of a new quality of life measure, a cancer patient may be asked
the same or similar general health questions at the beginning and end of a

questionnaire. The data from such studies give two ratings (e.g., answers to questions) on the same subject. The goal of these studies is to determine how well the ratings agree and to quantify their agreement as a way to assess the validity of measurement. Typically in these agreement studies, the ratings on the same subject are measured on an ordinal scale with equal numbers of categories. In certain circumstances, for example, during the development phase of an instrument, the two ratings on the same subject may not be on the same scale.

Two examples are presented in this paper. The first example is from the parent questionnaire from a study of childhood leukemia [Hinkle *et al.* (2004)]. One parent is asked questions about the child's health. In this data set, there are 84 parent surveys, one for each child. At the beginning of the survey questionnaire, a parent is asked, 'In general, compared to a year ago how would you rate your child's health? Much better, Somewhat better, About the same, or Worse.' At the end of the survey questionnaire, the subject's parents are asked 'Compared to others of your child's age and sex, how would you rate his/her overall health? Better, About the same, or Worse.' Thus, the answer to the first question is on a four-point scale: 1—Much better; 2—Somewhat better; 3—About the same; 4—Worse; and the answer to the second question is on a three-point scale: 1—Better; 2—About the same; 3—Worse. The difference between the two questions is that the second question has one less possible level than the first question; in particular, answers 1 (=Much better) and 2 (=Somewhat better) of the first question should correspond to answer 1 (= Better) of question 2. If respondents were thinking of the two questions in identical fashion, then we would expect that all subjects who give answer 3 to question 1 would give answer 2 to question 2; similarly, all subjects who give answer 4 to question 1 would give answer 3 to question 2. Finally, we would expect all subjects who give answer 1 or 2 to question 1 would give answer 1 to question 2. However, when we look at the data in Table 9.1, we see that this is not entirely the case.

Table 9.1: (4×3) table from answers to the two health status questions from the parent questionnaire from the childhood leukemia study

	Better	About the Same	Worse	Total
Much better	6	27	1	34
Somewhat better	2	22	3	27
About the same	1	9	10	20
Worse	1	1	1	3
Total	10	59	15	84

The second example is from the 2002 United States National General Social Survey [Smith (2003) and Davis and Smith (1992)], which has the basic purpose of gathering data on contemporary American society in order to monitor and explain trends and constants in attitudes, behaviours, and attributes. To be eligible for the survey, a subject had to be 18 years or older. In this data set, there are 1524 subjects. The survey has over 700 questions. At the beginning of the survey questionnaire, a subject is asked, 'Would you say your own health, in general, is Excellent, Good, Fair, or Poor?' At the end of the survey questionnaire, the subject is asked 'Would you say that in general your health is Excellent, Very Good, Good, Fair, or Poor?' Thus, the answer to the first question is on a four-point scale: 1—Excellent; 2—Good; 3—Fair; 4—Poor; and the answer to the second question is on a five-point scale: 1—Excellent; 2—Very Good; 3—Good; 4—Fair; 5—Poor. The difference between the two questions is that the subject has one more possible level (Very Good) for the second question. If the subjects are thinking of the two questions in identical fashion, then we would expect that all subjects who give answer 1 to question 1 would give answer 1 to question 2; similarly, all subjects who give answer 3 to question 1 would give answer 4 to question 2; and all subjects who give answer 4 to question 1 would give answer 5 to question 2. Finally, we would expect all subjects who give answer 2 to question 1 would give answers 2 or 3 to question 2. However, when we examine the data in Table 9.2, we note that this is not entirely the case.

Table 9.2: (4×5) table from answers to the two health status questions from the 2002 United States National General Social Survey (GSS)

	Excellent	Very Good	Good	Fair	Worse	Total
Excellent	435	69	10	2	0	516
Good	18	273	394	14	2	701
Fair	0	8	40	190	3	241
Worse	0	1	0	13	52	66
Total	453	351	444	219	57	1524

When evaluating these data, it is important to determine how well the answers to these two questions agree, but, because they are on different scales, and the resulting contingency table is not 'square,' the popular measures of agreement (i.e., Kappa or weighted Kappa) cannot be used. For two nominal ratings, Kraemer (1992) proposed a matrix of Kappa coefficients, in which a diagonal element of the matrix is the Kappa coefficient for a particular category relative to all other categories combined. By looking at the matrix, one can see where agreement is the highest, and where and if it is appropriate to combine categories for further analysis. In this paper, we propose an analogous analysis for ordinal data. In particular, we propose dichotomizing the two ratings at each cutpoint on the ordinal scale, and then examining the Kappa coefficient at each of the possible cutpoints. In the second example, in which the first rating (question) has four levels, we dichotomize at three cutpoints: 1 versus ≥ 2; ≤ 2 versus ≥ 3; and ≤ 3 versus 4. Similarly, for the second rating, we dichotomize at four cutpoints: 1 versus ≥ 2; ≤ 2 versus ≥ 3; ≤ 3 versus ≥ 4; and ≤ 4 versus 5. There are 12 (3×4) possible (2×2) tables formed by looking at all possible cutpoints, and thus 12 possible Kappa coefficients. In general, if there are R rows and C columns, there are $(R-1)(C-1)$ possible (2×2) tables and thus $(R-1)(C-1)$ Kappa coefficients.

This research was motivated by the agreement problem that arose in the Parent Questionnaire in the childhood leukemia study described in Table 9.1 (Example 1) and is further characterized using the health status questions from the National General Social Survey in Table 9.2 (Example 2). In Section 9.2, we introduce some notation and briefly outline the rationale behind the formation of the Kappa coefficients. Section 9.3 contains analyses of these examples.

9.2   Notation and Model

In an agreement study, subject i $(i = 1, \ldots, n)$ has two ratings. The n subjects are assumed to be independent. The first rating on subject i can take on R ordered levels, and is denoted by the random variable Y_{i1}. The second rating on subject i can take on C ordered levels, and is denoted by the random variable Y_{i2}. In general, $R \neq C$. In the first example, $R = 3$ and $C = 4$ and in the second example, $R = 4$ and $C = 5$. The joint distribution of (Y_{i1}, Y_{i2}) is multinomial with probabilities

$$p_{jk} = \Pr[Y_{i1} = j, Y_{i2} = k] \tag{9.1}$$

for $j = 1, \ldots, R$ and $k = 1, \ldots, C$. Let n_{jk} be the number of subjects in which the first rating is level j and the second rating is level k, that is, the number of subjects with $Y_{i1} = j$ and $Y_{i2} = k$. Considering all n independent subjects, the joint distribution of the data is multinomial [Bishop *et al.* (1975)]

$$f(n_{11}, \ldots, n_{RC} | p_{11}, \ldots, p_{RC}) = \frac{n!}{n_{11}! \cdots n_{RC}!} \, p_{11}^{n_{11}} \cdots p_{RC}^{n_{RC}} \, . \tag{9.2}$$

Because the ratings are ordinal, cumulative random variables are often used [McCullagh (1980)]. Suppose, for the first rating, we form the cumulative random variables $U_{ij} = 1$ if $Y_{i1} \leq j$; 2 if $Y_{i1} > j$, $j = 1, \ldots, R-1$, and, for the second rating, we form the cumulative random variables $T_{ik} = 1$ if $Y_{i2} \leq k$; 2 if $Y_{i2} > k$, $k = 1, \ldots, C-1$. Looking at all possible combinations of (U_{ij}, T_{ik}), we can form $(R-1)(C-1)$ possible (2×2) tables. The goal of this paper is to examine all these (2×2) tables, and identify where agreement is the highest, which will tell us where categories can be combined for further analysis.

For a given j and k, suppose we let n_{11jk} be the number of subjects with $Y_{i1} \leq j$ $(U_{ij} = 1)$ and $Y_{i2} \leq k$ $(T_{ik} = 1)$; n_{12jk} be the number of subjects with $Y_{i1} \leq j$ $(U_{ij} = 1)$ and $Y_{i2} > k$ $(T_{ik} = 2)$; n_{21jk} be the number of subjects with $Y_{i1} > j$ $(U_{ij} = 2)$ and $Y_{i2} \leq k$ $(T_{ik} = 1)$; n_{22jk} be the number of subjects with $Y_{i1} > j$ $(U_{ij} = 2)$ and $Y_{i2} > k$ $(T_{ik} = 2)$. Then, we can form the (2×2) table given in Table 9.3.

Table 9.3: (2×2) table of cell counts at cutpoints j and k

		Rating 2		
		$Y_{i2} \leq k$	$Y_{i2} > k$	Total
Rating 1	$Y_{i1} \leq j$	n_{11jk}	n_{12jk}	n_{1+jk}
	$Y_{i1} > j$	n_{21jk}	n_{22jk}	n_{2+jk}
	Total	n_{+1jk}	n_{+2jk}	n

The probabilities for Table 9.3 are $p_{11jk} = \Pr[Y_{i1} \leq j, Y_{i2} \leq k]$; $p_{12jk} = \Pr[Y_{i1} \leq j, Y_{i2} > k]$; $p_{21jk} = \Pr[Y_{i1} > j, Y_{i2} \leq k]$; $p_{22jk} = \Pr[Y_{i1} > j, Y_{i2} > k]$, and can be displayed in a (2×2) table as given in Table 9.4.

Table 9.4: (2×2) table of probabilities at cutpoints j and k

		Rating 2		
		$Y_{i2} \leq k$	$Y_{i2} > k$	Total
Rating 1	$Y_{i1} \leq j$	p_{11jk}	p_{12jk}	p_{1+jk}
	$Y_{i1} > j$	p_{21jk}	p_{22jk}	p_{2+jk}
	Total	p_{+1jk}	p_{+2jk}	1

The Kappa coefficient [Cohen (1960)] κ_{jk}, that is, the observed probability of agreement corrected for the agreement based on chance, for the (2×2) table in Table 9.4 is

$$\kappa_{jk} = \frac{p_{agree,jk} - p_{chance,jk}}{1 - p_{chance,jk}}, \tag{9.3}$$

where $p_{agree,jk}$ is the probability that the two ratings agree,

$$p_{agree,jk} = p_{11jk} + p_{22jk}, \tag{9.4}$$

and $p_{chance,jk}$ is the probability that two ratings agree if they are independent,

$$p_{chance,jk} = p_{1+jk}p_{+1jk} + p_{2+jk}p_{+2jk}. \tag{9.5}$$

Then, putting (9.4) and (9.5) in (9.3), we have

$$\kappa_{jk} = \frac{p_{11jk} + p_{22jk} - (p_{1+jk}p_{+1jk} + p_{2+jk}p_{+2jk})}{1 - (p_{1+jk}p_{+1jk} + p_{2+jk}p_{+2jk})}.$$

Using the underlying multinomial distribution in Eq. (9.2), one can show that the maximum likelihood estimate (MLE) of the probability p_{utjk} is

$$\hat{p}_{utjk} = \frac{n_{utjk}}{n},$$

for $u, t = 1, 2$. Given these probability estimates, the MLE of κ_{jk} is

$$\hat{\kappa}_{jk} = \frac{(n_{11jk} + n_{22jk})/n - (n_{1+jk}n_{+1jk} + n_{2+jk}n_{+2jk})/n^2}{1 - (n_{1+jk}n_{+1jk} + n_{2+jk}n_{+2jk})/n^2}.$$

Even though the $(R-1)(C-1)$ $\hat{\kappa}_{jk}$s are correlated, a confidence interval or a consistent estimate of the standard error of $\hat{\kappa}_{jk}$ can be obtained by using standard methods for (2×2) tables [Klar *et al.* (2002), Lee and Tu (1994) and Fleiss (1981)]. Assessing these $\hat{\kappa}_{jk}$s, we see where agreement is the highest and utilize this knowledge to find cutpoints at which the two questions have the highest agreement.

9.3   Examples and Interpretation

The parent questionnaire from the study of childhood leukemia [Hinkle *et al.* (2004)] provides data for the first example. At the beginning of the questionnaire, a parent is asked, 'In general, compared to a year ago, how would you rate your child's health? Much better, somewhat better, about the same, or worse.' At the end of the survey questionnaire, the subject's parents are asked 'Compared to others of your child's age and sex, how would you rate his/her overall health? Better, about the same, or worse.' The joint distributions of the paired responses from the two questions are depicted in Table 9.1. With rating 1 having 4 levels and rating 2 having 3 levels, there are 6 (= 3 × 2) possible (2×2) tables formed by looking at all possible cutpoints, and thus 6 possible Kappa coefficients. The goal is to look at all of these (2×2) tables and Kappa coefficients, and see where agreement is the highest to identify cutpoints at which the two questions have the highest agreement.

Table 9.5 gives the estimates of the 6 different Kappa coefficients, and 95% confidence intervals obtained from a SAS macro developed for this method. We note from Table 9.5 that the highest agreement occurs ($\hat{\kappa} = 0.463$) when the first question is dichotomized at ≤ 2 (much better or somewhat better) versus ≥ 3 (about the same or worse), and the second question is dichotomized at ≤ 2

(better or about the same) versus 3 (worse). Table 9.6 gives the (2×2) table that corresponds to this Kappa of 0.463. Using the cutpoints where agreement is highest, we can decide on where we can combine the data for further analysis.

Table 9.5: Table of six Kappa coefficients at all cutpoints using the childhood leukemia study. Estimates and 95% confidence intervals obtained from SAS Proc Freq

	1 versus ≥ 2	≤ 2 versus 3
1 versus ≥ 2	0.109 $(-0.058, 0.276)$	0.215 $(0.086, 0.344)$
≤ 2 versus ≥ 3	0.026 $(-0.059, 0.111)$	**0.463** **$(0.245, 0.681)$**
≤ 3 versus 4	-0.018 $(-0.066, 0.030)$	0.055 $(-0.136, 0.246)$

Table 9.6: (2×2) table corresponding to $\hat{\kappa}_{22} = 0.463$ in Table 9.5

		Question 2		
		Better or about the same	**Worse**	**Total**
Question 1	**Much better or somewhat better**	57	4	61
	About the same or worse	12	11	23
	Total	69	15	84

The questionnaire from the 2002 United States National General Social Survey [Smith (2003) and Davis and Smith (1992)] provides the data for our second example. At the beginning of the survey, a subject is asked, 'Would you say your own health, in general, is Excellent, Good, Fair, or Poor?' At the end of the survey questionnaire, the subject is asked 'Would you say that in general your health is Excellent, Very Good, Good, Fair, or Poor?' The joint distributions of the paired responses from the two questions are depicted in Table 9.2. With rating 1 having 4 levels and rating 2 having 5 levels, there are

12 ($= 3 \times 4$) possible (2×2) tables formed by looking at all possible cutpoints, and thus 12 possible Kappa coefficients. The goal is to assess all of these (2×2) tables and Kappa coefficients, and identify where agreement is the highest. This will tell us the cutpoints at which the categories can be combined.

Table 9.7 gives the estimates of the 12 different Kappa coefficients, and 95% confidence intervals. We see from Table 9.7 that the highest agreement occurs ($\hat{\kappa} = 0.858$) when the first question is dichotomized at ≤ 2 (excellent or good) versus ≥ 3 (fair or worse), and the second question is dichotomized at ≤ 3 (excellent, very good, or good) versus ≥ 4 (fair or worse). Table 9.8 gives the (2×2) table that corresponds to this Kappa of 0.858. Using the cutpoints where agreement is highest, we can decide on where we can combine the data for further analysis.

Table 9.7: Table of 12 Kappa coefficients at all cutpoints using the 2002 United States National General Social Survey. Estimates and 95% confidence intervals obtained from SAS Proc Freq

	1 versus ≥ 2	≤ 2 versus ≥ 3	≤ 3 versus ≥ 4	≤ 4 versus 5
1 versus ≥ 2	0.851 (0.822,0.879)	0.598 (0.561,0.635)	0.199 (0.174,0.224)	0.039 (0.029,0.049)
≤ 2 versus ≥ 3	0.193 (0.169,0.217)	0.415 (0.376,0.454)	**0.858** **(0.825,0.891)**	0.255 (0.199,0.311)
≤ 3 versus 4	0.038 (0.028,0.047)	0.094 (0.071,0.116)	0.334 (0.271,0.396)	0.839 (0.768,0.910)

Table 9.8: (2×2) table corresponding to $\hat{\kappa}_{23} = 0.858$ in Table 9.7

		Question 2		
		Excellent Very Good or Good	Fair or Poor	Total
Question 1	Excellent or Good	1199	18	1217
	Fair or Poor	49	258	307
	Total	1248	276	1524

9.4   Discussion

This chapter compares the degree of agreement between two different ratings consisting of different ordinal scales. This comparison is illustrated using questions that are routinely asked in a clinical setting. Using a matrix of Kappa coefficients we describe a method to identify cutpoints where agreement is highest and where categories can be combined for further analysis.

The method described in this paper may be applied in various settings when survey data are collected using different ordinal scales. For the situation when data of this type are elicited, we provide a formal method for further analysis. Two examples were provided where this method is relevant. A confidence interval or a consistent estimate of the standard error of $\hat{\kappa}_{jk}$ can be obtained by using standard methods. Assessing the estimated Kappa statistics to find the location where the agreement is the highest is helpful to find cutpoints at which the two questions have the highest agreement, and also can be useful in planning future agreement studies.

SAS macros are available upon request from the authors.

References

1. Bishop, Y. M. M., Fienberg, S. E., and Holland, P. W. (1975). *Discrete Multivariate Analysis: Theory and Practice*, MIT Press, Cambridge, MA.

2. Cohen, J. (1960). A coefficient of agreement for nominal scales, *Educational and Psychological Measurement*, **20**, 37–46.

3. Davis, J. A., and Smith, T.W. (1992). *The NORC General Social Survey: A User's Guide*, Sage, Newbury Park, CA.

4. Fleiss, J. L. (1981). *Statistical Methods for Rates and Proportions*, Second edition, John Wiley & Sons, New York.

5. Hinkle, A. S., Proukou, C., French, C. A., Kozlowski, A. M., Constine, L. S., Lipsitz, S. R., Miller, T. L., and Lipshultz, S. E. (2004). A clinic-based, comprehensive care model for studying late effects in long-term survivors of pediatric illnesses, *Pediatrics*, **113**, 1141–1145.

6. Klar, N., Lipsitz, S. R., Parzen, M., and Leong, T. (2002). An exact bootstrap confidence interval for Kappa in small samples, *Journal of the Royal Statistical Society, Series D*, **51**, 467–478.

7. Kraemer, H. C., Periyakoil, V. S., and Noda, A. (2002). Kappa coefficients in medical research, *Statistics in Medicine*, **21**, 2109–2129.

8. Kraemer, H. C. (1992). Measurement of reliability for categorical data in medical research, *Statistical Methods in Medical Research*, 183–199.

9. Lee, J. J., and Tu, Z. N. (1994). A better confidence interval for Kappa: On measuring agreement between two raters with binary outcomes, *Journal of Computational and Graphical Statistics*, **3**, 301–321.

10. McCullagh, P. (1980). Regression models for ordinal data, *Journal of the Royal Statistical Society, Series B*, **42**, 109–142.

11. Smith, T. W. (2003). *A Generation of Data: The General Social Survey, 1972-2002*, NORC, Chicago, IL.

PART IV
Survival Analysis

10

The Role of Correlated Frailty Models in Studies of Human Health, Ageing, and Longevity

Andreas Wienke,[1] **Paul Lichtenstein,**[2] **Kamila Czene,**[2] **and Anatoli I. Yashin**[3]

[1] *Martin-Luther-University Halle-Wittenberg, Halle, Germany*
[2] *Karolinska Institute, Stockholm, Sweden*
[3] *Duke University, Durham, NC, USA*

Abstract: Frailty models are becoming more and more popular in multivariate survival analysis. Shared frailty models in particular are often used despite their limitations. To overcome their disadvantages, numerous correlated frailty models were established during the last decade. In this study, we present different variants and extensions of the bivariate correlated gamma frailty model with special focus on the analysis of bivariate breast cancer onset data from the Swedish Twin Registry. Points of discussion are parametric versus semiparametric approaches, the inclusion of observed covariates, dependence of the frailty distribution on observed covariates, and a possible cure fraction.

Keywords and phrases: Multivariate survival analysis, shared frailty model, correlated frailty model, twins, breast cancer

10.1 Introduction

Models based on the hazard function have dominated survival analysis since the proportional hazards model was suggested in the seminal paper by Cox (1972). At least in part, this model is so popular because of the ease with which technical difficulties such as censoring and truncation are handled. This is due to the appealing interpretation of the hazard function as a risk that changes over time. Naturally, the concept allows the entering of covariates to describe their influence and to model different levels of risk for different subgroups. However, in general it is impossible to include all relevant risk factors, perhaps because we have no information on individual values, which is often the case in demography. Furthermore, we may not know all relevant risk factors or it is impossible to measure them without great financial costs, something that is common in medical, epidemiological, and biological studies. The neglect of

151

covariates leads to (unobserved) heterogeneity. That is, the population consists of individuals with different risks.

This chapter focuses on frailty models, which is a specific area in survival analysis. The notion of frailty provides a convenient way of introducing unobserved heterogeneity and associations into models for survival data. A frailty model is a random effects model for time-to-event data, where the random effect (the frailty) acts multiplicatively on the baseline hazard function. It can be used for univariate (independent) lifetimes, that is, to describe the influence of unobserved covariates in a proportional hazards model (heterogeneity). The univariate frailty model was introduced by Vaupel *et al.* (1979). Here, the variability of lifetimes is formulated as arising from two different sources: first, natural variability, which is included in the baseline hazard function; second, unobserved heterogeneity modelled as frailty. There are advantages in separating these two sources of variability: unobserved heterogeneity can give an alternative interpretation of some results such as crossing-over or levelling-off effects of hazard functions.

Frailty models have been used frequently for modelling dependence in multivariate time-to-event data; see, for example, Clayton (1978), Yashin *et al.* (1995), Hougaard (2000), and Wienke *et al.* (2002). The dependence usually arises because individuals in the same group (family, litter, study center) are related to each other or because of the multiple recurrence of an event for the same individual. The traditional proportional hazards model cannot be applied to these cases. A possible solution to this problem is the use of conditional proportional hazards given the frailty. The random effect explains the dependence in the sense that had we known the frailty, the events would have been independent. In other words, the lifetimes are conditionally independent given the frailty. We assume that, given unobserved frailty, the hazard for each survival time follows a proportional hazards model, with the frailty variable and the covariate effect acting multiplicatively on the baseline hazard. Consequently, specifications of the baseline hazard (in the case of parametric models) and distributional assumptions about the frailty are necessary.

The most common frailty distribution is the gamma distribution. It has been widely applied as a mixture distribution. From a computational and analytical point of view, the gamma distribution fits well into the proportional hazards framework, because it facilitates closed-form expressions of survival, density, and hazard functions. This is due to the simplicity of the Laplace transform, which allows for the use of traditional maximum likelihood procedures in parameter estimation. Note that no biological reason exists which would prefer the use of one frailty distribution over another. Nearly all arguments in favor of or against a distribution are mathematically based. In a very recent publication, Abbring and van den Berg (2003) proved that the frailty distribution among the survivors at a specific time t converges to a gamma distribution under some regularity assumptions, which speaks in favor of this distribution. We will use the gamma distribution in the present paper as well but would like to point out that the concept of correlated frailty is not limited to this frailty distribution. A useful generalization of the gamma distribution can be found in Peng *et al.* (1998). Furthermore, to keep the model as simple as possible, we restrict our analysis to bivariate lifetime models with single spell data.

The chapter is organized as follows. In Sections 10.2 and 10.3, we introduce the shared frailty and the correlated frailty model, respectively. In Section 10.4, we describe the correlated gamma frailty model in detail. Section 10.4.1 deals with the Swedish breast cancer twin data used as an illustrative example. Sections 10.4.2, 10.4.3, and 10.4.4 consider different variants and extensions of the correlated gamma frailty model. The chapter ends with a discussion in Section 10.5.

10.2   Shared Frailty Model

A shared frailty model in survival analysis is defined as follows. Suppose there are n clusters and that the ith cluster has n_i individuals and is associated with an unobserved random effect (frailty) Z_i ($1 \leq i \leq n$). Conditional on frailties Z_i, the survival times are assumed to be independent and their hazard functions to be of the form

$$\lambda(t, Z_i) = Z_i \lambda_{0j}(t),$$

where t denotes age or time and λ_{0j}, ($j = 1, \ldots, n_i$) is the baseline hazard function for the jth failure. The frailties Z_i are assumed to be identically and independently distributed random variables with a common density function $f(z, \theta)$, where θ is the parameter of the frailty distribution. A semiparametric shared frailty model is a model where the baseline hazard functions λ_{0j} are left unspecified. Observed covariates will be introduced into the model later.

For simplicity, we restrict our treatment of frailty models to the bivariate case ($n_i = 2$), because extensions to the multivariate case are straightforward. The assumption of a shared frailty model is that both individuals in a pair share the same frailty Z_i, and this is why the model is called the shared frailty model. It was introduced by Clayton (1978) (who did not use the notion of "frailty") and extensively studied by Hougaard (2000). The two lifetimes are assumed to be conditionally independent with respect to the shared (common) frailty. We derive the quantities based on this conditional formulation below. In the following, we will use Z as a shorthand for all Z_i.

Conditionally on Z, the hazard function of an individual in a pair is of the form $Z\lambda_{0j}(t)$, where the value of Z is common to both individuals in the pair, and thus is the cause for dependence between lifetimes within pairs. Independence of the lifetimes corresponds to a degenerate frailty distribution (no variability in Z). In all other cases, the dependence is positive. It is assumed that there is independence between different pairs. The conditional bivariate survival function is of the form

$$S(t_1, t_2 | Z) = S_{01}(t_1)^Z S_{02}(t_2)^Z = e^{-Z(\Lambda_{01}(t_1) + \Lambda_{02}(t_2))}, \qquad (10.1)$$

where $\Lambda_{0j}(t) = \int_0^t \lambda_{0j}(s)\, ds \; (j = 1, 2)$, and $S_{0j}(t) = e^{-\Lambda_{0j}(t)}$ are the cumulative baseline hazard and survival functions of the marginal distributions. Averaging (10.1) with respect to Z produces the marginal bivariate survival function

$$\begin{aligned} S(t_1, t_2) &= \mathbf{E}S(t_1, t_2 | Z) = \mathbf{E}S_{01}(t_1)^Z S_{02}(t_2)^Z \\ &= \mathbf{E}e^{-Z(\Lambda_{01}(t_1) + \Lambda_{02}(t_2))} = \mathbf{L}(\Lambda_{01}(t_1) + \Lambda_{02}(t_2)), \end{aligned}$$

where $\mathbf{L}$ denotes the Laplace transform of Z. Thus, the bivariate survival function is expressed as the Laplace transform of the frailty distribution, evaluated at the cumulative baseline hazard.

The standard assumption about the frailty distribution is that it is a gamma distribution with mean 1 and variance σ^2. In this case, we get

$$\begin{aligned} S(t_1, t_2) &= \mathbf{L}(\Lambda_{01}(t_1) + \Lambda_{02}(t_2)) \\ &= (1 + \sigma^2(\Lambda_{01}(t_1) + \Lambda_{02}(t_2)))^{-1/\sigma^2} \\ &= (S_1(t_1)^{-\sigma^2} + S_2(t_2)^{-\sigma^2} - 1)^{-1/\sigma^2}. \end{aligned}$$

The notion of shared frailty is different from the definition of individual frailty introduced by Vaupel *et al.* (1979) in his analysis of univariate duration data. This difference has gone largely unrecognized, perhaps because of the superficial similarity of the individual hazards in the two approaches. The frailty in the bivariate shared frailty model is only a part of the individual frailty, capturing only the components of frailty that both individuals share.

Asymptotic properties of the nonparametric maximum likelihood estimates in the shared gamma frailty model are well established. Murphy shows consistency [Murphy (1994)] and asymptotic normality [Murphy (1995)] in the model without observed covariates.

Shared frailty models explain correlations within groups or for recurrent events facing the same individual. However, this approach does have limitations. First, it forces unobserved factors to be the same within the group, which is not generally acceptable. For example, it is inappropriate to assume that both partners in a twin pair share all of their unobserved risk factors. Second, the dependence between survival times within the group is based on their marginal distributions. To see this, when covariates are present in a proportional hazards model with a gamma distributed frailty, the dependence parameter and the population heterogeneity are confounded, implying that the multivariate distribution of the lifetimes can be identified from the marginal distributions of these lifetimes. Elbers and Ridder (1982) show that this problem applies to any univariate frailty distribution with a finite mean. Third, in most cases, shared frailty will only induce a positive association within the group. However, there are some situations in which survival times for subjects within the same cluster are negatively associated.

To avoid these limitations, correlated frailty models are being developed for the analysis of multivariate failure time data; see, for example, Yashin and Iachine (1994), Pickles and Crouchley (1994), Xue and Brookmeyer (1996), Petersen (1998), and Wienke *et al.* (2003a,b), in which associated random variables are used to characterize the frailty effect for each cluster. In twin pairs, for example, one random variable is assigned to twin one and another to twin two, so that they are no longer constrained to have a common frailty. These two variables are associated and jointly distributed, and so, knowing one of them does not automatically imply the other. As a consequence, correlated frailty models provide not only variance parameters of the frailties as in shared frailty models, but they also contain additional parameters for modelling the correlation between frailties in each group. Also, these variables may be negatively associated, which would then induce a negative association between survival times.

10.3   Correlated Frailty Model

Consider some bivariate observations such as the lifetimes of twins, or age at onset of a disease in spouses, and so on. In the correlated frailty model, the frailty of each individual in a pair is defined by a measure of relative risk, that is, exactly as it was defined in the univariate case. For two individuals in a pair, frailties are not necessarily the same, as they are in the shared frailty model. We are assuming that the frailties are acting multiplicatively on the baseline hazard function and that the observations in the pairs are conditionally independent, given the frailties. Hence, the hazard of individual j ($j = 1, 2$) in pair i ($i = 1, \ldots, n$) has the form

$$\lambda(t, Z_{ij}) = Z_{ij}\lambda_{0j}(t), \qquad (10.2)$$

where λ_{0j} are some baseline functions and Z_{ij} are unobserved (random) effects or frailties. Bivariate correlated frailty models are characterized by the joint distribution of a two-dimensional vector of frailties (Z_{i1}, Z_{i2}).

In order to derive a marginal likelihood function, the assumption of conditional independence of life spans given frailty is always used. Let δ_{ij} be a censoring indicator for an individual j ($j = 1, 2$) in pair i ($i = 1, \ldots, n$). Indicator δ_{ij} is 1 if the individual has experienced the event of interest, and 0 otherwise. The contribution of the jth individual in the ith pair of the conditional likelihood is given by

$$L(t_{ij}, \delta_{ij}|Z_{ij}) = \left(Z_{ij}\lambda_{0j}(t_{ij})\right)^{\delta_{ij}} e^{Z_{ij}\Lambda_{0j}(t_{ij})}, \tag{10.3}$$

where t_{ij} stands for the lifetime or the censoring time of the individual and $\Lambda_{0j}(t)$ is the cumulative baseline hazard function. Then, assuming the conditional independence of life spans given frailty and integrating out the random effects, we obtain the marginal likelihood function as

$$L(t, \delta) = \prod_{i=1}^{n} \int \int_{R^+ \times R^+} \left(z_{i1}\lambda_{01}(t_{i1})\right)^{\delta_{i1}} e^{z_{i1}\Lambda_{01}(t_{i1})}$$

$$* \left(z_{i2}\lambda_{02}(t_{i2})\right)^{\delta_{i2}} e^{z_{i2}\Lambda_{02}(t_{i2})} f_Z(z_{i1}, z_{i2})\, dz_{i1}\, dz_{i2},$$

where $t = (t_1, \ldots, t_n)$, $t_i = (t_{i1}, t_{i2})$, $\delta = (\delta_1, \ldots, \delta_n)$, $\delta_i = (\delta_{i1}, \delta_{i2})$, and $f_Z(\cdot, \cdot)$ is the p.d.f. of the corresponding frailty distribution.

10.4 Correlated Gamma Frailty Model

This model was introduced by Yashin and Iachine (1994) and Pickles and Crouchley (1994) and applied to related lifetimes in many different settings; see, for example, Yashin et al. (1995), Yashin and Iachine (1997), Petersen (1998), Wienke et al. (2001, 2003b), and Zdravkovic et al. (2002). Applying the Laplace transform of the gamma distributed random variables, we can derive the unconditional model as

$$S(t_1, t_2) = S_1(t_1)^{1-(\sigma_1/\sigma_2)\rho} S_2(t_2)^{1-(\sigma_2/\sigma_1)\rho} (S_1(t_1)^{-\sigma_1^2} + S_2(t_2)^{-\sigma_2^2} - 1)^{-(\rho/\sigma_1\sigma_2)}. \tag{10.4}$$

Here and in the following sections, S is used as a generic symbol for a survival function. In the following, we apply different variants of the correlated gamma frailty model to Swedish breast cancer twin data. Because of the symmetric structure of the twin data, we use the simplification $S(t) = S_1(t) = S_2(t)$ and $\sigma^2 = \sigma_1^2 = \sigma_2^2$.

Parner (1998) proved consistency and asymptotic normality of the nonparametric maximum likelihood estimator in the multivariate correlated gamma-frailty model with observed covariates.

10.4.1   Swedish breast cancer twin data

First established in the late 1950s to study the importance of smoking and alcohol consumption on cancer and cardiovascular diseases whilst controlling for genetic propensity to disease, the Swedish Twin Registry has today developed into a unique source. Since its establishment, the registry has been expanded and updated on several occasions, and the focus has similarly broadened to most common complex diseases.

The present analysis is restricted to the so-called old cohort (born 1886–1925) because of small numbers of breast cancer in the younger cohorts. The data set was created by merging the Swedish Twin Registry with the Swedish Cancer Registry maintained by the National Board of Health and Welfare.

The church registers from all parishes of the relevant time period were manually checked to identify all twin births. Between 1959 and 1961, to all twins a questionnaire was sent which included a question about phenotypic similarities to assess the zygosity: 'Were you as children as alike as two peas in a pod?' When both partners agreed, they were defined as MZ twins. This zygosity classification was compared with laboratory methods (serological markers). The misclassification rate for this method was very low.

The event under study is the onset of breast cancer. If a woman did not develop breast cancer or she died during the follow-up, the corresponding observation is censored.

In order to adjust for year at birth, a variable for different birth periods was created. This variable was divided into three categories, 1886–1905, 1906–1915, and 1916–1925. The period between 1886 and 1905 served as the reference category. Information on dates about childbirth was obtained by means of linkage with the Swedish Multi Generation Register. This register contains information on all Swedish residents born on or after 1932 who did not die before 1961. The variable age at first birth was divided into four groups: younger than 25 years (reference category), 25 up to 30 years, 30 years and older and no children. The last category also contains all women with no information about childbirth, especially all women from the older birth cohorts, who gave birth before 1932.

The data set contains records of 5904 female twin pairs with both partners being alive in 1959–1961. Individuals were followed up from 1959–1961 to 31 December 2001. The final sample contained, therefore, 4056 MZ and 7752 DZ females, respectively, with 774 observed breast cancer cases.

For a comprehensive description of the Swedish Twin Registry database, with a focus on the recent data collection efforts and a review of the principal findings that have come from the Registry, see Lichtenstein *et al.* (2002).

10.4.2 Parametric and semiparametric models

In most applications of frailty models, a parametric approach is used, which means that the baseline hazard function is specified up to a finite-dimensional parameter. The main advantage of multivariate frailty models without covariates when compared with univariate models without covariates is that it is possible to relax the parametric assumption about the baseline hazard in a similar way as with the Cox regression model. In semiparametric frailty models, no parametric assumption about the form of the baseline hazard function is necessary. We deal with both a parametric and a semiparametric approach. In the parametric approach, we use a Gompertz and a Weibull model, respectively:

$$\lambda_0(t) = ae^{bt}, \qquad \lambda_0(t) = abt^{b-1}.$$

In the semiparametric model the univariate marginal survival is left unspecified. The data is right censored and left truncated which has to be included into the likelihood. The results of the maximum likelihood parameter estimation procedure are given in Table 10.1.

Table 10.1: Correlated gamma frailty model applied to breast cancer data

Model	Gompertz	Weibull	Semi-parametric
a	3.90e−7 (2.17e−7)	5.20e−16 (1.07e−15)	—
b	0.151 (0.011)	7.627 (0.507)	—
σ	6.930 (0.427)	5.046 (0.400)	7.403 (1.364)
ρ_{MZ}	0.131 (0.041)	0.157 (0.050)	0.126 (0.041)
ρ_{DZ}	0.116 (0.030)	0.139 (0.037)	0.111 (0.031)

In all cases, the estimates of correlation coefficients of frailty for MZ twins (ρ_{MZ}) tend to be slightly higher than for DZ twins (ρ_{DZ}). Higher correlations in MZ twins compared to DZ twins indicate the influence of genetic factors in susceptibility to breast cancer. However, the difference between the two correlations is not significant. Heterogeneity (σ^2) seems to be huge. Another important aspect is the similarity of the results in parametric and semiparametric analysis. The estimates are close to each other. Using the semiparametric analysis as a standard, the Gompertz parameterization shows advantage (estimates are closer to the estimates of the semiparametric analysis) compared to the Weibull parameterization.

It is necessary to keep in mind that the parameter ρ describes the correlation between the frailties in a pair and not the correlation of the respective lifetimes. Lindeboom and van den Berg (1994) analyzed the relation of correlation between frailties and between lifetimes. They derived explicit expressions for the correlation between the survival times and examined the properties of this correlation in the special case of a constant baseline hazard function.

10.4.3 Correlated gamma frailty model with covariates

One reason for the popularity of frailty models is that (observed) covariates can be easily included in the model. We demonstrate the use of the correlated gamma frailty model with covariates [Yashin and Iachine (1997)] by applying the model on the Swedish breast cancer twin data described above. We analyze the influence of birth cohort and age at first birth on the risk to develop breast cancer. The model takes into account the dependence of lifespans of relatives (twins). This approach enables the combined analysis of bivariate data on time to onset and observed covariates; and furthermore, to account for unobserved heterogeneity and to deal with censored observations. The model results from (10.2) and the unconditional bivariate survival function is given by

$$\begin{aligned} S(t_1, t_2 | X_1, X_2) &= S(t_1 | X_1)^{1-\rho} S(t_2 | X_2)^{1-\rho} (S(t_1 | X_1)^{-\sigma^2} \\ &\quad + S(t_2 | X_2)^{-\sigma^2} - 1)^{-(\rho/\sigma^2)}, \end{aligned}$$

where $S(t|X)$ denotes the marginal univariate survival function and X_1 and X_2 denote the vectors of observed covariates. We used a Gompertz model

$$S(t|X) = \left(1 + \sigma^2 \frac{a}{b}(e^{bt} - 1)e^{\beta X}\right)^{-(1/\sigma^2)}.$$

Here, β_1 and β_2 describe the effect of the birth cohort 1906–1915 and 1916–1925 compared to the birth cohort 1886–1905. The younger birth cohorts show

Table 10.2: Correlated gamma frailty model with observed covariates

Model	Without Covariates	With Covariates	Dispersion Frailty
a	3.90e-7 (2.17e-7)	3.30e-11 (—)	4.20e-11 (—)
b	0.151 (0.011)	0.201 (0.022)	0.196 (0.018)
σ	6.930 (0.427)	8.235 (0.655)	8.286 (0.553)
ρ_{MZ}	0.131 (0.041)	0.115 (0.038)	0.126 (0.040)
ρ_{DZ}	0.116 (0.030)	0.093 (0.029)	0.099 (0.031)
β_1		2.016 (0.403)	1.845 (0.360)
β_2		3.160 (0.533)	2.984 (0.465)
β_3		0.769 (0.388)	0.899 (0.368)
β_4		0.260 (0.389)	0.359 (0.365)
β_5		0.324 (0.387)	0.310 (0.314)
γ			−0.202 (0.092)

a significant higher risk ($\beta_1 = 2.016$, $\beta_2 = 3.160$) to breast cancer. The parameters β_3, β_4, and β_5 show the effect of age at first birth. Women giving birth at age between 25-30 show a significant increased risk ($\beta_3 = 0.769$) compared to women giving first birth at age before 25, whereas the risk for women giving birth at older ages (30 years and older) is slightly less increased ($\beta_4 = 0.260$). The risk for nulliparous women (including women from the older birth cohorts with births before 1932) is also increased ($\beta_5 = 0.324$). Table 10.2 shows that the inclusion of observed covariates into the model has only small effects on the estimates of the bivariate frailty distribution, σ^2, ρ_{MZ}, and ρ_{DZ}. Interestingly, the variance estimate of the frailty (σ^2) increases slightly after including observed covariates. This is the opposite of what we expected, because the observed covariates should account for at least a part of the unobserved heterogeneity in the model without observed covariates. This indicates the existence of important covariates that are not included in our model. A more detailed example of a correlated gamma frailty model with observed covariates applied to coronary heart disease can be found in Zdravkovic *et al.* (2004).

Traditionally, analysis of failure times using a frailty model deals with identically distributed frailties. However, such a homogeneous assumption about frailties could sometimes be suspect. For modelling heterogeneity in frailties, a dispersion frailty model can be used. This model was suggested by Wassell and Moeschberger (1993) and allows for different heterogeneity (variance of the frailty) in the study population depending on the value of observed covariates as

$$\sigma(X) = \sigma e^{\gamma X}.$$

Here, γ is an additional parameter to be estimated. It indicates whether there is heterogeneity in the frailties ($\gamma \neq 0$) or not ($\gamma = 0$). This model was applied to the Swedish breast cancer twin data and the results are given in the last column in Table 10.2. The parameter γ allowing for different frailty variances of women giving births at different ages is significantly far from zero. In the concrete situation above, nulliparous women show a slightly lower heterogeneity in frailty than the other women.

10.4.4   Cure-mixture models

A bivariate cure-mixture approach for modelling familiar association in diseases was established by Chatterjee and Shih (2001). For a pair of individuals

$$Y_j = \begin{cases} 1 & : \quad \text{if the } j\text{th individual is susceptible} \\ 0 & : \quad \text{otherwise,} \end{cases} \tag{10.5}$$

let T_j denote the age at onset for the jth individual when $Y_j = 1$ ($j = 1, 2$). In that case, the likelihood function is of the form

$$L(t_1, t_2, \delta_1, \delta_2)$$
$$= \delta_1 \delta_2 \phi_{11} S_{t_1,t_2}(t_1, t_2)$$
$$+ \delta_1 (1 - \delta_2) \Big(\phi_{11} S_{t_1}(t_1, t_2) + \phi_{10} S_{t_1}(t_1) \Big)$$
$$+ (1 - \delta_1) \delta_2 \Big(\phi_{11} S_{t_2}(t_1, t_2) + \phi_{01} S_{t_2}(t_2) \Big)$$
$$+ (1 - \delta_1)(1 - \delta_2) \Big(\phi_{11} S(t_1, t_2) + \phi_{10} S(t_1) + \phi_{01} S(t_2) + \phi_{00} \Big).$$

Here the following notations are used: $\phi_{11} = \mathbf{P}(Y_1 = 1, Y_2 = 1)$, $\phi_{10} = \mathbf{P}(Y_1 = 1, Y_2 = 0)$, $\phi_{01} = \mathbf{P}(Y_1 = 0, Y_2 = 1)$, and $\phi_{00} = \mathbf{P}(Y_1 = 0, Y_2 = 0)$. Chatterjee and Shih (2001) applied three different copulas in their approach: the shared gamma frailty model (Clayton's model), Frank's copula, and Hougaard's shared positive stable frailty model. Their model was extended by Wienke *et al.* (2003a), who substituted the shared gamma frailty model by the correlated gamma frailty model. A parametric model with a Gompertz baseline hazard was used. The likelihood function of a right-censored lifetime data is given by

$$L(t_1, t_2, \delta_1, \delta_2)$$
$$= \delta_1 \delta_2 \phi_{11} S_{t_1,t_2}(t_1, t_2) + \delta_1 (1 - \delta_2)(\phi_{11} S_{t_1}(t_1, t_2) + \phi_{10} S_{t_1}(t_1))$$
$$+ (1 - \delta_1) \delta_2 (\phi_{11} S_{t_2}(t_1, t_2) + \phi_{01} S_{t_2}(t_2)) + (1 - \delta_1)(1 - \delta_2)(\phi_{11} S(t_1, t_2)$$
$$+ \phi_{10} S(t_1) + \phi_{01} S(t_2) + \phi_{00}).$$

The model was applied to the Swedish breast cancer twin data and results are given in Table 10.3.

We consider two different cure models. In the first case, it is assumed that the susceptible status of the individuals in a pair is independent of the other; that is, $\mathbf{P}(Y_1 = p_1, Y_2 = p_2) = \mathbf{P}(Y_1 = p_1)\mathbf{P}(Y_2 = p_2)$ with $p_1, p_2 \in \{0, 1\}$. The cure fraction is given by the univariate probability $\phi = \mathbf{P}(Y_1 = 1) = \mathbf{P}(Y_2 = 1)$, which results in $\phi_{11} = \phi^2$, $\phi_{10} = \phi_{01} = \phi(1 - \phi)$, $\phi_{00} = (1 - \phi)^2$. In the second case, which is an extension of the first one, the restriction of independence between the susceptibility status of the two partners in a pair is relaxed and substituted by the weaker constraints $\phi_{10} = \phi_{01}$, $\phi_{11} + \phi_{10} + \phi_{01} + \phi_{00} = 1$. When comparing the likelihoods, it turns out that the cure model with an independent susceptible status of the twin partners shows a nonsignificantly better fit than the model without a cure fraction ($\chi_1^2 = 1.69$, $p = 0.19$). The more complicated cure model without an independence assumption between the susceptible status of the twin partners shows no improvement compared to the cure model assuming independence ($\chi_1^2 = 0.86$, $p = 0.35$). Interestingly, the estimate of the size of a susceptible fraction (due to breast cancer) with 0.213 (0.105) is closed to the estimate 0.22 (0.0093) in the parametric model found by Chatterjee and Shih (2001) in a study population that is completely different.

Table 10.3: Correlated gamma frailty model without and with a cure fraction

Parameter	Without Cure Fraction Estimates (std)	With Cure Fraction[1] Estimates (std)	With Cure Fraction[2] Estimates (std)
a	3.90e$-$7 (2.17e$-$7)	3.05e$-$6 (3.04e$-$6)	1.40e$-$6 (1.99e$-$6)
b	0.151 (0.011)	0.139 (0.013)	0.144 (0.011)
σ	6.930 (0.427)	2.592 (1.092)	3.920 (1.566)
ρ_{MZ}	0.131 (0.041)	0.918 (0.694)	1.000 (—)
ρ_{DZ}	0.116 (0.030)	0.843 (0.676)	0.940 (0.274)
ϕ_{11}	1.000 (—)	0.045 (—)	0.076 (0.087)
ϕ_{10}	0.000 (—)	0.168 (—)	0.310 (0.342)
ϕ_{00}	0.000 (—)	0.619 (—)	0.304 (0.769)
ϕ	1.000 (—)	0.213 (0.105)	0.386[3] (—)

[1]constrained by $\phi_{11} = \phi^2$, $\phi_{10} = \phi_{01} = \phi(1 - \phi)$, $\phi_{00} = (1 - \phi)^2$.
[2]constrained by $\phi_{10} = \phi_{01}$, $\phi_{11} + \phi_{10} + \phi_{01} + \phi_{00} = 1$.
[3]calculated by $\phi = \phi_{11} + \phi_{10}$.

The strong increase of the correlation estimates ρ_{MZ} and ρ_{DZ} after allowing for a cure fraction makes sense because in the model without a cure fraction the correlation is measured in all twin pairs, whereas in the model with a cure fraction the correlation is only measured in susceptible individuals. This is also the reason for the decline in the frailty variance σ^2.

The results of this study are slightly different from the numbers obtained in Wienke *et al.* (2003a) because the study population used in the present analysis contains a few more twin pairs with longer follow-up.

Multivariate cure models suffer from the same inherent identifiability problem with the right-censored observations as univariate cure models. For such observations, the event under study has not occurred either because the person is insusceptible or the person is susceptible, but follow-up did not last long enough to observe the event. The identifiability problem grows with increasing censoring, but is less of a problem with parametric modelling of the baseline hazard. In cure models with fixed censoring times (caused by ending the study), censoring is no longer noninformative even if censoring times and the survival times are independent. The proportion of censored observations contains important information about parameters in the model. For example, in the (usual ideal) case of no censoring, $\phi = 1$.

10.5   Discussion

Frailty models are becoming increasingly popular in multivariate survival analysis. We discuss the advantages and limitations of the commonly used shared frailty model. To overcome the disadvantages of shared frailty models, correlated frailty models as an extension were established during the last decade. In the present study, we examine correlated gamma frailty models in detail.

First, the relation between parametric and semiparametric correlated gamma frailty models is analysed. A parametric approach means that the baseline hazard function is specified up to a finite-dimensional parameter, for example, by a Gompertz or Weibull distribution. The main advantage of multivariate frailty models without covariates when compared with univariate frailty models without covariates is that it is possible to relax the parametric assumption about the baseline hazard similar to the Cox model, which means the univariate baseline hazard functions are left unspecified. The analysis of the Swedish breast cancer twin data shows the similarity of the results in parametric and semiparametric analysis, which supports the use of parametric models, because they are easier to handle than semiparametric models.

Second, observed covariates can be easily included in the model. This can be done in the same natural way as in the proportional hazards model by Cox (1972). We demonstrate the use of the correlated gamma frailty model with observed covariates by analyzing the influence of birth cohort and age at first birth on risk to develop breast cancer. The model takes into account the dependence of event times of relatives (twins). This approach enables the combined analysis of bivariate data on time to onset and observed covariates, and also to account for unobserved heterogeneity.

Third, the often-used assumption of identically distributed frailties can be relaxed by introducing a dispersion frailty model, which allows for heterogeneity in the frailty distribution of the study population. Here, the variance of the frailty depends on observed covariates.

Fourth, correlated frailty models can be easily extended to include a cure fraction to overcome the often unstated assumption that everybody in the study population is susceptible to the event under study and will eventually experience this event if the follow-up is sufficiently long. These models extend the understanding of time-to-event data by allowing for the formulation of more accurate and informative conclusions. These conclusions are otherwise unobtainable from an analysis which fails to account for a cured or insusceptible fraction of the population. If a cured component is not present, the analysis reduces to standard approaches of survival analysis.

All model variants allow us to deal with censored and truncated data in a simple way. The advantages of these models are illustrated by application to

Swedish breast cancer twin data. We conclude that the concept of correlated frailty provides a useful tool to model multivariate time-to-event data. This concept is open for further extensions in various directions. One promising example of research is the use of correlated log-normal frailty models, where the frailties are assumed to be log-normally distributed [Locatelli *et al.* (2004)]. The log-normal model is much more flexible than the gamma model, because it is not based on the additive composition of the two frailties. On the other hand, the log-normal distribution does not allow an explicit representation of the likelihood function, which requires more sophisticated estimation strategies.

References

1. Abbring, J., and van den Berg, G. J. (2003). The unobserved heterogeneity distribution in duration analysis, *Working Paper*, Free University Amsterdam, The Netherlands.

2. Chatterjee, N., and Shih, J. (2001). A bivariate cure-mixture approach for modeling familial association in diseases, *Biometrics*, **57**, 779–786.

3. Clayton, D. (1978). A model for association in bivariate life tables and its application in epidemiological studies of familial tendency in chronic disease incidence, *Biometrika*, **65**, 141–151.

4. Cox, D. R. (1972). Regression models and life-tables, *Journal of the Royal Statistical Society, Series B*, **34**, 187–220.

5. Elbers, C., and Ridder, G. (1982). True and spurious duration dependence: The identifiability of the proportional hazard model, *Review of Economic Studies*, **XLIX**, 403–409.

6. Hougaard, P. (2000) *Analysis of Multivariate Survival Data*, Springer-Verlag, New York.

7. Lichtenstein, P., de Faire, U., Floderus, B., Svartengren, M., Svedberg, P., and Pedersen, N. L. (2002). The Swedish Twin Registry: a unique resource for clinical, epidemiological and genetic studies, *Journal of Internal Medicine*, **252**, 184–205.

8. Locatelli, I., Lichtenstein, P., and Yashin, A. I. (2004). The heritability of breast cancer: A Bayesian correlated frailty model applied to Swedish twins data, *Twin Research*, **7**, 182–191.

9. Lindeboom, M., and van den Berg, G. J. (1994). Heterogeneity in models for bivariate survival: the importance of the mixing distribution, *Journal of the Royal Statistical Society, Series B*, **56**, 49–60.

10. Murphy, S. A. (1994). Consistency in a proportional hazards models incorporating a random effect, *The Annals of Statistics*, **22**, 712–731.

11. Murphy, S. A. (1995). Asymptotic theory for the frailty model, *The Annals of Statistics*, **23**, 182–198.

12. Parner, E. (1998). Asymptotic theory for the correlated gamma-frailty model, *The Annals of Statistics*, **26**, 183–214.

13. Peng, Y., Dear, K. B. G., and Denham, J. W. (1998). A generalized *F* mixture model for cure rate estimation, *Statistics in Medicine*, **17**, 813–830.

14. Petersen, J. H. (1998). An additive frailty model for correlated lifetimes, *Biometrics*, **54**, 646–661.

15. Pickles, A., and Crouchley, R. (1994). Generalizations and applications of frailty models for survival and event data, *Statistical Methods in Medical Research*, **3**, 263–278.

16. Vaupel, J. W., Manton, K. G., and Stallard, E. (1979). The impact of heterogeneity in individual frailty on the dynamics of mortality, *Demography*, **16**, 439–454.

17. Wassell, J. T., and Moeschberger, M. L. (1993). A bivariate survival model with modified gamma frailty for assessing the impact of interventions, *Statistics in Medicine*, **12**, 241–248.

18. Wienke, A., Holm, N., Skytthe, A. and Yashin A. I. (2001). The heritability of mortality due to heart diseases: A correlated frailty model applied to Danish twins, *Twin Research*, **4**, 266–274.

19. Wienke, A., Christensen, K., Skytthe, A., and Yashin, A. I. (2002). Genetic analysis of cause of death in a mixture model with bivariate lifetime data, *Statistical Modelling*, **2**, 89–102.

20. Wienke, A., Lichtenstein, P., and Yashin, A. I. (2003a). A bivariate frailty model with a cure fraction for modeling familial correlations in diseases, *Biometrics*, **59**, 1178–1183.

21. Wienke, A., Holm, N., Christensen, K., Skytthe, A., Vaupel, J., and Yashin, A. I. (2003b). The heritability of cause-specific mortality: A correlated gamma-frailty model applied to mortality due to respiratory

diseases in Danish twins born 1870–1930, *Statistics in Medicine*, **22**, 3873–3887.

22. Xue, X., and Brookmeyer, R. (1996). Bivariate frailty model for the analysis of multivariate survival time, *Lifetime Data Analysis*, **2**, 277–290.

23. Yashin, A. I., and Iachine, I. A. (1994). Environment determines 50% of variability in individual frailty: Results from Danish twin study, In *Population Studies of Aging*, **10**, Odense University, Research Report.

24. Yashin, A. I., and Iachine, I. A. (1997). How frailty models can be used for evaluating longevity limits: Taking advantage of an interdisciplinary approach, *Demography*, **34**, 31–48.

25. Yashin, A. I., Vaupel, J. W. and Iachine, I. A. (1995). Correlated individual frailty: an advantageous approach to survival analysis of bivariate data, *Mathematical Population Studies*, **5**, 145–159.

26. Zdravkovic, S., Wienke, A., Pedersen, N. L., Marenberg, M. E., Yashin, A. I., and de Faire, U. (2002). Heritability of death from coronary heart disease: A 36 years follow-up of 20,966 Swedish twins, *Journal of Internal Medicine*, **252**, 247–254.

27. Zdravkovic, S., Wienke, A., Pedersen, N. L., Marenberg, M. E., Yashin, A. I., and de Faire, U. (2004). Genetic influences on CHD-death and the impact of known risk factors: Comparison of two frailty models, *Behavior Genetics*, **34**, 585–591.

11

Prognostic Factors and Prediction of Residual Survival for Hospitalized Elderly Patients

M. L. Calle,[1] **P. Roura,**[2] **A. Arnau,**[2] **A. Yáñez,**[2] **and A. Leiva**[2]

[1] *Universitat de Vic, Catalonia, Spain*
[2] *Vic General Hospital, Catalonia, Spain*

Abstract: The aim of this study, corresponding to a research project on functional decline and mortality of frail elderly patients, is to build a predictive survival process that takes into account the functional and nutritional evolution of the patients over time. We deal with both survival data and repeated measures, but the usual statistical methods for the joint analysis of longitudinal and survival data are not appropriate in this case. As an alternative, we use the multistate survival model approach to evaluate the association between mortality and the recovery, or not, of normal functional and nutritional levels. Once the model is estimated and the prognostic factors of mortality identified, a predictive process is computed that allows predictions to be made of a patient's survival based on his or her history at a given time. This provides a more exact estimate of the prognosis for each group of patients that may be very helpful to clinicians in the making of decisions.

Keywords and phrases: Survival analysis, longitudinal data, predictive process, prognostic factors

11.1 Introduction

In any medical specialty, the regular measurement of health and quality of life indicators is known to be an effective tool that allows the perception of the function and patients' capacities to be incorporated into clinical decisions. This is particularly relevant in geriatrics, where evaluations of impairment and disability play a fundamental clinical role.

The goal of this work, which corresponds to a research project on the functional decline and mortality of frail elderly patients, is to build a predictive process that includes the functional and nutritional evolution of the patients

167

over time as prognostic factors of mortality. The data set includes survival times and repeated observations (the functional and nutritional levels of the patients at each visit) and their analysis requires a specific statistical methodology. The problem is that most available methods for the joint analysis of longitudinal and survival data, such as those used by Faucett and Thomas (1996), Wulfsohn and Tsiatis (1997), and Henderson, Diggle, and Dobson (2000), are not appropriate for our data. The reasons are, firstly, that these methods do not allow for the use of multivariate markers and, secondly, that due to the mortality of the patients, for many of them we have fewer than three measurements, insufficient for the proper use of the mixed model.

As an alternative, we propose to focus our analysis on two clinically relevant aspects of the health progression: whether the normal levels of functional and nutritional status are recovered, and the speed of recovery of these normal levels. We use a multistate survival model to evaluate the association of these two aspects with mortality. Once the model is estimated and the prognostic factors of mortality identified, we can obtain a predictive process of a patient's survival based on his or her history at a given time. These predictive probabilities are computed as described in Klein, Keiding, and Copelan (1994) and Klein and Moeschberger (1998, pp. 289–294).

The paper is organized as follows: In Section 11.2, we describe the cohort study and the follow-up process. In Section 11.3, we propose specific multistate models for the analysis of our data set. The resulting predictive process is developed in Section 11.3.1. A concluding discussion appears in Section 11.4.

11.2   Cohort Description and Follow-Up

For many elderly patients, an acute medical illness requiring hospitalization is followed by a progressive decline, resulting in high rates of mortality in this population during the year following discharge. However, few prognostic indices have focused on predicting posthospital mortality in older patients. In order to know more about this question, we analyze a cohort of frail elderly patients older than 75, who have had an acute disease and that, after being treated in an acute care unit, were admitted to the geriatric rehabilitation unit.

A multidimensional geriatric assessment was performed at baseline visit including information on demographics (age, sex, education, living site prior to admission and after discharge, etc.); cognitive, functional (measured by Barthel index), and nutritional (measured by Mini nutritional assessment) status; presence of depression; co-morbidity; and quality of life level. For any patient, information for all assessments was collected either from the patient himself or herself (when cognitive performance was intact) or from a knowledgeable informant.

It is a well-known clinical fact that, in this kind of cohort, the status of patients at admission is not enough for an accurate prognosis to be made. Instead, the evolution of their functional and nutritional status, especially in the first weeks after admission, might be very informative of the future mortality of these patients. For this reason, we planned a one-year prospective longitudinal follow-up. The patients were visited on admission to the geriatric unit and at around 1, 3, and 6 months after admission. Of course, not all patients were able to attend all 4 visits because of mortality during the follow-up. In addition to this, information on mortality up to 12 months after admission was obtained through telephone interviews.

The cohort included 165 patients with an average age of 83.3 years old (standard deviation of 5.1 years) and 31.5% were male. The average length of stay in the acute care unit was 15.2 days (SD 8.1) and 32% had a good or very good perception of his quality of life before the acute episode of illness. At 6 months, accumulated mortality was 29.1% (CI 0.95: 22.2–36.7) and the mortality accumulated at 12 months was 36.4 (CI 0.95: 29.0–44.2).

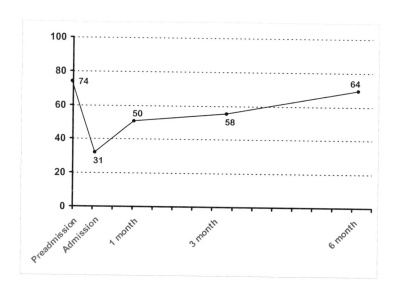

Figure 11.1: Mean profile of functional status

The functional status of the patients was measured with the so-called Barthel index which consists of a questionnaire dealing with daily activities (bowels and bladder continence, grooming, toilet use, feeding, transfers, mobility, dressing, and stairs). In addition to information collected at baseline, 1, 3, and 6 months, for this index the investigators estimated retrospectively the patient functional status 15 days before admission to the acute care unit (called preadmission assessment). Barthel index rules between 0 and 100 and a Barthel index lower than 50 indicates the patient is functionally dependent, whereas a Barthel index higher than 50 is considered to be normal for this kind of cohort. Figure 11.1 represents the mean profile of the functional status of this cohort. Most of the patients enter the rehabilitation unit with very low Barthel indexes but after a certain time some of them improve, with functional capacity reaching normal Barthel levels.

The nutritional status of patients was measured at each visit with the mini nutritional assessment (MNA) test. This assessment tool can be used to identify patients at risk of malnutrition. It is composed of 18 questions grouped in 4 categories: anthropometric assessment (weight, height, and weight loss), general assessment (lifestyle, medication, and mobility), dietary assessment (food and fluid intake and autonomy of feeding), and subjective assessment (self-perception of health and nutrition). A total score lower than 20 indicates a risk of malnutrition and a score higher than 20 can be considered as a normal nutritional level for this cohort. In Figure 11.2, we present the mean profile for the nutritional status of this cohort. As before, most patients enter the unit at risk of malnutrition but after a certain time the nutritional status of some patients improves.

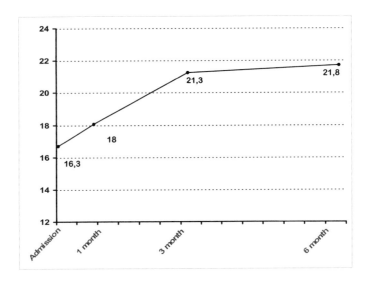

Figure 11.2: Mean profile of nutritional status

11.3 Multistate Survival Model

As explained in the introduction, the available methods for jointly analyzing longitudinal and survival data using mixed-effect models are not appropriate in this study. As an alternative approach, we focus our analysis on two important aspects of the patients' evolution. These two aspects are whether the normal levels of functional and nutritional status are recovered and the speed at which this recovery occurs. We use a multistate survival model approach to evaluate the association of these two aspects with mortality.

We consider two intermediate events defined as follows. We use E_1 to denote the event of a patient's recovery of normal functional levels and, in a similar way, E_2 denotes the event of a patient's recovery of normal nutritional levels. All possible paths for a patient who enters the rehabilitation unit are described in the multistate model represented in Figure 11.3. There are three survival times involved in this model: the survival time of interest, denoted by T, which is the elapsed time from admission to death; the elapsed time from admission to the occurrence of event E_1, which is denoted by T_B; and the elapsed time from admission to the occurrence of event E_2, which is denoted by T_N.

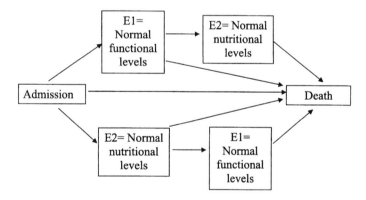

Figure 11.3: Multistate model with two intermediate events to describe all possible paths from admission to death

We use Z to denote all fixed covariates measured at admission and define two time-dependent covariates as $B(t) = \mathbf{1}\{T_B \leq t\}$ and $N(t) = \mathbf{1}\{T_N \leq t\}$ which are indicators of whether the normal functional and nutritional levels have been achieved at time t.

The multistate model in Figure 11.3 can be analyzed under the proportional hazards assumption with three Cox models [Cox (1972)]: a Cox model for the survival time T with $B(t)$ and $N(t)$ as time-dependent covariates

$$\lambda_T(t|Z, B(t), N(t)) = \lambda_{T0}(t)\exp\{\beta_T Z + \gamma_T B(t) + \theta_T N(t)\};$$

a Cox model for T_B, the time to normal functional levels, with $N(t)$ as time-dependent covariate

$$\lambda_B(t|Z, N(t)) = \lambda_{B0}(t)\exp\{\beta_B Z + \theta_B N(t)\};$$

and a Cox model for T_N given $B(t)$ as time-dependent covariate

$$\lambda_N(t|Z, B(t)) = \lambda_{N0}(t)\exp\{\beta_N Z + \gamma_N B(t)\}.$$

When fitting the first model, the result we obtained indicated that the parameter γ in (11.1) was not significatively different from zero; that is, time T_B to normal functional levels turned out to be not significant. Thus, our initial multistate model can be simplified as shown in Figure 11.4.

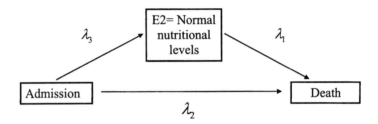

Figure 11.4: Multistate model with one intermediate event to describe all possible paths from admission to death

This new multistate model can be analyzed with only two Cox models: a Cox model for the survival time T with $N(t)$ as time-dependent covariate

$$\lambda_T(t|Z, N(t)) = \lambda_{T0}(t)\exp\{\beta_T Z + \theta_T N(t)\}, \tag{11.1}$$

and a Cox model for T_N

$$\lambda_N(t|Z) = \lambda_{N0}(t)\exp\{\beta_N Z\}. \tag{11.2}$$

The three hazard functions defined in the new multistate model (Figure 11.4) are obtained from models (11.1) and (11.2) as follows.

$$
\begin{aligned}
\lambda_1(t) &= \lambda_T(t|Z, N(t) = 1) = \lambda_{T0}(t)\exp\{\beta_T Z + \theta_T\} &\qquad (11.3)\\
\lambda_2(t) &= \lambda_T(t|Z, N(t) = 0) = \lambda_{T0}(t)\exp\{\beta_T Z\} &\qquad (11.4)\\
\lambda_3(t) &= \lambda_N(t|Z) = \lambda_{N0}(t)\exp\{\beta_N Z\}. &\qquad (11.5)
\end{aligned}
$$

The best fit for the model (11.1) shows that there are three fixed covariates associated with mortality: gender, nutritional status at admission, and functional status before the onset of the acute disease. The results are presented in Table 11.1. They show that at the moment of admission the risk of mortality of a man is approximately three times that for a woman and that patients with low nutritional levels at admission and with low functional levels before the onset of the acute disease have a higher risk of mortality. This fit also shows that the time taken to regain normal nutritional levels is associated with mortality.

Table 11.1: Risk coefficient estimates for model 11.1

	coef	exp(coef)	exp(−coef)	p
Gender	$\beta_{1T} = -1.1083$	0.330	3.03	0.000029
Barthel (pre-admission)	$\beta_{2T} = -0.0142$	0.986	1.01	0.003800
MNA (admission)	$\beta_{3T} = -0.0741$	0.929	1.08	0.027000
$N(t)$	$\theta_T = -0.9963$	0.369	2.71	0.015000

11.3.1 Predictive process

The results in Table 11.1 are useful in describing the effect of the fixed covariates on survival, but if our interest is rather in how the process of recovering normal nutritional levels influences the prognosis for a patient, it is more useful to compute what is called the predictive process. The predictive process is defined as the probability of death before time u given that the patient is alive at time t and given the history of this patient at time t:

$$\pi(u,t) = P[t < T \le u | H(t)]. \tag{11.6}$$

In our study, we have two possible histories:

$$H_1(t) = \{T > t,\ T_N \le t\} = \{T > t,\ N(t) = 1\}$$

and

$$H_2(t) = \{T > t,\ T_N > t\} = \{T > t,\ N(t) = 0\}.$$

The first one, H_1, corresponds to a patient who recovered normal nutritional levels before time t and the second one, H_2, to a patient whose nutritional levels continued to be lower than normal at time t.

The predictive process can be obtained in a closed form for both possible histories, H_1 and H_2, and will be denoted by $\pi_1(u,t)$ and $\pi_2(u,t)$, respectively.

The probability $\pi_1(u,t)$ of death before time u for a patient who at time t is alive and has recovered normal nutritional levels can be obtained by integrating the conditional density over all possible death times between t and u:

$$
\begin{aligned}
\pi_1(u,t) &= P[t < T \le u | H_1(t)] = P[t < T \le u | T > t, N(t) = 1] \\
&= \int_t^u \frac{f_1(s)}{S_1(t)}\, ds = \int_t^u \frac{S_1(s)\lambda_1(s)}{S_1(t)}\, ds \\
&= \int_t^u \exp\{-(H_1(s) - H_1(t))\}\lambda_1(s)\, ds.
\end{aligned}
$$

This expression can be estimated with the estimated risk factors obtained from fitting model (11.1) and using expression (11.3):

$$
\begin{aligned}
\pi_1(u,t) &\approx \sum_{t < t_i \le u} \exp\left\{ -\exp\left(\hat{\beta}_T Z + \hat{\theta}_T\right)\left(\hat{\Lambda}_{T0}(t_i) - \hat{\Lambda}_{T0}(t)\right)\right\} \\
&\qquad \times \exp\left(\hat{\beta}_T Z + \hat{\theta}_T\right)\hat{\lambda}_{T0}(t_i),
\end{aligned}
$$

where $\hat{\Lambda}_{T0}(t)$ is Breslow's estimate of the cumulative baseline hazard function corresponding to model (11.1).

The probability $\pi_2(u,t)$ of death before time u for a patient who at time t is alive and has not yet recovered normal nutritional levels can be obtained by considering two possibilities: that the patient dies at time s or that the patient recovers normal nutritional levels at time s and then dies between s and u:

$$
\begin{aligned}
\pi_2(u,t) &= P[t < T \le u | H_2(t)] = \int_t^u \left(\frac{f_2(s)}{S_2(t)} + \frac{f_3(s)}{S_3(t)}\pi_1(u,s)\right) ds \\
&= \int_t^u \big(\exp\{-(H_2(s) - H_2(t))\}\lambda_2(s) \\
&\qquad\qquad + \exp\{-(H_3(s) - H_3(t))\}\lambda_3(s)\pi_1(u,s)\big)\, ds.
\end{aligned}
$$

To approximate this expression, we use the estimated risk factors obtained from fitting models (11.1) and (11.2) and using the relationship between λ_2 and λ_T when $N(t) = 0$ given in expression (11.4) and the relationship between λ_3 and λ_N given in expression (11.5):

$$
\begin{aligned}
\pi_2(u,t) &\approx \sum_{t < t_i \le u} \Big(\exp\left\{ -\exp\left(\hat{\beta}_T Z\right)\left(\hat{\Lambda}_{T0}(t_i) - \hat{\Lambda}_{T0}(t)\right)\right\}\exp\left(\hat{\beta}_T Z\right)\hat{\lambda}_{T0}(t_i) \\
&\qquad \times \exp\left\{ -\exp\left(\hat{\beta}_N Z\right)\left(\hat{\Lambda}_{N0}(t_i) - \hat{\Lambda}_{N0}(t)\right)\right\} \\
&\qquad \times \exp\left(\hat{\beta}_N Z\right)\hat{\lambda}_{N0}(t_i)\pi_1(u,t_i)\Big),
\end{aligned}
$$

where $\hat{\Lambda}_{T0}(t)$ and $\hat{\Lambda}_{N0}(t)$ are Breslow's estimates of the cumulative baseline hazard function of T and T_N corresponding to models (11.1) and (11.2), respectively.

The predictive process depends on the time t at which the history is known and the point s at which we wish to make a prediction. By fixing or varying adequately the values of t and s, we can obtain different insights into the problem. In Figure 11.5, we show the predictive process when fixing $t = 2$ and varying s. This corresponds to the predicted residual survival times for patients two months after admission. It is clear that gender is an important risk factor with women having a higher predicted survival time than men. Also, recovering or not normal nutritional levels during the first two months appears to be a risk factor, though not a very strong one; that is, the survival curves for women in both categories are very similar as are the survival curves for men in both categories.

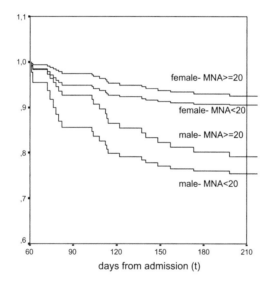

Figure 11.5: Predicted residual survival curves for patients two months after admission

Now we computed the predictive process with $t = 4$ and varying s. This gives the residual survival curves four months after being admitted (Figure 11.6). Here we note that the differences between patients who recovered and those who did not, have increased. In particular, though gender is still an important risk factor, now women who did not recover MNA during the first four months after admission have a similar predicted survival time to men who did recover. What these two pictures show is that the recovery, or not, of normal

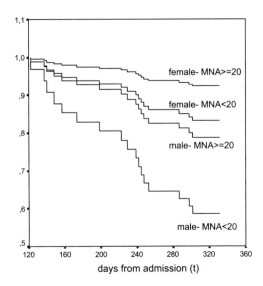

Figure 11.6: Predicted residual survival curves for patients four months after admission

nutritional levels is a dynamic prognostic factor and its impact on mortality varies over time.

This can be seen more clearly in Figure 11.7. In this graph, we have plotted the predictive process with a variable value of t and taking $s = 6 + t$. This corresponds to the probability of death during the next six months as a function of the time t from admission. As shown in the figure, it is clear that the differences between recovering or not recovering normal nutritional levels start to become apparent around two months after admission. During these first two months the predicted mortality is similar for both categories, whereas failure to recover nutritional levels after these two months is associated with a higher risk of mortality in the next six months for both men and women.

11.4 Discussion

Many medical studies could be improved by introducing information on the evolution of patients and it is worth working on methodologies that deal with this problem.

In this work, on the functional decline and mortality of frail elderly patients, we obtained a predictive process that illustrates the dynamic prognostic power of nutritional evolution of the patients. Although the data contain both

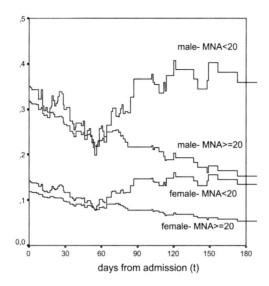

Figure 11.7: Probability of death during the next six months as a function of the time t from admission

survival and repeated observations, the available methods for the joint analysis of longitudinal and survival data were not appropriate in this case and, as an alternative we propose a multistate survival model. We observed that the recovery of normal nutritional levels during the first two months is critical. This methodology gives the clinicians a dynamic tool for prediction.

Acknowledgements. The data analyzed correspond to a research project on functional decline and mortality of frail patients. Dr. Espaulella from Hospital de la Santa Creu de Vic is the main researcher and the project received financial support in 2002 from the Acadèmia de ciències mèdiques de Catalunya i de Balears (a regional academic and scientific association). The authors have provided methodological support to the researchers. We gratefully acknowledge the comments and opinions we have received from the doctors and nurses at the Hospital de la Santa Creu de Vic, which have helped and encouraged us in the study and implementation of this methodology.

References

1. Cox, D. R. (1972). Regression models and life-tables (with discussion), *Journal of the Royal Statistical Society, Series B*, **34**, 187–220.

2. Faucett, C. L., and Thomas, D. C. (1996). Simultaneously modeling censored survival data and repeatedly measured covariates: A Gibbs sampling approach, *Statistical Methods in Medical Research*, **15**, 1663–1686.

3. Henderson, R., Diggle, P., and Dobson, A. (2000). Joint modeling of longitudinal measurements and event time data, *Biostatistics*, **3**, 33–50.

4. Klein, J. P., Keiding, N., and Copelan, E. A. (1994). Plotting summary predictions in multistate survival models. Probability of relapse and death in remission for bone marrow transplanted percents, *Statistics in Medicine*, **12**, 2315–2332.

5. Klein, J. P., and Moeschberger, M. L. (1998). *Survival Analysis. Techniques for Censored and Truncated Data*, Springer-Verlag, Inc, New York.

6. Wulfsohn, M. S., and Tsiatis, A. A. (1997). A joint model for survival and longitudinal data measured with error, *Biometrics*, **53**, 330–339.

12

New Models and Methods for Survival Analysis of Experimental Data

Ganna V. Semenchenko,[1] **Anatoli I. Yashin,**[2] **Thomas E. Johnson,**[3] **and James W. Cypser**[3]

[1] *Max Planck Institute for Demographic Research, Rostock, Germany*
[2] *Duke University, Durham, NC, USA*
[3] *University of Colorado at Boulder, Boulder, CO, USA*

Abstract: We propose an approach for analysis of survivorship data from observational and/or experimental studies that allows comparison of survival in the control and several experimental groups. Our approach is based on the model of heterogeneous mortality (frailty model), and we also assume that the difference between survivals for the control and experimental groups is in both the frailty distribution and baseline hazard. We explore the variety of survival patterns that can be captured by different specifications of the proposed model and illustrate the approach with an example of the model application to the analysis of data from stress-experiment with nematodes *Caenorhabditis elegans*. We show that the proposed model gives a good fit to the data and helps to advance our understanding of biological phenomena as they appear at both individual and population levels.

Keywords and phrases: Frailty model, hormesis, longevity, survival analysis

12.1   Introduction

The Gompertz model [Gompertz (1825)] is very often used to analyze survival in the experiments on laboratory animals. Parameters of this model are associated with the rate of aging and initial mortality, but these associations are biologically unjustified. It is well documented that mortality rates for humans [Manton and Stallard (1984) and Strehler and Mildvan (1960)] as well as for laboratory animals [Carey *et al.* (1992), Curtsinger *et al.* (1992), and Fukui *et al.* (1996)] decelerate at advanced ages and deviate from the Gompertz law. It is also discussed, that only for inbred populations in highly controlled homogeneous will the environments mortality rate follow the Gompertz curve

[Economos (1985), Sacher (1966), and Vaupel *et al.* (1979)]. Still, the theoretical challenge is to understand how different effects of environmental conditions or the application of treatment to the experimental group combine to produce different survival patterns [Boxenbaum *et al.* (1988), Lithgow *et al.* (1995), and Yakovlev *et al.* (1993)].

The notion of heterogeneity, as applied to a description of stochastic processes, first appeared in connection with an analysis of demographic processes [Keyfitz and Littman (1979)]. The authors drew attention to the fact that application of treatment produces different effects on homogeneous and heterogeneous populations. In a homogeneous population, the reduction in death rate and extension of lifespan are equal: a drop of one percent in the death rate is equivalent to an increase of one percent in the expectation of life. In a heterogeneous population, the reduction and extension can be very different. Thus, neglect of heterogeneity can lead to an overestimation of healthcare improvement.

In a homogeneous population, risk of dying is the same for all individuals of the given age. Due to this, population characteristics such as average lifespan, hazard, or survival function are true for every member of the population. In a heterogeneous population, such a generalization can be misleading.

In the model proposed in this chapter, the heterogeneity assumption means that the population consists of individuals with different susceptibility to death. This characteristic, which is also called frailty, influences the individual's risk of dying. Although lifespan is registered in most observational and experimental studies, aiming to investigate influences of different treatments on survival, it is often difficult to detect or measure an individual's frailty. The model of heterogeneous mortality [Vaupel *et al.* (1979)] allows us to take into account hidden heterogeneity of the population for survival analysis because of the assumption about probability distribution of an unobserved random variable—frailty. We propose an approach for analysis of survivorship data that allows comparison of survival in the control and several experimental groups.

12.2   Semiparametric Model of Mortality in Heterogeneous Populations Influenced by Exogenous Interventions

12.2.1   The heterogeneous mortality model

Let T and Z be the life span and the heterogeneity (frailty) variable such that the conditional hazard of death given Z is $Z\mu_0(x)$, where $\mu_0(x)$ is the baseline hazard, which corresponds to the risk of dying for the individual whose frailty is equal to 1. This means that the baseline hazard can only be observed in a homogeneous population, which is comprised of identical individuals.

Let us assume that Z is a gamma-distributed random variable ($Z \sim G(k, \lambda)$) with mean 1 and variance σ^2; that is, $k = \lambda$, and $\sigma^2 = 1/\lambda$.

Let $H(x) = \int_0^x \mu_0(u)\, du$ be the cumulative baseline hazard. Then for the observed mortality $\bar{\mu}(x)$, one can write [Vaupel *et al.* (1979)]

$$\bar{\mu}(x) = \frac{\mu_0(x)}{1 + \sigma^2 H(x)}. \tag{12.1}$$

The marginal survival function $S(x)$, can be presented as follows.

$$S(x) = \left(1 + \frac{1}{\lambda} H(x)\right)^{-k} = \left(1 + \sigma^2 H(x)\right)^{-(1/\sigma^2)}. \tag{12.2}$$

For a homogeneous population, $\sigma^2 = 0$, the expression (12.1) transforms into $\bar{\mu}(x) = \mu_0(x)$. It is easy to show, using the L'Hôpital rule, that $S(x) \to \exp(-H(x)) = S_0(x)$, for $\sigma^2 \to 0$ in (12.2), which corresponds to mortality and survival functions for a homogeneous population.

12.2.2 Changes in the baseline hazard and frailty distribution

In our further calculations, we followed the methodology suggested by Yashin *et al.* (1996). Such a methodology was also used for the analysis of data from stress experiments with *Drosophila melanogaster* [Semenchenko *et al.* (2004a)] and for investigation of influences of different stressors and antistressors on the survival of transgenic mice HER-2/neu [Semenchenko *et al.* (2004b)].

Let us consider two identical heterogeneous populations whose chances of survival correspond to the proportional hazards model [Eqs. (12.1) and (12.2)], and assume that the initial frailties are gamma-distributed with means 1 and variances σ_1^2, σ_2^2, respectively.

The first population—the control group—experiences standard living conditions without any interventions, and the second—experimental group—is subjected to some treatment at the age interval $[x_0, x^*]$. At the age x^*, the treatment is over.

To compare the survival functions after age x^* in the experimental and in the control group let us assume that in the control group, the baseline hazard $\mu_{01}(x)$ does not change and in the experimental cohort the baseline hazard $\mu_{02}(x)$ increases or decreases at the interval $[x_0, x^*]$. After age x^*, it can be represented as follows: $\mu_{02}(x) = \mu_0(x) + f(x)$. Note that if $f(x) \equiv 0$, the baseline hazard is on the level of the control group. A negative $f(x)$ manifests a decrease of the baseline hazard during the treatment, and a positive $f(x)$ represents an increase of the baseline hazard compared to the control group.

Changes in the baseline hazard can serve as a characteristic of changes in the intensity of occurrence of intracellular damages caused by treatment [Michalski et al. (2001)]. If the intensity of damage occurrence decreases, the baseline hazard also decreases. An increase of the intensity of damage occurrence leads to an increase of the baseline hazard. Thus, we can consider a beneficial effect of the treatment as a decrease of the baseline hazard, whereas a detrimental effect of the treatment is characterized by an increase of the baseline hazard. Because changes in the baseline hazard can be persistent, progressive, or even regressive, it is appropriate to consider them as a function of age when the treatment is over ($f(x)$ for $x \geq x^*$).

It follows from (12.2) that the marginal survival functions $S_i(x)$, $i = 1, 2$, for those who survived age x^* in both control and experimental groups are

$$S_i(x) = \left(1 + \frac{1}{\lambda_i^*} H_i^*(x)\right)^{-k_i}, \qquad i = 1, 2, \tag{12.3}$$

where $\lambda_i^* = (1/\sigma_i^2) + H_i(x^*)$, $H_i(x^*) = \int_0^{x^*} \mu_{0i}(u)du$, $H_1^*(x) = \int_{x^*}^x \mu_0(u)du$, $H_2^*(x) = \int_{x^*}^x \mu_0(u)du + F(x)$, $F(x) = \int_{x^*}^x f(u)du$, $k_i = 1/\sigma_i^2$, $i = 1, 2$.

Let us assume that under normal living conditions an individual's susceptibility to death does not change during her life and that any exogenous intervention can increase or decrease an individual's frailty. Note that in the control population the "natural" selection process does not change the shape parameter $k_1 = 1/\sigma_1^2$ of the frailty distribution. If the application of treatment does not influence an individual's frailty, this parameter also does not change in the experimental cohort; that is, $k_2 = 1/\sigma_2^2$.

Let us assume that $\sigma_1^2 = \sigma_2^2 = \sigma^2$ and that the application of a treatment can also change the shape parameter of the frailty distribution by a factor γ; that is, $k_2 = 1/\gamma\sigma^2$. So, for the survival in the control cohort after age x^*, one can write:

$$S_1(x) = \left(1 + \frac{k_1}{\lambda_1}\sigma^2 H_1(x)\right)^{-k_1} = \left(1 + m_1\sigma^2 H_1(x)\right)^{-(1/\sigma^2)}. \tag{12.4}$$

Then the survival in the experimental cohort ($x > x^*$) can be presented as follows.

$$S_2(x) = \left(1 + m_2\gamma\sigma^2 H_2(x)\right)^{-(1/\gamma\sigma^2)}. \tag{12.5}$$

In (12.4) and (12.5), m_1 and m_2 denote the mean values of frailty distribution at age x^* in the control and in the experimental populations, respectively. Factor γ shows the presence of changes in the frailty distribution that are not associated with changes of average frailty in the population during the treatment.

Changes in individual frailty characterize the ability of an organism to switch on new mechanisms of defense or repair in order to withstand harmful effects of treatment or to repair lesions that occurred due to treatment

[Yashin *et al.* (2002)]. Thus, the beneficial effect of the applied treatment can be due to a decrease of the average frailty of the population. This means that individual characteristics of every cohort member were improved and individual susceptibility to death was reduced. The detrimental effect produced by treatment can result in increased average frailty of the population. However, the application of treatment can produce different effects on different members of a heterogeneous population. Robust individuals can become more robust, and weak individuals can become more weak after the treatment, and this results in an increase of population heterogeneity. If the treatment is beneficial for weak individuals and detrimental for robust ones, the population becomes more homogeneous.

12.2.3   Semiparametric representation of the model

Additional assumptions about the parametric form of the baseline hazard in both control and experimental groups are needed in representations (12.4) and (12.5), as well as (12.2). Because it is impossible to observe the baseline hazard in a heterogeneous population, any assumption about its parametric form is biologically unjustified and should be avoided in an analysis of valuable experimental data.

It follows from (12.4) and from the definition of $F(x)$ that

$$H_2(x) = \frac{S_1(x)^{-\sigma^2} - 1}{\sigma^2 m_1} + F(x). \tag{12.6}$$

Replacing $H_2^*(x)$ in (12.5) with (12.6), we obtain the following equation for the survival $S_2(x)$, $(x > x^*)$ in the experimental group.

$$S_2(x) = \left(1 + r\gamma\left(S_1(x)^{-\sigma^2} - 1\right) + m_1 r\gamma\sigma^2 F(x)\right)^{-(1/\gamma\sigma^2)}, \tag{12.7}$$

where $r = m_2^*/m_1^*$, the ratio of mean values of the frailty distributions in experimental and control groups.

Assuming that an increase or decrease of the baseline hazard after the application of treatment can vary nonlinearly with age, in our calculations we use $f(x) = a e^{\beta(x-x^*)}$. Denoting $\alpha = a m_1^*$, Eq. (12.7) can be rewritten as

$$S_2(x) = \left(1 + r\gamma\left(S_1(x)^{-\sigma^2} - 1\right) + \gamma r\sigma^2\frac{\alpha}{\beta}\left(e^{\beta x} - 1\right)\right)^{-(1/\gamma\sigma^2)}. \tag{12.8}$$

We call this representation semiparametric because the survival function in the experimental group (12.8) contains $S_1(x)$, the observed survival function in the control group. However, parametric approximations of $S_1(x)$ [Thatcher *et al.* (1998)] can be used as well as nonparametric ones [Kaplan and Meier (1958)].

12.2.4   Interpretation of parameters

In the framework of this model several treatment groups can be considered and compared to one control group. The model (12.8) has four unknown parameters α, β, r, γ that are specific to each experimental group and its treatment and one parameter σ^2 that is common to all groups, the frailty variance in the control cohort.

Parameter σ^2 indicates the presence of hidden heterogeneity in the control population. When values of σ^2 are close to zero, the control population can be considered as homogeneous; large values of σ^2 characterize the control population as highly heterogeneous.

Dependences of the survival function in the experimental group on changes of the model's parameters are presented in Figures 12.1 and 12.2.

Effects of changes in the baseline hazard, controlled by parameters α and β, are presented in Figure 12.1. If $\beta = 0$ in the additive part of hazard for the treatment group $f(x) = a \exp(\beta x)$, changes in parameter α reflect permanent (constant) decrease or increase of the baseline hazard (Figure 12.1a), producing rectangularization or derectangularization of the survival curve (Figure 12.1b), respectively, depending on whether α is greater or less than zero. It can also be seen that permanent decrease or increase of the baseline hazard does not influence the "tail" of the survival curve.

Parameter β describes the amplification or disappearance of the α-effect, according to whether β is greater or less than zero. For each effect a small value of α was fixed. Absolute values of negative β characterize the rate at which the baseline hazard in the experimental group returns to the level of the control group (Figure 12.1c). Different patterns of survival curves, corresponding to the changes in parameter $\beta < 0$, for increased or decreased baseline hazard are presented in Figure 12.1d. It can be seen that these changes do not influence the "tail" of the survival function, as in the case of constant changes of the baseline hazard.

Positive values of β characterize an amplification of effects, produced by the treatment, during the life (Figure 12.1e). Amplified with age increase of the baseline hazard shifts the survival curve to the left along the age axis (compared to the control group), and amplified with age decrease shifts it to the right along the age axis (Figure 12.1f). In both cases the tail of the survival curve moves in the same direction. The shifts produced are not parallel; they resemble rotation around the initial level of increased or decreased survival.

Changes produced by the treatment on the frailty distribution and corresponding survival functions are presented in Figure 12.2. An increase or decrease in the mean of the frailty distribution (Figure 12.2a) produces a nearly parallel shift of the survival curve along the age axis with respective lengthening/shortening of its tail (Figure 12.2b). Parameter $r < 1$ shows an increase

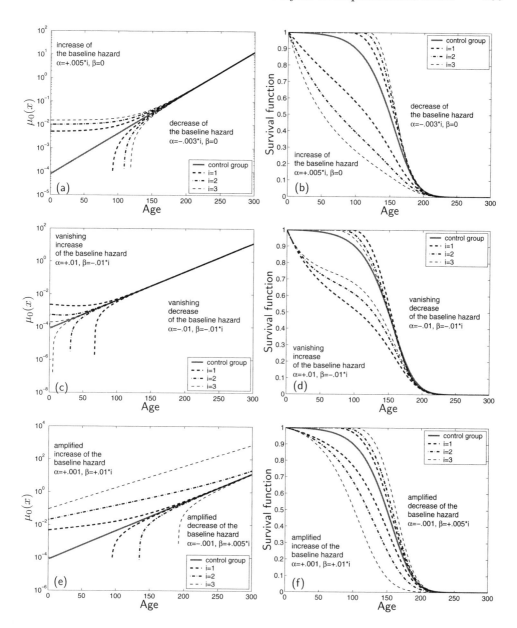

Figure 12.1: Dependence of survival function for the experimental group on changes in the baseline hazard

in the average robustness, whereas $r > 1$ indicates an accumulation of frail individuals in the population subjected to the treatment.

Parameter $\gamma \neq 1$ characterizes changes in frailty variance in the experimental groups compared to the control cohort (Figure 12.2c). A decrease in variance of the frailty distribution ($\gamma < 1$) indicates that the experimental group became less heterogeneous, and an increase in frailty variance ($\gamma > 1$) corresponds to an

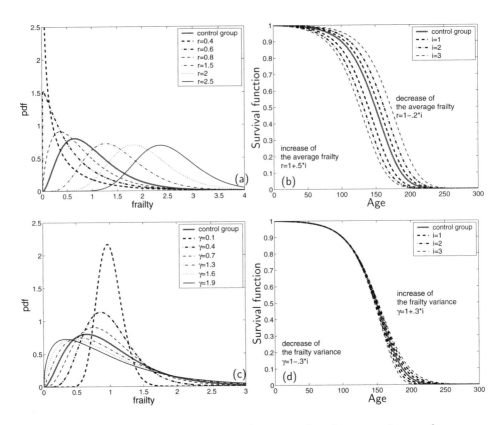

Figure 12.2: Dependence of survival function for the experimental group on changes in the frailty distribution

increase of heterogeneity of the experimental population after the application of a treatment. It can be seen in Figure 12.2d that changes in population heterogeneity mostly influence the tail of the survival function. The population, which is more heterogeneous, comprises more individuals with high chances of survival to advanced ages.

By fixing some parameters on the level of the control group, it is possible to consider a different specification of the proposed model. Thus, if the application of treatment does not influence survival of the experimental group, the control and experimental populations remain identical. The following combination of parameter values $\alpha = 0$, $r = 1$, $\gamma = 1$ corresponds to such a case. If the only effect produced by the treatment is a change in the mean value of the frailty distribution, parameter $r \neq 1$ and all others are fixed on the level of the control group. If the only difference between the control and experimental cohorts is in their heterogeneity, the combination $\gamma \neq 1$, $\alpha = 0$, $r = 1$ will describe this situation. In much the same way, changes in the baseline hazard can be described by the following combination of parameter values; $\alpha \neq 0$, $\beta \neq 0$, $r = 1$, $\gamma = 1$.

12.3   One Example of the Model Application to the Analysis of Poststress Survival Data

12.3.1   Heat shock of different duration applied to populations of nematodes *Caenorhabditis elegans*

Nematodes from the strain TJ1060 (spe-9;fer-15) were raised at temperature 25.5°C. At three days of age, the worms were divided into ten groups and exposed to 35°C heat shock for periods of 0, 1, 2, 4, 6, 8, 10, 12, 16, or 24 hours (synchronous start, asynchronous stop). Immediately following the heat shock, worms were permitted to recover for up to 24 hours at temperature 20°C on NGM agar. They were then transferred to liquid survival medium and maintained at temperature 20°C for the remainder of the experiment. Starting from day four, the number of alive and dead worms was counted daily for all groups. No survivors were observed after 16 and 24 hours of heating. The details of the experiment are described in Michalski *et al.* (2001). To illustrate the approach proposed in this paper, we analyzed data only for groups subjected to heat shock of duration no longer than 8 hours. Characteristics of the lifespan in these groups are presented in Table 12.1.

Table 12.1: Lifespan characteristics in the groups of nematodes *Caenorhabditis elegans* subjected to heat shock of different duration

	Control	Heat Shock Duration				
		1 Hour	2 Hours	4 Hours	6 Hours	8 Hours
Mean lifespan, days	19,47	21,58	20,64	18,58	10,54	7,15
	(±0,5)	(±0,6)	(±0,5)	(±0,6)	(±0,6)	(±0,3)
Variance	4,91	5,57	5,11	6,06	5,42	2,56
Minimal lifespan	6	7	6	4	4	4
Maximal lifespan	36	36	34	27	33	25
p-value		0,002	0,015	0,023	0,001	0,001

Heat shock of a short duration (1–2 hours) produced a hormetic effect on survival of worms, whereas a long duration (6–8 hours) decreased chances of survival. Despite the fact that the mean lifespan of worms subjected to heating for 4 hours does not differ from one of the control group, the difference in survival according to the log-rank test is statistically significant. Moreover, the variance of the lifespan distribution is the biggest in this group. This means that the cohort subjected to 4 hours of heating contains more individuals whose life span is greater or lower than the average one. In groups that survived 6 or 8 hours of heating, the maximal lifespan, is six- to tenfold greater than the average lifespan. This bears evidence of heterogeneity in reaction to the proposed treatment.

12.3.2   Technical details

To obtain the estimates of the model parameters, the observations of life spans in all treatment groups were used simultaneously. The maximum likelihood approach was implemented and parameters were estimated using a nonlinear optimization procedure [Fletcher (1987)]. Because the structure of the data corresponds to the number of dead and alive nematodes during discrete time periods, the log-likelihood function is derived from the binomial distribution, where binomial probabilities depend on model parameters:

$$\text{LogLik} = \sum_j (m_j \ln(q_j) + (n_j - m_j) \ln(1 - q_j)),$$

where m_j is the number of deaths on day j of life, and n_j is the number of individuals that were alive on day $j - 1$. Values q_j are related to survival functions for the experimental groups by the relationship

$$q_j = 1 - \frac{S(j+1)}{S(j)}.$$

Confidence intervals for the parameter estimates were calculated using the bootstrap method [Davison and Hinkley (1997)].

12.3.3   Results of fitting the model to the data

In order to describe effects produced by treatments on frailty distribution and baseline hazard, several specifications of the heterogeneous mortality model were considered. The first one deals with effects such as increase of average robustness or accumulation of frail individuals in the population. In the second, changes in mean frailty are accompanied by changes in the baseline hazard. The third takes into account the opportunity of changes in population heterogeneity during the treatment in addition to changes in the baseline hazard and mean values of the frailty distribution. All models are nested, so respective hypotheses were tested using the likelihood ratio statistics. It turned out that the third specification of the model fits the data better than the others ($p < 0.01$).

Parameter estimates of this specification are presented in Table 12.2. Using the estimate of frailty variance (parameter σ^2 in Table 12.2), Eq. (12.1) allows us to estimate the conditional baseline hazard for the control group, which is presented in Figure 12.3a. It can be seen that the baseline hazard deviates from the Gompertz law at advanced ages.

In order to explore predictive abilities of the the model, parameter estimation procedure was conducted in two stages, and first for the groups subjected

Table 12.2: Parameter estimates of the semiparametric model of heterogeneous mortality for groups of nematodes *Caenorhabditis elegans* subjected to heat shock of different duration

Parameter	1 Hour	2 Hours	Heat Shock Duration 4 Hours	6 Hours	8 Hours
$\alpha \times 10^{-1}$	0,3	0,2	0,4	5,4	7,1
	(0,25; 0,32)	(0,19; 0,22)	(0,38; 0,41)	(5,22; 5,47)	(7,05; 7,13)
$\beta \times 10^{-1}$	−0,9	−0,3	−0,8	1	3,9
	(−1; −0,88)	(−0,32; −0,27)	(−0,9; −0,72)	(0,92; 1,11)	(3,86; 4,07)
$r \times 10^{-1}$	3,6	4,5	6,3	2	1,6
	(3,45; 3,62)	(4,36; 4,54)	(6,16; 6,32)	(1,97; 2,08)	(1,52; 1,63)
γ	0,31	0,40	0,87	1,40	1,31
	(0,28; 0,33)	(0,37; 0,41)	(0,85; 0,9)	(1,38; 1,44)	(1,3; 1,33)
σ^2	Common for all groups 0,28 (0,27; 0,29)				

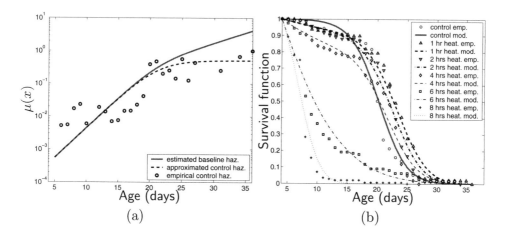

(a)   (b)

Figure 12.3: (a) Estimated baseline hazard for the control group of nematodes compared to the estimates of observed hazard and (b) empirical and modeled conditional survival functions for experimental groups of worms (survival function for the control group is approximated by gamma–Gompertz model with parameters $\alpha = 4.4\text{e-}4$ (3e-4; 5e-4), $\beta = 0.42$ (0.4; 0.43), $\sigma^2 = 0.83$ (0.81; 0.85))

to heating during 1, 4, and 8 hours. According to the proposed model, an increase in survival after 1 hour of heating (Table 12.1 and Figure 12.3b) is due to a decrease of the average frailty, despite the fact that it was accompanied by an increase of the baseline hazard before the age of about 17 days and a decrease of the population heterogeneity.

The effect of incomplete hormesis (the intersection of survival curves in the control and experimental groups), which was observed after four hours of heating, was caused by greater increase of the baseline hazard at young ages, accompanied by decrease of the average frailty and heterogeneity (both were less than in the first group).

The group subjected to eight hours of heating became the least frail and the most heterogeneous, however, long duration of heating not only increased the baseline hazard but also the rate of its amplification with age. A combination of these effects determined a concave pattern of survival function and its long "tail" in this group (Table 12.1 and Figure 12.3b).

Proceeding from these results, we assumed that after two and six hours of heating the mean values and variances of the frailty distributions, as well as baseline hazards, are in the intervals between the values, which characterize respective effects in the groups that survived heat shock during one, four, and eight hours. As the next step, we conducted parameter estimation for all groups simultaneously, and the results (Table 12.2) confirmed the assumption that the baseline hazard increases with an increase of the heat shock duration. Heat shock of short duration (one and two hours) made the population of nematodes less frail on average and less heterogeneous. With an increase of heat shock duration up to four hours, average frailty and its variance increased but remained less then in the control group. Further increase of heat shock duration (six and eight hours) decreased average frailty but increased heterogeneity of experimental populations compared to the control group. The fact that the estimate of the frailty variance for the group survived six hours of heating is greater than one for the group subjected to heat shock during eight hours, gives evidence that the longer duration of heating would lead to decrease of heterogeneity of the population of worms.

12.4   Discussion

The main reason for attempts to investigate influences of toxic substances on survival [Boxenbaum *et al.* (1988) and Neafsey *et al.* (1988)] was to explain the deviations of the hazard function from the Gompertz curve under assumption that "The Law" holds for mortality in the absence of treatment.

Further development of studies of survival under or after stress using mathematical models [Butov *et al.* (2001), Yakovlev *et al.* (1993), and Yashin *et al.* (2001)] helped to bind some biological and physiological mechanisms to population mortality. However, those models did not take into account heterogeneity in response to applied treatment.

The Cox regression model [Cox (1972)], which is also widely used in medical and biological studies, is a method of choice in the case of observed covariates.

When it is impossible to observe covariates, the specification for the two-sample problem allows us to estimate relative risk of death in the treatment group compared to the control population.

Application of a frailty model in the case of unobserved covariates is more appropriate [Vaupel *et al.* (1979)]. Still this approach requires additional assumptions for the parametric form of a baseline hazard [Michalski *et al.* (2001)]. These assumptions are biologically unjustified because of the impossibility of observing the baseline hazard in the heterogeneous population, and they also make the model unidentifiable from the viewpoint that the frailty variance depends on the choice of the baseline hazard. The semiparametric representation of the heterogeneous mortality model allows us to avoid unjustified assumptions and makes the model identifiable. Moreover, such a representation makes it possible to estimate the baseline hazard for the control group, knowing the variance of frailty distribution.

The main distinctive feature of our model in comparison to other gamma frailty models [Klein (1992), Michalski *et al.* (2001), Nielsen *et al.* (1992), and Vaupel *et al.* (1979)] is that we assume that treatment influences parameters of both frailty distribution and baseline hazard.

Changes in frailty distribution under stressful experimental conditions first were discussed and studied by modeling discrete frailty classes [Yashin *et al.* (2002)]. This model is based on the assumption that a population consists of three subpopulations of individuals: weak, normal, and robust. Stressful experimental conditions can influence an individual's frailty and change proportion of members in each subpopulation. If applied treatment is detrimental, robust individuals become normal, normal ones become weak, and weak individuals die. The hormetic effect is caused by an increase in robustness of individuals. If application of treatment is beneficial, weak individuals become normal, normal ones become robust. When some individuals from a normal subpopulation become weak and at the same time other normal individuals become robust, the effect of incomplete hormesis is observed. We incorporated this elegant idea into our semiparametric model of heterogeneous mortality assuming continuous distribution for the frailty variable. We believe that the application of sophisticated mathematical models advances our understanding of biological phenomena as they appear at both individual and population levels.

References

1. Boxenbaum, H., Neafsey, P., and Fournier, D. (1988). Hormesis, Gompertz functions and risk assessment, *Drug Metabolism Reviews*, **19**, 195–229.

2. Butov, A., Johnson, T., Cypser, J., Sannikov, I., Volkov, M., Sehl, M., and Yashin, A. (2001). Hormesis and debilitation effects in stress experiments using the nematode worm *Caenorhabditis elegans*: the model of balance between cell damage and hsp levels, *Experimental Gerontology*, **37**, 57–66.

3. Carey, J., Liedo, P., Orozco, D., and Vaupel, J. (1992). Slowing of mortality rates at older ages in large medfly cohorts, *Science*, **258**, 457–461.

4. Cox, D. (1972). Regression models and life-tables (with discussion), *Journal of the Royal Statistical Society, Series B*, **34**, 187–220.

5. Curtsinger, J., Fukui, H., Townsend, D., and Vaupel, J. (1992). Demography of genotypes: Failure of the limited life-span paradigm in drosophila melanogaster, *Science*, **258**, 461–463.

6. Davison, A. C., and Hinkley, D. V. (1997). *Bootstrap Methods and Their Application*, Cambridge University Press, Cambridge, England.

7. Economos, A. (1985). Rate of aging, rate of dying and non-Gompertzian mortality, *Encore Gerontology*, **31**, 106–111.

8. Fletcher, R. (1987). *Practical Methods of Optimization*, Second edition, John Wiley & Sons, New York.

9. Fukui, H., Ackert, L., and Curtsinger, J. (1996). Deceleration of age-specific mortality rates in *Drosophila melanogaster*, *Experimental Gerontology*, **31**, 517–531.

10. Gompertz, B. (1825). On the nature of the function expressive of the law of human mortality, and on the new mode of determining the values of life contingencies, *Philosophical Transaction, The Royal Society, London*, **115**, 513–585.

11. Kaplan, E., and Meier, P. (1958). Nonparametric estimation from incomplete observation, *Journal of the American Statistical Association*, **53**, 457–481.

12. Keyfitz, N., and Littman, G. (1979). Mortality in a heterogeneous population, *Population Studies*, **33**, 333–342.

13. Klein, J. P. (1992). Semiparametric estimation of random effects using the cox model based on the em algorithm, *Biometrics*, **48**, 795–806.

14. Lithgow, G., White, T., Melov, S., and Johnson, T. (1995). Thermotolerance and extended life span confered by single-gene mutations and induced by thermal stress, *Proceedings of the National Academy of Science USA*, **92**, 7540–7544.

15. Manton, K., and Stallard, E. (1984). *Recent Trends in the Mortality Analysis*, Academic, Orlando, Florida.

16. Michalski, A. I., Johnson, T. E., Cypser, J. R., and Yashin, A. I. (2001). Heating stress patterns in *Caenorhabditis elegans* longevity and survivorship, *Biogerontology*, **2**, 35–44.

17. Neafsey, P. J., Boxenbaum, H., Ciraulo, D. A., and Fournier, D. J. (1988). A gompertz age-specific mortality rate model for aging, hormesis and toxicity: Single dose studies, *Drug Metabolism Reviews*, **19**), 369–401.

18. Nielsen, G., Gill, R., Andersen, P., and Sørensen, T. (1992). A counting process approach to maximum likelihood estimation in frailty models, *Scandinavian Journal of Statistics*, **19**, 25–43.

19. Sacher, G. (1966). The Gompertz transformation in the study of the injury-mortality relationship: Application to late radiation effects and ageing, In *Radiation and Ageing. Proceedings of a Colloquium held in Semmering, Austria*, pp. 411–441, Taylor and Francis, London.

20. Semenchenko, G. V., Khazaeli, A. A., Curtsinger, J. W., and Yashin, A. I. (2004a). Stress resistance declines with age: Analysis of data from survival experiment with *Drosophila melanogaster*, *Biogerontology*, **5**, 17–30.

21. Semenchenko, A., Anisimov, V., and Yashin, A. (2004b). Stressors and antistressors: How do they influence survival in HER-2/neu transgenic mice? *Experimental Gerontology*, **39**, 1499–1511.

22. Strehler, B., and Mildvan, A. (1960). General theory of mortality and aging, *Science*, **132**, 14–21.

23. Thatcher, A., Kanisto, V., and Vaupel, J. (1998). The force of mortality at ages 80 to 120, In *Monographs on Population Aging*, Volume 5, Odense University press, Odense, Denmark.

24. Vaupel, J., Manton, K., and Stallard, E. (1979). The impact of heterogeneity in individual frailty on the dynamics of mortality, *Demography*, **16**, 439–454.

25. Yakovlev, A., Tsodikov, A., and Bass, L. (1993). A stochastic model of hormesis, *Mathematical Biosciences*, **116**, 197–219.

26. Yashin, A., Andreev, K., Curtsinger, J., and Vaupel, J. (1996). Death-after-stress-data in the analysis of heterogeneous mortality, In *Transactions of Symposium in Applied Statistics* (Ed., G. Christensen), pp. 24–32.

27. Yashin, A., Cypser, J., Johnson, T., Michalski, A., Boyko, S., and Novoseltsev, V. (2001). Ageing and survival after different doses of heat shock: the results of analysis of data from stress experiments with the nematode worm *Caenorhabditis elegans*, *Mechanisms of Ageing and Development*, **122**, 1477–1495.

28. Yashin, A., Cypser, J., Johnson, T., Michalski, A., Boyko, S., and Novoseltsev, V. (2002). Heat shock changes the heterogeneity distribution in populations of *Caenorhabditis elegans*: does it tell us anything about the biological mechanism of stress response? *The Journals of Gerontology, Series A*, **57**, B83–B92.

13

Uniform Consistency for Conditional Lifetime Distribution Estimators Under Random Right-Censorship

Paul Deheuvels and Gérard Derzko

Université Pierre et Marie Curie—Paris VI, Paris, France
Sanofi-Aventis, Montpellier, France

Abstract: We define nonparametric kernel-type estimators of the conditional distribution of a lifetime, in a random censorship framework. We show that these estimators have closed-form expressions, and establish their strong uniform consistency under minimal assumptions.

Keywords and phrases: Nonparametric estimation, lifetime distributions, regression estimation, kernel estimation, empirical processes, functional estimation, weak laws, laws of large numbers

13.1   Introduction and Results

13.1.1   Notation and statement of the problem

The present work is concerned with the estimation of a conditional lifetime distribution under random censorship from the right. The model we consider is based upon a sequence of observations (X_n, Y_n, U_n), $n = 1, 2, \ldots$, of a random vector (X, Y, U), where X denotes a positive lifetime of interest, Y a positive censoring time, and U a concomitant variable whose influence on the distributions of X and Y is to be assessed. Throughout, we will assume that X and Y are conditionally mutually independent, given U. The observed data set is given by the triplets (Z_i, δ_i, U_i), $i = 1, \ldots, n$, where $(Z_i := X_i \wedge Y_i, \delta_i := \mathbb{1}_{\{X_i \leq Y_i\}}, U_i)$, for $i = 1, \ldots, n$, constitutes a random sample of independent and identically distributed copies of $(Z := X \wedge Y, \delta := \mathbb{1}_{\{X \leq Y\}}, U)$. Our aim is to estimate the conditional distribution function $F(x|u) = \mathbb{P}(X \leq x|U = u)$ [respectively, $G(y|u) = \mathbb{P}(Y \leq y|U = u)$], provided that this last expression is meaningful.

We start by giving some notation and assumptions that are needed for the forthcoming definition of our estimators.

We mention that, in the uncensored case, corresponding to the limiting degenerate case where $Y = \infty$ with probability 1, our estimators reduce to that given by Stute (1986) for conditional empirical distribution functions. The latter estimators turn out to be a special version of the Nadaraya-Watson nonparametric regression estimator [see Nadaraya (1964, 1989), Watson (1964), Härdle (1990), Einmahl and Mason (2000), Deheuvels and Mason (2004), and the references therein]. In the case where U is independent of (X, Y), our estimators yield, as a special case, the usual product-limit estimator due to Kaplan and Meier (1958), for which there is a huge literature [see, e.g., Burke, Csörgő, and Horváth (1981, 1988), Deheuvels and Einmahl (2000), Földes, Rejtő, and Winter (1981), Gill (1980), Stute (1995), and the references therein].

Unless otherwise specified, the (possibly defective) distribution functions we will consider will be assumed to be right-continuous, and of the general form $\Psi(t) = \Psi_+(t) = \mathbb{P}(\{R \leq t\} \cap \mathcal{E}) = \lim_{\epsilon \downarrow 0} \Psi(t + \epsilon)$. At times, we will make use of the left-continuous version of Ψ, denoted by $\Psi_-(t) = \mathbb{P}(\{R < t\} \cap \mathcal{E}) = \lim_{\epsilon \downarrow 0} \Psi(t - \epsilon)$. Below, we will always assume that the distribution functions $F(x) = \mathbb{P}(X \leq x)$ and $G(y) = \mathbb{P}(Y \leq y)$, of X and Y, respectively, are continuous, so that $F(x) = F_\pm(x)$, $G(y) = G_\pm(y)$, and $F_\pm(0) = G_\pm(0) = 0$. This assumption entails that the distribution function $H(z) = \mathbb{P}(Z \leq z) = 1 - (1 - F(z))(1 - G(z))$ of Z is continuous, and such that $H(0) = 0$. In this framework, with probability 1 for each $n \geq 1$, the order statistics $0 < Z_{1,n} < \cdots < Z_{n,n}$ of $Z_1, \ldots, Z_n$ are distinct and positive. Unless otherwise specified, we will work on the event of probability 1 on which this property holds. There exists therefore (on the latter event) a rank sequence $\{r_{1,n}, \ldots, r_{n,n}\}$, defined as the unique permutation of $\{1, \ldots, n\}$ such that

$$Z_{i,n} = Z_{r_{i,n}} \quad \text{for} \quad i = 1, \ldots, n. \tag{13.1}$$

In the sequel, we will set accordingly

$$\delta_{i:n} = \delta_{r_{i,n}} \quad \text{and} \quad U_{i:n} = U_{r_{i,n}} \quad \text{for} \quad i = 1, \ldots, n. \tag{13.2}$$

We stress the fact that the $U_{i:n}$ for $1 \leq i \leq n$ are not to be confused with the order statistics of $U_1, \ldots, U_n$, which will not be used here. The latter should be denoted, in agreement with the notation above, by $U_{1,n} \leq \cdots \leq U_{n,n}$.

The conditioning random variable U will be assumed to have a measurable density $\kappa(u)$ on $\mathbb{R}$, and, therefore, a continuous distribution function $\mathcal{K}(u) = \int_{(-\infty, x]} \kappa(u) du$. We are specifically interested in conditioning on $\{U = u\}$ when u varies in a specified bounded interval $I := [A, B]$ of $\mathbb{R}$. We will assume, for technical purposes, the existence of a larger interval $J := [A', B'] \supset I$, such that $-\infty < A' < B < B' < \infty$, and $\kappa(\cdot)$ is continuous and positive (and thus, bounded away from 0) on J. Our primary concern is to estimate $F(x|u)$ when u varies in I. To give a precise meaning to this last expression, we assume further that (X, U) and (Y, U) have joint densities on $\mathbb{R}^+ \times \mathbb{R}$, denoted by $f(x, u)$ and $g(y, u)$, respectively. Moreover, we assume that $f(x, u)$ and $g(y, u)$ are continuous on $\mathbb{R}^+ \times J$. This allows us to set, for each $u \in J$ and $x, y \in \mathbb{R}^+$,

$$F(x|u) = \mathbb{P}(X \leq x|U = u) = \frac{1}{\kappa(u)} \int_0^x f(x, u)dx, \tag{13.3}$$

$$G(y|u) = \mathbb{P}(Y \leq y|U = u) = \frac{1}{\kappa(u)} \int_0^y g(y, u)dy, \tag{13.4}$$

$$\kappa(u) = \int_0^\infty f(x, u)dx = \int_0^\infty g(y, u)dy. \tag{13.5}$$

We note for further use that our assumptions on $\kappa(\cdot)$, $f(\cdot, \cdot)$, and $g(\cdot, \cdot)$, imply, via (13.3)–(13.5), that $F(\cdot|\cdot)$ and $G(\cdot|\cdot)$ are both continuous on $\mathbb{R}^+ \times J$. In this framework, we will make use of the following distribution functions, where, as usual, we set $Z = X \wedge Y$ and $\delta = \mathbb{I}_{\{X \leq Y\}}$. We set, for each $u \in J$ and $z \in \mathbb{R}^+$,

$$H^{(0)}(z|u) = \mathbb{P}(Z \leq z, \delta = 0|U = u) = \int_{(0,z]} (1 - F_-(t|u)) \, dG(t|u)$$

$$= \frac{1}{\kappa(u)} \int_{(0,z]} (1 - F_-(t|u)) \, g(t, u)dt, \tag{13.6}$$

$$H^{(1)}(z|u) = \mathbb{P}(Z \leq z, \delta = 1|U = u) = \int_{(0,z]} (1 - G_-(t|u)) \, dF(t|u)$$

$$= \frac{1}{\kappa(u)} \int_{(0,z]} (1 - G_-(t|u)) \, f(t, u)dt, \tag{13.7}$$

and

$$H(z|u) = \mathbb{P}(Z \leq z|U = u) = 1 - (1 - F(t|u))(1 - G(t|u))$$

$$= H^{(0)}(z|u) + H^{(1)}(z|u). \tag{13.8}$$

Even though the continuity of $F(\cdot|\cdot)$ and $G(\cdot|\cdot)$ implies that, in (13.6)–(13.8), $F(t|u) = F_\pm(t|u)$ and $G(t|u) = G_\pm(t|u)$ over $(t, u) \in \mathbb{R}^+ \times J$, it is of interest to use the above formulations in anticipation of the empirical versions of these equations given later on [see, e.g., (13.30)–(13.32) in the sequel]. We keep in mind that, under the previous assumptions, (13.6)–(13.8) jointly imply that $H(\cdot|\cdot)$, $H^{(0)}(\cdot|\cdot)$, and $H^{(1)}(\cdot|\cdot)$ are continuous on $\mathbb{R}^+ \times J$.

For each $u \in J$, let $\omega_X(u) = \sup\{t : F(t|u) < 1\}$, $\omega_Y(u) = \sup\{t : G(t|u) < 1\}$, and $\omega_Z(u) = \omega_X(u) \wedge \omega_Y(u) = \sup\{t : H(t|u) < 1\}$ denote the upper endpoints of the conditional distributions of X, Y, and Z, respectively, given that $U = u$. A direct consequence of (13.6)–(13.7) is that, for each specified $u \in J$,

$F(t|u)$ and $G(t|u)$ are uniquely defined for $t \in [0, \omega_Z(u))$ as the right-continuous joint solutions of the differential system

$$dF(t|u) = \frac{dH^{(1)}(t|u)}{1 - G_-(t|u)} \quad \text{and} \quad dG(t|u) = \frac{dH^{(0)}(t|u)}{1 - F_-(t|u)}, \quad (13.9)$$

or, equivalently, via (13.8),

$$\frac{dF(t|u)}{1 - F_-(t|u)} = \frac{dH^{(1)}(t|u)}{1 - H_-(t|u)} \quad \text{and} \quad \frac{dG(t|u)}{1 - G_-(t|u)} = \frac{dH^{(0)}(t|u)}{1 - H_-(t|u)}, \quad (13.10)$$

subject to the boundary conditions

$$F_-(0|u) = G_-(0|u) = 0. \quad (13.11)$$

Among other consequences, the fact that the above equations do not make sense when $t > \omega_Z(u)$ illustrates the property that our data set does not carry any detailed information on $F(t|u)$ and $G(t|u)$ for $t > \omega_Z(u)$. We will therefore restrict our interest to the values of $t \in [0, C]$, where C denotes a specified constant, fulfilling, uniformly over $u \in I$,

$$0 < C < \omega_Z(u). \quad (13.12)$$

By continuity of $H(\cdot|\cdot)$ on $\mathbb{R}^+ \times I$, we infer from (13.12) the existence of a constant $\gamma = \gamma(C, I) \in (0, \frac{1}{2})$ such that

$$1 - 2\gamma := \sup_{u \in I} H(C|u) < 1. \quad (13.13)$$

In the next section, we will describe a class of nonparametric estimators $F_{n,a}(x|u)$ of $F(x|u)$ [respectively, $G_{n,a}(y|u)$ of $G(y|u)$] depending upon a smoothing factor $a > 0$. We will establish their uniform consistency over $(x, u) \in [0, C] \times I$, viz., by showing, in Theorem 13.1.2 that, under suitable conditions imposed upon $a = a_n$, we have, almost surely as $n \to \infty$,

$$\sup_{0 \le x \le C} \sup_{u \in I} |F_{n,a}(x|u) - F(x|u)| \to 0, \quad (13.14)$$

and

$$\sup_{0 \le y \le C} \sup_{u \in I} |G_{n,a}(x|u) - G(x|u)| \to 0. \quad (13.15)$$

13.1.2 Definition of the estimators and uniform consistency

With the aim of estimating $F(x|u)$ and $G(y|u)$, we start by introducing a general kernel $K(\cdot)$, defined as a right-continuous function fulfilling the conditions $(K.1-3)$ below.

(K.1)   The total variation $\|dK\| := \int_{\mathbb{R}} |dK(t)|$ of K on $\mathbb{R}$ is bounded;

(K.2) $\int_{\mathbb{R}} K(t)dt = 1$;

(K.3)   There exists an $M < \infty$ such that $K(t) = 0$ for $|t| \geq M/2$.

We consider further two sequences of positive constants $\{a'_n : n \geq 1\}$ and $\{a''_n : n \geq 1\}$, such that

$$0 < a'_n \leq a''_n \quad \text{for each} \quad n \geq 1, \tag{13.16}$$

$$na'_n / \log n \to \infty \quad \text{and} \quad a''_n \to 0. \tag{13.17}$$

We set, for each $n \geq 1$, $\mathcal{A}_n = [a'_n, a''_n]$. The estimators that will be introduced in this section will be indexed by a positive bandwidth $a > 0$. In practice, one needs to select this factor in a way that is appropriate to the data set [see, e.g., Deheuvels and Mason (2004)]. This question, for the estimators, which will be introduced below, will be considered elsewhere. In this chapter, we will limit ourselves to show, in Theorem 13.1.2, that the uniform strong consistency of our estimators will hold independently of the choice of $a \in \mathcal{A}_n$. Our estimators of $F(x|u)$ and $G(y|u)$ are defined as follows.

First, we introduce a kernel density estimator of $\kappa(u)$ [refer to Parzen (1962) and Rosenblatt (1958)], defined, for each choice of $u \in \mathbb{R}$, $n \geq 1$, and of the bandwidth $a > 0$, by

$$\kappa_{n,a}(u) = \frac{1}{na} \sum_{i=1}^{n} K\left(\frac{u - U_i}{a}\right). \tag{13.18}$$

Second, we introduce, for each $n \geq 1$ and $a > 0$, an array of random (and possibly negative) weights $\{W_{i,n,a}(u) : 1 \leq i \leq n\}$, by setting, for $1 \leq i \leq n$,

$$W_{i,n,a}(u) = \frac{K\left(\frac{u-U_i}{a}\right)}{\sum_{j=1}^{n} K\left(\frac{u-U_j}{a}\right)} = \frac{1}{\kappa_{n,a}(u)} \left\{ \frac{1}{na} K\left(\frac{u - U_i}{a}\right) \right\}, \tag{13.19}$$

when $\kappa_{n,a}(u) \neq 0$, and

$$W_{i,n,a}(u) = \frac{1}{n}, \tag{13.20}$$

when $\kappa_{n,a}(u) = 0$. We then set

$$
\begin{aligned}
H_{n,a}(z|u) &= \sum_{i=1}^{n} W_{i,n,a}(u) \mathbb{1}_{\{Z_i \leq z\}} = \frac{\sum_{i=1}^{n} \mathbb{1}_{\{Z_i \leq z\}} K\left(\frac{u-U_i}{a}\right)}{\sum_{i=1}^{n} K\left(\frac{u-U_i}{a}\right)} \\
&= \frac{1}{\kappa_{n,a}(u)} \sum_{i=1}^{n} \mathbb{1}_{\{Z_i \leq z\}}\left\{ \frac{1}{na} K\left(\frac{u-U_i}{a}\right)\right\} =: \frac{R_{n,a}(z|u)}{\kappa_{n,a}(u)}, \quad (13.21)
\end{aligned}
$$

$$
\begin{aligned}
H_{n,a}^{(0)}(z|u) &= \sum_{i=1}^{n} W_{i,n,a}(u) \mathbb{1}_{\{Z_i \leq z\}}(1-\delta_i) = \frac{\sum_{i=1}^{n} \mathbb{1}_{\{Z_i \leq z\}}(1-\delta_i) K\left(\frac{u-U_i}{a}\right)}{\sum_{i=1}^{n} K\left(\frac{u-U_i}{a}\right)} \\
&= \frac{1}{\kappa_{n,a}(u)} \sum_{i=1}^{n} \mathbb{1}_{\{Z_i \leq z\}}(1-\delta_i)\left\{ \frac{1}{na} K\left(\frac{u-U_i}{a}\right)\right\} =: \frac{R_{n,a}^{(0)}(z|u)}{\kappa_{n,a}(u)},
\end{aligned}
$$

$$(13.22)$$

$$
\begin{aligned}
H_{n,a}^{(1)}(z|u) &= \sum_{i=1}^{n} W_{i,n,a}(u) \mathbb{1}_{\{Z_i \leq z\}}\delta_i = \frac{\sum_{i=1}^{n} \mathbb{1}_{\{Z_i \leq z\}}\delta_i K\left(\frac{u-U_i}{a}\right)}{\sum_{i=1}^{n} K\left(\frac{u-U_i}{a}\right)} \\
&= \frac{1}{\kappa_{n,a}(u)} \sum_{i=1}^{n} \mathbb{1}_{\{Z_i \leq z\}}\delta_i\left\{ \frac{1}{na} K\left(\frac{u-U_i}{a}\right)\right\} =: \frac{R_{n,a}^{(1)}(z|u)}{\kappa_{n,a}(u)}, \quad (13.23)
\end{aligned}
$$

whenever $\kappa_{n,a}(u) \neq 0$, and

$$
H_{n,a}(z|u) = \sum_{i=1}^{n} W_{i,n,a}(u) \mathbb{1}_{\{Z_i \leq z\}} = \frac{1}{n}\sum_{i=1}^{n} \mathbb{1}_{\{Z_i \leq z\}}, \quad (13.24)
$$

$$
H_{n,a}^{(0)}(z|u) = \sum_{i=1}^{n} W_{i,n,a}(u) \mathbb{1}_{\{Z_i \leq z\}}(1-\delta_i) = \frac{1}{n}\sum_{i=1}^{n} \mathbb{1}_{\{Z_i \leq z\}}(1-\delta_i), \quad (13.25)
$$

$$
H_{n,a}^{(1)}(z|u) = \sum_{i=1}^{n} W_{i,n,a}(u) \mathbb{1}_{\{Z_i \leq z\}}\delta_i = \frac{1}{n}\sum_{i=1}^{n} \mathbb{1}_{\{Z_i \leq z\}}\delta_i, \quad (13.26)
$$

when $\kappa_{n,a}(u) = 0$.

The following proposition turns out to follow, either directly [for (13.27)–(13.28) below], or after some routine adaptations of the proofs [for (13.29) below], from Corollary 1 and Theorem 3 of Einmahl and Mason (2005), and so the corresponding details are omitted.

Proposition 13.1.1 *Under the assumptions above, we have, almost surely*

$$\sup_{a \in \mathcal{A}_n} \sup_{u \in I} |\kappa_{n,a}(u) - \kappa(u)| = o(1), \tag{13.27}$$

$$\sup_{a \in \mathcal{A}_n} \sup_{u \in I} \sup_{z \in \mathbb{R}^+} |H_{n,a}(z|u) - H(z|u)| = o(1), \tag{13.28}$$

and, for $\ell = 0, 1$,

$$\sup_{a \in \mathcal{A}_n} \sup_{u \in I} \sup_{z \in \mathbb{R}^+} |H_{n,a}^{(\ell)}(z|u) - H^\ell(z|u)| = o(1). \tag{13.29}$$

In view of these preliminary results, it becomes very logical to define our estimators of $F(x|u)$ and $G(y|u)$, denoted, respectively, by $F_{n,a}(x|u)$ and $G_{n,a}(y|u)$, as the joint solutions, whenever they exist, of the differential system obtained by the formal replacements in (13.9)–(13.11) of $H^{(0)}(t|u)$, $H^{(1)}(t|u)$, and $H(t|u)$, respectively, by their empirical counterparts $H_{n,a}^{(0)}(t|u)$, $H_{n,a}^{(1)}(t|u)$, and $H_{n,a}(t|u)$, as defined in (13.21)–(13.26). By so doing, we are led to the differential system

$$dF_{n,a}(t|u) = \frac{dH_{n,a}^{(1)}(t|u)}{1 - G_{n,a-}(t|u)} \quad \text{and} \quad dG_{n,a}(t|u) = \frac{dH_{n,a}^{(0)}(t|u)}{1 - F_{n,a-}(t|u)}, \tag{13.30}$$

or, equivalently (see, e.g., Remark 13.1.1),

$$\frac{dF_{n,a}(t|u)}{1 - F_{n,a-}(t|u)} = \frac{dH_{n,a}^{(1)}(t|u)}{1 - H_{n,a-}(t|u)} \quad \text{and} \quad \frac{dG_{n,a}(t|u)}{1 - G_{n,a-}(t|u)} = \frac{dH_{n,a}^{(0)}(t|u)}{1 - H_{n,a-}(t|u)}, \tag{13.31}$$

subject to the boundary conditions

$$F_{n,a-}(0|u) = G_{n,a-}(0|u) = 0. \tag{13.32}$$

It turns out, rather surprisingly, that the solutions of the differential system (13.30)–(13.32) have simple closed-form expressions in terms of the random weights $\{W_{i,n,a}(u) : 1 \leq i \leq n\}$, and ranks $\{r_{i,n} : 1 \leq i \leq n\}$, as defined in (13.1) and (13.19)–(13.20). These are given as follows. For notational convenience, we define below a sequence of ranked random weights $\{w_{i,n,a}(u) : 1 \leq i \leq n\}$. Recalling the definition (13.2) of $\{U_{i:n} : 1 \leq i \leq n\}$, we set, for $u \in \mathbb{R}$, $a > 0$, and $1 \leq i \leq n$,

$$w_{i,n,a}(u) = W_{r_{i,n},n,a}(u) = \frac{K\left(\frac{u - U_{i:n}}{a}\right)}{\sum_{j=1}^n K\left(\frac{u - U_{j:n}}{a}\right)} = \frac{1}{\kappa_{n,a}(u)}\left\{\frac{1}{na}K\left(\frac{u - U_{i:n}}{a}\right)\right\}, \tag{13.33}$$

whenever $\kappa_{n,a}(u) \neq 0$, and

$$w_{i,n,a}(u) = W_{r_{i,n},n,a}(u) = \frac{1}{n}, \tag{13.34}$$

when $\kappa_{n,a}(u) = 0$. Next, recalling the definitions (13.21)–(13.24), of $H_{n,a}(z|u)$, and (13.33)–(13.34), of $w_{i,n,a}(u)$, we introduce a random index, defined, for each $u \in \mathbb{R}$, $a > 0$, and $n \geq 1$ by

$$N_{n,a}(u) = \min\left\{i \in \{1,\ldots,n\} : \sum_{j=1}^{i} w_{j,n,a}(u) = 1\right\}$$

$$= \min\left\{i \in \{1,\ldots,n\} : H_{n,a}(Z_{i,n}|u) = 1\right\}. \qquad (13.35)$$

Because of the fact [obvious, via (13.21)–(13.24)] that $H_{n,a}(Z_{n,n}|u) = 1$, the index $N_{n,a}(u) \in \{1,\ldots,n\}$ always exists. The following simple lemma gives a useful limiting property of this statistic.

Lemma 13.1.1 *Under the assumptions above, we have, almost surely for all n sufficiently large,*

$$\inf_{a \in \mathcal{A}_n} \inf_{u \in I} Z_{N_{n,a}(u),n} \geq C. \qquad (13.36)$$

PROOF. In view of (13.35), it is enough to show that the inequality

$$\sup_{a \in \mathcal{A}_n} \sup_{u \in I} H_{n,a}(C|u) < 1$$

holds ultimately in $n \to \infty$ with probability 1. This, however, is a direct consequence of (13.12)–(13.13), when combined with (13.28). ∎

   We are now ready to state the first main result of this chapter, giving explicit closed-form expressions for the solutions $F_{n,a}(x|u)$ and $G_{n,a}(y|u)$ of the differential system (13.30)–(13.32). In the statement of the theorem, we use the conventions that $\sum_{\emptyset}(\cdot) = 0$ and $\prod_{\emptyset}(\cdot) = 1$.

Theorem 13.1.1 *For each $u \in \mathbb{R}$, $n \geq 1$, and $a > 0$, the solutions $F_{n,a}(x|u)$ and $G_{n,a}(y|u)$ of the differential system (13.30)–(13.31), subject to the boundary conditions (13.32), are uniquely defined over $t \in [0, Z_{N_{n,a}(u),n})$, and coincide on this interval with the functions defined on $\mathbb{R}^+$ by*

$$F_{n,a}(t|u) = 1 - \prod_{i:Z_{i,n} \leq t} \left\{\frac{1 - \sum_{j=1}^{i} w_{j,n,a}(u)}{1 - \sum_{j=1}^{i-1} w_{j,n,a}(u)}\right\}^{\delta_{i:n}} \qquad when \quad t < Z_{N_{n,a}(u),n},$$

$$= 1 \quad when \quad t \geq Z_{N_{n,a}(u),n}, \qquad (13.37)$$

and

$$G_{n,a}(t|u) = 1 - \prod_{i:Z_{i,n} \leq t} \left\{\frac{1 - \sum_{j=1}^{i} w_{j,n,a}(u)}{1 - \sum_{j=1}^{i-1} w_{j,n,a}(u)}\right\}^{1-\delta_{i:n}} \qquad when \quad t < Z_{N_{n,a}(u),n},$$

$$= 1 \quad when \quad t \geq Z_{N_{n,a}(u),n}. \qquad (13.38)$$

The proof of Theorem 13.1.1 is postponed until Section 13.2.

Remark 13.1.1 (1) It is obvious from the definition (13.25) of $N_{n,a}(u)$ that $F_{n,a}(\cdot|\cdot)$ and $G_{n,a}(\cdot|\cdot)$ are properly defined by (13.37)–(13.38), and fulfill

$$H_{n,a}(t|u) = 1 - \big(1 - F_{n,a}(t|u)\big)\big(1 - G_{n,a}(t|u)\big) \quad \text{for} \quad t < Z_{N_{n,a}(u),n}. \quad (13.39)$$

On the other hand, the equality on the left-hand side of (13.39) may not be true for some $t \geq Z_{N_{n,a}(u),n}$. If that is the case, we see that the equivalence between the differential systems (13.30) and (13.31) fails to hold in the interval $[Z_{N_{n,a}(u),n}, \infty)$.

(2) As a consequence of (1), there exists almost surely an $n_0 = n_0(C, I)$ such that, for all $n \geq n_0$, (13.39) holds uniformly over $t \in [0, C]$, $u \in I$, and $a \in \mathcal{A}_n$, with $F_{n,a}(t|u) < 1$ and $G_{n,a}(t|u) < 1$ being properly defined by (13.37)–(13.38). We will make a repeated implicit use of this observation in the remainder of this chapter.

Our second theorem gives a general uniform consistency result of our estimators.

Theorem 13.1.2 *Under the assumptions above, we have, almost surely*

$$\sup_{a \in \mathcal{A}_n} \sup_{u \in I} \sup_{x \in [0,C]} |F_{n,a}(x|u) - F(x|u)| = o(1), \quad (13.40)$$

and

$$\sup_{a \in \mathcal{A}_n} \sup_{u \in I} \sup_{x \in [0,C]} |G_{n,a}(y|u) - G(y|u)| = o(1). \quad (13.41)$$

The proof of Theorem 13.1.2 will be given in Section 13.2. The study of rates of consistency for these estimators will be investigated elsewhere.

13.2 Proofs

13.2.1 Construction of the estimators

In the present subsection, we give a proof of Theorem 13.1.1, together with additional details on the construction of our estimators. We recall that the distribution function $H(z) = \mathbb{P}(Z \leq z) = 1 - (1 - F(z))(1 - G(z))$ is continuous, and that the order statistics $Z_{1,n}, \ldots, Z_{n,n}$ of $Z_1, \ldots, Z_n$ are almost surely distinct and fulfilling

$$0 < Z_{1,n} < \cdots < Z_{n,n}. \quad (13.42)$$

For convenience, we will set, in the sequel,

$$Z_{0,n} = 0 \quad \text{and} \quad Z_{n+1,n} = \infty. \tag{13.43}$$

The strict inequalities in (13.42) allow us to define, on the event where (13.42) holds, a unique permutation $\{r_{1,n}, \ldots, r_{n,n}\}$ of $\{1, \ldots, n\}$, such that, for $i = 1, \ldots, n$,

$$Z_{r_{1,n}} = Z_{i,n}. \tag{13.44}$$

In view of (13.42)–(13.44), we set, for $i = 1, \ldots, n$,

$$\delta_{i:n} = \delta_{r_{i,n}}. \tag{13.45}$$

Let now $\pi_{1:n}, \ldots, \pi_{n:n}$ be any sequence of (possibly negative) weights fulfilling $\pi_{1:n} + \cdots + \pi_{n:n} = 1$, and set

$$n_\pi = \min\Big\{ i \in \{1, \ldots, n\} : \sum_{j=1}^{i} \pi_{j:n} = 1 \Big\}. \tag{13.46}$$

Keeping in mind that $1 \le n_\pi \le n$, we set further

$$\mathcal{H}_{n;\pi}^{(0)}(z) = \sum_{j:Z_{j,n}\le z} \pi_{j:n}(1 - \delta_{j:n}), \tag{13.47}$$

and

$$\mathcal{H}_{n;\pi}^{(1)}(z) = \sum_{j:Z_{j,n}\le z} \pi_{j:n}\delta_{j:n}. \tag{13.48}$$

Throughout, we make use of the convention that $\sum_\emptyset(\cdot) = 0$. In particular, in (13.51)–(13.52) below, we set $\sum_{j=1}^{0} \pi_{j:n} = 0$. We next define $\mathcal{F}_{n;\pi}(z)$ and $\mathcal{G}_{n;\pi}(z)$ for $z \in \mathbb{R}^+$ as follows.

– When $\sum_{i=1}^{n_\pi} \delta_i = 0$, we set, for all $z \in \mathbb{R}^+$,

$$\mathcal{F}_{n;\pi}(z) = 0 \quad \text{and} \quad \mathcal{G}_{n;\pi}(z) = \mathcal{H}_{n;\pi}^{(0)}(z). \tag{13.49}$$

– When $\sum_{i=1}^{n_\pi} (1 - \delta_i) = 0$, we set, for all $z \in \mathbb{R}^+$,

$$\mathcal{F}_{n;\pi}(z) = \mathcal{H}_{n;\pi}^{(1)}(z), \quad \text{and} \quad \mathcal{G}_{n;\pi}(z) = 0. \tag{13.50}$$

– When $0 < \sum_{i=1}^{n_\pi} \delta_i < n_\pi$, we set

$$\mathcal{F}_{n;\pi}(z) = \begin{cases} 1 - \displaystyle\prod_{i:Z_{i,n}\le z} \left\{ \dfrac{1 - \sum_{j=1}^{i} \pi_{j:n}}{1 - \sum_{j=1}^{i-1} \pi_{j:n}} \right\}^{\delta_{i:n}} & \text{for } z < Z_{n_\pi,n}, \\[4mm] 1 & \text{for } z \ge Z_{n_\pi,n}. \end{cases} \tag{13.51}$$

$$\mathcal{G}_{n;\pi}(z) = \begin{cases} 1 - \displaystyle\prod_{i:Z_{i,n}\le z} \left\{ \dfrac{1 - \sum_{j=1}^{i} \pi_{j:n}}{1 - \sum_{j=1}^{i-1} \pi_{j:n}} \right\}^{1-\delta_{i:n}} & \text{for } z < Z_{n_\pi,n}, \\[4mm] 1 & \text{for } z \ge Z_{n_\pi,n}. \end{cases} \tag{13.52}$$

Theorem 13.2.1 *The differential system*

$$d\mathcal{G}_n(z) = \frac{d\mathcal{H}_{n;\pi}^{(0)}(z)}{1 - \mathcal{F}_{n-}(z)}, \quad \text{and} \quad d\mathcal{F}_n(z) = \frac{d\mathcal{H}_{n;\pi}^{(1)}(z)}{1 - \mathcal{G}_{n-}(z)}. \tag{13.53}$$

with limit conditions

$$\mathcal{F}_{n-}(0) = \mathcal{G}_{n-}(0) = 0, \tag{13.54}$$

has a pair of right-continuous solutions, uniquely defined on $[0, Z_{n_\pi,n})$ by $\mathcal{F}_n(z) = \mathcal{F}_{n;\pi}(z)$ and $\mathcal{G}_n(z) = \mathcal{G}_{n;\pi}(z)$.

PROOF. We will limit ourselves to the case where $n_\pi = n$. The proof of the theorem when $1 \le n_\pi < n$ turns out to follow from simple modifications of our arguments, and the details will be therefore omitted. Set $S_n = \delta_1 + \cdots + \delta_n$.

– When $S_n = 0$, we infer from (13.51)–(13.52) that $\mathcal{F}_{n;\pi}(z) = 0$ for all $z < Z_{n,n}$, whereas, for $i = 0, \ldots, n$ and $Z_{i,n} \le z < Z_{i+1,n}$,

$$\mathcal{G}_{n;\pi}(z) = \sum_{j=1}^{i} \pi_{j:n} = \sum_{j=1}^{i} \pi_{j:n}(1 - \delta_{j:n}) = \mathcal{H}_{n;\pi}^{(0)}(z).$$

It is now straightforward that the so-defined $\mathcal{F}_{n;\pi}(z)$ and $\mathcal{G}_{n;\pi}(z)$ are solutions on $[0, Z_{n,n})$ of the differential system (13.53). The arguments are very similar when $S_n = n$ and shall be omitted.

– We now turn to the only remaining case where $0 < s := S_n < 1$, and define a sequence of indices $1 \le j_1 < \cdots < j_s \le n$ in such a way that $\delta_{i:n} = 1$ iff $i \in \{j_1, \ldots, j_s\}$. Obviously, for $Z_{j_{m-1},n} \le z < Z_{j_m,n}$,

$$1 - \mathcal{F}_{n;\pi}(z) = 1 - \mathcal{F}_{n;\pi}(Z_{j_{m-1},n}), \tag{13.55}$$

whereas, for $z = Z_{j_m,n}$,

$$1 - \mathcal{F}_{n;\pi}(Z_{j_m,n}) = \left\{1 - \mathcal{F}_{n;\pi}(Z_{j_{m-1},n})\right\}\left\{\frac{1 - \sum_{i=1}^{j_m} \pi_{i:n}}{1 - \sum_{i=1}^{j_m-1} \pi_{i:n}}\right\}$$

$$= \mathcal{F}_{n;\pi}(Z_{j_{m-1},n}) + \left\{1 - \mathcal{F}_{n;\pi}(Z_{j_{m-1},n})\right\}\left\{\frac{\pi_{j_m:n}}{1 - \sum_{i=1}^{j_m-1} \pi_{i:n}}\right\}.$$

Now, we use the observation that

$$\left\{1 - \mathcal{F}_{n;\pi}(Z_{j_{m-1},n})\right\}\left\{1 - \mathcal{G}_{n;\pi}(Z_{j_{m-1},n})\right\} = 1 - \sum_{i=1}^{j_{m-1}} \pi_{i:n},$$

so that

$$\mathcal{F}_{n;\pi}(Z_{j_m,n}) = \mathcal{F}_{n;\pi}(Z_{j_{m-1},n}) + \frac{\pi_{j_m:n}}{1 - \mathcal{G}_{n;\pi}(Z_{j_{m-1},n})}\left\{\frac{1 - \sum_{i=1}^{j_{m-1}} \pi_{i:n}}{1 - \sum_{i=1}^{j_m-1} \pi_{i:n}}\right\}$$

$$= \mathcal{F}_{n;\pi}(Z_{j_{m-1},n}) + \frac{d\mathcal{H}_{n;\pi}^{(1)}(Z_{j_m,n})}{1 - \mathcal{G}_{n;\pi}(Z_{j_{m-1},n})}.$$

This, in turn, suffices to show that $\mathcal{F}_{n;\pi}$ satisfies the differential system (13.53) on $(Z_{j_{m-1},n}, Z_{j_m,n}]$. By combining this property with a straightforward induction, and a similar argument for $\mathcal{G}_{n;\pi}$, we readily conclude the proof of Theorem 13.2.1. ∎

PROOF OF THEOREM 13.1.1. It suffices to apply Theorem 13.2.1 in the particular case where the weights are given by $\pi_{i:n} = w_{i,n,a}(u)$ for $1 \leq i \leq n$. ∎

13.2.2 A useful auxiliary result

In this section, we will show that the proof of Theorem 13.1.2 turns out to be a simple consequence of Proposition 13.1.1, when combined with a useful auxiliary result of independent interest, stated in Proposition 13.2.1. Consider, in general, two pairs of right-continuous distribution functions $\mathcal{F}_\ell$ and $\mathcal{G}_\ell$, $\ell = 1, 2$. Set, for $z \in \mathbb{R}$ and $\ell = 1, 2$,

$$\mathcal{H}_\ell^{(0)}(z) = \int_{(0,z]} \big(1 - \mathcal{F}_{\ell-}(t)\big) d\mathcal{G}_\ell(t), \tag{13.56}$$

$$\mathcal{H}_\ell^{(1)}(z) = \int_{(0,z]} \big(1 - \mathcal{G}_{\ell-}(t)\big) d\mathcal{F}_\ell(t), \tag{13.57}$$

$$\mathcal{H}_\ell(z) = 1 - \big(1 - \mathcal{F}_\ell(z)\big)\big(1 - \mathcal{G}_\ell(z)\big)$$

$$= \mathcal{H}_\ell^{(0)}(z) + \mathcal{H}_\ell^{(1)}(z). \tag{13.58}$$

We have the following proposition.

Proposition 13.2.1 *Let $c > 0$ and $\theta > 0$ be such that, for $\ell = 0, 1$,*

$$\sup_{0 \leq t \leq c} |\mathcal{H}_1^{(\ell)}(t) - \mathcal{H}_2^{(\ell)}(t)| \leq \theta. \tag{13.59}$$

Assume further that, for some $0 < \rho < 1$,

$$\mathcal{H}_1(c) \vee \mathcal{H}_2(c) \leq \rho < 1. \tag{13.60}$$

Then, we have

$$\sup_{0 \leq x \leq c} |\mathcal{F}_1(x) - \mathcal{F}_2(x)| \leq \frac{4\theta}{(1-\rho)^2}. \tag{13.61}$$

PROOF. Under (13.59), we infer from (13.58) the inequalities

$$\sup_{0 \leq t \leq c} |\mathcal{H}_{1\pm}(t) - \mathcal{H}_{2\pm}(t)|$$

$$\leq \sup_{0 \leq t \leq c} |\mathcal{H}_1^{(0)}(t) - \mathcal{H}_2^{(0)}(t)| + \sup_{0 \leq t \leq c} |\mathcal{H}_1^{(1)}(t) - \mathcal{H}_2^{(1)}(t)| \leq 2\theta. \tag{13.62}$$

Moreover, we infer from (13.60) and (13.58) that, uniformly over $0 \le t \le c$, and $\ell = 0, 1$,

$$0 \le \mathcal{H}_{1\pm}^{(\ell)}(t) \vee \mathcal{H}_{2\pm}^{(\ell)}(t) \le \mathcal{H}_1(t) \vee \mathcal{H}_2(t) \le \rho < 1. \qquad (13.63)$$

Observe that, for $\ell = 1, 2$, $\mathcal{F}_\ell(t)$ and $\mathcal{G}_\ell(t)$ are joint solutions over $t \in [0, c]$ of the differential system

$$\frac{d\mathcal{F}_\ell(t)}{1 - \mathcal{F}_{\ell-}(t)} = \frac{d\mathcal{H}_\ell^{(1)}(t)}{1 - \mathcal{H}_{\ell-}(t)} \quad \text{and} \quad \frac{d\mathcal{G}_\ell(t)}{1 - \mathcal{G}_{\ell-}(t)} = \frac{d\mathcal{H}_\ell^{(0)}(t)}{1 - \mathcal{H}_{\ell-}(t)}, \qquad (13.64)$$

subject to the boundary conditions

$$\mathcal{F}_{\ell-}(0) = \mathcal{G}_{\ell-}(0) = 0. \qquad (13.65)$$

Thus, making use of (13.64) and integrating by parts, we may write, for $0 \le x \le c$,

$$
\begin{aligned}
\Delta(x) \; := \; & \left\{ -\log\left(1 - \mathcal{F}_1(x)\right) \right\} - \left\{ -\log\left(1 - \mathcal{F}_2(x)\right) \right\} \\
= \; & \int_{(0,x]} \left\{ \frac{d\mathcal{F}_1(t)}{1 - \mathcal{F}_{1-}(t)} \right\} - \int_{(0,x]} \left\{ \frac{d\mathcal{F}_2(t)}{1 - \mathcal{F}_{2-}(t)} \right\} \\
= \; & \int_{(0,x]} \left\{ \frac{d\mathcal{H}_1^{(1)}(t)}{1 - \mathcal{H}_{1-}(t)} \right\} - \int_{(0,x]} \left\{ \frac{d\mathcal{H}_2^{(1)}(t)}{1 - \mathcal{H}_{2-}(t)} \right\} \\
= \; & \int_{(0,x]} \left\{ \frac{\left(1 - \mathcal{H}_{2-}(t)\right) - \left(1 - \mathcal{H}_{1-}(t)\right)}{\left(1 - \mathcal{H}_{2-}(t)\right)\left(1 - \mathcal{H}_{1-}(t)\right)} \right\} d\mathcal{H}_1^{(1)}(t) \\
& + \int_{(0,x]} \left\{ \frac{1}{1 - \mathcal{H}_{2-}(t)} \right\} d\left\{ \mathcal{H}_1^{(1)}(t) - \mathcal{H}_2^{(1)}(t) \right\} \\
= \; & \int_{(0,x]} \left\{ \frac{\mathcal{H}_{1-}(t) - \mathcal{H}_{2-}(t)}{\left(1 - \mathcal{H}_{2-}(t)\right)\left(1 - \mathcal{H}_{1-}(t)\right)} \right\} d\mathcal{H}_1^{(1)}(t) + \frac{\mathcal{H}_1^{(1)}(x) - \mathcal{H}_2^{(1)}(x)}{1 - \mathcal{H}_{2-}(x)} \\
& - \int_{(0,x]} \left\{ \mathcal{H}_1^{(1)}(t) - \mathcal{H}_2^{(1)}(t) \right\} \left\{ \frac{d\mathcal{H}_2(t)}{\left(1 - \mathcal{H}_{2-}(t)\right)^2} \right\}.
\end{aligned}
$$

This, in turn, readily implies, via (13.62) and (13.63), that

$$\sup_{0 \le x \le c} |\Delta(x)| \le \frac{2\theta}{(1 - \rho)^2} + \frac{\theta}{1 - \rho} + \frac{\theta}{(1 - \rho)^2} \le \frac{4\theta}{(1 - \rho)^2}. \qquad (13.66)$$

Next, we infer from Taylor's formula that, for each choice of $0 \le u \le v < 1$, there exists a $w \in [u, v]$ for which

$$\left\{ -\log(1 - v) \right\} - \left\{ -\log(1 - u) \right\} = \frac{v - u}{1 - w} > v - u.$$

We have, therefore, for any $0 \leq u, v \leq 1$,

$$|v - u| \leq \left| \left\{ -\log(1 - v) \right\} - \left\{ -\log(1 - u) \right\} \right|,$$

so that we infer readily (13.61) from (13.66), by setting $u = \mathcal{F}_1(x)$ and $v = \mathcal{F}_2(x)$ in this last inequality.   ∎

PROOF OF THEOREM 13.1.2. It is a straightforward consequence of Propositions 13.1.1 and 13.2.1, in combination with Theorem 13.1.2.   ∎

13.2.3 Concluding comments

The well-known results [see, e.g., Deheuvels and Mason (2004) and the references therein] concerning the consistency of Nadaraya–Watson regression estimators (which are obtained as a special case of our estimators, as mentioned in Section 13.1), show readily that the conditions of our theorems are sharp.

References

1. Burke, M. D., Csörgő, S., and Horváth, L. (1981). Strong approximations of some biometric estimates under random censorship, *Z. Wahrsch. Verw. Gebiete*, **56**, 87–112.

2. Burke, M. D., Csörgő, S., and Horváth, L. (1988). A correction to and an improvement of strong approximations of some biometric estimates under random censorship, *Probability Theory and Related Fields*, **56**, 87–112.

3. Deheuvels, P., and Einmahl, J. H. J. (2000). Functional limit laws for the increments of Kaplan-Meier product-limit processes and applications, *The Annals of Statistics*, **28**, 1301–1335.

4. Deheuvels, P., and Mason, D. M. (2004). General asymptotic confidence bands based on kernel-type function estimators, *Statistical Inference for Stochastic Processes*, **7**, 225–277.

5. Einmahl, U., and Mason, D. M. (2000). An empirical approach to the uniform consistency of kernel-type function estimators, *Journal of Theoretical Probability*, **13**, 1–37.

6. Einmahl, U., and Mason, D. M. (2005). Uniform in bandwidth consistency of kernel-type function estimators, *Annals of Probability*, **33**, 1380–1403.

7. Földes, A., Rejtő, L., and Winter, B. B. (1981). A LIL type result for the product-limit estimator, *Z. Wahrsch. Verw. Gebiete*, **56**, 75–86.

8. Gill, R. D. (1980). *Censoring and Stochastic Integrals*, Mathematisch Centrum Tracts, Amsterdam, The Netherlands.

9. Härdle, W. (1990). *Applied Nonparametric Regression*, Cambridge University Press, Cambridge.

10. Kaplan, E. L., and Meier, P. (1958). Nonparametric estimation for incomplete observations, *Journal of the American Statistical Association*, **53**, 457–481.

11. Nadaraya, E. A. (1964). On estimating regression, *Theory of Probability and Its Applications*, **9**, 141–142.

12. Nadaraya, E. A. (1989). *Nonparametric Estimation of Probability Densities and Regression Curves*, Kluwer, Dordrecht, The Netherlands.

13. Watson, G. S. (1964). Smooth regression analysis, *Sankhyā, Series A*, **26**, 359–372.

14. Stute, W. (1986). On almost sure convergence of conditional empirical distribution functions, *The Annals of Statistics*, **14**, 891–901.

15. Stute, W. (1995). The central limit theorem under random censorship, *The Annals of Statistics*, **23**, 86–107.

14

Sequential Estimation for the Semiparametric Additive Hazard Model

L. Bordes and C. Breuils

University of Technology of Compiègne, LMAC, Compiègne, France
University of Metz, LMAM, Metz, France

Abstract: In this chapter, we investigate the asymptotic behavior of the sequential version of the regression parameter estimator for the additive hazard model. We mainly establish that the Lin and Ying (1994) nonsequential estimator is strongly consistent (in the sense of complete convergence) and that this estimator, indexed by any regular sequence (sequential estimator), has the same asymptotic behavior as the nonsequential estimator. An example of a fixed-width confidence-type sequential estimator is illustrated by simulations.

Keywords and phrases: Semiparametric additive hazard model, sequential estimation, right-censored survival data, complete convergence

14.1 Introduction

In semiparametric survival studies, Cox's (1972) proportional hazards model (PHM) is certainly the most popular among lifetime regression models. However, several studies [see, for example, Huffer and McKeague (1991)] showed that the hazard rate proportionality assumption is not satisfied and it is therefore necessary to use alternative models. The additive hazards regression model [Cox and Oakes (1984)], studied by Lin and Ying (1994), like the PHM, allows easy interpretation of the covariates effect. Formally, the hazard rate function $\lambda(t; Z)$ of a duration T, given a covariate process Z, is defined at time $t \in \mathbb{R}^+$, by

$$\lambda(t; Z) = \lambda_0(t) + \beta_0^T Z(t), \tag{14.1}$$

where λ_0 is a baseline hazard rate function (a nuisance parameter in this study) and $\beta_0 \in \mathbb{R}^p$ a vector of regression parameters.

In many studies, the cost of the study is linked to the total duration of the experiments or to the number of experiments. This is the reason why we need to propose an earlier stop of the study without deteriorating the quality of the estimators [see Lai (2001) for a recent overview on sequential trials]. This naturally leads us to define stopping rules (i.e., criteria), which once they are satisfied, lead to estimators having some prespecified properties. In this chapter, we consider sequential versions of the Lin and Ying (1994) regression estimator.

Let T be the failure time of interest, Z be a covariate vector (that possibly depends on time t), and C be a censoring time that is conditionally independent of T given Z. We are given data on $X = \min(T, C), \delta = I(T \leq C)$ (where $I(\cdot)$ is the set characteristic function), and also on covariates $Z \equiv \{Z(s); s \leq X\}$. The problem is to account for the covariate effect by assuming that the conditional hazard function of T given Z follows model (14.1). Suppose we are given n such independent observations $(X_1, \delta_1, Z_1), \ldots, (X_n, \delta_n, Z_n)$. For simplicity we shall assume that the covariate processes are real-valued. Lin and Ying (1994) proposed to estimate β_0 by $\hat{\beta}_n$, solving $U_n(\hat{\beta}_n, \tau) = 0$, where

$$U_n(\beta, t) = \frac{1}{n} \sum_{i=1}^{n} \int_0^t (Z_i(s) - E_n(s)) (dN_i(s) - Y_i(s)\beta Z_i(s)ds),$$

with τ the (deterministic) upper bound of the time interval of study, and

$$
\begin{aligned}
N_i(s) &= I(X_i \leq s, \delta_i = 1), \qquad Y_i(s) = I(X_i \geq s), \\
\overline{Z}_n^{(k)}(s) &= \frac{1}{n} \sum_{i=1}^{n} Z_i^k(s) Y_i(s), \quad k \in \{0, \ldots, 3\}, \quad E_n = \overline{Z}_n^{(1)} / \overline{Z}_n^{(0)}.
\end{aligned}
$$

From the linearity of U_n with respect to β, the estimator of β_0 has an explicit form

$$\hat{\beta}_n \equiv \hat{\beta}_n(\tau) = \mathcal{I}_n^{-1}(\tau) \times \Theta_n(\tau),$$

where

$$\mathcal{I}_n(\tau) = \int_0^\tau \left(\overline{Z}_n^{(2)}(s) - \overline{Z}_n^{(1)}(s) E_n(s) \right) ds$$

and

$$\Theta_n(\tau) = \frac{1}{n} \sum_{i=1}^{n} \int_0^\tau (Z_i(s) - E_n(s)) \, dN_i(s).$$

It is also interesting to note that $\hat{\beta}_n = \arg\max_{\beta \in \mathbb{R}} C_n(\beta, \tau)$, where $C_n(\beta, \tau) = \beta \Theta_n(\tau) - \beta^2 \mathcal{I}_n(\tau)/2$ is concave (at least asymptotically) and twice continuously differentiable with respect to β. Let us recall that a random sequence of integers $(T_n)_{n \geq 1}$ is regular if there exists a deterministic sequence of integers $(t_n)_{n \geq 1}$ such that (i) $t_n \to +\infty$ as $n \to +\infty$, and (ii) $T_n/t_n \to 1$ in probability, as $n \to +\infty$.

Lin and Ying (1994) proved that $\sqrt{n}(\hat{\beta}_n - \beta_0)$ is asymptotically Gaussian with zero mean and covariance $\sigma_0^2(\tau)$ consistently estimated by $\hat{\sigma}_n^2(\tau) = \mathcal{I}_n^{-2}(\tau)\mathcal{V}_n(\tau)$, where

$$\mathcal{V}_n(\tau) = \frac{1}{n} \sum_{i=1}^n \int_0^\tau (Z_i(s) - E_n(s))^2 \, dN_i(s).$$

In Section 14.3, we introduce general assumptions for which we prove the following results.

(A) $\hat{\beta}_n$ converges completely (see Section 14.4.1) to β_0, as $n \to +\infty$;

(B) For any regular sequence $(T_n)_{n \geq 1}$, $\sqrt{n}(\hat{\beta}_n - \beta_0)$ and $\sqrt{T_n}(\hat{\beta}_{T_n} - \beta_0)$ have the same asymptotic behavior;

(C) $\hat{\sigma}_{T_n}^2(\tau)$ is a consistent estimator of $\sigma_0^2(\tau)$.

14.2   Example and Numerical Study

One of the most popular sequential estimators arises from fixing the length of a α-level confidence set [see, for example, Ghosh *et al.* (1997)] leading to a regular sequence $(N_d)_{d>0}$ of stopping rules defined by

$$N_d = \inf\{n \geq n_0; n \geq \bar{\sigma}_n^2(\tau)u_\alpha^2/d^2\}, \qquad (14.2)$$

where u_α is the quantile of order $1 - \alpha/2$ of a standard Gaussian distribution, n_0 an initial sample size, $2d > 0$ an upper bound of the length of the asymptotic confidence set, and $\bar{\sigma}_n^2 = \max(\hat{\sigma}_n^2, \varepsilon_n)$, where $(\varepsilon_n)_{n \geq 1}$ is a sequence of real numbers decreasing to 0. One can show [see, for example, Ghosh *et al.* (1997) and Breuils (2003)] that such a sequence is regular with respect to the deterministic sequence $(n_d)_{d>0}$, where

$$n_d = \inf\{n \geq n_0; n \geq \sigma_0^2(\tau)u_\alpha^2/d^2\}. \qquad (14.3)$$

Note that here, asymptotics must be understood in the sense that $d \to 0^+$; that is, the smaller the length of the confidence set is, the more accurate is the estimator. Under assumptions given in the next section, we obtain:

(i) $\hat{\beta}_{N_d}$ converges in probability to β_0, as $d \to 0^+$;

(ii) $\sqrt{N_d}(\hat{\beta}_{N_d} - \beta_0)$ converges in distribution to $\mathcal{N}(0, \sigma_0^2(\tau))$, as $d \to 0^+$, where $\mathcal{N}(\mu, \sigma^2)$ denotes a Gaussian distribution with mean μ and variance σ^2;

(iii) $\hat{\sigma}_{N_d}^2(\tau)$ converges in probability to $\sigma_0^2(\tau)$, as $d \to 0^+$.

Moreover, by assuming that the whole data are identically distributed, we prove that

(iv) $\sqrt{N_d} - \sqrt{n_d}$ is asymptotically Gaussian, as $d \to 0^+$.

Now, we provide some results obtained by Monte Carlo simulations, taking a Weibull law for both baseline hazard rate and censorship laws. The covariates are supposed to be time independent and uniformly distributed on $[0, 1]$.

Table 14.1: N_d behavior for various values of d ($\beta_0 = 1$, censorship rate: 48%)

d	EM.($\hat{\beta}_{N_d}$)(StD.)	EM.(N_d)(StD.)	M.1	M.2	C.I.
1	0.90(0.34)	95(33)	5.97	6.43	91
0.9	0.97(0.29)	126(35)	6.41	8.17	87
0.8	0.99(0.25)	164(39)	6.71	8.60	93
0.7	0.95(0.19)	203(45)	6.39	6.70	90
0.6	0.98(0.15)	283(42)	6.56	6.06	92
0.5	0.99(0.13)	415(47)	6.71	6.64	94
0.4	1.00(0.11)	641(69)	6.65	7.51	92
0.3	0.99(0.07)	1149(90)	6.72	6.15	97
0.2	1.00(0.05)	2585(138)	6.65	6.64	94
0.15	1.00(0.04)	4575(181)	6.69	5.71	97

The given results are Empirical Means (EM.), Standard Deviations (StD.) of estimators from 100 simulations. In Table 14.1, we study the sequential rule behavior as d is positively decreasing to 0. We can observe that the required sample size is increasing. This study affords two ways to estimate the asymptotic variance: M.2 is the variance of the $\sqrt{N_d}(\hat{\beta}_{N_d} - \beta_0)$ (which cannot be computed for real data) and M.1 is the mean of estimated variances, which seems more stable as d varies. The last column "C.I." gives the percentage (based on 100 simulations) of coverage of the confidence interval. We can see the behavior of $N_{0.5}$ when β_0 decreases ($d = 0.5$) in Table 14.2. The required sample sizes decrease, which is explained by the fact that the theoretical risks are closer to λ_0 as β_0 goes to 0. The column "Cens. (%)" indicates the censoring percentages.

Table 14.2: $N_{0.5}$ with respect to β_0

β_0	EM.$(\hat{\beta}_{N_{0.5}})$(StD.)	EM.$(N_{0.5})$(StD.)	M.1	M.2	Cens. (%)	C.I.
5	5.01(0.13)	5013(201)	81.11	85.92	12.7	95
4	3.99(0.12)	3345(146)	54.03	48.25	15.8	94
3	3.00(0.12)	2034(120)	33.00	28.96	20.9	98
2	2.01(0.13)	1069(80)	17.33	19.07	29.9	92
1.5	1.49(0.15)	701(77)	11.35	14.20	37.5	92
1	1.02(0.11)	413(48)	6.68	4.73	48.6	98
0.5	0.49(0.12)	190(35)	3.04	2.77	65.3	93
0	0(0.09)	24(17)	0.29	0.29	93.5	100

14.3   Assumptions and Theoretical Results

We consider the following assumptions.

A1.   There exist deterministic functions γ_i defined on $[0, \tau]$, satisfying

$$\forall k \in \{0, \ldots, 3\}, \ \sup_{s \in [0,\tau]} \left| \mathbb{E}\overline{Z}_n^{(k)}(s) - \gamma_k(s) \right| \to 0, \ \text{as } n \to +\infty,$$

with γ_0 bounded away from 0 on $[0, \tau]$,

$$0 < \mathcal{I}_0(\tau) = \int_0^\tau (\gamma_2(s) - e_1(s)\gamma_1(s))ds < +\infty$$

and

$$
\begin{aligned}
0 < \mathcal{V}_0(\tau) \ = \ & \int_0^\tau \lambda_0(s)(\gamma_2(s) - e_1(s)\gamma_1(s))ds \\
& + \beta_0 \int_0^\tau (\gamma_3(s) - 2e_1(s)\gamma_2(s) + e_1^2(s)\gamma_1(s))ds < +\infty,
\end{aligned}
$$

where $e_i = \gamma_i/\gamma_0$ for $i = 1, 2$;

A2. τ is positive real number such that $\int_0^\tau \lambda_0(s)ds < +\infty$;

A3. $\{Z_i(t); t \in [0, \tau]\}_{i \geq 1}$ has bounded variations (uniformly in $i \geq 1$); that is, there exists $0 < B < \infty$ such that

$$\forall i \geq 1, \quad \int_0^\tau |Z_i(ds)| \leq B;$$

A4. The random triples $(T_i, C_i, Z_i(\cdot))$ are identically distributed.

Note that the first assumption in A1 is automatically fulfilled if A4 is true because in this case, we have equality between $\mathbb{E}\overline{Z}_n^{(k)}(s)$ and $\gamma_k(s)$ for all $s \in [0, \tau]$. The last assumptions in A1 ensure a nondegenerate asymptotic distribution for $\sqrt{n}(\hat{\beta}_n - \beta_0)$. Assumption A2 specifies that the probability to observe a failure near the upper bound of the interval of study is large enough. A3 is an assumption that is met in practical survival analysis studies and A4 is purely a technical assumption. Our main result is then as follows.

Theorem 14.3.1 *Under A1–A3, we have results* (**A**), (**B**)*, and* (**C**) *of Section 14.1. If A4 is also satisfied, and if N_d and n_d are defined by (14.2) and (14.3), respectively, then $\sqrt{N_d} - \sqrt{n_d}$ is asymptotically Gaussian with zero mean.*

PROOF. For all $n \geq 1$, the map $\beta \mapsto C_n(\tau, \beta)$ we introduced in Section 14.1, defined on a bounded open subset $\mathcal{B} \subset \mathbb{R}$ containing β_0, is twice continuously differentiable and concave (for n large enough; see C1 and C2 below). We also denote by $U_n(\tau, \beta)$ and $\mathcal{I}_n(\tau) = \mathcal{I}_n(\beta, \tau)$ the first- and second-order derivatives of C_n with respect to β. By Theorems 2.1, 2.2, and 2.3 in Bordes and Breuils (2006), we need to prove Condition C1–C4 below (under A1–A3), and C5 if A4 is also satisfied:

C1. $|\mathcal{I}_n(\tau) - \mathbb{E}\mathcal{I}_n(\tau)| \xrightarrow{c} 0$, and $|\mathcal{V}_n(\tau) - \mathbb{E}\mathcal{V}_n(\tau)| \xrightarrow{c} 0$, as $n \to \infty$;

C2. $\mathbb{E}\mathcal{I}_n(\tau) \longrightarrow \mathcal{I}_0(\tau) > 0$ and $\mathbb{E}\mathcal{V}_n(\tau) \longrightarrow \mathcal{V}_0(\tau)$, as $n \to \infty$;

C3. $(U_n(\beta_0))_{n \geq 1}$ converges completely to 0, as $n \to \infty$;

C4. For all regular sequences of integer-valued random variables $(T_n)_{n \geq 1}$, we have
$$\sqrt{T_n} U_{T_n}(\beta_0) \xrightarrow{D} \mathcal{N}(0, \mathcal{V}_0(\tau)), \quad \text{as } n \to \infty;$$

C5. For all regular sequences of integer-valued random variables $(T_n)_{n \geq 1}$, we have
$$\sqrt{T_n} \left(\begin{array}{c} \mathcal{V}_{T_n}(\hat{\beta}_{T_n}) - \mathcal{V}_0(\tau) \\ \mathcal{I}_{T_n}(\hat{\beta}_{T_n}) - \mathcal{I}_0(\tau) \end{array} \right) \xrightarrow{D} \mathcal{N}(0, \Gamma_0(\tau)), \quad \text{as } n \to \infty. \quad (14.4)$$

First note that C4 with $T_n = n$ follows directly from Lin and Ying (1994), and C2 is straightforward under A1. The main part of this proof consists in showing C1, C3, C4, and C5. Let us recall [see, for example, Andersen *et al.* (1993)] that processes M_i, defined for $t \in [0, \tau]$ by

$$M_i(t) = N_i(t) - \int_0^t Y_i(s)(\lambda_0(s) + \beta_0 Z_i(s))ds,$$

are martingales with respect to the natural filtration.

PROOF OF C3: First note that for $\beta = \beta_0$, $U_n(\beta_0, \cdot)$ is a martingale, because we have

$$U_n(\beta_0, t) = \frac{1}{n} \sum_{i=1}^{n} \int_0^t (Z_i(s) - E_n(s)) \, dM_i(s).$$

Because by A3 covariates Z_i are uniformly bounded by a constant B, we have

$$
\begin{aligned}
|\Delta U_n(\beta_0, t)| &\leq \frac{1}{n} \sum_{i=1}^{n} \left| \Delta \int_0^t (Z_i(s) - E_n(s)) \, dN_i(s) \right| \\
&\leq \frac{1}{n} \sum_{i=1}^{n} |Z_i(X_i) - E_n(X_i)| \, \Delta N_i(t) \leq \frac{2B}{n},
\end{aligned}
$$

and, using A2 and A3 there exists a constant K such that

$$| \langle U_n(\beta_0, \cdot) \rangle (t) | \leq \frac{K}{n}.$$

Then, applying Proposition 14.4.3, we get the complete convergence of the sequence $(\sup_{t \in [0, \tau]} |U_n(\beta_0, t)|)_{n \geq 1}$ to 0.

PROOF OF C1: For t in $[0, \tau]$, we write

$$
\begin{aligned}
\mathcal{I}_n(t) - \mathbb{E}\mathcal{I}_n(t) &= \int_0^t \left(\overline{Z}_n^{(2)}(s) - \mathbb{E}\overline{Z}_n^{(2)}(s) \right) ds \\
&\quad + \int_0^t \left(\mathbb{E}\left(\overline{Z}_n^{(1)}(s) E_n(s) \right) - \overline{Z}_n^{(1)}(s) E_n(s) \right) ds,
\end{aligned}
$$

whose complete convergence can then be easily deduced from Lemma 14.4.1. For $\mathcal{V}_n$, straightforward calculations lead to

$$
\mathcal{V}_n(t) - \mathbb{E}\mathcal{V}_n(t) = \frac{1}{n} \sum_{i=1}^{n} \int_0^t (Z_i(s) - E_n(s))^2 \, dM_i(s) \tag{14.5}
$$

$$
+ \int_0^t \left(H_n^{(1)}(s) - \mathbb{E}H_n^{(1)}(s) \right) \lambda_0(s) ds \tag{14.6}
$$

$$
+ \beta_0 \int_0^t \left(H_n^{(2)}(s) - \mathbb{E}H_n^{(2)}(s) \right) ds, \tag{14.7}
$$

where

$$H_n^{(1)}(s) = \overline{Z}_n^{(2)}(s) - \overline{Z}_n^{(1)}(s) E_n(s)$$

and

$$H_n^{(2)}(s) = \overline{Z}_n^{(3)}(s) - 2E_n(s)\overline{Z}_n^{(2)}(s) + \overline{Z}_n^{(1)}(s)(E_n(s))^2.$$

L. Bordes and C. Breuils

Again Lemma 14.4.1 allows us to prove the uniform complete convergence of $H_n^{(k)} - \mathbb{E}H_n^{(k)}$ to 0 on $[0, \tau]$ for $k = 1, 2$; then, using A2, we get the complete convergence of (14.6) and (14.7) to 0. Following the proof of C3, we finally show that (14.5) converges completely to 0.

PROOF OF C4:   Let us define $\tilde{U}_n$ on $[0, \tau]$ by

$$\sqrt{n}\tilde{U}_n(\beta_0, t) = \frac{1}{\sqrt{n}} \sum_{i=1}^{n} \int_0^t (Z_i(s) - e_1(s))\, dM_i(s).$$

Lemma 14.3.1 $(\sqrt{n}\tilde{U}_n(\beta_0, \cdot))$ and $(\sqrt{n}U_n(\beta_0, \cdot))$ are completely asymptotically equivalent.

PROOF. First note that for $t \in [0, \tau]$, we have

$$B_n(t) = \sqrt{n}(U_n(\beta_0, t) - \tilde{U}_n(\beta_0, t)) = \frac{1}{\sqrt{n}} \sum_{i=1}^{n} \int_0^t (E_n(s) - e_1(s))\, dM_i(s),$$

and, as in the proof of C3, we check that the assumptions of Proposition 14.4.3 are fulfilled. Indeed, $B_n(\cdot)$ is a martingale, such that $\Delta B_n(\cdot)$ is a $O(n^{-1/2})$, and we have

$$P\left(\langle B_n \rangle (t) > n^{-1/4}\right)$$
$$= P\left(\int_0^t (E_n(s) - e_1(s))^2 \frac{1}{n} \sum_{i=1}^{n} d < M_i > (s) > n^{-1/4}\right)$$
$$\leq P\left(\sup_{s \in [0,\tau]} |E_n(s) - e_1(s)| > Bn^{-1/8}\right).$$

We then use Lemma 14.4.1(ii) to obtain the second assumption of Proposition 14.4.3 and to complete the proof of the result. ∎

Lemma 14.3.2 For $t \in [0, \tau]$, $(\sqrt{n}\tilde{U}_n(\beta_0, t))_{n \geq 1}$ satisfies the Anscombe condition (see Section 14.4.1).

PROOF. For t in $[0, \tau]$ and k an integer, we have

$$\left| \sqrt{n+k}\, \tilde{U}_{n+k}(\beta_0, t) - \sqrt{n}\, \tilde{U}_n(\beta_0, t) \right|$$
$$\leq \left| \frac{1}{\sqrt{n+k}} - \frac{1}{\sqrt{n}} \right| \left| \sum_{i=1}^{n} \int_0^t (Z_i(s) - e_1(s))\, dM_i(s) \right| \qquad (14.8)$$
$$+ \frac{1}{\sqrt{n+k}} \left| \sum_{i=n+1}^{n+k} \int_0^t (Z_i(s) - e_1(s))\, dM_i(s) \right|. \qquad (14.9)$$

By applying the Rebolledo theorem to (14.8) and the Kolmogorov inequality to (14.9), we show that the Anscombe condition is fulfilled and the lemma is proved [for details of such a proof see Bordes and Breuils (2006)]. ∎

To achieve the proof of C4, we use a result by Breuils (2003) [see also Bordes and Breuils (2006)]. By the Rebolledo theorem, it is easy to see that $(\sqrt{n}U_n(\beta_0, \cdot))$ and $(\sqrt{n}\tilde{U}_n(\beta_0, \cdot))$ have the same asymptotic Gaussian distribution. Therefore, both Lemmas 14.3.1 and 14.3.2 allow us to apply Proposition 14.4.1 which proves C4.

PROOF OF C5. Here we assume that A1–A4 are satisfied; in this case, the primary assumption in A1 is satisfied because $\mathbb{E}\overline{Z}_n^{(k)} = \gamma_k$ for $0 \leq k \leq 3$. In the sequel, we use the $o_c(1)$ notation to specify that a "remaining term" converges completely to 0. Straightforward but lengthy calculations allow us to show, using Lemma 14.4.1 repeatedly, that for $t \in [0, \tau]$ we have

$$\mathcal{Z}_n(t) = \sqrt{n}\left(\begin{array}{c} \mathcal{I}_n(t) - \mathcal{I}_0(t) \\ \mathcal{V}_n(t) - \mathcal{V}_0(t) \end{array}\right) = \tilde{\mathcal{Z}}_n(t) + o_c(1),$$

with

$$\tilde{\mathcal{Z}}_n(t) = \left(\begin{array}{c} \sum_{i=0}^{2} \int_0^t k_i(s) W_n^{(i)}(s)ds \\ \sum_{i=0}^{3} \int_0^t h_i(s) W_n^{(i)}(s)ds + \sum_{i=4}^{6} \int_0^t h_i(s) dW_n^{(i)}(s) \end{array}\right),$$

where for $0 \leq k \leq 3$, $W_n^{(k)}(t) = \sqrt{n}(\overline{Z}_n^{(k)}(t) - \gamma_k(t))$, and

$$W_n^{(k)}(t) = n^{-1/2} \sum_{i=1}^{n} \int_0^t (Z_i(s))^{k-4} dM_i(s)$$

for $4 \leq k \leq 6$. Functions h_i and k_i are defined by

$$\begin{array}{llll} h_0 = \lambda_0 e_1^2 + 2\beta_0 e_1 e_2 - 2\beta_0 e_1^3, & h_1 = 3\beta_0 e_1^2 - 2\beta_0 e_2 - 2e_1 \lambda_0, \\ h_2 = \lambda_0 - 2\beta_0 e_1, & h_3 = \beta_0, & h_4 = e_1^2, & h_5 = -2e_1, & h_6 = 1, \end{array}$$

and $k_0 = e_1^2$, $k_1 = -2e_1$, $k_2 = 1$.

Let us define on $[0, \tau]$, the $\mathbb{R}^7$-valued process $W_n = (W_n^{(0)}, \ldots, W_n^{(6)})^T$. By A4 and the definition of the $W_n^{(i)}$s, we can see that

$$W_n = \frac{1}{\sqrt{n}} \sum_{i=1}^{n} W_{n,i},$$

where the $W_{n,i}$s are independent and identically distributed processes. Because we proved that $\mathcal{Z}_n(\tau)$ is asymptotically completely equivalent to $\tilde{\mathcal{Z}}_n(\tau)$, an $\mathbb{R}^2$-valued linear functional of $W_n(\cdot)$, it follows that $\tilde{\mathcal{Z}}_n(\tau)$ is a sum of centered, independent, and identically distributed random variables with finite variance under A2–A3. By the classical central limit theorem, $\tilde{Z}_n(\tau)$ has an asymptotic centered Gaussian distribution with a variance–covariance matrix $\Gamma_0(\tau)$. Moreover, $\tilde{Z}_n(\tau)$ satisfies the Anscombe condition (as a sum of centered independent and identically distributed random vectors with finite variance–covariance matrix), and so by Proposition 14.4.1, Condition C5 is fulfilled and, hence, Theorem 14.3.1 is proved. ∎

14.4 Technical Tools

14.4.1 Complete convergence, Anscombe condition, and exponential inequality

First we recall that a sequence $(X_n)_{n\geq 1}$ of real-valued random variables converges completely to a random variable X (denoted by $X_n \xrightarrow{c} X$) if for all $\varepsilon > 0$ we have

$$\sum_{n\geq 1} P(|X_n - X| > \varepsilon) < +\infty.$$

Two sequences $(X_n)_{n\geq 1}$ and $(Y_n)_{n\geq 1}$ of real-valued random variables are completely asymptotically equivalent if their difference converges completely to 0.

We say that $(X_n)_{n\geq 1}$ satisfies the Anscombe condition or is uniformly continuous in probability, if for all $\varepsilon > 0$ there exists an integer $n_0 \geq 1$ and a real number $\delta > 0$ such that

$$P\left(\max_{0\leq k\leq \delta n} |X_{n+k} - X_n| > \varepsilon\right) < \varepsilon, \ \forall n \geq n_0.$$

Proposition 14.4.1 *Let $(X_n)_{n\geq 1}$ and $(Y_n)_{n\geq 1}$ be two asymptotically completely equivalent sequences. If $(X_n)_{n\geq 1}$ satisfies the Anscombe condition, and $(T_n)_{n\geq 1}$ is a regular sequence, then*

$$Y_{T_n} - Y_{t_n} \xrightarrow{P} 0.$$

Moreover, if $(X_n)_{n\geq 1}$ converges to X in distribution, $(Y_{T_n})_{n\geq 1}$ converges to X in distribution too.

PROOF. See Breuils (2003) or Bordes and Breuils (2006). ∎

We consider $(\Omega, \mathcal{A}, P)$ a probability space. For $\omega \in \Omega$, we define

$$\mathcal{F}_{n,\omega} = \{f_n(\omega, t) = (f_{n,1}(\omega, t), \ldots, f_{n,n}(\omega, t)), t \in [0, \tau]\},$$

a subset of $\mathbb{R}^n$ corresponding to a triangular array of processes. We focus our interest on the random element defined by

$$\Delta_n(\omega) = \sup_{t\in[0,\tau]} |S_n(\omega, t) - \mathbb{E}S_n(\cdot, t)|, \qquad \omega \in \Omega,$$

where $S_n(\omega, t) = \sum_{i=1}^{n} f_{n,i}(\omega, t)$. We write $\mathbb{F}_{n,\omega} = \left(F_{n,\omega}^{(1)}, \ldots, F_{n,\omega}^{(n)} \right)$, the envelope of $\mathcal{F}_{n,\omega}$, and it satisfies $|f_{n,i}(\omega, t)| \leq F_{n,\omega}^{(i)}$ for all $t \in [0, \tau]$ and $1 \leq i \leq n$; we write $\delta_n(\omega) = |\mathbb{F}_{n,\omega}|_2$, where $|\cdot|_2$ denotes the Euclidean norm in $\mathbb{R}^n$.

Proposition 14.4.2 *Let $\mathcal{F}_{n,\omega}$ be a subset of $\mathbb{R}^n$. We assume that (i) $\delta_n(\omega) = \mathcal{O}(n^{-1/2})$ uniformly in $\omega \in \Omega$, and (ii) $\mathcal{F}_{n,\omega}$ is Euclidean [see Pollard (1990)]. Then, there exist constants $0 < c_1 \leq 5$ and $c_2 > 0$ such that*

1. $P(\Delta_n \geq \varepsilon) \leq c_1 \exp(-c_2 n \varepsilon^2)$, *for all $n \geq 1$,*

2. $\Delta_n \xrightarrow{c} 0$, *as $n \to \infty$.*

PROOF. Follows from Pollard (1990, Chapter 7); see Breuils (2003) and Bordes and Breuils (2064). ∎

Proposition 14.4.3 *Let $(\tilde{M}_n)_{n \geq 1}$ be a sequence of local martingales, locally uniformly integrable, with value $\bar{0}$ at 0. We suppose that for $n \geq 1$, we have*

$$\sup_{t \in [0, \tau]} |\Delta \tilde{M}_n(t)| \leq \frac{c}{\sqrt{n}},$$

where $c > 0$. If we have

$$\sum_{n \geq 1} P\left(\left\langle \tilde{M}_n \right\rangle (\tau) \geq n^{-1/4} \right) < +\infty,$$

then $(\sup_{t \in [0, \tau]} |\tilde{M}_n(t)|)_{n \geq 1}$ converges completely to 0.

PROOF. Follows from a result by Shorack and Wellner (1986, p. 900); see Breuils (2003) and Bordes and Breuils (2006). ∎

14.4.2 Technical results

Lemma 14.4.1 *Under A1–A3, we have:*
(i) *There exist real numbers $c > 0$, $d > 0$, and an integer $n_0 \geq 1$, such that for all $\varepsilon > 0$, $0 \leq k \leq 3$, and $n \geq n_0$:*

$$P\left(\sup_{s \in [0, \tau]} \left| \overline{Z}_n^{(k)}(s) - \gamma_k(s) \right| > \varepsilon \right) \leq c \, \exp(-dn\varepsilon^2);$$

moreover, both $\sup_{s \in [0, \tau]} \left| \overline{Z}_n^{(k)}(s) - \mathbb{E}\overline{Z}_n^{(k)}(s) \right|$ and $\sup_{s \in [0, \tau]} \left| \overline{Z}_n^{(k)}(s) - \gamma_k(s) \right|$ converge completely to 0;
(ii) *There exist real numbers $c' > 0$, $d' > 0$, and an integer $n_0' \geq 1$, such that for all $\varepsilon > 0$, and $n \geq n_0'$:*

$$P\left(\sup_{s \in [0, \tau]} |E_n(s) - e_1(s)| > \varepsilon \right) \leq c' \exp(-d'n\varepsilon^2).$$

PROOF. Let us prove (i). By the triangular inequality applied to $\overline{Z}_n^{(k)}(s) - \gamma_k(s)$ and A1, it is enough to prove the result for $\sup_{s \in [0,\tau]} |\overline{Z}_n^{(k)}(s) - \mathbb{E}\overline{Z}_n^{(k)}(s)|$. Moreover, we prove that the family $\mathcal{F}_{n\omega}$ defined by

$$\mathcal{F}_{n\omega} = \{(f_{n,1}(\omega, t), \ldots, f_{n,n}(\omega, t)), t \in [0, \tau]\},$$

for $i \in \{1, \ldots, n\}$, $f_{n,i}(\omega, t) = n^{-1} Y_i(t) Z_i^k(t)$, is Euclidean by arguments similar to those of Bilias *et al.* (1997). This family has an envelope $\mathbb{F}_{n,\omega}$ with an Euclidean norm less than $Cn^{-1/2}$ (with $C > 0$) and thus satisfies assumptions of Proposition 14.4.2 giving constants c_k and d_k. Finally, we take $c = \max c_k$ and $d = \min d_k$. The last two results of (i) follow immediately.

Result (ii) is straightforward by using the triangular inequality with result (i) and the fact that, by A1 and A3, $1/\gamma_0$ and E_n are, respectively, bounded. ∎

References

1. Andersen, P. K., Borgan, O., Gill, R. D., and Keiding, N. (1993). *Statistical Models Based on Counting Processes*, Springer-Verlag, New York.

2. Bilias, Y., Gu, M., and Ying, Z. (1997). Towards a general asymptotic theory for Cox model with staggered entry, *The Annals of Statistics*, **25**, 662–682.

3. Bordes, L., and Breuils, C. (2006). Sequential estimation for semiparametric models with application to the proportional hazards model, *Journal of Statistical Planning and Inference*, in press.

4. Breuils, C. (2003). Analyse de Durées de Vie : Analyse Séquentielle du Modèle des Risques Proportionnels et Tests d'homogénéité, *Ph.D. Dissertation* (in French) University of Compiègne, **D1484**. (downloadable at `http://tel.ccsd.cnrs.fr`).

5. Cox, D. R. (1972). Regression models with life-tables (with Discussion), *Journal of the Royal Statistical Society, Series B*, **34**, 187–220.

6. Cox, D. R., and Oakes, D. (1984). *Analysis of Survival Data*, Chapman & Hall, London, U.K.

7. Ghosh, M., Mukhopadhay, N., and Sen, P. K. (1997). *Sequential Estimation*, John Wiley & Sons, New York.

8. Huffer, F. W., and McKeague, I. W. (1991). Weighted least square estimation for Aalen's additive risk model, *Journal of the American Statistical Association*, **86**, 114–129.

9. Lai, T. L. (2001). Sequential analysis: Some classical problems and new challenges (with Discussion), *Statistica Sinica*, **11**, 303–408.

10. Lin, D. Y., and Ying, Z. (1994). Semiparametric analysis for the additive risk model, *Biometrika*, **81**, 61–71.

11. Pollard, D. (1990). *Empirical Processes: Theory and Applications*, NSF-CBMS Regional Conference Series in Probability and Statistics, **2**.

12. Shorack, G. R., and Wellner, J. A. (1986). *Empirical Processes with Applications to Statistics*, John Wiley & Sons, New York.

15

Variance Estimation of a Survival Function with Doubly Censored Failure Time Data

Chao Zhu and Jianguo Sun

University of Missouri, Columbia, MO, USA

Abstract: Doubly censored failure time data often occur in epidemiological or disease progression studies. In this situation, several authors have investigated the problem of estimating a survival function and proposed methods for the problem. However, there appears to be no existing research studying variance estimation of an estimated survival function. This chapter discusses pointwise estimation of variances of an estimated survival function and several methods are presented. The evaluation and comparison of the methods are conducted using numerical studies and a set of real doubly censored failure time data. The results suggest that the proposed methods work well under practical situations.

Keywords and phrases: AIDS incubation time, disease progression studies, pointwise estimation of variance, survival function

15.1 Introduction

Doubly censored failure time data arise in many studies of disease progression that involve two events, an initial event and an end event such as disease onset and subsequent death [De Gruttola and Lagakos (1989) and Sun (2004)]. By doubly censored data, we mean that the survival time of interest is defined as the elapsed time between the initial and end events and observations on the occurrences of both events can be either right- or interval-censored [Finkelstein (1986), Kalbfleisch and Prentice (2002), and Sun (2005)]. If the initial event can be exactly observed, we then have right- or interval-censored failure time data depending on observations on the end event. This chapter discusses pointwise estimation of variances of the estimated survival function and several methods are presented.

An example of doubly censored data that motivated this research occurs in the analysis of follow-up studies of patients who have been or are at risk of being infected by the Type-1 human immunodeficiency virus (HIV-1) and thus are also at risk of developing the acquired immune deficiency syndrome (AIDS). In this case, one variable of great interest is AIDS incubation time [De Gruttola and Lagakos (1989)], the survival time of interest defined as the time from HIV-1 infection (initial event) to the diagnosis of AIDS (end event). The HIV-1 infection time is often interval-censored partly due to the recruitment of HIV-1 positive patients into the studies and the fact that the infection times of these patients can usually only be determined retrospectively to lie in some intervals. In the meantime, observations on the diagnosis of AIDS could be right- or interval-censored too.

A number of authors have considered the analysis of doubly censored failure time data. For example, De Gruttola and Lagakos (1989) and Gómez and Calle (1999) proposed some algorithms for estimation of the survival function. Goggins et al. (1999), Pan (2001), and Sun et al. (1999) investigated regression analysis of doubly censored data under the proportional hazards model and Sun (2001a) developed a nonparametric test for survival comparison based on doubly censored data. However, there does not seem to be research discussing variance estimation of estimated survival functions except that one sometimes suggests using the Fisher information matrix. It is well known that the Fisher information matrix approach could usually work only for the case with a finite number of parameters and it does not seem to provide a reasonable choice in the presence of interval censoring [Goodall et al. (2004)]. In the following, several methods are presented and studied for the pointwise estimation of variances of estimated survival functions. More references on doubly censored data can be found in Sun (2004).

The remainder of the chapter is organized as follows. Section 15.2 introduces some notation and assumptions that will be used throughout the chapter and also gives a brief review of variance estimation of survival functions with right-censored data. In Section 15.3, four approaches are presented for pointwise variance estimation of estimated survival functions when only doubly censored data are available. The first two are generalizations of methods given in Sun (2001b) for interval-censored failure time data. For evaluation and comparison of the proposed methods, simulation studies are conducted and their results are reported in Section 15.4, which indicate that they work well under realistic situations. Also in Section 15.4, we apply the methods to the AIDS example that motivated this study and some concluding remarks are given in Section 15.5.

15.2 Preliminaries

Consider a survival study in which there are n independent subjects and each experiences two related events, initial and end events. Let X_i and $T_i > 0$ represent the time to the initial event (HIV infection time in the case of AIDS) and the time to the end event (diagnosis of AIDS), respectively, for $i = 1, \ldots, n$. The random variable $S_i = T_i - X_i$ corresponds to the survival time of interest (AIDS incubation time). Assume that $\{1, 2, \ldots, k+1\}$ is the possible range of X_i, T_i and S_i, $i = 1, \ldots, n$, for a simple presentation. That is, we assume that all of the random variables are discrete and there are only finite possible failure time points, which is often the case when data arise from clinical trials or longitudinal studies. A more practical way would be to assume that X_i, T_i, and S_i belong to a set of times whose indices are from $\{1, 2, \ldots, k+1\}$. In this case, the following proposed methods can be developed in the same way. When the underlying variable is continuous, the approach here also applies if observed data are discrete. In this case, $k + 1$ represents infinity.

For each subject, suppose that intervals $A_i = [a_{i1}, a_{i2}]$ and $I_i = [a_{i3}, a_{i4}]$ are observed to which X_i and T_i belong, respectively, where $a_{ij} \in \{1, 2, \ldots, k+1\}$ and $a_{i1} \leq a_{i2} \leq a_{i3} \leq a_{i4}$, $i = 1, \ldots, n$ and $j = 1, 2, 3, 4$. That is, we have interval-censored data on the X_is and T_is and observed data on the S_is are doubly censored and have the form $\{(A_i, I_i); i = 1, \ldots, n\}$. If $a_{i1} = a_{i2}$, $i = 1, \ldots, n$, then the occurrence of the initial event is exactly observed and we have the usual interval-censored data for the S_is [Finkelstein (1986) and Sun (2005)]. Furthermore, if $a_{i3} = a_{i4}$ or $a_{i4} = k+1$ for all subjects, we then observe right-censored failure time data [Kalbfleisch and Prentice (2002)]. Let $v_1 < \cdots < v_r$ denote the possible mass points for the X_is and $u_1 < \cdots < u_m < u_{m+1} = k+1$ the possible mass points for the S_is. Define $\alpha_{lj}^i = I(a_{i1} \leq v_l \leq a_{i2}, a_{i3} \leq v_l + u_j \leq a_{i4})$, $w_l = \Pr(X_i = v_l)$, and $f_j = \Pr(S_i = u_j)$, $l = 1, \ldots, r$, $j = 1, \ldots, m$. Then the full likelihood function L can be written as

$$L(w_l's, f_j's) = \prod_{i=1}^{n} \sum_{l=1}^{r} \sum_{j=1}^{m+1} \alpha_{lj}^i w_l f_j .$$

Let $H(x) = \Pr\{X_i \leq x\}$ and $S(t) = \Pr\{S_i > t\}$ denote the cumulative distribution function of the X_is and the survival function of the S_is, respectively. Also let $\hat{S}(t)$ and $\hat{H}(x)$ denote the joint nonparametric maximum likelihood estimators of S and H, which have no closed forms and can be obtained by, for example, the self-consistency algorithm of De Gruttola and Lagakos (1989). In the following, our main interest focuses on the problem of estimating the point-wise variances of $\hat{S}(t)$. As did other authors [De Gruttola and Lagakos (1989), Sun (2004), Gómez and Calle (1999), Goggins *et al.* (1999), Pan (2001), Sun *et al.* (1999), and Sun (2001b)], we will assume that X_i and S_i are independent. Also we will assume that the censoring mechanisms yielding the A_is and I_is are independent of the failure variables X_is and S_is.

Note that for right-censored data, $\hat{S}(t)$ has a closed form and is given by

$$\hat{S}_{KM}(t) = \prod_{j|u_j \leq t} \frac{n_j - d_j}{n_j} ,$$

the so-called Kaplan–Meier estimator [Kalbfleisch and Prentice (2002)], where $d_j = \# \{i; a_{i3} - a_{i1} = a_{i4} - a_{i1} = u_j\}$, the failure numbers at u_j, and $n_j = \# \{i; a_{i3} - a_{i1} \geq u_j\}$, the risk numbers at u_j^-. In this case, the most commonly used variance estimator of $\hat{S}_{KM}(t)$ is given by the so-called Greenwood formula [Kalbfleisch and Prentice (2002)]

$$V_G(t) = \hat{S}_{KM}^2(t) \sum_{j|u_j \leq t} \frac{d_j}{n_j(n_j - d_j)} .$$

Corresponding to the Greenwood formula, which tends to underestimate the variance, Simon and Lee (1982) and Zhao (1996) suggested using, respectively,

$$V_{SL}(u_j) = \frac{\hat{S}_{KM}^2(u_j)\{1 - \hat{S}_{KM}(u_j)\}}{(n_j - c_j)}$$

and

$$V_Z(u_j) = \frac{\hat{S}_{KM}^2(u_j)\{1 - \hat{S}_{KM}(u_j)\}}{(n_j - d_j)}$$

for the variance estimation of $\hat{S}$ at u_j, where $c_j = \# \{i; a_{i3} - a_{i1} = u_j\}$, the number of tied observations at u_j.

15.3   Variance Estimation

This section presents four methods for pointwise variance estimation of $\hat{S}(t)$. The first one is conceptually simple and based on the bootstrap approach [Efron (1981)], but may be computationally intensive. In contrast, the other three use the imputation approach [Pan (2001) and Wei and Tanner (1991)] and are computationally simpler than the first one.

15.3.1   Simple bootstrap method

Let M be a prespecified integer. For each l $(1 \leq l \leq M)$, let $(A_1^{(l)}, I_1^{(l)}), \ldots, (A_n^{(l)}, I_n^{(l)})$ be an independent sample of size n drawn with replacement from the observation set $\{(A_i, I_i)\}$ and $\hat{S}^{(l)}(t)$ denote the maximum likelihood estimator of $S(t)$ based on $\{(A_1^{(l)}, I_1^{(l)}), \ldots, (A_n^{(l)}, I_n^{(l)})\}$. Then for given t, one can estimate the variance of $\hat{S}(t)$ by the sample variance

$$V_B(t) = \frac{1}{M-1} \sum_{l=1}^{M} [\hat{S}^{(l)}(t) - \bar{S}(t)]^2 \,,$$

where

$$\bar{S}(t) = \frac{\sum_{l=1}^{M} \hat{S}^{(l)}(t)}{M} \,.$$

15.3.2 Generalized Greenwood formula

Let M be a prespecified integer as before. For each l ($1 \le l \le M$), first we draw a right-censored survival sample of size n using the following algorithm.

Step 1. Let $\{X_i^{(l)}; \ i = 1, \ldots, n\}$ be an independent sample of size n such that $X_i^{(l)}$ is drawn from the conditional probability function

$$\hat{h}_i(x) = \Pr\{X_i^{(l)} = x\} = \frac{\hat{H}(x) - \hat{H}(x-)}{\hat{H}(a_{i2}) - \hat{H}(a_{i1}-)}, \qquad x \in [a_{i1}, a_{i2}]$$

given $X_i \in [a_{i1}, a_{i2}]$, $i = 1, \ldots, n$.

Step 2. For the given $X_i^{(l)}$s, let $\{(S_i^{(l)}, \delta_i^{(l)}); \ i = 1, \ldots, n\}$ be an independent right-censored number of size n such that if $a_{i4} = k + 1$, let $S_i^{(l)} = a_{i3} - X_i^{(l)}$ and $\delta_i^{(l)} = 0$ and if $a_{i4} < k + 1$, let $S_i^{(l)}$ be a random sample drawn from the conditional survival probability function

$$f_i(s) = \Pr\{S_i^{(l)} = s\} \ = \ \frac{\hat{S}(s-) - \hat{S}(s)}{\hat{S}((a_{i3} - X_i^{(l)})-) - \hat{S}(a_{i4} - X_i^{(l)})}$$

$$s \in [a_{i3} - X_i^{(l)}, a_{i4} - X_i^{(l)}]$$

and $\delta_i^{(l)} = 1$, $i = 1, \ldots, n$, where $\delta_i^{(l)}$ is the censoring indicator.

Let $d_j^{(l)}$ and $n_j^{(l)}$ denote the failure and risk numbers d_j and n_j defined above, but based on the data set $\{(S_i^{(l)}, \delta_i^{(l)}); \ i = 1, \ldots, n\}$, and $\hat{S}_{KM}^{(l)}(t)$ and $V_G^{(l)}(t)$ the Kaplan–Meier estimator of S and the Greenwood estimator V_G also based on the data set $\{(S_i^{(l)}, \delta_i^{(l)}); \ i = 1, \ldots, n\}$, respectively, $l = 1, \ldots, M$. Then the variance of $\hat{S}(t)$ can be estimated by

$$V_{GG}(t) = \frac{1}{M} \sum_{l=1}^{M} V_G^{(l)}(t) + \left(1 + \frac{1}{M}\right) \frac{\sum_{l=1}^{M} \{\hat{S}_{KM}^{(l)}(t) - \bar{S}_{KM}(t)\}^2}{M-1} \,,$$

where

$$\bar{S}_{KM}(t) = \frac{\sum_{l=1}^{M} \hat{S}_{KM}^{(l)}(t)}{M} \; .$$

It is easy to see that if right-censored data are available, the proposed estimate V_{GG} reduces to the Greenwood formula V_G.

15.3.3 Imputation methods I and II

For given l and the generated data set $\{(S_i^{(l)}, \delta_i^{(l)}); \; i = 1, \ldots, n\}$, by using the notation given above, let

$$V_{SL}^{(l)}(u_j) = \frac{\hat{S}_{KM}^{(l)2}(u_j)\{1 - \hat{S}_{KM}^{(l)}(u_j)\}}{(n_j^{(l)} - c_j^{(l)})}$$

and

$$V_Z^{(l)}(u_j) = \frac{\hat{S}_{KM}^{(l)2}(u_j)\{1 - \hat{S}_{KM}^{(l)}(u_j)\}}{(n_j^{(l)} - d_j^{(l)})} \; ,$$

where as c_j, $c_j^{(l)}$ denotes the number of tied observations at u_j, $l = 1, \ldots, M$, $j = 1, \ldots, m$. Then following V_{SL} and V_Z, we can also estimate the variance of $\hat{S}(u_j)$ by

$$V_{GSL}(u_j) = \frac{1}{M} \sum_{l=1}^{M} V_{SL}^{(l)}(u_j) + \left(1 + \frac{1}{M}\right) \frac{\sum_{l=1}^{M}\{\hat{S}_{KM}^{(l)}(u_j) - \bar{S}_{KM}(u_j)\}^2}{M - 1}$$

or

$$V_{GZ}(u_j) = \frac{1}{M} \sum_{l=1}^{M} V_Z^{(l)}(u_j) + \left(1 + \frac{1}{M}\right) \frac{\sum_{l=1}^{M}\{\hat{S}_{KM}^{(l)}(u_j) - \bar{S}_{KM}(u_j)\}^2}{M - 1} \; ,$$

which will be referred to as imputation I and imputation II.

As mentioned above, the simple bootstrap method is clearly conceptually simpler than other three methods, but it is computationally more demanding than the others. This is because the former requires estimation of the survival function based on doubly censored data, which could be really slow. In contrast, the other methods only need the estimation with right-censored data, which does not need iterations. In both the simulation and the example below, the self-consistency algorithm proposed by De Gruttola and Lagakos (1989) was used for the estimation with doubly censored data. To apply the above methods, one needs to choose M and our simulation experience suggests that $M = 30$ seems large enough for all situations considered. Of course, for a particular example, one may want to try different values of M to obtain stable variance estimation.

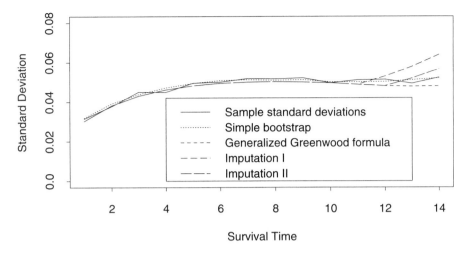

Figure 15.1: Estimated standard deviations with $b = 1$

15.4 Numerical Results

We conducted a simulation study to investigate the performance of the proposed variance estimators. In the study, we assumed that a failure could occur only at $1, 2, \ldots, 20$ and infinity; that is, $k = 20$. In the simulation, the failure time S_i of interest was assumed to follow an exponential distribution with the hazard λ_0. To generate doubly censored data, we first generated the initial event time X_i from the uniform distribution $U\{1, 2, \ldots, a\}$; given this value of X_i, a_{i1} and a_{i2} were generated by subtracting from X_i (for a_{i1}) and adding to X_i (for a_{i2}) two random numbers generated from the uniform distribution $U\{0, 1, \ldots, b\}$, respectively, where a and b are some integers. For the T_is, we assumed that right-censored data are available and defined $T_i = X_i + S_i$ with a common right-censoring time point 20. The results reported below are based on the sample size $n = 100$, $M = 30$, $a = 8$, and 300 replications.

Figure 15.1 shows the sample means of the estimated standard deviations given by four methods presented in the previous section with $b = 1$ and $\lambda_0 = 1/12$, which corresponds to roughly 30% right-censoring on the S_is. For comparison, the sample standard deviations based on estimated survival functions are also calculated and included in the figure. It can be seen that all estimates are close to each other except at the tail, where there exists relatively less information about the survival time of interest. As expected, while approaching the tail, the estimates given by the bootstrap, imputation I and II start to overestimate the variances, and the generalized Greenwood formula underestimates.

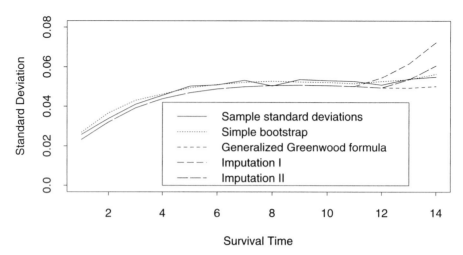

Figure 15.2: Estimated standard deviations with $b = 2$

Figure 15.2 displays the same estimates as Figure 15.1 except with $b = 2$ and gives similar conclusions to Figure 15.1. We also considered other set-ups and obtained similar results. In summary, the results suggest that all four methods seem to work reasonably well and give similar variance estimates except at the tail. In particular, the simple bootstrap method seems little better than the other three without considering computational effort. Also, it should be noted that the simple bootstrap method may need relatively large M to obtain stable estimates compared to the other three methods.

To illustrate the proposed methods, we applied them to a set of doubly censored data from an AIDS study on hemophiliacs [De Gruttola and Lagakos (1989), Goggins *et al.* (1999), and Sun *et al.* (1999)]. The original study consisted of individuals with Type A or B hemophilia who were at risk for HIV-1 infection through the contaminated blood factor they received during their treatment. The subjects were classified into two groups, lightly and heavily treated groups, according to the amount of blood. The data include observed intervals for HIV infection and AIDS diagnosis times, respectively, and one of the objectives was to compare the AIDS incubation distributions between the two groups. For illustration, here we will focus on observed data from the subjects in the heavily treated group.

Figure 15.3 presents the estimated survival function for AIDS incubation time along with the estimated 95% confidence bands given by the simple bootstrap method and generalized Greenwood formula. The confidence bands based on imputations I and II were also obtained and are similar to those shown in Figure 15.3 except at the tail as seen in Figures 15.1 and 15.2, and so were omitted. To check the dependence of the results on M, we tried a number of values of M including 10, 20, 30, 50, 100, and 200. It seems that the estimated

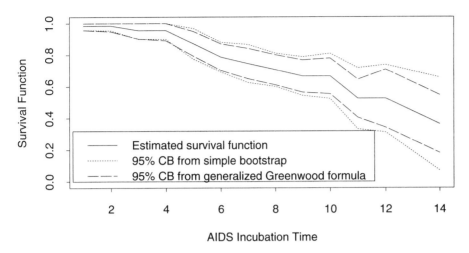

Figure 15.3: Estimated survival function and 95% confidence bands

standard deviations by the generalized Greenwood formula and imputation I and II are quite stable when M is close to 30. In contrast, the results given by the simple bootstrap method are still changing for large M although the change is somewhat mild. Note that the dependence of the results on M could also depend on the sample size.

15.5   Concluding Remarks

This chapter discussed variance estimation of estimated survival functions for doubly censored data and four methods were presented for the problem. Among them, the simple bootstrap method seems little better than the others, but it requires more computational effort and larger M than the others. The three approaches based on imputation tend to give very close estimates except at the tail, where the generalized Greenwood formula tends to underestimate the variance. In contrast, imputations I and II tend to overestimate the variance at the tail. The bootstrap method and generalized Greenwood formula are generalizations of the methods given in Sun (2001b) for interval-censored failure time data.

For simplicity, the discussion was confined to discrete situations, which is the case for many clinical and epidemiological studies with periodic follow-ups. In these situations, subjects under study are usually given or assigned prespecified finite numbers of clinical visit or observation times although actual visit or observation times may differ from subject to subject. This includes the situation where the underlying variable is continuous, but observed data appear on a discrete scale as is the case in the example discussed in Section 15.4. It is straightforward to generalize the presented methods to situations where all concerned variables are continuous with doubly censored data.

Throughout this chapter, we assumed that there are no covariates. For regression analysis, several methods have been proposed under the proportional hazards model [Goggins *et al.* (1999), Pan (2001), and Sun *et al.* (1999)] and all proposed methods focused on estimation of regression parameters. In other words, no research or method exists for variance estimation of baseline hazard or survival function. It would be useful to generalize the methods proposed above to regression situations. This is needed, for example, if one wants survival prediction. The same is true for truncated and doubly censored failure time data, which often occur in cohort or longitudinal studies [Turnbull (1976)].

Acknowledgements. The research of the second author was supported in part by a grant from the U.S. National Institutes of Health.

References

1. De Gruttola, V. G., and Lagakos, S. W. (1989). Analysis of doubly-censored survival data, with application to AIDS, *Biometrics*, **45**, 1–11.

2. Efron, B. (1981). Censored data and the bootstrap, *Journal of the American Statistical Association*, **76**, 312–331.

3. Finkelstein, D. M. (1986). A proportional hazards model for interval-censored failure time data, *Biometrics*, **42**, 845–854.

4. Goggins, W. B., Finkelstein, D. M., and Zaslavsky, A. M. (1999). Applying the Cox proportional hazards model for analysis of latency data with interval censoring, *Statistics in Medicine*, **18**, 2737–2747.

5. Gómez, G., and Calle, M. L. (1999). Nonparametric estimation with doubly censored data, *Journal of Applied Statistics*, **26**, 45–58.

6. Goodall, R. L., Dunn, D. T., and Babiker, A. G. (2004). Interval-censored survival time data: Confidence intervals for the non-parametric survivor function, *Statistics in Medicine*, **23**, 1131–1145.

7. Kalbfleisch, J. D., and Prentice, R. L. (2002). *The Statistical Analysis of Failure Time Data*, Second edition, John Wiley & Sons, New York.

8. Pan, W. (2001). A multiple imputation approach to regression analysis for doubly censored data with application to AIDS studies, *Biometrics*, **57**, 1245–1250.

9. Simon, R., and Lee, Y. J. (1982). Nonparametric confidence limits for survival probabilities and median survival time, *Cancer Treatment Reports*, **66**, 37–42.

10. Sun, J. (2001a). Nonparametric test for doubly interval-censored failure time data, *Lifetime Data Analysis*, **7**, 363–375.

11. Sun, J. (2001b). Variance estimation of a survival function for interval-censored survival data, *Statistics in Medicine*, **20**, 1249–1257.

12. Sun, J. (2004). Statistical analysis of doubly interval-censored failure time data, In *Handbook of Statistics – 23: Advances in Survival Analysis* (Eds., N. Balakrishnan and C. R. Rao), pp. 105–122, North-Holland, Amsterdam, The Netherlands.

13. Sun J. (2005). Interval censoring, In *Encyclopedia of Biostatistics*, Second edition, pp. 2603–2609, John Wiley & Sons, New York.

14. Sun, J., Liao, Q., and Pagano, M. (1999). Regression analysis of doubly censored failure time data with applications to AIDS studies, *Biometrics*, **55**, 909–914.

15. Turnbull, B. W. (1976). The empirical distribution function with arbitrarily grouped censored and truncated data, *Journal of the Royal Statistical Society, Series B*, **38**, 290–295.

16. Wei, G. C. G., and Tanner, M. A. (1991). Applications of multiple imputation to the analysis of censored regression data, *Biometrics*, **47**, 1297–1309.

17. Zhao, G. (1996). The homogenetic estimate for the variance of survival rate, *Statistics in Medicine*, **15**, 51–60.

PART V
CLUSTERING

16

Statistical Models and Artificial Neural Networks: Supervised Classification and Prediction Via Soft Trees

Antonio Ciampi and Yves Lechevallier

McGill University, Montreal, QC, Canada
INRIA-Rocquencourt, Le Chesnay, France

Abstract: It is well known that any statistical model for supervised or unsupervised classification can be realized as a neural network. This discussion is devoted to supervised classification and therefore the essential framework is the family of feedforward nets.

Ciampi and Lechevallier have studied two- and three-hidden-layer feedforward neural nets that are equivalent to trees, characterized by neurons with "hard" thresholds. Softening the thresholds has led to more general models. Also, neural nets that realize additive models have been studied, as well as networks of networks that represent a "mixed" classifier (predictor) consisting of a tree component and an additive component. Various "dependent" variables have been studied, including the case of censored survival times.

A new development has recently been proposed: the soft tree. A soft tree can be represented as a particular type of hierarchy of experts. This representation can be shown to be equivalent to that of Ciampi and Lechevallier. However, it leads to an appealing interpretation, to other possible generalizations and to a new approach to training. Soft trees for classification and prediction of a continuous variable will be presented. Comparisons between conventional trees (trees with hard thresholds) and soft trees will be discussed and it will be shown that the soft trees achieve better predictions than the hard tree.

Keywords and phrases: Prediction trees, probabilistic nodes, hierarchy of experts

16.1 Introduction

The task of learning from data has been the object of two independent but converging traditions: machine learning, which emphasizes algorithmic approaches, and statistical modeling, which emphasizes choice of a model for the probability distribution of the observed data. From the point of view of statistical learning theory, the well-known distinction between supervised and unsupervised learning corresponds to the problems of conditional and unconditional density estimation, respectively.

Traditional parametric modeling uses data to search for an optimal value of a parameter that varies within a space of specified dimension. Complex data, such as those encountered in contemporary data analysis can seldom be fully studied by this traditional approach. Statistical learning theory [Hastie, Tibshirani, and Friedman (2001)] aims to extract information from complex data by a new, flexible approach known as adaptive modeling. Typically, dictionaries—that is, "super-families" of models of unspecified dimension—replace parametric models. And model searches are conducted within dictionaries relying on various heuristics, often inspired by simple cognitive strategies. Although the goal of statistical learning remains the modeling of a probability distribution, the approach becomes increasingly algorithmic. Also, the goal of finding a global optimum is often reduced to the search for a suboptimal but meaningful solution such as a reasonably stable local optimum.

In this chapter, we are concerned with supervised learning and, in particular, with the prediction problem. The aim is to construct from data the regression function $E[y|x]$, which is the expectation of the variable to predict y given the vector of predictors x. Two common examples of regression functions are *ordinary linear regression*, in which y is a continuous variable and $E[y|x]$ is assumed linear in the x; and *generalized linear regression*, in which linearity is assumed for a monotone transformation of $E[y|x]$, as in logistic and Poisson regressions. In the statistical modeling tradition, variable selection algorithms for multivariable regression may be considered as the ancestors of adaptive modeling in supervised learning.

Much of contemporary research in statistical supervised learning focuses on approaches shared with machine learning, such as trees and, to a lesser extent, feedforward Artificial Neural Networks (ANN). Neural networks appear particularly attractive because they are universal approximators [Hornik, Stinchcombe, and White (1989)]. However, this very desirable property is of little use in practice. Indeed, before training an ANN, one needs to choose its architecture. This is not done by use of mathematical results, but rather by trial and error and reliance on past experience. This lack of mathematical definition may well be one of the main reasons why ANNs have been to date less attractive to statisticians.

Indeed, statisticians have directed their attention to the sampling properties of ANNs and to some training algorithms for simple architectures [Venable and Ripley (2002)], but not so much to the design of innovative architectures.

On the other hand, owing to the universal approximation property, any statistical model can be realized as an ANN. Therefore, one can use a statistical model that produces reasonably good predictions as the basis on which to build the architecture of an ANN. Once trained, this ANN should produce predictions at least as good as the original statistical model. In the last few years, we have pursued this theme in the context of supervised learning [Ciampi and Lechevallier (1995a,b, 1997, 2000, 2001), Ciampi and Zhang (2002), and Ciampi, Couturier, and Li (2002)]. In this chapter, we present some of the results obtained in the endeavor. In Section 16.2, we state more formally the correspondence between statistical models and ANNs. We also demonstrate the realization of linear, generalized linear, and tree-shaped prediction models as specific ANN architectures. Furthermore, we show how these specific architectures can be made more flexible and to produce indeed ANNs which should be at least as good as the original ones. In Section 16.3, we introduce a simple approach to the design of an ANN that has statistical models as building blocks, and explore its advantages and shortcomings. A subtler approach to combining models, developed in Section 16.4, is based on the notion of hierarchy of experts. In Section 16.5, we propose a new architecture, the soft tree, which can be seen as a special case of hierarchy of experts, but one that can be constructed directly from data. This constructive approach is extended in Section 16.5 to a more general hierarchy of experts. Section 16.6 contains a few concluding remarks.

16.2 The Prediction Problem: Statistical Models and ANNs

For the purpose of this work, the prediction problem can be formulated as follows. Suppose we have obtained a data matrix $D = [Y|X]$, whose columns represent measurements on n randomly sampled units of the variable y and of the vector of predictors x. Assume a statistical model for the conditional distribution of y given x as

$$y|x \sim f(y; \theta(x), \phi),$$

where θ is a parameter that can be influenced by x, and ϕ is a possibly infinite-dimensional parameter that does not depend on x and may be considered as a nuisance parameter. Often, we have $\theta(x) = \mu(x)$, the expected value of y given x. The task is to estimate from D a functional form for $\theta(x)$, $\hat{\theta}(x)$.

The ANN modeling approach to the prediction problem is summarized in Figure 16.1. The "input" data vector x enters the ANN through the input layer and then flows through the inner layers towards the output layer. Each unit or (artificial neuron) transforms an input into an output through a specified function, known as the *activation function* of the neuron. Neurons are disposed in layers. Usually the neurons of a layer share the same activation function. The first layer is the input layer; its neurons receive as input one of the components of x and the output repeats the input (identity activation function). Each neuron in the inner layers is connected to some or all of those in the immediately preceding layer; the lines in the figure represent the connections. The input of each inner layer neuron is a linear combination of the outputs of the neurons directly connected to it. The coefficients of the linear combination are called *connection weights* and have to be determined from the data. They can be considered as constituting a high-dimensional vector parameter w. It should be noted here that, from the point of view of the classical statistical modeler, trained to strive for parsimony of parameterization and interpretability of parameters, the role of w as "parameter" is highly unusual: the ANN does not appear parsimonious, but rather overparameterized. The activation function of the inner layers' neurons is usually a sigmoid function (e.g., the logistic function). At the output of the outer layer neurons (in Figure 16.1, there is only one), one reads the output $out(x|w)$, which represents the prediction. The activation function of the neurons of the outer layer depends on the specific problem.

In the training phase, connection weights are determined from data. In general, the optimal weights vector parameter $\hat{w}$ is determined by maximizing

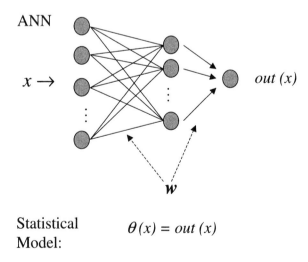

Figure 16.1: ANN and prediction models

a "cost function" $c(Y, out(X|\boldsymbol{w}))$. Backpropagation is the most popular maximization algorithm: it has an intuitive appeal in terms of learning theory, but it is by no means the only way to approach the maximization problem.

It is natural to identify $out(x)$ with $\theta(x)$, and, when training is completed, $out(x|\hat{\boldsymbol{w}})$ with $\hat{\theta}(x)$. Although the choice of the cost function can be dictated by a number of pragmatic considerations, a statistically natural one is to identify the cost function with the deviance, that is, the negative of twice the log-likelihood of the data. It is clear that with these choices, the neural network family is simply a highly flexible model family and ANN training is just one approach to likelihood maximization.

We shall now see how some familiar statistical models can be represented as ANNs.

16.2.1   Generalized linear models as ANNs

Consider the generalized linear model family:

$$
\begin{aligned}
f(y|x) &= f(y|\theta(x)), & (16.1) \\
\eta(\mu(x)) &= \eta(\theta(x)) = \beta x, & (16.2)
\end{aligned}
$$

where η is the link function and f is a density of the exponential family [McCullagh and Nelder (1989)]. For ease of notation, we do not explicitly indicate the dispersion parameter, inasmuch as it does not play a role in the estimation of the regression coefficients.

Several useful regression models are included in this general definition: one simply has to specify the link and the density f. For example, the normal linear regression model corresponds to the choice of the identity link and of a normal density. Two other examples, particularly useful in health statistics, are the logistic regression model, with the logit link function and the binomial distribution, and the Poisson regression model, with the logarithmic link and Poisson distribution. The Poisson regression model can be easily adapted to treat censored survival data when the survival time is assumed to be exponentially distributed.

Figure 16.2 represents the generalized linear model as an ANN.

The architecture consists of one inner layer, with identity activation function for its neurons; the weights of the connections from the input to the inner layer are fixed and equal, for example, all equal to 1; and the output neuron has an activation function equal to the inverse of the link function. Clearly, the only weights to learn are those of the connections between the inner layer and the output neuron, so that $\boldsymbol{w}$ is identified with β, the vector of the regression coefficients. In particular, for ordinary linear regression we have

$$
out(x|\beta) - \theta(x) = \mu(x) = \beta x, \qquad (16.3)
$$

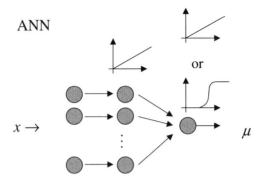

Figure 16.2: Linear predictor

and for logistic regression we have

$$out(x|\beta) = \theta(x) = \mu(x) = p(x) = \frac{e^{\beta x}}{1 + e^{\beta x}}. \tag{16.4}$$

A likelihood-based cost function is then

$$c(Y, out(X, \beta)) = -2 \log L = -2 \sum_{i=1}^{n} \log f(y_i | out(x_i | \beta)). \tag{16.5}$$

Thus it can be seen that from an ANN perspective, the choice of the density function and of the link function corresponds to the choice of the cost function and of the activation function of the output neuron, respectively.

As long as we wish to limit ourselves to fitting generalized linear models, the correspondence we have outlined amounts to nothing more than a formal remark; in particular, backpropagation is not especially useful in this situation, as there are simple and powerful algorithms to learn the parameters, which require no iterations for the linear model and generally few iterations for the generalized linear models. However, suppose we want to allow little deviations from linearity. Then we can use logistic thresholds in the inner layer, allow variable connection weights between the input and the inner layer, but choose an initialization of these weights so that the logistic activation functions behave virtually as identity functions at the first step of the training. Also, at initialization, the weights of the connections of the inner layer with the output layer can be taken as the regression coefficients of the regression estimated by the appropriate statistical procedure. During training, these initial weights may change very little or not at all, in which case the linear model is consistent with the data, or they may change substantially, indicating that the linear assumption is not valid. Therefore, the data will decide whether a deviation from the linear model is warranted. We stress, however, that if such deviation is warranted, it will be of a particular nature: the final model will be linear in some logistic transformation of the original predictors. Therefore, it will still be "close" to a linear model, in the sense that it will be a simple case of additive model.

Another way to enlarge the generalized linear model ANN (GLM-ANN) is to add a second hidden layer, initialize the training process so that the new ANN is indistinguishable from the GLM-ANN, and then let the data determine whether the generalization is warranted. In principle, the result can be any ANN with one hidden layer. The "linear" initialization underlies the approach developed in Ciampi and Zhang (2002) for training an ANN. It has a number of advantages on the standard random initialization, at least when the variable to predict is a binary variable. In this case, training is achieved in a shorter time than with random initialization and the predictive accuracy is not inferior to that obtained by the more costly initialization; furthermore, one demonstrably improves the predictive accuracy of the "initial" linear regression model. A similar approach was developed in Ciampi and Lechevallier (2000, 2001) for censored survival data, using the formal equivalence of censored exponential regression with a Poisson model referred to above.

16.2.2 Generalized additive models as ANNs

Generalized additive models are an extension of the generalized linear model that has proved very useful in a variety of applications [Hastie and Tibshirani (1990)]. The linear assumption in Eq. (16.2) is replaced by the additive assumption

$$\eta(\mu(x)) = \theta(x) = \sum g_i(x_i), \qquad (16.6)$$

where the gs are arbitrary continuous functions, to be determined from the data through flexible modeling.

An ANN, as shown in Figure 16.3, can also represent the most general additive model. Here, instead of having an inner layer of neurons, we have an inner layer of ANNs; in other words, the architecture is that of a network of networks.

Each component x_i of the predictor vector x serves as input to a standard ANN whose internal connection weights have to be learned from the data. The output of the ith inner layer ANN is denoted by $g_i(x_i)$; because of the universal approximation property of ANNs, the form of this function is totally flexible. The outputs of the inner layer ANNs flow towards the output of the network of networks, with fixed, equal connection weights. As for the linear case, the form of the activation function of the output neuron and the choice of the cost function determine the type of additive model. The output functions for

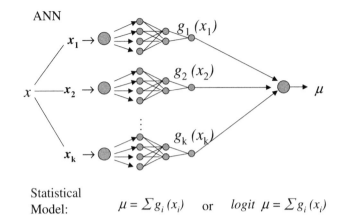

Figure 16.3: Additive predictor

ordinary and for logistic additive regression are, respectively,

$$out(x|\beta) = \theta(x) = \mu(x) = \sum_{i=1}^{n} \beta x_i \qquad (16.7)$$

and

$$out(x|\beta) = \theta(x) = \mu(x) = p(x) = \frac{e^{\sum g_i(x_i)}}{1 + e^{\sum g_i(x_i)}}. \qquad (16.8)$$

The ANN for additive modeling can be enlarged, in a manner similar to that discussed at the end of the previous section. We can, for instance, add another inner layer between the layer of networks and the output layer, initialize it in a way that it is indistinguishable from the additive model ANN, and then let the data determine departures from the initial model.

16.2.3   Classification and regression trees as ANNs

Tree-structured prediction is becoming increasingly popular in a vast domain of applications. A prediction tree is a graph such as the one shown in Figure 16.4, with which the following statistical model is associated.

$$\mu(x) = \mu_1 I\,[x_1 > a_1]\,I\,[x_1 > a_2] + \mu_2 I\,[x_1 > a_1]\,I\,[x_1 \le a_2] + \mu_3 I\,[x_1 \le a_2]\,.$$
$$(16.9)$$

Here $I[x \in A]$ is the characteristic function of the set A; that is, $I[x \in A](x)$ is 1 if x is in A and 0 otherwise. Also this model has an ANN representation, which was proposed in Ciampi and Lechevallier (1995b, 1997) and Ciampi and Zhang (2002) and is shown in Figure 16.4.

This ANN has two inner layers, with activation functions $I[x \le 0]$. The first inner layer has as many neurons as there are inner nodes in the tree: it creates the questions at the nodes, in the sense that each neuron has output 1 or 0 depending on whether the question defining the branching has answer *yes* or *no*. The second inner layer has as many neurons as there are leaves and the output of each neuron is 1 or 0 depending on whether the subject with predictor x is assigned to the corresponding leaf. The output layer simply realizes Equation (16.9).

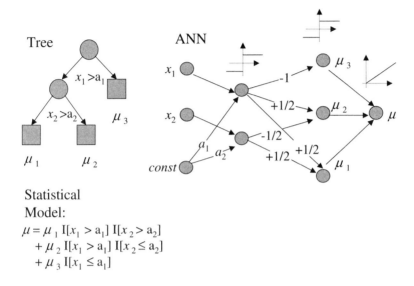

Statistical
Model:
$$\mu = \mu_1 \, I[x_1 > a_1] \, I[x_2 > a_2]$$
$$+ \mu_2 \, I[x_1 > a_1] \, I[x_2 \leq a_2]$$
$$+ \mu_3 \, I[x_1 \leq a_1]$$

Figure 16.4: Prediction tree and its associated ANN

As in Section 16.2.1, the main interest of the correspondence between tree and ANN is that it can be used to train a neural net that can in fact improve on the tree. The problem with the description of Figure 16.4(b) is that we have "hard thresholds" as activation functions for the inner layer neurons, which makes optimization hard and impossible with techniques based on differentiation of the activation function, such as backpropagation. However, by appropriate choice of the initial conditions, one can replace hard thresholds with very steep soft thresholds without changing the numerical value of the cost function at initialization. As training proceeds, the weights may evolve so that the activation functions become quite far from the initial steep threshold, in which case the indication given by the data is that a tree model can be improved upon. Our experience shows that this behavior is observed in practical applications and that substantial improvement on the tree may result [Ciampi and Lechevallier (1995b, 1997) and Ciampi and Zhang (2002)]. Unfortunately, when thresholds become soft, the interpretation of the model is not clear. However, it is possible to interpret the output of the neurons of the first inner layer: if we still consider an inner layer neuron as corresponding to a node in the tree, then the output of such a neuron is between 0 and 1; it is close to 1 if the input is large and close to 0 if it is small. It is suggestive to interpret this output as a probabilistic answer to the question defining the node, which could be restated as, "Is x_1 large?" For instance, if x_1 is very large or very small for a subject, then that subject goes left or right; for "intermediate" values of x_1, the subject goes to the left with the probability given by the output of the neuron and to the right with complementary probability. We are implicitly assuming that there is a latent binary variable, taking values 1 for "large" and 0 for "small," for which x_1 is an indicator.

We will see later that this interpretation can be developed more fully but only after we propose an alternative representation of the tree as an ANN.

16.3   Combining Prediction Models: Hierarchy of Experts

We have seen that an additive model can be represented as a network with an inner layer consisting of networks. There is, however, the important restriction that each neuron of the input layer, corresponding to a one-dimensional component of x, is connected to only one of the inner networks. What if we drop this restriction and allow full connectivity between the outer and the inner layer? We proposed this in Ciampi and Lechevallier (2000), and suggested that each inner network might represent a statistical model; for example, we might have two inner networks, one representing a linear model, and the other a tree. The output of the whole network would then appropriately weight the two models and suggest whether a tree or a linear model is more consistent with the data. Again, our experience shows that, when the data warrant it, the ANN based on the combination of two statistical models does better than the individual models themselves and the associated ANNs [Ciampi and Lechevallier (2000)].

Although the idea of a network of networks has proved useful in the direct form proposed in Ciampi and Lechevallier (2000), we have recently pursued an interesting alternative to the development of a network of networks: we can arrange several networks in a hierarchical structure called *hierarchy of experts* [Jordan and Jacobs (1994)]. Figure 16.5 represents such a structure.

At the core of the graph, there is a tree structure. However, data flow from the leaves to the root of the tree. The leaves of the tree, represented by darkly filled squares, are neural networks, receiving input x. Each node, represented as usual by a circle, is a neuron with sigmoid activation function, receiving input from its children and sending its output towards its parent node. Next to each branch there is a neural network, represented by a lightly filled box and known as a gating network or, more briefly, *gater*. A gater also receives x as input, and outputs a number p between 0 and 1. The role of the gater is to

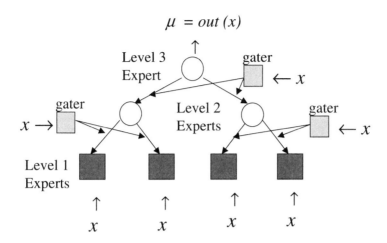

Figure 16.5: Alternative architecture: hierarchy of experts

weight the outputs of the children with its own output. Conventionally the left branch receives weight p and the right branch receives weight $1 - p$. Then these weighted outputs serve as input to the parent node. The output of the root node is the output of the whole system.

The name of this architecture is explained by the following suggestive interpretation. A leaf of the tree represent a "first-level" expert, who looks at the data and makes a prediction. This prediction is examined by a "second-level" expert, who also examines the data but only to decide how to weight the predictions of the first-level experts. Second-level experts submit their own predictions, based on the weighted predictions of their subordinates, to third-level experts; and so on, until a "super expert," represented by the root of the tree, makes the final prediction.

The idea of mixing ANNs based on statistical models can easily be realized with the hierarchy of experts architecture. For example, one can place classical statistical models at the leaves, and use as gaters networks with constant output: this will be equivalent to the network of networks architecture discussed at the beginning of this section. More generally, using linear or additive ANNs as gaters allows greater flexibility, because models are weighted by weights that may depend on the predictors.

Hierarchy of experts has great flexibility and can be used to mimic a wide variety of situations. One such situation is the following: leaf networks represent "experts" working with different sets of variables: for example, one expert might make a tentative diagnosis based on standard blood tests, another on genetic tests, yet another on an X-ray examination, and so on. Then the role of a "super expert" is to combine these different points of view and, based on the totality of the information, to weight the partial diagnoses and issue a comprehensive one.

In spite of many impressive features, the hierarchy of experts remains an *architecture*, that is, a structure that should be designed a priori before using the data for learning the weights of its components. This is a limitation that we are attempting to overcome by developing algorithms that can construct a hierarchy of experts directly from data. The key idea at the root of this development is the soft tree.

16.4   The Soft Tree

In Section 16.2.3, we have discussed an ANN architecture based on a tree; we also pointed out that during training, the resulting predictor may differ quite markedly from the original tree structure and may indeed lose the advantage of interpretability. The hierarchy of the experts offers an alternative approach to the design of a network based on a tree, which remains interpretable even if the data suggest departures from the original tree structure. Indeed, a hard tree can be easily represented as a hierarchy of experts with very specific features. The expert at the leaves should be imagined as making the same prediction for all subjects, regardless of the values of the predictor variables x; in other words, the outputs of the leaf networks do not depend on the input. Furthermore, each gater should be thought of as a hard threshold on a single variable, characteristic of the corresponding node. In terms of the expert interpretation, the super expert simply chooses one of the predictions of its subordinate experts, and does so on the basis of just one variable.

As in Section 16.2.3, one can replace hard thresholds with soft thresholds, initialize all the gaters so that at the beginning of the learning process they behave as hard thresholds, and then train the networks while allowing departures from the hard thresholds. The resulting structure is a tree with *soft nodes*, or, for brevity, a *soft tree*. It is represented in Figure 16.6.

The process for creating such a structure may be entirely constructive: the data are used a first time to determine the hard tree structure on which to base the architecture of hierarchy of experts, and a second time to soften the hard thresholds, if warranted to improve prediction. It could be easily implemented as an algorithm. However, we have developed a more efficient alternative approach, which determines recursively both the variable at each node and the gater associated with it. The details of the algorithms to predict a binary response are discussed in Ciampi, Couturier, and Li (2002). In what follows, we outline the main ideas.

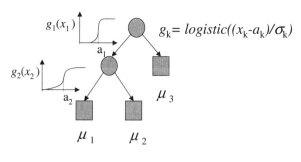

Statistical Model:
$$\mu = \mu_1 \, g_1[x_1 > a_1] \, g_2[x_2 > a_2]$$
$$+ \mu_2 \, g_1[x_1 > a_1] \, (1\text{-}g_2[x_2 > a_2])$$
$$+ \mu_3 \, (1\text{-}g_1[x_1 > a_1])$$

Figure 16.6: Example of soft tree

16.4.1 General concepts in tree construction

The construction algorithm proposed in Ciampi, Couturier, and Li (2002) rests on some intuitive concepts that are simple generalizations of their counterparts for a tree with ordinary hard thresholds [see Hornik, Stinchcombe, and White (1989)]; we will refer to the latter as a *hard tree*. Consider first a simple binary split with a soft threshold based on the variable x_1, say: thus a subject goes to the left branch with probability $g(x_1)$ and to the right branch with complementary probability $1 - g(x_1)$. The trivial tree consisting of the root node is only a statistical model corresponding to the hypothesis that the distribution of $y|x$ does not depend on x. The tree with the two nodes of the split is also a statistical model, according to which the distribution of $y|x$ is a mixture of distributions of the form

$$f(y|x) = g(x_1)f_1(y) + (1 - g(x_1))f_2(y). \tag{16.10}$$

We define the *information content* of the split as the Likelihood Ratio Statistic (LRS) for comparing these two models. This definition is easily generalized to a tree of general structure T. In fact, we can construct an LRS for comparing the root node model with the model associated with the leaves of T, that is, a formula for the conditional density that generalizes (16.10) in a direct way

$$f(y|x) = \sum_{l=1}^{L} G_l(x) f_l(y), \tag{16.11}$$

where $f_l(y)$ denotes the probability density associated with the ℓth leaf, the sum is over the L leaves of T, and the coefficient of $f_\ell(y)$s is obtained from basic properties of probability, as a product of "soft threshold" functions $g_\ell(x_\ell)$ and of complements of such functions associated with the nodes that are ancestors of the ℓth leaf. Thus the information content of a tree is

$$IC(T : Root|data) = LRS(T : Root|data). \qquad (16.12)$$

Other concepts used in (soft) tree-growing are Information Gain (IG) and Information Loss (IL). If $T*$ is a rooted subtree of T (a subtree containing the root node), then the IG of T with respect to $T*$ and the IL of $T*$ with respect to T are

$$IG(T : T * |data) = LRS(T : T * |data) = IC(T|data) - IC(T * |data)$$

and

$$IL(T* : T|data) = LRS(T* : T|data) = IC(T * |data) - IC(T|data).$$

Given a tree T, we define the best one-split augmentation of T as the tree obtained from T by adding to one split one leaf such that the augmented tree has the highest information gain with respect to T.

16.4.2   Constructing a soft tree from data

We can now write the general outline of our soft tree construction algorithm:

GENERAL ALGORITHM:
1. FIX admissibility conditions and selection rules (AIC or BIC)
2. STEP 0: INITIALIZE:
Estimate the parameter for the trivial tree T_0=$Root$
....
3. STEP k :ENLARGE TREE BY 1 SPLIT
Find best 1-split augmentation of T_k
4. UPDATE: $T_k \leftarrow T_{k+1}$
5. If IG($T* : T$) is small enough
THEN STOP
ELSE, GO TO 3.

In order to perform STEP k, we need to repeatedly estimate the parameters of the soft tree T_k and of all its one-split augmentations. The parameters of a soft tree describe the constant leaf predictors; on the other hand, there are also parameters describing the soft nodes. If we model the gater at a node by a logistic function

$$f_k(x) = \frac{e^{a_k+b_k x}}{1 + e^{a_k+b_k x}},$$

we have two parameters to estimate for each node: a_k and b_k. If L is the number of leaves and we have K parameters per leaf, we have a total of $(2 + K)L - 2$ parameters, or $3L - 2$ for $K = 1$, the case of a single continuous or binary response variable.

We estimate the parameters by an EM-type algorithm, described below. Indeed, the actual likelihood of a soft tree of a given structure is rather hard to write down and maximize directly. On the other hand, it is easy to "complete" the data and to write a "complete data" likelihood, based on the following idea. Suppose that there is an unobserved binary variable at each node k, such that $\zeta_k = 1$ means "go left" and $\zeta_k = 0$ means "go right." Then we can complete the observed data by adding hypothetical values of ζ_k so that the soft tree becomes a hard tree: when this is done, the task of writing and maximizing the likelihood is trivial or, at least, reducible to a well-known one.

EM ALGORITHM FOR ESTIMATING THE PARAMETERS OF A SOFT TREE
1. INITIALIZE:
Assign initial values to all parameters $\theta^{(0)}$
2. E-STEP:
Calculate $\mathrm{E}[\zeta_k \mid y; \theta^{(r)}]$ and substitute this to ζ_k in the complete likelihood
3. M-STEP:
Maximize complete likelihood to obtain $\theta^{(r+1)}$
4. UPDATE: $\theta^{(r)} \leftarrow \theta^{(r+1)}$
5. IF update parameters are "close enough" to old parameter,
THEN STOP
ELSE GO TO 2

The algorithms of tree construction and parameter estimation are quite general in the form presented here, however, several technical difficulties had to be overcome in practice. Different types of response variable present different problems. We now have a stable algorithm for the case of binary and continuous responses. An improved version of this approach, which can handle continuous, binary and multinomial responses, is now under development and the results seem promising.

16.4.3 An example of data analysis

We summarize here the results of the construction of a soft tree predictor from a well-known data set in the public domain: the Pima Indians Diabetes data [Venable and Ripley (2002)]. Data are available on 532 subjects of Pima Indian heritage, all females and of age 21 or older, living near Phoenix, Arizona. The goal is to predict a binary variable that indicates the presence of Type II diabetes (WHO definition), from the following predictors: number of pregnancies (npreg), plasma glucose concentration (Glu), diastolic blood pressure (bp), triceps skin fold thickness (skin), body mass index (BMI), diabetes pedigree function (Ped), and age. Figure 16.7 shows a soft tree constructed from these data according to the algorithm outlined in Section 16.4.2.

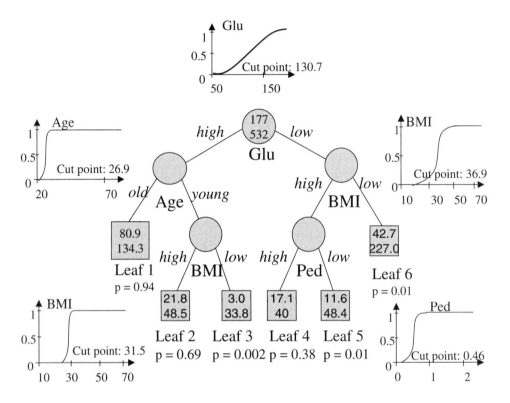

Figure 16.7: Soft tree for Pima Indians data

Notice that the soft nodes vary in degree of "softness," as shown by the gater functions at the nodes: for instance, the first node, determined by plasma glucose concentration is very soft, and the lowest node based on BMI is nearly hard. For purpose of comparison, we also constructed a hard tree from the same data, shown in Figure 16.8.

Is one model clearly better than the other? Model comparison is summarized in Table 16.1, which contains four common cross-validated measures of predictive accuracy [Harrell (2002)] for the soft and the hard trees: deviance, area under the receiving operator characteristic (ROC) curve, Brier's score, and misclassification error. Except for the Brier's score, which is the same for the two predictors, the measures reveal a clear advantage of the soft tree.

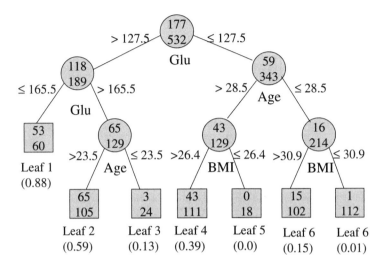

Figure 16.8: Hard tree for Pima Indians data

Table 16.1: Model comparison for Pima Indians data

	Soft tree	Hard tree
Deviance	448.23	453.67
Area under the ROC curve	86.54	85.81
Brier's score	0.14	0.14
Misclassification error	19.55%	21.05%

1. Split at random the data into a learning set and a test set (10% of the data).
2. Build two predictors, hard and soft tree, on the black *learning set*.
3. On the *test set*, compare the accuracy of the two predictors
Repeat the random splitting 100 times.

Table 16.2: Test set classification error

	Soft tree		Hard tree		
	Mean	Std	Mean	Std	p-values
Breast cancer	3.998	2.499	5.31	2.715	< 0.0001
Pima Indian	22.86	5.58	26.12	5.797	< 0.0001
Heart disease	22.37	7.429	33.73	7.803	< 0.0001
Liver disease	37.74	7.556	50.63	8.634	< 0.0001
Diabetes 2	15.68	5.34	14.62	5.47	0.0007
Prostate cancer	36.92	6.92	39.19	6.65	0.0013

16.4.4   An evaluation study

The analysis of the Pima Indian data is part of an evaluation study presented in Ciampi and Couturier (2002). We chose six public domain data sets with a binary response: breast cancer, Pima Indian, heart disease, liver disease, diabetes 2, and prostate cancer. By the following resampling approach, we compared soft and hard trees on these data.

The results are summarized in Tables 16.2 and 16.3, in which the comparison is based on the classification error. Clearly, as could be expected, the soft tree performs statistically better than the hard tree.

Table 16.3: Proportion of time the hard tree test set classification error (E_H) is greater than the soft node test set classification error (E_S)

	$E_H > E_S(\%)$	$E_H >= E_S(\%)$
Breast cancer	58	84
Pima Indian	69	77
Heart disease	82	86
Liver disease	86	93
Diabetes 2	3	78
Prostate cancer	54	66

The results of the comparisons based on other measures of predictive accuracy point in the same direction, and are not shown here.

16.5 Extending the Soft Tree

The soft tree model can be easily extended in order to increase predictive accuracy while sacrificing as little as possible of interpretability and parsimony. The idea is suggested by the hierarchy of expert paradigm, and on the other hand by some generalized tree-growing algorithms for trees with hard nodes [Ciampi (1991), Chaudhuri *et al.* (1995), and Chipman, George, and McCulloch (2002)]. One can replace the constant predictor at the leaves by a (generalized) linear predictor, that is, a regression equation. The algorithm outlined in Section 16.4.2 has to be modified by allowing at each split some simple form of stepwise variable selection.

Although we are still in the process of developing stable algorithms, we will present here some new results. We have analyzed another public domain data set, the car mileage data [Venable and Ripley (2002)]. These data contain city-cycle fuel consumption in miles per gallon, to be predicted in terms of the following predictors: cylinders, displacement, horsepower, weight, acceleration, model year. Hard, soft, and extended soft trees were constructed from these data. They are shown in Figures 16.9–16.11.

The cross-validated prediction mean square error was calculated for each of the predictors, obtaining 11.64 for the hard tree, 10.23 for the soft tree, and 9.68 for the extended soft tree. Clearly, at least for these data, the extended

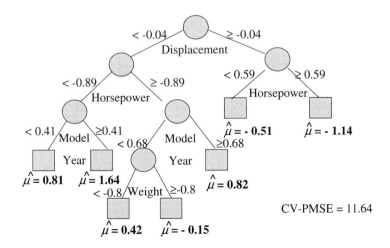

Figure 16.9: Hard tree for car mileage data

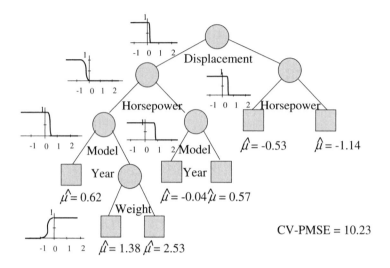

Figure 16.10: Soft tree for car mileage data

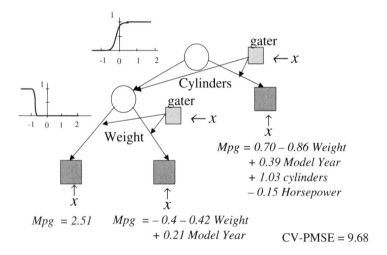

Figure 16.11: Extended soft tree

soft tree appears to be superior and the soft tree better than the hard tree. An empirical evaluation study based on several publicly available data sets is under way.

16.6   Conclusions

We have summarized some work and presented some new results based on the interplay of statistical modeling and artificial neural networks. The simple remark that ANNs and statistical models are equivalent opens up new directions of methodological development. Statistical models can be used to advantage for designing ANNs and initializing ANN training algorithms. On the other hand, ANN thinking may suggest new statistical modeling approaches. Indeed, new adaptive modeling approaches such as the soft tree begin to emerge; they can be seen as true "hybrids" of statistical models and ANNs.

ANNs and statistical models share the same goal, learning from data. But this goal is pursued with different emphasis: ANNs privilege predictive accuracy, whereas statistical modeling privileges interpretability and parsimony. The approach we have been developing aims at striking a compromise between the two principal aims. The soft tree, which we have discussed in some detail, is a primary example: it aims to be nearly as accurate as an ANN and nearly as interpretable/parsimonious as a statistical model. After a first successful attempt, the basic soft tree model has been extended to increase predictive accuracy while sacrificing as little as possible of interpretability and parsimony. This has been done, as we have shown, by replacing the constant predictor at the leaves of the soft tree by a regression equation. We are currently working at refining the present algorithm. Careful evaluation is also in progress. Soft trees for more complex response variables are under development (survival time, longitudinal response, etc.).

The process we have outlined can be extended much further. One possible goal could be the construction of a more general hierarchy of experts from data. Gating networks, which are for now of the simplest kind, can also be made a little more complex, while remaining interpretable. For instance, a simple gate could be one that responds to "total number of symptoms or features" out of a specified list. This and other ideas will be explored in future research.

References

1. Chaudhuri, P., Lo W.-D., Loh, W.-Y., and Yang, C.-C. (1995). Generalized regression trees, *Statistica Sinica*, **5**, 641–666.

2. Chipman, H., George, E., and McCulloch, R. (2002). Bayesian treed models, *Machine Learning*, **48**, 299–320.

3. Ciampi, A. (1991), Generalized regression trees, *Computational Statistics & Data Analysis*, **12**, 57–78.

4. Ciampi, A., Couturier, A., and Li, S. (2002). Prediction trees with soft nodes for binary outcomes, *Statistics in Medicine*, **21**, 1145–1165.

5. Ciampi, A. and Lechevallier Y. (1995a). Réseaux de neurones et modèles statistiques, *La revue de Modulad*, **15**, 27–46.

6. Ciampi, A., and Lechevallier, Y. (1995b). Designing neural networks from statistical models: A new approach to data exploration, In *Proceedings of the 1st International Conference on Knowledge Discovery and Data Mining*, pp. 45–50, AAAI Press, Menlo Park, California.

7. Ciampi, A., and Lechevallier Y. (1997). Statistical models as building blocks of neural networks, *Communication in Statistics*, **26**, 991–1009.

8. Ciampi, A., and Lechevallier, Y. (2000). Constructing artificial neural networks for censored survival data from statistical models, In *Data Analysis, Classification and Related Methods* (Eds., H. Kiers, J.-P. Rasson, P. Groenen, and M. Schader), pp. 223–228, Springer-Verlag, New York.

9. Ciampi, A., and Lechevallier, Y. (2001). Training an artificial neural network predictor from censored survival data, In *10th International Symposium on Applied Stochastic Models and Data Analysis* (Eds., G. Govaerts, J. Janssen, and N. Limnios), Vol. 1, pp. 332–337, Université de Technologie de Compiègne, France.

10. Ciampi, A., and Zhang F. (2002). A new approach to training backpropagation artificial neural networks: Empirical evaluation on ten data sets from clinical studies, *Statistics in Medicine*, **21**, 1309–1330.

11. Hastie, T. J., and Tibshirani, R. J. (1990). *Generalized Additive Models*, Chapman and Hall, New York.

12. Hastie, T., Tibshirani, R., and Friedman, J. H. (2001). *The Elements of Statistical Learning: Data Mining, Inference and Prediction*, Springer-Verlag, New York.

13. Harrell, F. E., Jr. (2002). *Regression Modeling Strategies*, Springer-Verlag, New York.

14. Hornik, K., Stinchcombe, M., and White H. (1989). Multilayer feedforward networks are universal approximators, *Neural Networks*, **2**, 359–366.

15. Jordan, M. I., and Jacobs, R. A. (1994). Hierarchical mixtures of experts and the EM algorithm, *Neural Computation*, **6**, 181–214.

16. McCullagh, P., and Nelder, J. (1989). *Generalized Linear Models*, Second edition, Chapman and Hall, London, U.K.

17. Venable, W. N., and Ripley, B. D. (2002). *Modern Applied Statistics with S*, Fourth edition, Springer-Verlag, New York.

17

Multilevel Clustering for Large Databases

Yves Lechevallier and Antonio Ciampi

INRIA-Rocquencourt, Le Chesnay, France
McGill University, Montreal, QC, Canada

Abstract: Standard clustering methods do not handle truly large data sets and fail to take into account multilevel data structures. This work outlines an approach to clustering that integrates the Kohonen Self-Organizing Map (SOM) with other clustering methods. Moreover, in order to take into account multilevel structures, a statistical model is proposed, in which a mixture of distributions may have mixing coefficients depending on higher-level variables. Thus, in a first step, the SOM provides a substantial data reduction, whereby a variety of ascending and divisive clustering algorithms becomes accessible. As a second step, statistical modeling provides both a direct means to treat multilevel structures and a framework for model-based clustering. The interplay of these two steps is illustrated on an example of nutritional data from a multicenter study on nutrition and cancer, known as EPIC.

Keywords and phrases: Clustering, classification on very large databases, data reduction

17.1 Introduction

Appropriate use of a clustering algorithm is often a useful first step in extracting knowledge from a data base. Clustering, in fact, leads to a *classification*, that is, the identification of homogeneous and distinct subgroups in data [Gordon (1981) and Bock (1993)], where the definition of homogeneous and distinct depends on the particular algorithm used: this is indeed a simple structure, which, in the absence of a priori knowledge about the multidimensional shape of the data, may be a reasonable starting point towards the discovery of richer, more complex structures.

In spite of the great wealth of clustering algorithms, the rapid accumulation of large databases of increasing complexity poses a number of new problems that traditional algorithms are not equipped to address. One important feature

Table 17.1: French center sample

Center	Number	Frequency
Ile-de-France	1201	24.75
Nord-Pas-de-Calais	452	9.32
Alsace-Lorraine	478	9.85
Rhone-Alpes	1018	20.98
Languedoc-Roussillon	625	12.88
Aquitaine	443	9.13
Bretagne-Pays-de-Loire	635	13.09

of modern data collection is the ever-increasing size of a typical database: it is not so unusual to work with data bases containing from a few thousand to a few million individuals and hundreds or thousands of variables. Now, most clustering algorithms of the traditional type are severely limited as to the number of individuals they can comfortably handle (from a few hundred to a few thousand). Another related feature is the multilevel nature of the data: typically a database may be obtained from a multicountry, multicenter study, so that individuals are nested into centers which are nested into countries. This is an example of an elementary known structure in the data that should not be ignored when attempting to discover new unknown structures.

This work arises from the participation of one of its authors in the EPIC project. EPIC is a multicenter prospective cohort study designed to investigate the effect of dietary, metabolic, and other lifestyle factors on the risk of cancer. The study started in 1990 and now includes 23 centers from ten European countries. By now, dietary data are available on almost 500,000 subjects. Here we initiate a new methodological development towards the discovery of dietary patterns in the EPIC database. We look for general dietary patterns, but taking into account, at the same time, geographical and socioeconomic variation due to country and centers.

For simplicity, we consider only data from a subsample of the EPIC population consisting of 4852 French women distributed in seven centers.

Also, we limit ourselves to an analysis of data from a 24-hour recall questionnaire concerning intake of 16 food groups. Thus, we will only discuss clustering for two-level systems: subjects (first level) and center (second level), in our case.

The approach we propose is based on two key ideas:

(1) A preliminary data reduction using a Kohonen Self-Organizing Map (SOM) is performed. As a result, the individual measurements are replaced by the means of the individual measurements over a relatively small number

of microregimens corresponding to Kohonen neurons. The microregimens can now be treated as new cases and the means of the original variables over microregimens as new variables. This reduced data set is now small enough to be treated by classical clustering algorithms. A further advantage of the Kohonen reduction is that the vector of means over the microregimens can safely be treated as multivariate normal, owing to the central limit theorem. This is a key property, in particular, because it permits the definition of an appropriate dissimilarity measure between microregimens.

(2) The multilevel feature of the problem is treated by a statistical model that assumes a mixture of distributions, each distribution representing, in our example, a regimen or dietary pattern. Although more complex dependencies can be modeled, here we will assume that the centers only affect the mixing coefficients, and not the parameters of the distributions. Thus we look for general dietary patterns assuming that centers differ from each other only in the distribution of the local population across the general dietary patterns.

Although the idea of a preliminary Kohonen reduction followed by the application of a classical clustering algorithm is not entirely new [Murthag (1995), Ambroise *et al.* (2000) and Thiria *et al.* (1997)], this work differs from previous attempts in several respects, the most important of which are:

(a) The Kohonen chart is trained by an initialization based on principal component analysis;

(b) The choice of clustering algorithm is guided by the multilevel aspect of the problem at hand;

(c) The clustering algorithm is based on a statistical model.

Thus this work continues the authors research program which aims to develop data analytic strategies integrating KDDM and classical data analysis methods [Ciampi and Lechevallier (1995, 1997)].

17.2   Data Reduction by Kohonen SOMs

We consider p measurements performed on n subjects grouped in C classes, $\{G_c, c = 1, \ldots, C\}$. We denote these measurements by $(G^{(i)}, x^{(i)})$, $i = 1, \ldots, n$, where for the ith subject $G^{(i)}$ denotes the class (the center, in our example), and $x^{(i)}$ the p-vector of measurements (the 16 food-group intake variables); or, in matrix form, $\mathbf{D} = [\mathbf{G}|\mathbf{X}]$.

In this section we describe the first step of the proposed approach, which consists in reducing the $n \times p$ matrix $\mathbf{X}$ to a $m \times p$ matrix, $m \ll n$. To do this, we first pass the data matrix $\mathbf{X}$ through a Kohonen SOM consisting of m units (neurons) disposed in a rectangular sheet with connections along two perpendicular axis.

17.2.1   Kohonen SOMs and PCA initialization

We recall that in a Kohonen SOM the neurons of the rectangular sheet are associated with a grid of prototypes in the p-dimensional space which represents the row-vectors of the data matrix: the sheet is supposed to represent the grid with a minimum distortion, so that a SOM can be seen as a nonlinear version of classical data reduction techniques such as a Principal Component Analysis (PCA). In order to specify a SOM, one needs to specify initial values of the sheet's connection weights and of the position of the prototypes. Then, the data points are repeatedly sent through the SOM, each passage causing an update of both the connection weights and the position of the prototypes, that is, an alteration of both the sheet in two-dimensional space and the grid in p-dimensional space. Normally, this process converges, in that the changes at each passage become negligible.

In the original approach, initial weights were chosen at random; however, as the efficacy of the algorithms crucially depends on the initialization, much effort has been devoted to improving this first step. The distinguishing feature of our construction consists in designing the sheet with the help of the results of PCA performed on $\mathbf{X}$. It is advantageous to choose the dimensions of the grid, a and b ($m = ab$), such that

$$\frac{a}{b} = \frac{\sqrt{\lambda_1}}{\sqrt{\lambda_2}},$$

where λ_1 and λ_2 denote the first and second eigenvalues of the PCA; see Figure 17.1. Also, the initial connection weights and position of the prototypes are obtained from the two first eigenvectors of the PCA. The details are described in Elemento (1999), where it is also shown that PCA initialization presents substantial practical advantages over several alternative approaches.

17.2.2   Binning of the original data matrix using a Kohonen map

As a result of the training process, the SOM associates with each subject a unique neuron–prototype pair, which we shall refer to as a *microregimen*. Each microregimen, B_r, $r = 1, \ldots, m$, can be considered as a *bin* in which similar individuals are grouped. We shall denote by n_r the number of subjects in B_r and by $n_{r,c}$ the number of subjects in $B_r \cap G_c$. Also, let $\bar{x}_r$ and $\bar{x}_r^{(c)}$ denote

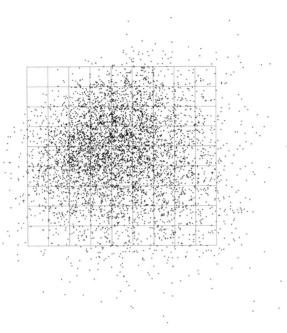

Figure 17.1: Initialization by PCA

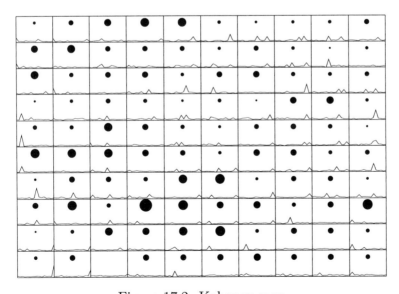

Figure 17.2: Kohonen map

the vectors of the means of $x^{(i)}$ taken over B_r and over $B_r \cap G_c$, respectively. Figure 17.2 gives a graphical representation of the bins [Hébrail and Debregeas (1998)]: in each bin, the dot is proportional to bin size and the graph is a profile of the input variables.

Already at this stage, an exploratory analysis of the two-way table $\{n_{r,c}; r = 1, \ldots, m, c = 1, \ldots, C\}$, would be instructive: for example, Correspondence Analysis (CA) of the table, ordering its rows and columns according to the factor scores and eventually clustering rows and columns, is likely to shed some light on the relationship between centers and microregimens.

Our goal, however, is to look for macroregimens, (dietary patterns in our example), by clustering microregimens. To proceed further, we assume here that the expected value of x and its variance–covariance matrix may depend on the microregimens but not on the centers. It follows that if $n_{r,c}$ is large enough, then, by the central limit theorem, $\bar{x}_r^{(c)}$ is approximately multivariate normal $\mathcal{N}_p(\mu_r, (1/n_{r,c})/\Sigma_r)$, and the maximum likelihood estimates of μ_r and Σ_r are

$$\bar{x}_r = \frac{1}{n_r} \sum_{i \in B_r} x^{(i)} \quad \text{and} \quad V_r = \frac{1}{n_r} \sum_{i \in B_r} (x^{(i)} - \bar{x}_r)^T (x^{(i)} - \bar{x}_r).$$

17.2.3 Dissimilarity for microregimens

From these considerations, a natural definition for a dissimilarity between two bins B_r and B_s follows. This is the Likelihood Ratio Statistic (LRS) comparing the hypothesis that $\bar{x}_r^{(c)}$ and $\bar{x}_s^{(c)}$ have different distributions with the hypothesis that they have the same distribution; viz.,

$$d(B_r, B_s) = 2 \sum_{s=1}^{C} \log \left\{ \frac{\mathcal{N}_p(\bar{x}_r^{(c)}|\bar{x}_r, \frac{1}{n_{r,c}} V_r) \mathcal{N}_p(\bar{x}_s^{(c)}|\bar{x}_s, \frac{1}{n_{s,c}} V_s)}{\mathcal{N}_p(\bar{x}_r^{(c)}|\bar{x}_{r \cup s}, \frac{1}{n_{r,c}} V_{r \cup s}) \mathcal{N}_p(\bar{x}_s^{(c)}|\bar{x}_{r \cup s}, \frac{1}{n_{s,c}} V_{r \cup s})} \right\}, \quad (17.1)$$

where $\mathcal{N}_p(.|\mu, \Sigma)$ is the density function of a multivariate normal $\mathcal{N}_p(\mu, \Sigma_r)$ and

$$\bar{x}_{r \cup s} = \frac{n_r \bar{x}_r + n_s \bar{x}_s}{n_r + n_s} \quad (17.2)$$

and

$$V_{r \cup s} = \frac{1}{n_r + n_s} [n_r V_r + n_s V_s + n_r n_s (\bar{x}_r - \bar{x}_s)(\bar{x}_r - \bar{x}_s)^T]. \quad (17.3)$$

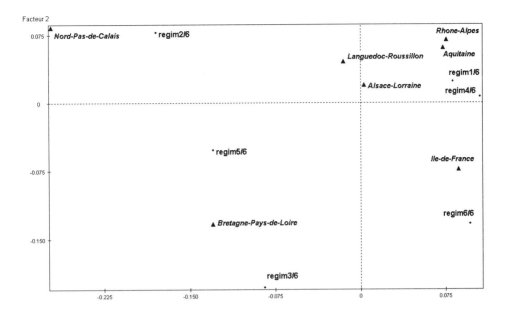

Figure 17.3: Relation between center and regimens

17.3   Clustering Multilevel Systems

Although the dissimilarity of Eqs. (17.1) and (17.2) is very natural in our context, some other ones can be usefully defined, such as those proposed in the symbolic data analysis literature [Bock and Diday (1999)]. Once the choice of dissimilarity has been made, several standard algorithms can be applied to the bins. Because the number of bins ($m \ll n$) may be chosen to be relatively small, a panoply of ascending approaches becomes accessible. Moreover, several dissimilarity-based divisive approaches are available. Among these, some conceptual clustering algorithms [Chavent (1998)] seem particularly promising as the one used in this work; see the next section, for example.

Suppose now that a clustering algorithm has been deployed. As a result, the m microregimens are grouped to produce $k \ll m$ macroregimens. Furthermore, the two-way table $\{m_{i,c}; i = 1, \ldots, k, \ c = 1, \ldots, C\}$ obtained by crossing centers with macroregimens can be analyzed by CA as outlined in the previous section. Finally, proportions of subjects following different regimens in each center would usefully summarize local characteristics, and a description of the clusters would give insight on the nature of the macroregimens found in the general population.

17.3.1 A two-level statistical model

A statistical model may now be proposed. This can be useful for efficiently extracting information from the data, as it suggests a family of model-based clustering algorithms that explicitly account for the multi-level structure of the data. For a two-level system, we suppose that the reduced data vector $\bar{x}_r^{(c)}$ has as distribution a mixture of k multivariate normal distributions, each corresponding to a macroregimen, or dietary pattern in our example. Thus the density can be written as

$$f(\bar{x}_r^{(c)}) = \sum_{i=1}^{k} \alpha_i(G_c) \mathcal{N}_p(\bar{x}_r^{(c)}|\mu_i, \Delta_i). \qquad (17.4)$$

A more complex model would include dependence of the μs and the Δs on c. The interest of such a model is limited, although it could eventually be used to check the adequacy of the one we propose. The simpler model is of greater interest, especially for our dietary data example, because it allows identification of general patterns that are to be found in all centers albeit in different proportions. For instance, we may expect that the Mediterranean diet is not an exclusive characteristic of Mediterranean regions; although more frequently encountered in these regions, it can be chosen as a way of eating normally, perhaps for health reasons, by people living in all areas of France, and indeed, of Europe.

It is easy to see how this two-level model can be generalized to three- and multilevel systems by introducing, for example, a country level and treating centers-within-country by random effects. This, however, will not be pursued here.

17.3.2 Estimating parameters by the EM algorithm

In many situations, a reasonable description of the data is amply sufficient. Then the statistical model of (17.3) serves as useful guidance, but the exploratory approach outlined above is all that is needed: indeed, it produces both a reasonable guess for the number of clusters and rough estimates of means, variance–covariance matrices, and mixing coefficients. On the other hand, when more precise estimates are desired, these rough ones can be used to initialize an iterative algorithm for maximum likelihood estimation. Here, as we are dealing with a mixture model, the EM algorithm seems an appropriate choice, with the dependence of the mixing coefficients on the center introducing only a minor additional complication.

The EM is applied as follows.

(a) The complete data are $\left(\bar{x}_r^{(c)}, \rho(r)\right)$, where $\rho(r)$ is the (actually unknown) regimen to which the rth microregimen belongs;

(b) The log-likelihood of the complete data is

$$l = \log L = \sum_{c=1}^{C} \sum_{r=1}^{m} \sum_{i=1}^{k} \log[\alpha_i^{(t)}(G_c) + \mathcal{N}_p(\bar{x}_r^{(c)}|\mu_i, \tfrac{1}{n_{r,c}}\Delta_i)].$$

(c) At step t, let

$$p^{(t)}(c|i, \bar{x}_r^{(c)}) = \frac{\alpha_i^{(t)}(G_c)\mathcal{N}_p(\bar{x}_r^{(c)}|\mu_i^t, \tfrac{1}{n_{r,c}}\Delta_i^t)}{\sum_{j=1}^{k} \alpha_j^{(t)}(G_c)\mathcal{N}_p(\bar{x}_r^{(c)}|\mu_j^t, \tfrac{1}{n_{r,c}}\Delta_j^t)}.$$

Then the iterative equations from the EM approach can be shown to be

$$\mu_i^{(t)} = \frac{1}{n}\sum_{c=1}^{C}\sum_{r=1}^{m} p^{(t-1)}(c|i, \bar{x}_r^{(c)}))\bar{x}_r^{(c)},$$

$$\Delta_i^{(t)} = \frac{1}{n}\sum_{c=1}^{C}\sum_{r=1}^{m} p^{(t-1)}(c|i, m^{(r,c)})(\bar{x}_r^{(c)}) - \mu_i^{(t-1)})^T(\bar{x}_r^{(c)}) - \mu_i^{(t-1)}),$$

$$p^{(t)}(c|i, \bar{x}_r^{(c)}) = \frac{1}{n_c}\sum_{s=1}^{m} p^{(t-1)}(c|i, \bar{x}_s^{(c)})).$$

17.4 Extracting Dietary Patterns from the Nutritional Data

We return now to the subset of the EPIC database describing dietary habits of 4852 French women. Figure 17.2 summarizes the Kohonen SOM analysis of the data based on a 10×10 sheet. Because one bin is empty, 99 distinct regimens were identified. Both a standard ascending algorithm [Murthag (1995)] and a conceptual clustering algorithm [Chavent (1998)] applied to the microregimens, suggest four, six, or nine classes or dietary patterns. The results of the six-class analysis are summarized in Figure 17.4 which shows the first factorial plane of the CA representing the relationship between centers and dietary pattern; Figure 17.4, which shows the Zoom Star graphs [Noirhomme-Fraiture and Rouard (1998)] of the eight most discriminating variables describing dietary patterns; and Table 17.4 which gives a rough estimate of the proportions of subjects following the six dietary patterns, overall and by center.

An example of interpretation is as follows: regimen 1 is characterized by high consumption of meat and vegetables; regimen 2 by high soup and low vegetable consumption; regimen 3 by high fish and low meat consumption (respectively, 13% and 3% of the total weight of food intake); regimen 4 by high meat and

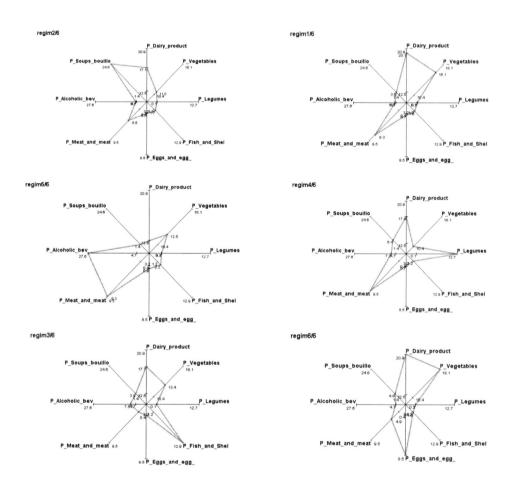

Figure 17.4: The six regimens by Zoom Stars

Table 17.2: Proportion of the six regimens: overall and by center

Regimens	Overall	Alsace -Lorraine	Aquitaine	Bretagne Loire	Ile-de -France	Languedoc -Roussillon	Nord -Pas -de-Calais	Rhone -Alpes
regim 1	0,56	0,58	0,59	0,49	0,58	0,54	0,46	0,61
regim 2	0,19	0,18	0,18	0,20	0,14	0,21	0,28	0,18
regim 3	0,08	0,08	0,07	0,12	0,09	0,08	0,08	0,06
regim 4	0,03	0,02	0,04	0,03	0,03	0,04	0,02	0,03
regim 5	0,10	0,10	0,08	0,11	0,10	0,08	0,13	0,09
regim 6	0,04	0,04	0,04	0,05	0,05	0,04	0,03	0,04

low fish consumption; regimen 5 by high alcohol and meat consumption; and regimen 6 by high consumption of dairy products, eggs, and vegetables and low consumption of fish, alcoholic beverage, and vegetables. Also, the Nord-Pas-de-Calais region is positively associated with regimens 2 and 5 and negatively with regimen 1; similarly, there is a positive association of Bretagne-Pays-de-Loire with regimen 3 and a negative association with regimen 1; and finally, Rhone-Alpes is positively associated with regimen 1.

Acknowledgements. We wish to thank Dr. F. Clavel for having shared the French data with us, and Dr. E. Riboli for general assistance in becoming familiar with EPIC.

References

1. Ambroise, C., Seže, G., Badran, F., and Thiria, S. (2000). Hierarchical clustering of self-organizing maps for cloud classification, *Neurocomputing*, **30**, 47–52.

2. Bock, H. H. (1993). Classification and clustering: Problems for the future, In *New Approaches in Classification and Data Analysis* (Eds., E. Diday, Y. Lechevallier, M. Schader, P. Bertrand, and B. Burtschy), pp. 3–24, Springer-Verlag, Heidelberg.

3. Bock, H. H., and Diday, E. (Eds.) (1999). Analysis of symbolic data, exploratory methods for extracting statistical information from complex data, In *Studies in Classification, Data Analysis and Knowledge Organization*, Springer-Verlag, Heidelberg.

4. Chavent, M. (1998). A monothetic clustering algorithm, *Pattern Recognition Letters*, **19**, 989–996.

5. Ciampi, A., and Lechevallier, Y. (1995). Designing neural networks from statistical models: A new approach to data exploration, In *Proceedings*

      of the *First International Conference on Knowledge Discovery and Data Mining*, pp. 45–50, AAAI Press, Menlo Park, California.

6. Ciampi, A., and Lechevallier, Y. (1997). Statistical models as building blocks of neural networks, *Communications in Statistics*, **26**, 991–1009.

7. Elemento, O. (1999). Apport de l'analyse en composantes principales pour l'initialisation et la validation de cartes de Kohonen, In *Septièmes Journées de la Société Francophone de Classification*, Nancy, France.

8. Gordon, A. D. (1981). *Classification: Methods for the Exploratory Analysis of Multivariate Data*, Chapman & Hall, London, UK.

9. Hébrail, G., and Debregeas, A. (1998). Interactive interpretation of Kohonen maps applied to curves, In *Proceedings of the Fourth International Conference on Knowledge Discovery and Data Mining*, pp. 179–183, AAAI press, Menlo Park, California.

10. Murthag, F. (1995). Interpreting the Kohonen self-organizing feature map using contiguity-constrained clustering, *Pattern Recognition Letters*, **16**, 399–408.

11. Noirhomme-Fraiture, M., and Rouard, M. (1998). Representation of sub-populations and correlation with Zoom Star, In *Proceedings of NNTS'98*, Sorrento, Italy.

12. Thiria, S., Lechevallier, Y., Gascuel, O., and Canu, S. (1997). *Statistique et Méthodes Neuronales*, Dunod, Paris.

18

Neural Networks: An Application for Predicting Smear Negative Pulmonary Tuberculosis

A. M. Santos,[1] **B. B. Pereira,**[2] **J. M. Seixas,**[2] **F. C. Q. Mello,**[2] **and A. L. Kritski**[2]

[1] *Federal University of Maranhão, Maranhão, Brazil*
[2] *Federal University of Rio de Janeiro, Rio de Janeiro, Brazil*

Abstract: Smear negative pulmonary tuberculosis (SNPT) accounts for 30% of pulmonary tuberculosis (PT) cases reported yearly. Rapid and accurate diagnosis of SNPT could provide lower morbidity and mortality, and case detection at a less contagious status. The main objective of this work is to evaluate a prediction model for diagnosis of SNPT, useful for outpatients who are attended in settings with limited resources. The data used for developing the proposed models werecomprised of 136 patients from health care units. They were referred to the University Hospital in Rio de Janeiro, Brazil, from March 2001 to September 2002, with clinical–radiological suspicion of SNPT. Only symptoms and physical signs were used for constructing the neural network (NN) modelling, which was able to correctly classify 77% of patients from a test sample. The achievements of the NN model suggest that mathematical modelling, developed for classifying SNPT cases could be a useful tool for optimizing application of more expensive tests, and to avoid costs of unnecessary anti-PT treatment. In addition, the main features extracted by the neural model are shown to agree with current analysis from experts in the field.

Keywords and phrases: Neural networks, cross-validation, clustering, tuberculosis, medical diagnosis

18.1   Introduction

Tuberculosis is a serious public health problem and it is estimated by the World Health Organization (WHO) that approximately 1.8 billion individuals are infected by Mycobacterium tuberculosis [WHO (2002)]. In Brazil, approximately 35 to 45 million individuals are currently infected by this disease.

Sputum smear and Mycobacterium tuberculosis culture have been advocated as valuable tools for diagnosis of pulmonary tuberculosis. However, the sputum smear staining lacks sensitivity, and culture confirmation requires several weeks; few tuberculosis-control programmes in low-income countries have access to facilities that allow culture performance in their primary-care diagnostic.

Approximately 20% to 50% of patients with pulmonary tuberculosis are smear negative, and 10% of these patients are culture negative. However, these smear-negative cases pose a relevant public health hazard due to their transmission rate of Mycobacterium tuberculosis of 17% among exposed individuals [Sarmiento *et al.* (2003)].

Much attention has recently been paid to the problem of smear negative pulmonary tuberculosis (SNPT) particularly due to the HIV epidemic, because the co-infection increases the risks of tuberculosis atypical presentation and associated morbidity and mortality. Quite appropriately, the discussion regarding SNPT has focused on low-income countries, home of the vast majority of individuals with tuberculosis and HIV infection and where the availability of culture diagnostics is limited. So, rapid and accurate diagnosis of SNPT could provide lower morbidity and mortality, and case detection at a less contagious status [Long (2001)].

Diagnosis of SNPT is usually based upon clinical presentation and radiological indicators that present a limited accuracy. In this context, there is a need for new approaches for the diagnosis of SNPT. For clinical use, these new tools should be used under routine conditions in the health care units.

In the medical literature, several statistical models have been suggested for pulmonary tuberculosis diagnostics. El-Solh *et al.* (1999) established a model for identification of PT using neural networks. Mello *et al.* (2006) use multivariate logistic regression and classification trees to predict the patient's probability of PT. Santos (2003) uses neural networks and classification trees to identify patients with clinical–radiological suspicion of SNPT.

Statistical models can be used for prediction of infection or of the disease. They also can be used to simulate epidemic situations providing clues for preventive interventions. If formulated in a systematic way and implemented with high-qualified data, these models can be representative of the clinical problem under evaluation and could be useful for physicians in their clinical regular practice, as well as for public health policy administration [Kritski and Ruffino-Netto (2000)].

In this work, we use artificial neural network for developing and evaluating a prediction model for diagnosing SNPT, useful for patients attended in health care units within areas of limited resources. In addition, we analyze the information that is extracted by the model and compare it to expert analysis for diagnosis. This analysis aims at helping doctors to understand the way the model works and to make them more confident in its practical application.

The chapter is arranged as follows. Section 18.2 describes the methods used in this work and specifically describes the networks used. This section also describes the data set in the study as well as the selection criteria for both the training and testing sets used for developing the artificial neural model and testing its generalization capacity. In Section 18.3, the methodology used to identify the relevant variables is presented. Results and conclusions are presented in Sections 18.4 and 18.5, respectively.

18.2   Materials and Methods

In this section, we first describe the data set used for artificial neural network design. In Section 18.2.2, the topology of the artificial neural networks used in this work is defined. Clustering techniques were applied for splitting the data set into a training and testing sets and this is described in Section 18.2.3. The section concludes with a study of the relevance of the explanatory variables that feed into networks.

18.2.1   Data set

The data set refers to 136 patients who agreed to participate in the study. They were referred to Hospital Clementino Fraga Filho, a University Hospital of Federal University of Rio de Janeiro, Brazil, from March, 2001 to September, 2002, with clinical–radiological suspicion of SNPT. The data consisted of information from anamnesis interview and included demographic and risk factors typically known for tuberculosis diagnosis.

These patients were under suspicion of active pulmonary tuberculosis, presenting negative smear. Forty-three percent of these patients actually showed PT in activity.

Firstly, 26 clinical variables were considered for model development. These included: age, cough, sputum, sweat, fever, weight loss, chest pain, shudder, dyspnea, diabetes, alcoholism, and others. In the sequence, the data set was described using just 12 or 8 clinical variables. Those variables were selected by experts active in tuberculosis research.

18.2.2   Neural network design

In this work, we use a multilayer feedforward architecture with a backpropagation algorithm [Haykin (1999)]. The network has three layers and each layer receives inputs only from its preceding layer. Adjacent layers are fully connected, that is, every neuron in a layer is connected to every neuron in an adjacent layer.

Several factors are important in a network design for pattern classification problems. These include the network architecture as well as the training methodology used. All the networks investigated in this study used a single hidden layer. It has been shown that neural networks of this type can handle the majority of problems [Hornik (1991)].

As already mentioned, from 26 to 8 input variables were fed into the network input nodes, which correspond to the patients' clinical variables. Variables were normalized by the following transformation:

$$x_i^* = \frac{x_i - \bar{x}}{\max(x_i - \bar{x})}, \qquad i = 1, 2, \ldots, 136, \tag{18.1}$$

where x_i is the original variable and $\bar{x}$ its arithmetic mean. Variable normalization is required for matching input variation with the dynamic range of activation function of the neurons. In our case, a hyperbolic tangent was chosen as the function for activating all neurons.

The binary variables were codified as -1 or 1, where -1 represents the absence of the observed attribute and 1 the presence of the attribute. The qualitative variables with three categories were codified as -1 (absence of observed attribute), 1 (presence of the observed attribute) and 0 (ignored).

The network has a single output neuron, with training targets defined as 1 if the patient is with active PT and -1 otherwise.

It is known that parsimonious models with few hidden neurons are preferable, because they tend to show better generalization ability, reducing the overfitting problem. The number of neurons in the hidden layer was defined through experimentation. Networks having three and four hidden neurons proved to work well for this problem.

The performance of the neural network (NN) was evaluated through the classification for the testing set, which is referred to here as accuracy. Other descriptive statistics were also used to evaluate the performance of NN in study, they are: *sensitivity* and *specificity*, because those measured are of general use in medicine. Sensitivity of the neural model will tell us how the model is classifying the patients with PT in activity, and the specificity will tell how the model is classifying patients without PT in activity.

We will use the notation $(i - h - o)$ to refer to a neural network with i inputs, h hidden neurons and o neurons in the output layer.

18.2.3   Data selection for network design

Building the training and testing sets is one of the main tasks in designing an artificial neural network, especially in practical situations where statistical restrictions are present.

Both training and testing sets should be constituted from the available data set. In practical applications, the amount of available data for model development may be small. In such a situation, the training and testing sets should be carefully selected, so that representative samples of the problem are obtained.

At first, the original data were randomly divided into the training and testing sets. Given the statistical limitations of the available data, a division in the form of 80% of the patients for the training set and 20% for the testing set would be preferable. With this strategy, model development was made varying the number of hidden neurons. It was observed that some neural networks exhibited poor performance. This was due to poor statistical representation of the training set with respect to patterns belonging to the testing set. If any region of the domain of the input of the network does not have an appropriate number of patterns included in the training set, this region will not be learned efficiently and, consequently, patterns in the testing set that belong to region will be probably classified erroneously [Alencar (2003)].

Efficient alternatives for data selection are cross-validation [Stone (1974)] and cluster analysis [Morrison (1990)].

Cross validation

Cross-validation has been successful in neural network designs. For this, the original data set $\mathcal{D}$ is divided randomly into k mutually exclusive subsets $\mathcal{D}_v$, $v = 1, \ldots, k$. The subsets should be the most homogeneous possible and the number of cases of each subset should be approximately the same. Frequently, k is taken to be ten and the division of the data into k subsets is through the k-fold cross-validation method.

After the division of the original data $\mathcal{D}$, as showed in Figure 18.1, the neural networks are trained, using as training set $\mathcal{D} - \mathcal{D}_v$ (the cases that belong to $\mathcal{D}$ but not to $\mathcal{D}_v$) and as test set $\mathcal{D}_v$. In Figure 18.1, the first subset is the testing set, and the others form the training set. Next, the second subset is the testing set and the others as training set, and so on. We can observe that each subset enters the training set as well as the testing set.

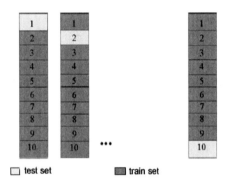

Figure 18.1: Example of cross-validation for $k = 10$

In this study, the data set was split into six subsets, containing approximately the same number of patterns. Four of the six subsets were used for training of the NN, and the remaining ones were used for testing the generalization capacity of the classifier. This procedure was repeated until all possible combinations of the six subsets were used for training the NN. In total, 15 different training and testing subsets were formed. Each training subset comprised on an average 92 patterns, and the testing subset 44.

Cluster analysis

Cluster analysis is a technique used to detect the existence of clusters in given data. This grouping process can be seen as an unsupervised learning technique.

Generally speaking, cluster analysis methods are of two types: (*a*) Partitioning methods: algorithms that divide the data set into k clusters, where the integer k needs to be specified by the user; (*b*) Hierarchical methods: algorithms yielding an entire hierarchy of clusterings of the data set. Agglomerative methods start by forming local clusters from each object in the data set and then successively merge clusters until only one large cluster remains that is the whole set of data. Divisive methods start by considering the whole data set as one cluster, and then split up clusters until each object is separate.

To avoid the possibility of some regions not being represented, training and testing sets were also obtained data clustering. Firstly, for obtaining the groups, we used the agglomerative hierarchical method. The hierarchical methods do not present an intuitive indicator for the number of clusters present in the data set. An alternative is the construction of the *dendrogram*, which is a tree whose leaves are data objects, and branches can be seen as the identified clusters [Morrison (1990)].

The dendrogram was constructed using Ward's method [Kaufman and Rousseeuw (1990)]. In the first step, the patterns were grouped according to the 26 explanatory variables. Analyzing the dendrogram, three main clusters were identified. Restricting the data space to 12 or 8 explanatory variables, three main clusters were also identified.

An artificial neural network method was also used to obtain homogeneous groups. This method is the *modified ART* (adaptive resonance theory) architecture, presented by Vassali, Seixas, and Calôba (2002). This method is based essentially on the Kohonen layer and competitive learning [Haykin (1999)].

In the modified ART, each neuron of such a layer has assigned to it a vector of synaptic weights with unitary norm. The classification of an input vector x is performed by the neuron that exhibits the smallest distance (according to the Euclidean metric) to this vector, among all neurons, provided that this distance is smaller than a predefined radius r_0. This neuron becomes the winner and will be the only neuron to be trained, according to the equation

$$\boldsymbol{w}_{n+1} = (1 - \eta)\boldsymbol{w}_n + \eta\boldsymbol{x}, \tag{18.2}$$

where η is the learning coefficient and $\boldsymbol{w}$ is the weight vector.

The distance between an incoming vector and a given weight vector can be obtained by computing the inner product between these two vectors as

$$< \boldsymbol{x}, \boldsymbol{w} > = 1 - \frac{d(\boldsymbol{x}, \boldsymbol{w})^2}{2}. \tag{18.3}$$

This is possible because vectors are normalized ($|\boldsymbol{x}| = |\boldsymbol{w}| = 1$). Vector normalization is performed by adding one more element to each original vector, so that this extra component provides the information concerning the norm of the original vector.

It should be clear that this operation is equivalent to a clustering procedure, where each neuron is assigned to a cluster. In fact, after a number of training steps, it is expected that the weight vector assigned with a neuron will converge to the centroid of the corresponding cluster [Vassali, Seixas, and Calôba (2002)].

An interesting feature that has been added to this network was the vigilance radius r_0, which can impose a limited region for the neuron's action. Geometrically, it is equivalent to imposing a maximum volume on each cluster, so that an incoming vector that does not exhibit similarity to any of the existing neurons will not be classified. During the training phase, whenever this happens, a new neuron is created, and its corresponding weight vector is the incoming vector itself. If this happens during the production phase, the incoming vector cannot be assigned to any class and it is declared to be unknown [Vassali, Seixas, and Calôba (2002)].

In the sequence, the modified ART method was applied. Initially, the norm of each vector of explanatory variables $\boldsymbol{x}_i$ was made unitary. Considering p explanatory variables, the normalization component, denoted as x_{ip+1}, was added as

$$x_{ip+1} = (M - \sum_{j=1}^{p} x_{ij}^2)^{1/2}, \qquad i = 1, 2, \ldots, 136, \tag{18.4}$$

where

$$M = \max \|\boldsymbol{x}_i\|. \tag{18.5}$$

So, the normalized data vector became

$$\boldsymbol{x}_i = \frac{1}{\sqrt{M}}(x_{i1}, x_{i2}, \cdots, x_{ip+1})', \qquad i = 1, 2, \ldots, 136. \tag{18.6}$$

The modified ART method requests a vigilance radius for each cluster to be formed. To obtain the vigilance radius, we calculated the Euclidean distance between the patterns in the data set. The choice for this radius was based on the more frequent distance. As result of this, three clusters were again recognized in the data set, despite describing the input space with 26, 12, or 8 exploratory variables.

Although both clustering methods under investigation pointed out three clusters in the data set, they were not the same. In this case, the training set was obtained by randomly selecting 75% of the patients in each cluster and 25% of patients was selected to form the testing set.

After having formed the training and the testing sets from both the clustering and cross-validation approaches, we trained several NN and evaluated their performance. The data sets that exhibited the best performance were chosen to form the final model. Table 18.1 presents these data sets. We can observe that amount of patients with PT in activity (PT^+) and without PT (PT^-) is different in the considered data sets.

Table 18.1: Composition of the training and testing sets selected.

Method	Variables	Train PT$^-$	Train PT$^+$	Train Sum	Test PT$^-$	Test PT$^+$	Test Sum
	26	52	39	91	25	20	45
Cross-validation	12	50	40	90	27	19	46
	8	49	42	91	28	19	45
	26	57	45	102	20	14	34
Clustering	12	59	42	101	18	17	35
	8	55	41	96	22	18	40

18.3 Relevance of Explanatory Variables

For network design, we should select the relevant explanatory variables. Using only relevant information, the dimensionality of the input data space can be reduced, which favors compact designs. The inclusion of variables that poorly contribute to the design target may reduce the generalization power.

Several methods for input variable selection have been proposed. Some authors use the Akaike Information Criterion [Akaike (1974)] and Bayesian Information Criterion [Schwarz (1978)] as the procedure for selection of the input variables. Here, the relevance of an input variable is measured by using statistic R_j; see Seixas, Calôba, and Delpino (1996). This statistic measures the variation, produced in the output of network when the value of an input variable is substituted by its mean, for all the events that belong to the training set. Therefore, R_j is given by

$$R_j = \frac{1}{N_{pat}} \sum_{i=1}^{N_{pat}} (y(\boldsymbol{x}_i, \omega) - y(\boldsymbol{x}_i, \omega)|_{x_{j,i} = \bar{x}_j}))^2, \tag{18.7}$$

where N_{pat} is the number of events in the training set and $y(\boldsymbol{x}_i, \omega)$ corresponds to the output of the network.

18.4 Results

After selecting the training and testing sets, the NNs were trained. Different numbers of neurons on the hidden layer were considered. Neural networks with three, four and five hidden neurons were tested. Alternative parameters were used (learning rate, momentum, and number of iterations) of the backpropagation algorithm. The NNs with the smallest classification errors in the test set were selected.

According to Table 18.2, the NN with 12 input variables presented the largest accuracy (77%), as well as the largest specificity (83%). However, the neural network developed with the training set obtained by cross-validation possessed the largest sensitivity (84%); that is, this network better classifies the individuals with active PT.

Table 18.2: Classification efficiencies

| | Cross Validation | | | Clustering | | |
Networks	Accuracy (%)	Specificity (%)	Sensitivity (%)	Accuracy (%)	Specificity (%)	Sensitivity (%)
(26-4-1)	71	76	65	71	65	79
(12-4-1)	72	63	84	77	83	71
(8-4-1)	71	68	76	70	61	82

To identify the relevant variables, considering the neural network with the largest accuracy, the relevance of each variable was computed. For this, Eq. (18.7), defined in Section 18.3, was used.

According to Figure 18.2, the neural network identified 11 relevant variables for the problem under study, except the variable extrapulmonary tuberculosis.

18.5   Conclusions

The proposed NN model suggests that mathematical modelling, for classifying SNPT cases, could be a useful tool for optimizing utilization of more expensive tests, and to avoid costs of unnecessary anti-PT treatment. Besides, the neural model was able to identify the important variables for the problem under study, as described by experts of the field.

In the case under study, the sample size was one of the main limitations for design network. We used cross-validation and clustering methods to overcome this limitation of NN model development. These techniques made it possible to identify a training set that could allow good response generalization for testing set.

The neural network model achieved good classification performance, exhibiting sensitivity from 71 to 82% and specificity from 60 to 83%. However, only symptoms and physical signs were used for constructing the neural network.

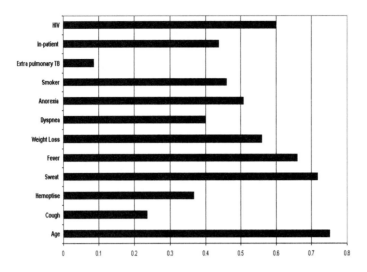

Figure 18.2: Relevance for data description using 12 variables

The validation of the network performance in an independent sample of patients is necessary to confirm these findings.

Acknowledgements. The authors thank the staff and students of the Tuberculosis Research Unit, Faculty of Medicine, Federal University of Rio de Janeiro, for making available the data used in this work and CAPES, CNPq, FAPERJ and FAPEMA for financially supporting this project.

References

1. Akaike, H. (1974). A new look at the statistical model identification, *IEEE Transactions on Automatic Control*, **19**, 716–723.

2. Alencar, G. A. (2003). Artificial neural networks as rain attenuation predictors in earth-space paths, *Ph.D. Thesis*, Federal University of Rio de Janeiro, Brazil.

3. El-Solh, A. A., Hsiao, C.-B., Goodnough, S., Serghani, J., and Grant, B. J. B. (1999). Predicting active pulmonary tuberculosis using an artificial neural network, *Chest*, **116**, 968–973.

4. Haykin, S. (1999). *Neural Networks: A Comparative Foundation*, Prentice-Hall, Upper Saddle River, New Jersey.

5. Hornik, K. (1991). Approximation capabilities of multilayer feedforward networks, *Neural Networks*, **4**, 251-257.

6. Kaufman, L., and Rousseeuw, P. (1990). *Finding Groups in Data*, John Wiley & Sons, New York.

7. Kritski, A. L., and Ruffino-Netto, A. (2000). Health sector reform in Brazil: Impact on tuberculosis control, *International Journal of Tuberculosis and Lung Disease*, **4**, 622–626.

8. Long, R. (2001). Smear-negative pulmonary tuberculosis in industrialized countries, *Chest*, **120**(2), 330–334.

9. Mello, F. C, Bastos, L. G, Soares, S. L, Rezende, V. M, Conde, M. B, Chaisson, R. E, Kritski, A. L, Ruffino-Netto, A., and Werneck, G. L. (2006). Predicting smear negative pulmonary tuberculosis with classification trees and logistic regression: a cross-sectional study, *BMC Public Health*, **6**.

10. Morrison, D. F. (1990). *Multivariate Statistical Methods*, Third edition, McGraw-Hill, New York.

11. Santos, A. M. (2003). Neural networks and classification trees: an application for predicting smear negative pulmonary tuberculosis, *Ph.D. Thesis*, Federal University of Rio de Janeiro, Brazil.

12. Sarmiento, O., Weigle, K., Alexander, J., Weber, D. J., and Miller, W. (2003). Assessment by meta-analysis of PCR for diagnosis of smear-negative pulmonary tuberculosis, *Journal of Clinical Microbiology*, **41**, 3233-3240.

13. Schwarz, G. (1978). Estimating the dimension of a model, *Annals of Statistics*, **6**, 461–464.

14. Seixas, J. M., Calôba, L. P., and Delpino, I. (1996). Relevance criteria for variable selection in classifier designs, In *International Conference on Engineering Applications of Neural Networks*, 451–454.

15. Stone, M. (1974). Cross-validatory choice and assessment of statistical predictions, *Journal of the Royal Statistical Society, Series B*, **36**, 111–147.

16. Vassali, M. R., Seixas, J. M. d., and Calôba, L. P. (2002). A neural particle discriminator based on a modified art architecture, In *Proceedings of the 2002 IEEE International Symposium on Circuits and Systems*, Volume 2, 121–124.

17. WHO (2002). Stop TB, annual report 2001.

19

Assessing Drug Resistance in HIV Infection Using Viral Load Using Segmented Regression

Hua Liang,[1] **Wai-Yuan Tan,**[2] **and Xiaoping Xiong**[3]

[1] *University of Rochester Medical Center, Rochester, NY, USA*
[2] *The University of Memphis, Memphis, TN, USA*
[3] *St. Jude Children's Research Hospital, Memphis, TN, USA*

Abstract: In this chapter, we have assessed the time to development of drug resistance in HIV-infected individuals treated with antiviral drugs by using longitudinal viral load HIV-1 counts. Through log-transformed data of HIV virus counts over time, we have assumed a linear changing-point model and developed procedures to estimate the unknown parameters by using the Bayesian approach. We have applied the method and procedure to the data generated by the ACTG 315 involving treatment by the drug combination (3TC, AZT, and Ritonavir). Our analysis showed that the mean time to the first changing point (i.e., the time the macrophage and long-lived cells began to release HIV particles) was around 15 days whereas the time to development of drug resistance by HIV was around 75 days. The Bayesian HPD intervals for these changing points are given by $(8.7, 21.3)$ and $(42, 108)$, respectively. This analysis indicated that if we use the combination of three drugs involving two NRTI inhibitors (3TC and AZT) and one PI inhibitor (Ritonavir) to treat HIV-infected individuals, in about two and half months, it would be beneficial to change drugs to avoid the problem of drug resistance.

Keywords and phrases: AIDS clinical trial, Gibbs sampler, HIV dynamics, longitudinal data, random change points, nonlinear mixed-effects models

19.1 Introduction

It has been well documented that plasma HIV RNA level (viral load) is a very effective predictor for clinical outcomes in HIV-infected individuals [Saag *et al.* (1996) and Mellors *et al.* (1995, 1996)], and has thus become a primary surrogate marker in most AIDS clinical trials. To assess the effects of drugs and also to monitor the progression of the disease in HIV-infected individuals treated with anti-retroviral drugs, it appears necessary to study the HIV dynamics during treatment through HIV viral loads and how the dynamics are related to the changing numbers of HIV virus load over time.

To illustrate the basic HIV dynamics in HIV-infected individuals, consider an HIV-infected individual treated with highly active antiretroviral therapy (HAART) involving two nucleoside reverse transcriptase inhibitors (NRTI) such as 3TC and AZT and one protease inhibitor (PI) such as Ritonavir. Then, it has been shown that within the first week, the total number of HIV counts per ml of blood can be approximated by an exponential function. It follows that in the first week, the log of the HIV virus load decreases linearly and sharply with large negative slope [Ho *et al.* (1995), Wei *et al.* (1995), and Tan (2000, Chapter 8)]. After the first week, however, the picture is very different and shows multiphases of decline and increase. In log scale, within the first two to three months after the first week, the picture is again linear but the curve is very flat due presumably to the release of HIV by macrophage and other long-lived cells from the lymph nodes [Perelson *et al.* (1997) and Tan (2000, Chapter 8)]; at some point between the third and eighth months, for some individuals the virus load increases sharply, reaching the level before treatment, due presumably to the development of drug resistance of HIV to the drugs. By using a comprehensive stochastic model of HIV pathogenesis involving flow of HIV from the lymph nodes and development of drug resistance, Tan (2000, Chapter 8) has demonstrated through computer simulation how these changes and outcomes are predicted by the model. To illustrate these points, we give in Figure 19.1 a scatter plot of viral load (in $\log_{10}$ scale) at different treatment times from an AIDS clinical study conducted by the AIDS Clinical Trials Group (ACTG 315). In this study, 48 HIV-1 infected patients were treated with potent antiviral therapy consisting of Ritonavir, 3TC, and AZT [see Lederman *et al.* (1998) and Wu *et al.* (1999) for more details on this study]. Viral load was monitored simultaneously at treatment days 0, 2, 7, 10, 14, 28, 56, 84, 168, and 336.

From Figure 19.1, we observe that the viral load of most patients declines rapidly within the first two weeks with large negative slope; after two weeks, however, the trend of decline decreases and becomes flat. At about ten weeks, the viral loads rebound mostly upward to the end of treatment. From this, it is logical to assume that the effect of treatment can be divided into three stages: rapid decline, slow decline, and rebound. We are interested in the rate of decline/rebound and the time of changing points. From the biological perspective, one may link the time of the first changing point as the time when the macrophage or other long-lived HIV-infected cells from lymphoid tissues release free HIV to the blood; one may link the second time of changing point as the time when HIV has developed resistance to the drugs. These time points have important clinical implications because this is the time to change drugs to avoid the problem of drug resistance.

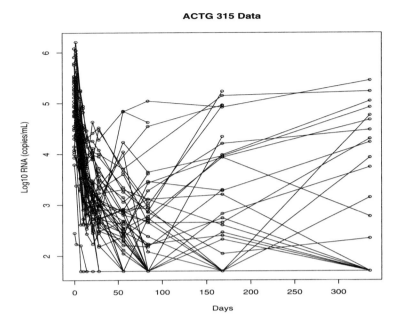

Figure 19.1: Viral load data for ACTG 315 study

For better understanding of the HIV pathogenesis and for better treatment management and care of AIDS patients, it is important to identify when the patients' viral load or CD4 cell counts decline, and when to change the declining trend, and rebound. For assessing HIV infection, Lange *et al.* (1992) considered a fully Bayesian analysis of CD4 cell counts. Kiuchi *et al.* (1995) used a similar approach to examine change points in the series of T4 counts prior to AIDS. Putter *et al.* (2002) and Han *et al.* (2002) have considered a population HIV dynamic model using the Bayesian approach. But none of these studies has ever attempted to estimate the time to drug resistance. By using data from the clinical trial ACTG 315, in this chapter we develop a Bayesian procedure to estimate the time of these changing points.

In this chapter, we propose a three-segment model with random change point to describe viral load trajectory data. We are concerned with the decline/ rebound rates and the location of changing points. This chapter is organized as follows. In Section 19.2, we propose the model structure, prior distributions and conditional posterior distributions. In Section 19.3, we describe the multilevel Gibbs sampling procedures to estimate the unknown parameters and the times of changing points. In Section 19.4, we present the analysis and results for the ACTG 315 data by using the models and methods given in previous sections. Finally, in Section 19.5, we present some conclusions and discussions.

19.2   The Model

For monitoring the disease progression in HIV-infected individuals, the data are usually the number of RNA virus copies over different time points. As illustrated in Section 19.1, in log scale these data sets are best described by a piecewise linear model with at most two unknown changing points. The first changing point is the time at which some HIV are released by macrophage or other long-lived cells from the lymphoid tissues [Perelson *et al.* (1997)]. The second changing point is the time at which the HIV in the HIV-infected individual develops resistance to the drugs. For those individuals in which the HIV has not yet developed resistance to the drugs, the log of the RNA virus copies per ml then showed a two-segment linear curve with one changing point; the first linear segment is a sharp linear declining curve with large negative slope showing a rapid decline of the HIV numbers due to the inhibition effect of the drugs whereas the second linear segment is a less rapid linearly declining curve with small negative slope due to additional new release of HIV of macrophage from lymphoid tissues [Perelson *et al.* (1997)]. When the HIV in the HIV-infected individual has developed drug resistance, then one would expect a three-piece linear model with two changing points; the third linear segment is a linear ascending curve with positive slope and the second changing point is the time when the HIV develops resistance to the drugs. A typical picture describing this situation is shown in Figure 19.2.

To describe the model, suppose that there are n HIV-infected individuals treated by the same drug combination. For the ith individual, let t_{Li} and t_{Ri} denote the time of the first and second changing points, respectively. Assuming a mixed model to account for the variation between individuals, then $\{t_{Li}, i = 1, \ldots, n\}$ is a random sample from an unknown density with mean t_L and $\{t_{Ri}, i = 1, \ldots, n\}$ is a random sample from an unknown density with mean t_R. It is generally believed that t_L occurs at about two weeks [Perelson *et al.* (1997)] and t_R occurs some time between the third and eleventh months [Tan (2000, Chapter 8)]. For the ith individual, the three linear segments are separated by t_{Li} and t_{Ri}. For this individual, the first line segment is $\eta_{0i} + \eta_{1i}t$, showing a rapid decline in log(RNA) after treatment. The second line segment is $\eta_{2i} + \eta_{3i}t$, showing a less rapid decline after some unknown time point t_{Li} due to the release of HIV from macrophage or other long-lived cells from the lymphoid tissues. The third segment is $\eta_{4i} + \eta_{5i}t$, showing an increase of the

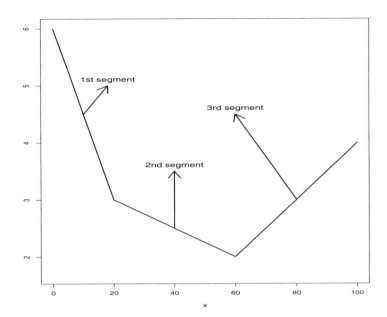

Figure 19.2: Illustrative plot of three segments used to explore viral load trajectory

log(RNA) after some unknown time point t_{Ri}, because of the drug resistance. Notice that the first two segments agree at t_{Li}, whereas the last two segments agree at t_{Ri}. Denote by $\Delta_{1i} = \eta_{3i} - \eta_{1i}$ and $\Delta_{2i} = \eta_{5i} - \eta_{3i}$. Then, by combing these three line segments we can express the piecewise linear model by the following equation:

$$y_{ij} = \eta_{0i} + \eta_{1i}t_{ij} + \Delta_{1i}(t_{ij} - t_{Li})_+ + \Delta_{2i}(t_{ij} - t_{Ri})_+ + \varepsilon_{ij}, \qquad (19.1)$$

where $s_+ = \max(s, 0)$ and ε_{ij} is the random measurement error for measuring y_{ij}.

It is assumed that the ε_{ij}s are independently distributed normal random variables with means 0 and variance σ_i^2, independently of $\{\eta_{ri}, \ r = 0, 1, \Delta_{ui}, u = 1, 2, t_{Li}, t_{Ri}\}$ for all $i = 1, \ldots, n$. That is, $\varepsilon_{ij} \sim N(0, \sigma_i^2)$, independently distributed of the random variables η_{0i}, η_{1i}, Δ_{1i}, Δ_{2i}, t_{Li}, and t_{Ri} for all $i = 1, \ldots, n$.

In the above model, because of variation between individuals, the $\{\eta_{ji}, j = 0, 1\}$ and the $\{\Delta_{ri}, r = 1, 2\}$ are random variables. As in Wu *et al.* (1999), we use a mixed-effects model to account for variation between individuals. Also, following Lange *et al.* (1992) and Kiuchi *et al.* (1995), we will model these variables by using first-order linear equations:

$$\eta_{0i} = \alpha_0 + \beta_{0i},$$

$$
\begin{aligned}
\eta_{1i} &= \alpha_1 + \beta_{1i}, \\
\Delta_{1i} &= \alpha_2 + \beta_{2i}, \\
\Delta_{2i} &= \alpha_3 + \beta_{3i},
\end{aligned}
$$

In the above equations, the αs denote population effects, and the βs individual effects to account for variations between individuals. Let $\boldsymbol{\beta}_i = (\beta_{0i}, \beta_{1i}, \beta_{2i}, \beta_{3i})^{\mathrm{T}}$. As in Lange *et al.* (1992) and Kiuchi *et al.* (1995), we assume that the $\boldsymbol{\beta}_i$s are independently and identically distributed as a Gaussian vector with mean 0 and unknown covariance matrix $\mathbf{V}$, that is, $\boldsymbol{\beta}_i \sim N(0, \mathbf{V})$, independently.

19.2.1   The likelihood function

In the above model, the $\{\mathbf{t}_{LR,i} = (t_{Li}, t_{Ri})^{\mathrm{T}}, \boldsymbol{\beta}_i\}$ are random variables. The unknown parameters are $\{\boldsymbol{\alpha} = (\alpha_0, \alpha_1, \alpha_2, \alpha_3)^{\mathrm{T}}, \mathbf{V}, \sigma_i^2\}$. Let $\boldsymbol{\beta}$ denote the collection of all $\boldsymbol{\beta}_i$, $\boldsymbol{\sigma}^2$ the collection of all σ_i^2, and $\mathbf{t}_{LR}$ the collection of all $\mathbf{t}_{LR,i} = (t_{Li}, t_{Ri})^{\mathrm{T}}$. Let $N(y|\mu, \sigma^2)$ denote the density of a normal distribution with mean μ and variance σ^2, and let $\mathbf{y} = (y_{ij}, i = 1, \ldots, n, j = 1, \ldots, n_i)^{\mathrm{T}}$. Then the conditional likelihood given $(\boldsymbol{\alpha}, \boldsymbol{\beta}, \mathbf{t}_{LR})$ is

$$
\mathcal{L}(\mathbf{y}|\boldsymbol{\alpha}, \boldsymbol{\beta}, \mathbf{t}_{LR}) = \prod_{i=1}^{n} \prod_{j=1}^{m_i} N(y_{ij}|\mu_{ij}, \sigma_i^2),
$$

where μ_{ij} is the right-hand side of (19.1) apart from ε_{ij}.

Let $p(\mathbf{t}_{LR,i})$ denote the probability density function of $\mathbf{t}_{LR,i}$. Then the joint density of $\{\mathbf{y}, \boldsymbol{\beta}, \mathbf{t}_{LR}\}$ given the parameters $\{\boldsymbol{\alpha}, \mathbf{V}, \boldsymbol{\sigma}^2\}$ is

$$
\mathcal{P}(\mathbf{y}, \boldsymbol{\beta}, \mathbf{t}_{LR}|\boldsymbol{\alpha}, \mathbf{V}, \boldsymbol{\sigma}^2) = \prod_{i=1}^{n} \prod_{j=1}^{m_i} N(y_{ij}|\mu_{ij}, \sigma_i^2) \prod_{i=1}^{n} \{N(\boldsymbol{\beta}_i|0, \mathbf{V}) p(\mathbf{t}_{LR,i})\}.
$$

In the above distribution, $p(\mathbf{t}_{LR,i})$ is a density of discrete random variables. To specify this density, we assume that the t_{Li}s are independently distributed of the t_{Ri}s. Because we have very little information about t_{Li} except that the expected value of t_{Li} probably occurs at about two weeks [Perelson *et al.* (1997)], we assume that the t_{Li} is a discrete uniform random variable on the set $\{8, 9, \ldots, 18\}$; similarly, because we have no information about t_{Ri} except that the plots of the data seemed to suggest that its expected value probably occurs between 60 and 90 days, we assume that t_{Ri} is a discrete uniform random variable on the set $\{60, 65, \ldots, 90\}$.

19.2.2   The prior distribution

For the prior distribution of the parameters $\{\boldsymbol{\alpha}, \boldsymbol{\sigma}^2, \mathbf{V}\}$, we assume that a priori these parameters are independently distributed of one another. As in Lange *et al.* (1992), we assume that $\boldsymbol{\alpha}$ is a normal vector with prior mean μ_α and prior covariance matrix D_α. For specifying these hyperparameters, we will adopt an empirical Bayes approach by using some data to estimate its values; for details, see Section 19.4. For the prior distribution of σ_i^2s, it is assumed that the σ_i^2s are independently and identically distributed as an inverted gamma distribution $IG(\lambda_1, \lambda_2)$ with $\lambda_1 = 10$ and $\lambda_2 = 0.06$. For the prior distribution of $\mathbf{V}$, we assume that the $\mathbf{V}$ is distributed as an inverted Wishart random matrix. Denote by $S \sim W(\Sigma, f)$ that the symmetric random matrix S is distributed as a Wishart distribution with matrix Σ and degrees of freedom f. Then, $\mathbf{V}^{-1} \sim W((\rho\boldsymbol{\Gamma})^{-1}, \rho)$. In $\boldsymbol{\Gamma}$, the left upper 2×2 submatrix is initiated by the covariance matrix of random term from modeling (19.9); the right-bottom 2×2 submatrix is an identity matrix and the other elements are zeros. We also take $\rho = 2$.

Let $N(\boldsymbol{\alpha}|\mu_\alpha, D_\alpha)$ denote the density of $\boldsymbol{\alpha}$, $IG(z|f_1, f_2)$ the density of an inverted Gamma distribution with parameters (f_1, f_2), and $W(\mathbf{V}^{-1}|(\rho\boldsymbol{\Gamma})^{-1}, \rho)$ the density of $\mathbf{V}^{-1}$. Using the above prior distributions, the joint density of $\{\mathbf{y}, \boldsymbol{\alpha}, \boldsymbol{\beta}, \mathbf{t}_{LR}, \boldsymbol{\sigma}^2, \mathbf{V}\}$ is

$$\mathcal{P}(\mathbf{y}, \boldsymbol{\alpha}, \boldsymbol{\beta}, \mathbf{t}_{LR}, \boldsymbol{\sigma}^2, \mathbf{V})$$
$$= \prod_{i=1}^{n}\prod_{j=1}^{m_i} N(y_{ij}|\mu_{ij}, \sigma_i^2) N(\boldsymbol{\alpha}|\mu_\alpha, \mathbf{D}_\alpha) \prod_{i=1}^{n} N(\boldsymbol{\beta}_i|0, \mathbf{V})$$
$$\times \prod_{i=1}^{n} IG(\sigma_i^2|\lambda_1, \lambda_2) \prod_{i=1}^{n} p(\mathbf{t}_{LR,i}) W(\mathbf{V}^{-1}|(\rho\boldsymbol{\Gamma})^{-1}, \rho). \quad (19.2)$$

19.2.3 The posterior distributions

From the joint density given in Eq. (19.2), one may readily derive the conditional posterior distributions of the parameters and the conditional distributions of $\{\boldsymbol{\beta}_i, \mathbf{t}_{LR,i}\}$. For this purpose, we introduce the following notations: $X_{ij} = \{1, t_{ij}, (t_{ij} - t_{Li})_+, (t_{ij} - t_{Ri})_+\}$, $\mathbf{X}_i = (X_{i1}^T, \ldots, X_{im_i}^T)^T$, $\boldsymbol{\varepsilon}_i = (\varepsilon_{i1}, \ldots, \varepsilon_{im_i})^T$, $\mathbf{y}_i = (y_{i1}, \ldots, y_{im_i})^T$. Then, (19.1) can be described as

$$y_{ij} = X_{ij}(\boldsymbol{\alpha} + \boldsymbol{\beta}_i) + \varepsilon_{ij} \quad \text{or} \quad \mathbf{y}_i = \mathbf{X}_i\boldsymbol{\alpha} + \mathbf{X}_i\boldsymbol{\beta}_i + \boldsymbol{\varepsilon}_i.$$

Then, with $\boldsymbol{\varepsilon}_i = \mathbf{y}_i - (\mathbf{X}_i\boldsymbol{\alpha} + \mathbf{X}_i\boldsymbol{\beta}_i)$,

$$\mathcal{L}(\mathbf{y}|\boldsymbol{\alpha}, \boldsymbol{\beta}, \mathbf{t}_{LR}, \boldsymbol{\sigma}^2) \propto \exp\left\{-\sum_{i=1}^{n}\frac{\boldsymbol{\varepsilon}_i^T\boldsymbol{\varepsilon}_i}{2\sigma_i^2}\right\}.$$

By direct calculation, one can readily derive the posterior distributions of the parameters. For implementing the Gibbs sampling method to estimate the unknown parameters and $\{\boldsymbol{\beta}_i, \mathbf{t}_{LR,i}\}$, we summarize these distributions as follows.

(a) Denote $\mathbf{r}_{\alpha,i} = \mathbf{y}_i - \mathbf{X}_i \boldsymbol{\beta}_i$. Then the conditional posterior distribution of $\boldsymbol{\alpha}$ given $\{\mathbf{y}, \mathbf{t}_{LR}, \boldsymbol{\beta}, \mathbf{V}, \boldsymbol{\sigma}^2\}$ is a Gaussian random vector with means $\hat{\boldsymbol{\alpha}}$ and covariance matrix $\hat{\Sigma}_\alpha$, where

$$\hat{\boldsymbol{\alpha}} = \left(\sum_{i=1}^{n} \frac{\mathbf{X}_i^{\mathrm{T}} \mathbf{X}_i}{\sigma_i^2} + \mathbf{D}_\alpha^{-1} \right)^{-1} \left(\sum_{i=1}^{n} \frac{\mathbf{X}_i^{\mathrm{T}} \mathbf{r}_{\alpha,i}}{\sigma_i^2} + \mathbf{D}_\alpha^{-1} \mu_\alpha \right)$$

and

$$\hat{\Sigma}_\alpha = \left(\sum_{i=1}^{n} \frac{\mathbf{X}_i^{\mathrm{T}} \mathbf{X}_i}{\sigma_i^2} + \mathbf{D}_\alpha^{-1} \right)^{-1}.$$

That is,

$$\boldsymbol{\alpha} | \{\mathbf{y}, \mathbf{t}_{LR}, \boldsymbol{\beta}, \mathbf{V}, \boldsymbol{\sigma}^2\} \sim N(\hat{\boldsymbol{\alpha}}, \hat{\Sigma}_\alpha). \tag{19.3}$$

(b) Denote $\mathbf{r}_{\beta,i} = \mathbf{y}_i - \mathbf{X}_i \boldsymbol{\alpha}$. Then,

$$\boldsymbol{\beta}_i | \{\mathbf{y}, \mathbf{t}_{LR}, \mathbf{V}, \boldsymbol{\alpha}, \boldsymbol{\sigma}^2\} \sim N(\hat{\boldsymbol{\beta}}_i, \hat{\Sigma}_\beta), \tag{19.4}$$

where

$$\hat{\boldsymbol{\beta}}_i = \left(\frac{\mathbf{X}_i^{\mathrm{T}} \mathbf{X}_i}{\sigma_i^2} + \mathbf{V}^{-1} \right)^{-1} \left(\frac{\mathbf{X}_i^{\mathrm{T}} \mathbf{r}_{\beta,i}}{\sigma_i^2} + \mathbf{V}^{-1} \mu_\alpha \right)$$

and

$$\hat{\Sigma}_\beta = \left(\frac{\mathbf{X}_i^{\mathrm{T}} \mathbf{X}_i}{\sigma_i^2} + \mathbf{V}^{-1} \right)^{-1}.$$

(c) Denote $\mathbf{r}_{\sigma^2,i} = \mathbf{y}_i - \mathbf{X}_i \boldsymbol{\alpha} - \mathbf{X}_i \boldsymbol{\beta}_i$. Then,

$$\sigma_i^2 | \{\mathbf{y}_i, \boldsymbol{\alpha}, \boldsymbol{\beta}_i, \mathbf{V}, \mathbf{t}_{LR}\} \sim IG \left\{ \lambda_1 + \frac{m_i}{2}, \left(\frac{1}{\lambda_2} + \frac{1}{2} \mathbf{r}_{\sigma^2,i}^{\mathrm{T}} \mathbf{r}_{\sigma^2,i} \right)^{-1} \right\}. \tag{19.5}$$

(d) Denote $\mathbf{a}_i = \boldsymbol{\alpha} + \boldsymbol{\beta}_i - \mu_\alpha$. Then,

$$\mathbf{V}^{-1} | \{\boldsymbol{\alpha}, \boldsymbol{\beta}_i, \boldsymbol{\sigma}, \mathbf{t}_L, \mathbf{t}_R\} \sim W \left\{ \left(\sum_{i=1}^{n} \mathbf{a}_i \mathbf{a}_i^{\mathrm{T}} + \rho \Gamma \right)^{-1}, n + \rho \right\}. \tag{19.6}$$

(e) Denote the exponent in the expression $\prod_{j=1}^{m_i} N(y_{ij} | \mu_{ij}, \sigma_i^2)$ from $\mathcal{L}(\mathbf{y} | \boldsymbol{\alpha}, \boldsymbol{\beta}, \mathbf{t}_{LR})$ as $\mathcal{G}$. Then, the conditional distribution of $\mathbf{t}_{Li}$ given $\{\mathbf{y}, \mathbf{t}_R, \boldsymbol{\alpha}, \boldsymbol{\beta}_i, \boldsymbol{\sigma}^2, \mathbf{V}\}$ is

$$\mathbf{t}_{Li} | \{\mathbf{y}, \mathbf{t}_{Ri}, \boldsymbol{\alpha}, \boldsymbol{\beta}_i, \boldsymbol{\sigma}^2, \mathbf{V}\} \sim \frac{\exp\{-\mathcal{G}(\mathbf{t}_{Li})\} p(\mathbf{t}_{Li})}{\sum_{\mathbf{t}_{Lk}} \exp\{-\mathcal{G}(\mathbf{t}_{Lk})\} p(\mathbf{t}_{Lk})}. \tag{19.7}$$

(f) In the exactly same way as (e), we obtain the conditional distribution of $\mathbf{t}_{Ri}$ given $\{\mathbf{y}, \mathbf{t}_L, \boldsymbol{\alpha}, \boldsymbol{\beta}_i, \boldsymbol{\sigma}^2, \mathbf{V}\}$ as

$$\mathbf{t}_{Ri} | \{\mathbf{y}, \mathbf{t}_{Li}, \boldsymbol{\alpha}, \boldsymbol{\beta}_i, \boldsymbol{\sigma}^2, \mathbf{V}\} \sim \frac{\exp\{-\mathcal{G}(\mathbf{t}_{Li})\} p(\mathbf{t}_{Ri})}{\sum_{\mathbf{t}_{Lk}} \exp\{-\mathcal{G}(\mathbf{t}_{Rk})\} p(\mathbf{t}_{Rk})}. \tag{19.8}$$

19.3 The Gibbs Sampling Procedure

In the Bayesian approach, one derives the Bayesian estimates via the posterior means and derives the HPD intervals of the parameters from the marginal posterior distributions. With the conditional posterior distributions given by Eqs. (19.3) to (19.8), one may generate random samples from the marginal distributions via the multi-level Gibbs sampling method. General theories of these procedures are given by Sheppard (1994), Liu and Chen (1998), and Kitagawa (1998). Detailed procedures and their proofs are given in Chapter 3 of Tan (2002). This is an iterative algorithm by sampling from the conditional distributions alternatively and sequentially with updated parameter values. At convergence, this then gives samples from the marginal distributions. For the model here, each cycle in this algorithm loops through the following steps.

Step 1. Starting with initial values $\Theta_0^\alpha = (\sigma_0^{-2}, \beta_0, \mathbf{V}_0, \mathbf{t}_{L0}, \mathbf{t}_{R0})^{\mathrm{T}}$, one draws a sample from the density $f_\alpha(\alpha|\mathbf{y}, \Theta_0^\alpha)$ given by (19.3). Denote the sample value of α by α_1.

Step 2. With $\Theta_0^\beta = (\sigma_0^{-2}, \alpha_1, \mathbf{V}_0, \mathbf{t}_{L0}, \mathbf{t}_{R0})^{\mathrm{T}}$, one draws a sample from the density $f_\beta(\beta_i|\mathbf{y}, \Theta_0^\beta)$ given by (19.4). Denote the sample value of β_i by $\beta_{i1}, i = 1, \dots, n$, and let $\beta_1 = \{\beta_i, i = 1, \dots, n\}^{\mathrm{T}}$.

Step 3. With $\Theta_0^{\sigma^2} = (\alpha_1, \beta_1, \mathbf{V}_0, \mathbf{t}_{L0}, \mathbf{t}_{R0})^{\mathrm{T}}$, one draws a sample of σ_i^2 from the density $f_\sigma(\sigma_i^2|\mathbf{y}, \Theta_0^{\sigma^2})$ given by (19.5). Denote the sample value of σ_i^2 by $\sigma_{i1}, i = 1, \dots, n$, and let $\sigma_1 = \{\sigma_{i1}, i = 1, \dots, n\}^{\mathrm{T}}$.

Step 4. With $\Theta_0^{(V)} = (\sigma_1, \alpha_1, \beta_1, \mathbf{t}_{L0}, \mathbf{t}_{R0})^{\mathrm{T}}$, one draws a sample of $\mathbf{V}$ from the density $f_V(\mathbf{V}^{-1}|\mathbf{y}, \Theta_0^{(V)})$ given by (19.6). Denote the sample value of $\mathbf{V}$ by $\mathbf{V}_1$.

Step 5. With $\Theta_0^{(L)} = (\sigma_1, \alpha_1, \beta_1, \mathbf{t}_{R0})^{\mathrm{T}}$, one draws a sample of $\mathbf{t}_{Li}$ from the density $f_L(\mathbf{t}_{Li}|\mathbf{y}, \Theta_0^{(L)})$ given by (19.7). Denote the sample value of $\mathbf{t}_{Li}$ by $\mathbf{t}_{Li,1}$, and let $\mathbf{t}_{L1} = \{\mathbf{t}_{Li,1}, i = 1, \dots, n\}^{\mathrm{T}}$.

Step 6. With $\Theta_0^{(R)} = (\sigma_1, \alpha_1, \beta_1, \mathbf{t}_{L1})^{\mathrm{T}}$, one draws a sample of $\mathbf{t}_{Ri}$ from the density $f_R(\mathbf{t}_{Ri}|\mathbf{y}, \Theta_0^{(R)})$ given by (19.8). Denote the sample value of $\mathbf{t}_{Ri}$ by $\mathbf{t}_{Ri,1}$, and let $\mathbf{t}_{R1} = \{\mathbf{t}_{Ri,1}, i = 1, \dots, n\}^{\mathrm{T}}$.

Step 7. With Θ_0^α in Step 1 replaced by $\Theta_0^\alpha = (\sigma_1^{-2}, \beta_1, \mathbf{V}_1, \mathbf{t}_{L1}, \mathbf{t}_{R1})^{\mathrm{T}}$, repeat the above cycle until convergence is reached.

As shown in Chapter 3 of Tan (2002), at convergence one generates a sample of size one from the marginal distribution of each parameter and of $\{\mathbf{t}_L, \mathbf{t}_R\}$ respectively. By repeating the above procedure, one generates a random sample of size m from the marginal posterior distribution for each parameter and for $\{\mathbf{t}_L, \mathbf{t}_R\}$, respectively. Then one may compute the sample means and the sample variances and covariances for these parameters. These estimates are optimal in the sense that under the squared loss function, the posterior mean values minimize the Bayesian risk function.

19.4   Analysis of the ACTG 315 Data

Using data from the ACTG 315 clinical trial on HAART, in this section we will derive a full Bayesian analysis to estimate the times to changing points and to drug resistance. In this analysis, we will adopt an empirical Bayesian approach to estimate the prior means and prior variances of the parameters $\boldsymbol{\alpha}$. Because the first change point generally occurs in about two weeks, we use the first two week's data to conduct linear mixed effects modelling via

$$y_{ij} = \eta_{0i} + \eta_{1i} t_{ij} + \varepsilon_{ij}. \tag{19.9}$$

The estimated values of α_0 and α_1 given here are taken as the means of our prior distributions of α_0 and α_1. The prior distribution of α_2 and α_3 are both assumed to be $N(\bullet|0,1)$. The covariance matrix of α_0 and α_1 obtained from (19.9) is taken as the left-upper submatrix of $\mathbf{D}$. The random estimated values are taken as the prior distributions of β_{0i} and β_{1i}.

With the posterior distributions given in Section 19.2 and with the Gibbs sampling procedure in Section 19.3, one can readily develop a full Bayesian analysis to estimate the relevant parameters and the times to changing points. To implement the MCMC sampling scheme, we follow the method proposed by Raftery and Lewis (1992). The procedure works as follows. After an initial number of 1000 burn-in iterations, every tenth MCMC sample is retained from the next 200,000 samples. Thus, we obtain 20,000 samples of targeted posterior distributions of the unknown parameters. The stability of the posterior means is checked informally by examining the graphics of the runs. Figure 19.3 shows the number of MCMC iterations and convergence diagnostics.

Figure 19.4 shows us a population trend of the viral load trajectory with $\eta_1 = -0.12(0.005)$, $\eta_3 = -0.011(0.006)$, and $\eta_5 = 0.003(0.003)$, $t_L = 15$, and $t_R = 75$. Denote the time period from entry time to 15 days as the first stage, and the time period from 15 days to 75 days as the second stage. Figure 19.4 then implies that the decline rate at the beginning stage is about ten times that

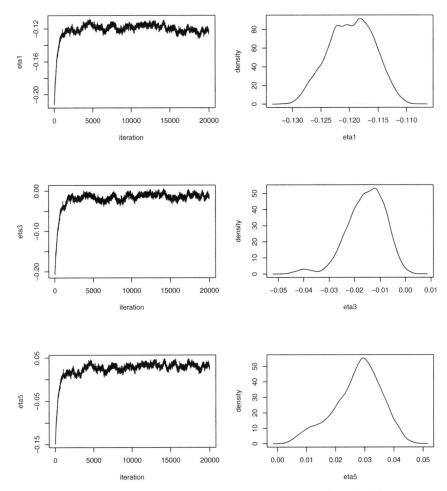

Figure 19.3: Diagnostic plots. Left panel: the number of MCMC iterations and posterior means; right panel: the densities of the posterior means

of the decline rate of the second stage. After 75 days, the viral load trajectory slightly rebounds.

To characterize the patterns of viral dynamics, we select four subjects and examine the trajectories of their viral load. Given in Table 19.1 are the estimates of the parameters for these four subjects. Given in Figure 19.5 are the plots of fitted values for these four subjects based on the three-segment model and the Bayesian approach. These results indicate that the individual estimates of η_1, t_L, and t_R are quite similar to the corresponding ones of the population estimates respectively. However, the individual estimates of η_3 and η_5 varied widely so that the individual estimates may be totally different from the ones of the population. Figure 19.5 shows that the viral load trajectory of patient 10 is comparable to that of the population but with a stronger rebound in the later stage; but the patterns of viral load trajectory in subjects 8 and 20 are very different from that of the population in that in the second segment, their viral loads continued declining (patient 8) or flat (patient 20) instead of a rebound as in the population pattern, suggesting that drug resistance in these patients had not yet been developed. Figure 19.5 also shows a large difference between individual viral load trajectory in patient 48 and that from the population; for this patient, the viral loads rapidly declined in the first stage, then rapidly rebounded in the second segment, and kept flatly rebound in the third segment to the end of the treatment. These results indicate that for the clinicians to manage treatment and care of AIDS patients, it is necessary to study the viral load trajectory of each individual. Because the HIV pathogenesis is a stochastic dynamic process, this calls for individual-based models to assess effects of treatment and drug resistance.

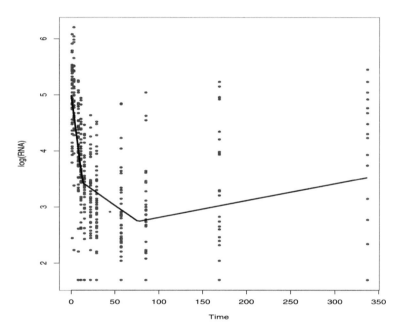

Figure 19.4: The estimated population mean curve obtained by using ACTG 315 data and Bayesian approach. The observed values are indicated by plus

Table 19.1: Estimates of the parameters of four subjects

ID	η_0	η_1	η_3	η_5	t_L	t_R
8	4.947	-0.12	-0.003	-0.005	14	75
10	5.38	-0.112	-0.017	0.009	15	76
30	4.741	-0.118	-0.019	0	15	76
48	4.838	-0.144	0.032	0.002	14	76

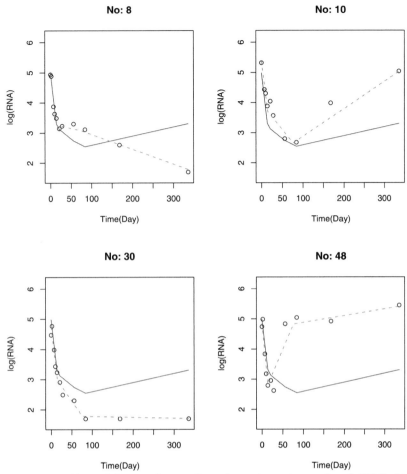

Figure 19.5: Profiles of four arbitrarily selected patients for ACTG 315 data. The dotted and solid lines are estimated individual and population curves. The observed values are indicated by the circle signs

---

19.5 Conclusion and Discussion

To treat HIV-infected individuals with antiretroviral drugs, a major obstacle is the development of drug resistance. In order to avoid the problem of drug resistance, it is therefore of considerable interest to estimate the time at which some resistance to the drugs have developed by the HIV. To answer this question, we have developed here a full Bayesian approach by assuming a three-segment linear model with two unknown changing points for the log of RNA viral load. In this model, the first changing point is the time when the macrophage or other long-lived cells release HIV to the blood from lymph nodes [Perelson *et al.* (1997)]; the second changing point is the time when the HIV develops resistance to the drugs [Tan (2000, Chapter 8)]. This statistical model is motivated and dictated by the dynamic models of HIV pathogenesis under treatment and by the observed and simulated data on HIV pathogenesis [Perelson *et al.* (1997) and Tan (2000, Chapter 8)]. The Bayesian approach is useful because it can incorporate prior information from an empirical study or other related or previous studies. This is important because current clinical data are not enough to identify all viral dynamic parameters.

In this chapter, we have applied the above Bayesian procedure to analyze the ACTG 315 data. These data treated patients with HAART involving 3TC and AZT (NRTI) and ritonavir (PI). For each patient, the data gave RNA viral load per ml of blood at different time points after treatment. Using this data and the log transformation, we have estimated the expected time to the first changing point as 15 days after treatment and the time to development of drug resistance as 75 days after treatment. The Bayesian HPD intervals for these changing points are $(8.7, 21.3)$ and $(42, 108)$, respectively. For the three-line segments, the estimates of the slope are -0.12, -0.011, and 0.003, respectively. The variances of these estimates are 0.005, 0.006, and 0.003 respectively. From these estimates, it is clear that most patients have very much the same slope for the first segment; but the opposite is true for the other two segments. Observing the log plots of RNA load, one may explain this by noting: (i) for some patients, the second segment is very short or hardly noticeable, whereas for other patients, the second segment is long. (ii) Although drug resistance have developed in some patients (about 21 patients), in other patients drug resistance had not developed or was hardly noticeable. Thus, for the second and third segments, there is considerable variation among individuals.

We have estimated the time to drug resistance by using a Bayesian approach, however, in treating HIV-infected individuals with antiretroviral drugs, many important problems cannot be answered by this or any other statistical model. In particular, to monitor the disease progression, to assess efficacy of the drugs, and to search for optimal treatment protocols, it is important to estimate effects of different drugs and how these effects are affected by many risk factors such as CD4 T cell counts and CD8 T cell counts; also it is important to estimate the numbers of infectious as well as noninfectious virus loads. Because the drug efficacy depends on pharmacokinetics and the bioavailability of the drugs, it is also of considerable interest to study how the pharmaco-kinetics affects effects of treatment and drug resistance. Because the HIV pathogenesis is a stochastic dynamic process, this calls for stochastic dynamic models and state space models. Using the ACTG 315 data, we are currently developing stochastic dynamic models and state space models to answer these questions.

Acknowledgements. Liang's research was partially supported by grants from the National Institute of Allergy and Infectious Diseases (R01 AI062247 and R01 AI059773). Xiong's research was partially supported by the American Lebanese Syrian Associated Charities (ALSAC).

References

1. Han, C., Chaloner, K., and Perelson, A. S. (2002). Bayesian analysis of a population HIV dynamic model, In *Case Studies in Bayesian Statistics*, Volume 6, Springer-Verlag, New York.

2. Ho, D. D., Neumann, A. U., Perelson, A. S., Chen, W., Leonard, J. M., and Makowitz, M. (1995). Rapid turnover of plasma virus and CD4 lymphocytes in HIV-1 infection, *Nature*, **373**, 123–126.

3. Kitagawa, G. (1998). A self organizing state space model, *Journal of the American Statistical Association*, **93**, 1203–1215.

4. Kiuchi, A. S., Hartigan, J. A., Holford, T. R., Rubinstein, P., and Stevens, C. E. (1995). Change points in the series of T4 counts prior to AIDS, *Biometrics*, **51**, 236–248.

5. Lange, N., Carlin, B. P., and Gelfand, A. E. (1992). Hierarchical Bayes models for the progression of HIV infection using longitudinal CD4 T-cell numbers (with discussion), *Journal of the American Statistical Association*, **87**, 615–632.

6. Lederman, M.M., Connick, E., Landay, A., Kuritzkes, D. R., Spritzler J, St Clair, M., Kotzin, B. L., Fox, L., Chiozzi, M. H., Leonard, J. M., Rousseau, F., Wade, M., D'Arc Roe, J., Martinez, A., and Kessier, H. (1998). Immunological responses associated with 12 weeks of combination antiretroviral therapy consisting of Zidovudine, Lamivudine, and Ritonavir: Results of AIDS clinical trial group protocol 315, *Journal of Infectious Diseases*, **178**, 70–79.

7. Liu, J. S., and Chen, R. (1998). Sequential Monte Carlo method for dynamic systems, *Journal of the American Statistical Association*, **93**, 1032–1044.

8. Mellors, J. W., Kingsley, L. A., and Rinaldo, C. R. (1995). Quantitation of HIV-1 RNA in plasma predicts outcome after seroconversion, *Annals of Internal Medicine*, **122**, 573–579.

9. Mellors, J. W., Rinaldo, C. R., and Gupta, P. (1996). Prognosis in HIV-1 infection predicted by the quantity of virus in plasma, *Science*, **272**, 1167–1170.

10. Perelson, A. S., Essunger, O., Cao, Y. Z., Vesanen, M., Hurley, A., Saksela, K., Markowitz, M., and Ho, D. D. (1997). Decay characteristics

of HIV infected compartments during combination therapy, *Nature*, **387**, 188–191.

11. Putter, H., Heisterkamp, S. H., Lange, J. M. A., and De Wolf, F. (2002). A Bayesian approach to parameter estimation in HIV dynamical models, *Statistics in Medicine*, **21**, 2199–2214.

12. Raftery, A. E., and Lewis, S. (1992). How many iterations in the Gibbs sample? In *Bayesian Statistics – 4* (Eds., J. Bernardo, J. Berger, A. Dawid, and A. Smith), pp. 763–773, Oxford University Press, Oxford, UK.

13. Saag, M. S., Holodniy, M., Kuritzkes, D. R., O'Brien, W. A., Coombs, R., Poscher, M. E., Jacobsen, D. M., Shaw, G. M., Richman, D. D., and Volberding, P. A. (1996). HIV viral load markers in clinical practice, *Nature Medicine*, **2**, 625–629.

14. Shephard, N. (1994). Partial non-Gaussian state space model, *Biometrika*, **81**, 115–131.

15. Tan, W. Y. (2000). *Stochastic Modeling of AIDS Epidemiology and HIV Pathogenesis*, World Scientific, River Edge, New Jersey.

16. Tan, W. Y. (2002). *Stochastic Models with Applications to Genetics, Cancers, AIDS and Other Biomedical Systems*, World Scientific, River Edge, New Jersey.

17. Wei, X., Ghosh, S. K., Taylor, M. E., Johnson, V. A., Emini, E. A., Deutsch, P., Lifson, J. D., Bonhoeffer, S., Nowak, M. A., Hahn, B. H., Saag, M. S., and Shaw, G. M. (1995). Viral dynamics in human immunodeficiency virus type 1 infection, *Nature*, **373**: 117-122.

18. Wu, H., and Ding, A. (1999). Population HIV-1 dynamics in vivo: Applicable models and inferential tools for virological data from AIDS clinical trials, *Biometrics*, **55**, 410–418.

19. Wu, H., Kuritzkes, D. R., and McClernon, D. R. (1999). Characterization of viral dynamics in human immunodeficiency virus type 1-infected patients treated with combination antiretroviral therapy: Relationships to host factors, cellular restoration and virological endpoints, *Journal of Infectious Diseases*, **179**, 799–807.

20

Assessment of Treatment Effects on HIV Pathogenesis Under Treatment By State Space Models

Wai-Yuan Tan,[1] **Ping Zhang,**[1] **Xiaoping Xiong,**[2] **and Pat Flynn**[2]

[1]*The University of Memphis, Memphis, TN, USA*
[2]*St. Jude Children's Research Hospital, Memphis, TN, USA*

Abstract: In this chapter, we have developed a method to estimate the efficiency of the drugs and the numbers of infectious and noninfectious HIV in HIV-infected individuals treated with antiretroviral drugs. As an illustration, we have applied the method to some clinical and laboratory data of an AIDS patient treated with various antiviral drugs. For this individual, the estimates show that the HAART protocol has effectively controlled the number of infectious HIV virus to below 400/ml copies although the total number of HIV copies was very high in some intervals.

Keywords and phrases: Productively infected CD4$^{(+)}$ T cells, numbers of infectious and noninfectious HIV, multilevel Gibbs sampling method, observation model, stochastic equation

20.1   Introduction

To control HIV, recently important progress has been made through the combination of three drugs: two of nucleoside reverse transcriptase inhibitors (NRTIs) such as AZT and 3TC with a nonnucleoside reverse transcriptase inhibitor (NNRTI) such as efavirenz or a protease inhibitor (PI) such as indinavir, referred to as the Highly Active Anti-Retroviral Therapy (HAART); see Bajaria *et al.* (2002). However, many recent studies on HAART have indicated that this treatment protocol, despite its effectiveness, is still far from perfect and life-long treatment is required [Betts *et al.* (2001), Chun *et al.* (1999), Garcia *et al.* (1999), and Pitcher *et al.* (1999)]. For monitoring HIV progression under treatment by antiviral drugs and to alert for possible development of drug resistance, it is therefore important to estimate the relative effects of NRTIs, NNRTIs, and PIs, as well as the numbers of infectious HIV virus and noninfectious HIV viruses over time. To date, methods for estimating these parameters and state variables are nonexistent. By applying the state space model and the multilevel Gibbs sampling procedures, the objective here is to develop efficient procedures to estimate these parameters and the state variables as well as other unknown parameters.

In Section 20.2, we will describe how to derive a stochastic model for HIV pathogenesis in HIV-infected individuals under treatment by antiretroviral drugs. In Section 20.3, we will derive a state space model for HIV pathogenesis in HIV-infected individuals under treatment by antiretroviral drugs by using data from the observed RNA virus counts over time. In Section 20.4, we will develop a general procedure via the multilevel Gibbs sampling method to estimate the unknown parameters and the state variables. As an application of our models, in Section 20.5 we will apply the results to the data of a patient from St. Jude Children's Research Hospital treated by various antiviral drugs.

20.2   A Stochastic Model for HIV Pathogenesis Under Treatment

To assess effects of different drugs and to estimate relevant state variables, in this section we will extend the Perelson et al. (1996) model into a more complex stochastic dynamic model for HIV pathogenesis in HIV-infected individuals treated with antiretroviral drugs including HAART. Under this model, free HIV viruses infect actively dividing CD4$^{(+)}$ T cells to generate productively infected CD4$^{(+)}$ T cells (denoted by T_P cells). At the death of a T_P cell, a large number ($N(t)$) of free HIV is generated, which will further infect other CD4$^{(+)}$ T cells. [Because $N(t)$ is very large, we will assume $N(t)$ as a deterministic function of t.] As in Perelson et al. (1996), we will ignore latently HIV-infected CD4$^{(+)}$ T cells because the contribution to HIV of these cells is very small. Because different drugs and drug combinations are used over different time periods in practical situations, we partition the time interval into nonoverlapping subintervals and follow Perelson et al. (1996) to assume that the number of uninfected CD4$^{(+)}$ T cells is a constant in each subinterval. This is justified by the observations that before the start of the treatment, the HIV pathogenesis is at a steady-state condition and that the uninfected CD4 T cells have a relatively long lifespan; see Cohen et al. (1998).

To derive the stochastic model, consider the situation in which an HIV-infected individual is treated by antiretroviral drugs including HAART. Let V_0 and V_1 denote noninfectious and infectious HIV, respectively. Let $\{V_0(t), V_1(t)\}$

denote the numbers of V_0 HIV and V_1 HIV per ml of blood at time t and $T_P(t)$ the number of productively HIV-infected CD4$^{(+)}$ T cells (T_P cells) at time t per ml of blood. Then we are entertaining a three-dimensional Markov process $\underset{\sim}{X}(t) = \{T_P(t), V_0(t), V_1(t)\}'$ with continuous time $\Omega = [0, \infty)$ and with discrete state space $S = \{(i, j, k), i, j, k = 0, 1, \ldots, \infty\}$. For this stochastic process, the traditional approach is too complicated to be of much use. Hence, we propose here an alternative approach by using stochastic differential equations.

20.2.1 Stochastic differential equations of state variables

To derive stochastic equations for the state variables, we define the following stochastic variables.

$D_P(t)$ = Number of deaths of T_P cells per ml of blood during $[t, t + \triangle t)$;

$D_{Vi}(t)$ = Number of free V_i HIV per ml of blood that have lost infectivity, or die, or have been removed during $[t, t + \triangle t)$, $i = 0, 1$;

$F(t)$ = Number of V_1 per ml of blood that have lost through infection of CD4$^{(+)}$ T cells during $[t, t + \triangle t)$. This is the number of V_1 HIV per ml that have entered the CD4$^{(+)}$ T cells but whose viral RNA have not yet been converted to viral DNA;

$F_1(t)$ = Number of productively infected CD4$^{(+)}$ T cells (T_P cells) per ml generated by the infection of actively dividing CD4$^{(+)}$ T cells by free HIV during $[t, t + \triangle t)$;

$R_j(t)$ = Number of noninfectious free HIV per ml of blood (i.e., V_0) generated by the death of the jth T_P cell during $[t, t + \triangle t)$ under treatment by PI inhibitors.

To specify the probability distribution of these variables, let $\mu_T(t)$ and $\mu_{Vi}(t)$ denote the death rate of T_P cells and the rate by which free V_i HIV are being removed, die, or have lost infectivity at time t, respectively. Let $k(t)$ be the HIV infection rate of CD4$^{(+)}$ T cells in the absence of NRTIs and NNRTIs, and let $k_T(t) = k(t)T(t)$, where $T(t)$ is the number of uninfected CD4$^{(+)}$ T cells per ml of blood at time t. Denote by $\xi_R(t)$ the probability that the $RNA \rightarrow DNA$ process is blocked by the NRTIs and/or NNRTIs at time t inside the uninfected CD4$^{(+)}$ T cells and let $\xi_P(t)$ denote the probability that free HIV released in the blood at time t by the death of a productively infected T cell in the blood is noninfectious. Then the conditional probability distribution of the above random variables given the state variables is given by:

- $[F(t), D_{V1}(t)] \mid V_1(t) \sim \text{Multinomial}[V_1(t); k_T(t)\Delta t, \mu_{V1}(t)\Delta t]$;

- $F_1(t) \mid F(t) \sim \text{Binomial}\{[c(t)F(t)]; [1 - \xi_R(t)]\}$, where $[c(t)F(t)]$ is the largest integer $\leq c(t)F(t)$ and where $c(t)$ is the proportion of activated CD4 T cells at time t among all uninfected CD4 T cells;

- $D_P(t) \mid T_P(t) \sim \text{Binomial}\ [T_P(t); \mu_T(t)\Delta t]$;

- $\{R_j(t), j = 1, \ldots, D_P(t)\} \mid D_P(t) > 0 \sim \text{Binomial}\ [N(t); \xi_P(t)]$ independently $(R_j(t) = 0$ if $D_P(t) = 0.)$;

- $D_{V0}(t) \mid V_0(t) \sim \text{Binomial}\ [V_0(t); \mu_{V0}(t)\Delta t]$.

Given $\boldsymbol{X}(t)$, conditionally $\{D_P(t), [F(t), D_{V1}(t)], D_{V0}(t)\}$ are independently distributed from one another; given $F(t)$, conditionally $F_1(t)$ is independently distributed from other variables.

By the conservation law and by using these distribution results, we obtain the following stochastic differential equations for $\{T_P(t), V_j(t), j = 0, 1\}$, respectively.

$$
\begin{aligned}
dT_P(t) &= T_P(t + \Delta t) - T_P(t) = F_1(t) - D_P(t) = \{c(t)k_T(t)[1 - \xi_R(t)]V_1(t) \\
&\quad - T_P(t)\mu_T(t)\}\Delta t + \varepsilon_1(t)\Delta t, \qquad\qquad (20.1) \\
dV_0(t) &= V_0(t + \Delta t) - V_0(t) = \sum_{j=1}^{D_P(t)} R_j(t) - D_{V0}(t) = R(t) - D_{V0}(t) \\
&= \{N(t)\xi_P(t)T_P(t)\mu_T(t) - \mu_{V0}(t)V_0(t)\}\Delta t + \varepsilon_3(t)\Delta t, \qquad (20.2) \\
dV_1(t) &= V_1(t + \Delta t) - V_1(t) = \sum_{j=1}^{D_P(t)} [N(t) - R_j(t)] - F(t) - D_{V1}(t) \\
&= \{N(t)[1 - \xi_P(t)]\mu_T(t)T_P(t) - k_T(t)V_1(t) - \mu_{V1}(t)V_1(t)\}\Delta t + \\
&\quad + \varepsilon_3(t)\Delta t. \qquad\qquad (20.3)
\end{aligned}
$$

In Eqs. (20.1) to (20.3), the random noises $\{\varepsilon_j(t)\Delta t, \ j = 1, 2, 3\}$ are derived by subtracting the conditional mean values from the random variables, respectively, and have expectation zero. It can easily be shown that these random noises are uncorrelated with the state variables $T_P(t)$ and $V_j(t), = 0, 1$; furthermore, one may also assume that the random noises $\varepsilon_j(t)$ are uncorrelated with the random noises $\varepsilon_l(\tau)$ for all j and l if $t \neq \tau$.

20.2.2   The probability distribution of state variables

Let Θ be the collection of all parameters. Letting $\Delta t \sim 1$ correspond to a small interval such as 0.1 day, then the state variables are $\boldsymbol{X} = \{\underset{\sim}{X}(t), t = 0, 1, \ldots, t_M\}$, where t_M is the termination time of the study. For implementing the multilevel Gibbs sampling procedure, we define the unobserved state variables $\underset{\sim}{U}(t) = \{F(t), D_P(t), R(t)\}$ and let $\boldsymbol{U} = \{\underset{\sim}{U}(t), t = 0, 1, \ldots, t_M - 1\}$. By using the above distribution results, we obtain the conditional density of $\underset{\sim}{U}(t)$ given $\underset{\sim}{X}(t)$ as

$$P\{\underset{\sim}{U}(t)|\underset{\sim}{X}(t)\} = C_1(t)[\mu_T(t)]^{D_P(t)}[1 - \mu_T(t)]^{T_P(t)-D_P(t)}[k_T(t)]^{F(t)}$$

$$\times [1 - k_T(t)]^{V_1(t)-F(t)}[\xi_P(t)]^{R(t)}[1 - \xi_R(t)]^{D_P(t)N-R(t)}, \tag{20.4}$$

where $C_1(t) = \binom{V_1(t)}{F(t)}\binom{T_P(t)}{D_P(t)}\binom{ND_P(t)}{R(t)}$ and $R(t) = 0$ if $D_P(t) = 0$.

The conditional density of $\underset{\sim}{X}(t+1)$ given $\{\underset{\sim}{U}(t), \underset{\sim}{X}(t)\}$ is

$$P\{\underset{\sim}{X}(t+1)|\underset{\sim}{U}(t), \underset{\sim}{X}(t)\} = \binom{[c(t)F(t)]}{A_1(t)}[\xi_R(t)]^{A_2(t)}[1 - \xi_R(t)]^{A_1(t)}$$

$$\times \binom{V_0(t)}{B_1(t)}[\mu_{V_0}(t)]^{B_1(t)}[1 - \mu_{V_0}(t)]^{V_0(t)-B_1(t)}$$

$$\times \binom{V_1(t) - F(t)}{B_2(t)}[\frac{\mu_{V_1}(t)}{1 - k_T(t)}]^{B_2(t)}$$

$$\times [1 - \frac{\mu_{V_1}(t)}{1 - k_T(t)}]^{V_1(t)-F(t)-B_2(t)}, \tag{20.5}$$

where

$$\{A_1(t) = T_P(t+1) - T_P(t) + D_P(t), A_2(t) = [c(t)F(t)] - A_1(t)\}$$

and

$$\{B_1(t) = V_0(t)-V_0(t+1)+R(t), B_2(t) = V_1(t)-V_1(t+1)+ND_P(t)-R(t)-F(t)\}.$$

The joint density of $\{\boldsymbol{X}, \boldsymbol{U}\}$ given Θ is

$$P\{\boldsymbol{X}, \boldsymbol{U}|\Theta\} = P\{\underset{\sim}{X}(0)|\Theta\} \prod_{t=1}^{t_M} P\{\underset{\sim}{X}(t)|\underset{\sim}{U}(t-1), \underset{\sim}{X}(t-1)\}$$

$$\times P\{\underset{\sim}{U}(t-1)|\underset{\sim}{X}(t-1)\}. \tag{20.6}$$

20.3 A State Space Model For HIV Pathogenesis Under Antiretroviral Drugs

Based on the observed number of RNA virus counts over time, in this section we develop a state space model for the HIV pathogenesis under treatment by antiretroviral drugs including HAART. For this state space model, the state variables are $X\underset{\sim}{}(t) = \{T_P(t), V_j(t),\ j = 0,1\}$. Thus the stochastic system model is represented by the stochastic Eqs. (20.1) to (20.6) given above for these variables. The observation model is given by the statistical model based on the observed number of RNA virus copies per ml of blood over time.

To derive the observation model, let y_j be the observed total number of HIV RNA virus load at time $t_j, j = 1, \ldots, n$. Then the conditional mean of y_j given $V(t_j) = V_0(t_j) + V_1(t_j)$ and the conditional variance of y_j given $V(t_j)$ are $V(t_j)$ and $\sigma^2 V(t_j)$, respectively [Tan and Xiang (1998) and Tan (2000, Chapter 3)], where $\sigma^2 > 0$. Let $e_j = (y_j - V(t_j))/\sqrt{V(t_j)}$. Following Tan and Xiang (1998), we assume that the e_js are independently distributed as normal variables with means 0 and variance σ^2. From this, the observation model is given by

$$y_j = V(t_j) + e_j\sqrt{V(t_j)}, \qquad j = 1, \ldots, n, \qquad (20.7)$$

where $e_j \sim N(0, \sigma^2),\ j = 1, \ldots, n$, independently.

Let $\boldsymbol{Y} = \{y_j, j = 1, \ldots, n\}$ and

$$f_Y\{y_j | X(t_j)\} = \{2\pi\, V(t_j)\sigma^2\}^{1/2} \exp\{-\frac{1}{2V(t_j)\sigma^2}[y_j - V(t_j)]^2\}. \qquad (20.8)$$

Then the joint density of $\{\boldsymbol{X}, \boldsymbol{U}, \boldsymbol{Y}\}$ given Θ is

$$P\{\boldsymbol{X}, \boldsymbol{U}, \boldsymbol{Y}|\Theta\} = P\{X\underset{\sim}{}(0)|\Theta\} \prod_{j=1}^{n} f_Y\{Y(j)|V(t_j)\} \prod_{t=t_{j-1}+1}^{t_j} P\{U\underset{\sim}{}(t-1)|X\underset{\sim}{}(t-1)\}$$
$$\times P\{X\underset{\sim}{}(t)|X\underset{\sim}{}(t-1), U\underset{\sim}{}(t-1)\}. \qquad (20.9)$$

20.4 Estimation of Unknown Parameters and State Variables

As in Tan (2000, Chapter 8), one may assume $\{c(t) = c, N(t) = N, \mu_T(t) = \mu_T, \mu_{V_i}(t) = \mu_V, i = 0,1\}$. To estimate the time-dependent parameters $\{\xi_R(t), \xi_P(t), k_T(t)\}$, we partition the time interval $[0, t_M)$ into k nonoverlapping subintervals $\{L_j = [s_{j-1}, s_j), j = 1, \ldots, k\}$ with $(s_0 = 0, s_k = t_M)$ and assume these parameters as constants in each subinterval. Now, we will use least squares methods to estimate $\Theta_1 = \{c, N\}$ and use the multilevel Gibbs sampling method to estimate $\Theta_2 = \{\mu_T, \mu_V, \sigma^2, \xi_R(t), \xi_P(t), k_T(t), t = 1, \ldots, k\}$, and then iterate between these two procedures until convergence. The least squares method is described in Tan and Wu (1998) by using some statistical packages from IMS.

The multilevel Gibbs sampling procedures are given in Tan (2002, Chapter 9) and Tan, Zhang, and Xiong (2004). The proof of convergence of these procedures is available from Tan (2002, Chapter 3) and Tan, Zhang, and Xiong (2004).

Let $P\{\Theta_2\}$ be the prior density of the parameters Θ_2. For $i = 1, \ldots, k$ and $r = 1, 2$, let

$$\bar{R}(i) = \sum_{j=s_{i-1}+1}^{s_i} R(j), \bar{D}_P(i) = \sum_{j=s_{i-1}+1}^{s_i} D_P(j),$$

$$\bar{F}(i) = \sum_{j=s_{i-1}+1}^{s_i} F(j), \bar{T}_P(i) = \sum_{j=s_{i-1}+1}^{s_i} T_P(j),$$

$$\bar{V}_l(i) = \sum_{j=s_{i-1}+1}^{s_i} V_l(j), l = 0, 1, \bar{A}_r(i) = \sum_{j=s_{i-1}+1}^{s_i} A_r(j),$$

$$\bar{B}_r(i) = \sum_{j=s_{i-1}+1}^{s_i} B_r(j), \bar{C}_r(i) = \sum_{j=s_{i-1}+1}^{s_i} C_r(j), r = 1, 2.$$

By using the densities given above, the conditional density of Θ_2 given $\{Y, X, U, \Theta_1\}$ is

$$P\{\Theta_2 | X, U, Y, \Theta_1\}$$

$$\propto P\{\Theta\} \mu_T^{\bar{D}_P} (1 - \mu_T)^{\bar{T}_P - \bar{D}_P} \mu_V^{\bar{B}} (1 - \mu_V)^{\bar{V} - \bar{B}} \prod_{j=1}^{n} [\xi_R(j)]^{\bar{A}_2(j)}$$

$$\times [1 - \xi_R(j)]^{\bar{A}_1(j)} [\xi_P(j)]^{\bar{R}(j)} [1 - \xi_P(j)]^{N\bar{D}_P(j) - \bar{R}(j)}$$

$$\times \left(\frac{k_T(j)}{1 - \mu_V} \right)^{\bar{F}(j)} \left(1 - \frac{k_T(j)}{1 - \mu_V} \right)^{\bar{V}_1(j) - \bar{F}(j) - \bar{B}_2(j)}, \qquad (20.10)$$

where

$$\bar{D}_P = \sum_{j=1}^{k} \bar{D}_P(j), \bar{T}_P = \sum_{j=1}^{k} \bar{T}_P(j), \bar{V} = \sum_{r=0}^{1} \sum_{j=1}^{k} \bar{V}_r(j), \bar{B} = \sum_{r=1}^{2} \sum_{j=1}^{k} \bar{B}_r(j).$$

Equation (20.10) will be used to generate Θ_2 given $\{X, U, Y, \Theta_1\}$ in the multilevel Gibbs sampling procedures.

20.5   An Illustrative Example

In this section, we apply the above method to a patient from St. Jude Children's Hospital treated by various drugs including HAART. This patient is a perinatal

AIDS treated by various anti-retroviral drugs. For this patient, the observed RNA virus copies per ml blood over time since HIV infection are given in Table 20.1. The history of drug treatment is given in Table 20.2. To analyze data from this patient, we partition the time period into k subintervals L_i as given in Table 20.3 and assume $\{\xi_R(t) = \xi_R(i), \xi_P(t) = \xi_P(i), k_T(t) = k_T(i)\}$ for $t \in L_i$.

Using the procedures in Section 20.4, we have developed a FORTRAN program to compute the estimates of the unknown parameters and the state variables. Applying this program to the data in Table 20.1, the estimates of $\{\mu_T, \mu_V, c, N\}$ are $\{\hat{\mu}_T = 0.0490 \pm 1.9819 \times 10^{-2}, \hat{\mu}_V = 0.3014 \pm 0.1336 \times 10^{-2}, \hat{\sigma}^2 = 5.0500 \pm 0.9514, \hat{c} = 0.03 \pm 0.4426 \times 10^{-2}, \hat{N} = 2,000 \pm 0.3987\}$. The estimates of the time-dependent parameters $\{\xi_R(i), \xi_P(i), k_T(i), i = 1, \ldots, k\}$ are given in Table 20.3. The estimates of the numbers of the infectious HIV and noninfectious HIV per ml of blood over time and the number of T_P cells per ml of blood over time are all plotted in Figure 20.1. Given in the third column in Table 20.1 are the predicted total numbers of HIV by using the model and the jackknife procedure of Efron (1982).

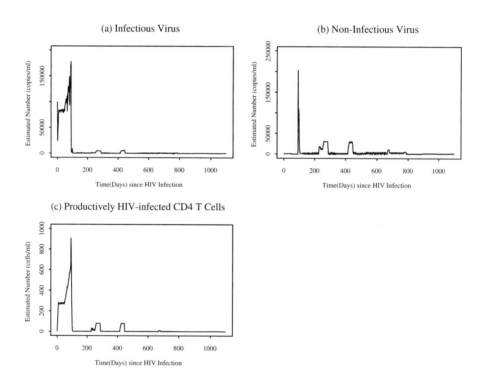

Figure 20.1: Plots showing the estimated numbers of infectious and noninfectious virus, and productively HIV-infected CD4 T cells per ml of blood

Table 20.1: The observed numbers of HIV RNA virus load of an HIV-infected patient

Days Since HIV Infection	RNA Copies/ml	Predicted RNA Copies/ml ± Std Error	Predicted Infectious RNA Copies/ml ± Std Error
80	150000	149104±58003	149104±58003
88	160000	167419±68292	167419±68292
92	210000	208541±170760	4659±4114
93	120000	116406±137000	2032±2490
95	110000	111653±7433	1931±1295
99	43000	43647±21277	9202±5024
120	1200	1364±2806	54±253
179	950	615±1461	92±313
204	≤400	532±1493	18±232
232	20000	20109±9440	1418±720
248	14000	14026±7412	743±398
260	36000	36286±17361	5037±2390
291	≤400	467±1272	39±269
331	≤400	551±1254	31±186
353	≤400	528±1455	19±164
437	34000	33805±18528	5068±2839
465	4400	4383±2672	332±214
527	≤400	517±1349	24±142
592	4100	3938±2807	575±370
671	12000	12088±6343	1110±618
746	3300	3389±2208	391±271
774	5700	5799±3098	854±483
802	≤400	487±1471	29±176
894	≤400	758±1591	56±185
984	1600	1897±1920	279±364
1073	1100	1354±1956	169±367

(1) The predicted numbers by using the model as given in Table 20.1 are very close to the observed numbers. This indicates that the fitting of the data by the model is extremely good; for more details, see Zhang (2004, Chapter 2).

(2) It appears that the estimates of $\{\mu_T, \mu_V\}$ are consistent with the estimates of Ho *et al.* (1995), indicating that both the productively HIV-infected CD4 T cells and the HIV are short lived. Similarly, the estimate of N is consistent with the estimate given by Tan and Wu (1998) and the estimate of c is close to the observation by Phillips (1996).

Table 20.2: The history of drug treatment

Days Partition	Drug Treatment	Inhibitor
$[0, 49)$	Zidovudine	NRTI
$[49, 91)$	No Drugs	No Inhibitor
$[91, 98)$	Ritonavir	PR Inhibitor
$[98, 122)$	Ritonavir, Lamivudine	NRTIs + PI
	Zidovudine	
$[122, 414)$	Ritonavir, Lamivudine, Zidovudine	NRTIs + PI
	Trimethoprim-sulfamethoxazole	
$[414, 668)$	Nelfinavir, Lamivudine, Zidovudine	NRTIs + PI
	Trimethoprim-sulfamethoxazole	
$[668, 773)$	Nelfinavir, Lamivudine, Zidovudine	NRTIs + PI
$[773, 1100)$	Didanosine, Efavirenz, Stavudine	NRTIs + NNRTI

(3) From Figure 20.1 (a), we observe that in most time periods after 440 days since HIV infection, the number of infectious HIV is very small. Apparently, the HAART protocols (i.e., the combination of two NRTIs and one PI) have successfully suppressed HIV reproduction. From the estimates of $\{\xi_R(t), \xi_P(t)\}$ in Table 20.3, it is observed that at least one of the drugs worked very well when HAART was applied. This may help explain why the HAART protocol is very effective in suppressing HIV replication.

(4) From the estimates of infectious HIV virus copies as given in Table 20.1 and Figure 20.1(a), we observe that the drug combination involving two NRTIs (Didanosine and Starvudine) and one NNRTI (Efavirenz) is at least as efficient as the three drug combinations in HAART involving two NRTIs (Lamivudine and Zidovudine) and one PI (Ritonavir or Nelfinavir) in suppressing HIV replication. This suggests that controlling HIV infection of CD4 T cells by HIV may be of primary importance.

20.6   Conclusions and Discussion

In this chapter, we have developed a state space model for the HIV pathogenesis under treatment by HAART based on data of RNA HIV virus copies over time. This is an individual-based model applicable to cases when the observed RNA HIV virus copies are available over time. Because different individuals have different genetic backgrounds, it is expected that different drugs and different

Table 20.3: The estimate of parameters

Periods Days After Infection	Estimate of $\{\xi_P(t)\}$ $\pm$ Std Error	Estimate of $\{\xi_R(t)\}$ $\pm$ Std Error	Estimate of $\{k_T(t)\}$ $\pm$ Std Error
$[0, 49)$	0.01 $\pm$ 6.0064E-04	0.845 $\pm$4.1930E-03	2.85E-02 $\pm$5.8051E-04
$[49, 91)$	0.0 $\pm$0.0	0.0 $\pm$1.1166E-02	5.101E-03 $\pm$1.7281E-04
$[91, 98)$	0.9775 $\pm$5.4589E-04	0.0 $\pm$1.2851E-02	6.05E-02 $\pm$9.6712E-04
$[98, 102)$	0.5 $\pm$4.0100E-03	0.9998 $\pm$1.2023E-03	6.67E-01 $\pm$2.1950E-03
$[102, 122)$	0.865 $\pm$0.3496	0.9885 $\pm$0.3225	1.5E-01 $\pm$6.8427E-02
$[122, 188)$	0.7535 $\pm$0.3341	0.9975 $\pm$0.3901	5.8152E-02 $\pm$2.7205E-02
$[188, 226)$	0.806 $\pm$0.3573	0.9971 $\pm$0.4263	1.985E-01 $\pm$9.9543E-02
$[226, 236)$	0.915 $\pm$0.4316	0.856 $\pm$0.3164	2.15E-02 $\pm$1.0879E-02
$[236, 251)$	0.935 $\pm$0.4411	0.8985 $\pm$0.3363	3.95E-02 $\pm$2.0148E-02
$[251, 284)$	0.8245 $\pm$0.3886	0.81 $\pm$0.2907	8.652E-02 $\pm$4.2733E-02
$[284, 311)$	0.7505 $\pm$0.3539	0.9975 $\pm$0.4543	1.251E-01 $\pm$6.2958E-02
$[311, 337)$	0.81 $\pm$0.4041	0.9975 $\pm$0.4820	1.51E-01 $\pm$8.3933E-02
$[337, 414)$	0.845 $\pm$0.4266	0.997 $\pm$0.4831	1.935E-01 $\pm$0.1101
$[414, 444)$	0.8085 $\pm$0.4084	0.8112 $\pm$0.3092	7.7E-02 $\pm$4.1171E-02
$[444, 465)$	0.9 $\pm$0.4544	0.9975 $\pm$0.4857	5.7455E-02 $\pm$3.1137E-02
$[465, 528)$	0.85 $\pm$0.4291	0.9973 $\pm$0.4847	1.9358E-01 $\pm$0.1098
$[528, 668)$	0.804 $\pm$0.4069	0.985 $\pm$0.4066	1.45E-01 $\pm$8.5151E-02
$[668, 679)$	0.7945 $\pm$0.4015	0.956 $\pm$0.4375	0.395 $\pm$0.2017
$[679, 773)$	0.845 $\pm$0.4270	0.9865 $\pm$0.4698	8.5295E-02 $\pm$4.7300E-02
$[773, 786)$	0.805 $\pm$0.4074	0.9785 $\pm$0.3630	7.286E-02 $\pm$4.3805E-02
$[786, 894)$	0.845 $\pm$0.4270	0.997 $\pm$0.4836	1.756E-01 $\pm$9.9170E-02
$[894, 1100]$	0.765 $\pm$0.3873	0.9885 $\pm$0.4679	7.55E-02 $\pm$4.2816E-02

treatment regimens are usually applied to different patients. This makes the individual-based model extremely useful and appropriate.

To monitor HIV progression in HIV-infected individuals treated by HAART or other protocols, it is important to estimate the number of infectious HIV and noninfectious HIV. In this chapter, by using the state space model, we have developed procedures to estimate both the unknown parameters and the numbers of infectious HIV virus and noninfectious HIV virus per ml of blood. We have applied these procedures to the data of a patient treated with various antiviral drugs and HAART at St. Jude Children's Research Hospital in Memphis, TN. For this patient, in most time periods the HAART treatment appeared to have controlled the number of infectious HIV to the undetectable level very effectively. Besides these results, we also make the following observations.

(1) We have provided here some examples indicating that in monitoring the disease status, using the total number of HIV to measure the success or failure of the drugs is very misleading and may be erroneous. For example, at 232, 248, and 260 days since HIV infection, the total number of observed HIV copies per ml of blood are 20,000, 14,000, and 36,000, respectively. However, most of the HIV are noninfectious and the estimated number of infectious HIV are 1418, 743, and 5307 copies per ml of blood, respectively, indicating the effectiveness of the treatment. These results suggest that for clinical applications and for providing guidelines for medical doctors to follow, it is important to estimate both the numbers of infectious HIV and noninfectious HIV.

(2) It has been reported in the literature that when the drugs are stopped, in 3 to 14 days the number of HIV rebounds, reaching the level before treatment; see Chun *et al.* (1999). We have obtained here similar results. For example, during the period $[49, 91)$ when the treatment had been stopped, both the number of productively HIV-infected CD4$^{(+)}$ T cells (i.e., T_P cells) and infectious HIV (i.e., V_1) copies are very high, reaching the highest number in a few days (200,000 copies HIV per ml of blood). However, our estimates also indicated that when the HAART treatment was reintroduced, in a few days the total number of HIV copies was reduced significantly whereas the number of infectious HIV had reduced to below 1931 copies per ml of blood by day 95 since HIV infection. This result provides some clues and justification of the use of a structural on and off HAART protocol as discussed in Bajaria *et al.* (2002).

(3) The estimates of $\{\xi_P(t), \xi_R(t)\}$ indicate that in most time periods, at least one type of drug has efficiency over 94%; thus although one might be anticipating possible problems such as drug resistance of HIV to one of the drugs and noncompliance by the patient due to high side-effects of the drugs, the HAART can still successfully control the HIV infection, suggesting the usefulness of the combination therapy.

(4) The successful suppression of HIV replication by the drug combination (Didanosine, Stavudine, and Efavirenz) suggests that one may replace the

protease inhibitors Ritonavir and Nelfinavir by the NNRTI drug Efavirenz. This has important clinical implications because the PIs Ritonavir and Nelfinavir have serious side-effects and toxicity for most patients.

To validate the model, we have used the jackknife procedure as given in Efron (1982) to derive the predicted value of each observation. This procedure deletes one observation each time and uses the remaining data (i.e., the data with the observation in question being deleted) and the model to derive the predicted value of the observed numbers of RNA HIV copies. The results are given in the third column of Table 20.1. These results indicated that the predicted numbers are very close to the observed ones.

Although the models and the methods developed here are useful to estimate the unknown parameters and state variables and to monitor the HIV dynamics under HAART, some further research is needed to address some important issues regarding the methods. Specifically, we need to do more research to answer the following questions.

(1) In this chapter, we have partitioned the time period into nonoverlapping subperiods and assume that the parameters $\{\xi_R(t), \xi_P(t), k_T(t)\}$ are constants in each subperiod. This partition is dictated by the treatment regimens and by the assumption that the number of noninfected CD4$^{(+)}$ T cells is a constant in each subperiod. In order for the latter assumption to prevail, the subperiods cannot be too long and more subperiods are needed in intervals where the number of HIV changes wildly. In our future research, we will examine the impact of this partitioning and look for optimal ways of selecting a partition.

(2) In many practical problems, it is important to assess the impact of many risk variables such as CD4 T cell counts over time and CD8 T cell counts over time. We have not addressed these problems here.

In this chapter, we have proposed a state space model based on RNA HIV copies over time. To make the procedures here widely applicable and useful, we need to develop user-friendly software for the computation. Also, we need to apply the model and methods to some data of the structural on-and-off HAART protocol as described in Bajaria *et al.* (2002); this will be our future research work.

References

1. Bajaria, S. H., Webb, G., Cloyd, M., and Kirschner, D. E. (2002). Dynamics of naive and memory CD4+ T lymphocytes in HIV-1 disease progression, *JAIDS*, **30**, 41–58.

2. Betts, M. R., Ambrozak, D. R., and Douek, D. C. (2001). Analysis of total human immunodeficiency virus (HIV)-specific CD4$^{(+)}$ and CD8$^{(+)}$

T-cell responses: Relationship to viral load in untreated HIV infection, *Journal of Virology*, **75**, 11983–11991.

3. Chun, T-W., Davey, R. T., and Engel, D. (1999). Re-emergence of HIV after stopping therapy, *Nature*, **401,** 874–875.

4. Cohen, O., Weissman, D. and Fauci, A. S. (1998). The immunopathpgenesis of HIV infection, In *Fundamental Immunology, Fourth edition* (Ed., W.E. Paul), Chapter 44, pp. 1511–1534, Lippincott-Raven, Philadelphia.

5. Dybul, M., Chun T-W., and Yoder, C. (2001). Short-cycle structural intermittent treatment of chronic HIV infection with highly active antiretroviral therapy: Effects on virologic, immunologic, and toxicity parameters, *Proceedings of the National Academy of Sciences USA* **98**, 15161–15166.

6. Efron, B. (1982). *The Jacknife, the Bootstrap and Other Resampling Plans*, SIAM, Philadelphia.

7. Garcia, P., Plana, M., and Vidal, C. (1999). Dynamics of viral load rebound and immunological changes after stopping effective antiretroviral therapy, *AIDS*, **13,** F79–86.

8. Ho, D. D., Neumann, A. U., and Perelson, A. S. (1995). Rapid turnover of plasma virus and CD4 lymphocytes in HIV-1 infection, *Nature*, **373**, 123–126.

9. Perelson, A. S., Neumann, A. U., and Markowitz, M. (1996). HIV-1 dynamics in vivo: Virion clearance rate, infected cell life-span,and viral generation time, *Science*, **271**, 1582–1586.

10. Phillips, A. N. (1996). Reduction of HIV concentration during acute infection: Independence from a specific immune response, *Science*, **271**, 497–499.

11. Pitcher, C. J., Quittner, C., and Peterson, D. M. (1999). HIV-1 specific CD4$^{(+)}$ T cells are detectable in most individuals with active HIV-1 infection, but decline with prolonged viral suppression, *Nature Medicine*, **5**, 518–525.

12. Tan, W. Y. (2000). *Stochastic Modeling of AIDS Epidemiology and HIV Pathogenesis*, World Scientific, River Edge, New Jersey.

13. Tan, W. Y. (2002). *Stochastic Models With Applications to Genetics, Cancers, AIDS and Other Biomedical Systems*, World Scientific, River Edge, New Jersey.

14. Tan, W. Y., and Wu, H. (1998). Stochastic modeling of the dynamic of CD4$^{(+)}$ T cell infection by HIV and some Monte Carlo studies, *Mathematical Bioscience*, **147**, 173–205.

15. Tan, W. Y., and Xiang, Z. H. (1998). State space models for the HIV epidemic with variable infection in homosexual populations by state space models, *Journal of Statistical Planning and Inference*, **78**, 71–87.

16. Tan, W. Y., Zhang, P., and Xiong, X. (2004). A state space model for HIV pathogenesis under anti-viral drugs and applications, In *Deterministic and Stochastic Models of AIDS Epidemic and HIV with Interventions* (Eds., W. Y. Tan and H. Wu), Chapter 14 World Scientific, River Edge, New Jersey.

17. Zhang, P. (2004). Stochastic modeling of HIV pathogenesis under therapy and AIDS vaccination, *Ph.D. Thesis*, Department of Mathematical Sciences, The University of Memphis, Memphis, Tennessee.

PART VI
Safety and Efficacy Assessment

21

Safety Assessment Versus Efficacy Assessment

Mary A. Foulkes

Center for Biologics Evaluations and Research, FDA, Rockville, MD, USA

Abstract: Many statistical methods have been developed that focus primarily on efficacy. Safety evaluation frequently involves many additional considerations. Randomized controlled trials, especially later phase 3 trials, are infrequently designed based on safety outcomes. Most of these trials are designed based on efficacy outcomes, and therefore have limited power to detect important differences in safety outcomes. Recently, there have been calls to design trials with sufficient power to address known safety concerns. When prevention trials introduce an experimental preventive intervention (e.g., a vaccine) to an otherwise healthy (although at-risk) population, safety considerations can substantially affect the benefit:risk ratio and thus the utility and acceptability of the intervention. Observation of safety outcomes is often less controlled than for efficacy outcomes, particularly for safety concerns that emerge during the course of the trial. When either safety or efficacy outcomes are missing, specific assumptions are required for analysis (e.g., missing completely at random, MCAR), but often these assumptions may not apply. The statistical methods that rely on these assumptions have largely been developed with a focus on efficacy outcomes. Illustrative examples, including meta-analyses, will be presented and the underdeveloped areas highlighted.

Keywords and phrases: Patient safety, clinical evaluations

21.1   Introduction

Most clinical trials are designed with a focus on efficacy assessment. Recently, there have been calls for longer-term safety studies with large placebo groups to determine the natural rate of a particular disease, and for larger vaccine trials with the capability of estimating rates of rare adverse events (AEs) [Ellenberg *et al.* (2004)]. Usually, safety and efficacy are evaluated separately within the same subjects, and then at benefit:risk ratio assessed. Counterterrorism preparedness, however, has opened the possibilities of evaluation of safety of therapeutics or preventive interventions (as demonstrated in more than one animal species, as well as in humans), and regulatory decisions made without definitive efficacy evaluations in humans, for example, for post exposure treatments for soman gas exposure [Couzin (2003)]. This puts the careful evaluation of safety into sharper focus. Prospective safety evaluation based on studies that are large enough, long enough, and detailed enough present different experimental design, analysis, and inference issues than do efficacy evaluations. Differences (some subtle and some not so subtle) and the opportunities for novel approaches to the evaluation of safety and evaluation of efficacy will be examined.

21.2 Design Issues

21.2.1 Outcomes

In order to arrive at inferences and conclusions that are reproducible, interpretable, and generalizable, precise definitions of terms, including processes by which the data may be obtained, are critical to acquiring information on outcomes in a reproducible fashion. Experimental or observational study design, either early in product/intervention development or later in general use, requires the specific definition of an outcome of interest. Efficacy outcomes are, by design, defined a priori with specific methods of measurement, observed on a planned schedule (e.g., monthly), and capable of being observed on every subject regardless of experimental treatment. Safety outcomes are often not.

AE reporting (particularly outside of a controlled trial, e.g., passive postmarketing surveillance) relies on medical/clinical personnel to observe, recognize and report suspected AEs. The occurrence of adverse events is actively queried in a controlled trial at follow-up visits, which occurred on an established schedule. By contrast, passive spontaneous AE reports are recorded often without any coding conventions, on an irregular, undefined schedule, notoriously incomplete in their detail and application of rigorous, a priori definitions. So an overall evaluation of all available safety data needs to take into account the context of the AE report, and address both the information that is available and that which is not. Unexpected safety issues often emerge during the course of a controlled trial, and require analyses that are necessarily data-driven. The more forethought and predefined analyses the better, for example, "Decide before looking at the data on order [rules of intensity grade] based on certainty of diagnosis and anticipated adverse experience" [Chuang-Stein et al. (1992)]. Adjudication of safety outcomes rarely involves the process of oversight that primary efficacy outcomes adjudication committee reviews provide [Jovanovic,

Algra, and van Gijn (2004) and Walter *et al.* (1997)], except in those cases where the safety outcome is the primary outcome [Bombardier *et al.* (2000) and Wingard *et al.* (2000)].

Safety and efficacy cannot, in some cases, be completely separated and evaluated based on disjoint sets of variables. The same instrument can measure both safety and efficacy, for example, in psychopharmacological trials [Bender *et al.* (2004)].

21.2.2 Power

Comparisons for each individual data item lack power for the safety comparisons of interest. Clinical trials, for example, are designed to provide sufficient power to address a primary hypothesis, most frequently the primary efficacy hypothesis. This establishes the overall sample size, but it may not be adequate to address safety issues that emerge during the conduct of a trial or later. Rare reactions, reactions with delayed onset, or reactions in specific subpopulations are all difficult to detect, and difficult to assess associations with exposure to a specific medical intervention or product. The sample size needed to detect differences between treatment groups in background rates of anticipated adverse events, such as differences in rates of torsade de pointe arrhythmias in cardiac patients, are not necessarily considered. If the safety question of interest depends upon having sufficient power to detect a rare event, the approximate sample sizes needed as a function of that event rate are shown in this table:

	Sample Size	
Rate of Event	80% Power	90% Power
0.01	160	230
0.001	1,600	2,300
0.0001	16,000	23,000

With smallpox vaccine, for example, for every million people immunized, there would be anexpected one to two deaths and 15 life-threatening complications, and about 60 less serious events (such as encephalitis) [Fauci (2003)]. These represent event rates considerably smaller than 0.0001, and would require very large trials to detect.

If, however, the safety question of interest were whether a particular adverse event rate increased with chronic exposure, the issue of power and sample size also involves duration of follow-up. O'Neill (1995) presented an example that, with 1000 subjects exposed to a drug and followed for six months and 20% of those followed for an additional six months (with an expected gastrointestinal bleeding rate of 1% in a six month period), the power was insufficient to detect a sixfold increase in that rate of gastrointestinal bleeding.

21.2.3 Population

Efficacy trial enrollment may be purposefully restricted to those at highest risk, to improve efficiency and demonstrate an effect. However, to the extent that the trial enrollees do not reflect the ultimate target population, unanticipated safety issues may emerge when a new intervention or product is introduced to a less restrictive population. Safety issues might not be uniform across all population subgroups, for example, across age groups or gender. The diversity of the population initially studied, which will necessarily be constrained by the size of the studies, may limit the detection of some safety issues until effects are observable in a more diverse population.

21.2.4 Comparison

A strength of the experimental design in controlled trials is the appropriate comparison group for the efficacy assessment. The appropriate comparison group for safety assessments is not always well defined, or even known. In randomized trials, there may be no placebo or untreated group, which would in some cases be the appropriate comparison group. In observational studies, it may be difficult to determine whether the noncases (those without the adverse event) were exposed to the intervention or product.

21.3   Analytic Issues

21.3.1   Compliance

Compliance may be more of a concern in evaluation of safety data, where it may be difficult to attribute an adverse event occurring to a noncompliant subject. Comparisons of efficacy outcomes relying (at least initially) on "intention-to-treat" analysis (ITT) may be less directly dependent on individual compliance [Institute of Medicine Committee on Data Standards for Patient Safety (2003)]. Safety analyses can sometimes focus on "as treated" subgroups of subjects, for example, subjects who received one, two, or three doses, which destroys the randomized comparison groups and, as with all postbaseline characteristic subgroups, may introduce bias. Safety evaluations are performed with caution and the concern is more with minimizing risk than maximizing benefits, with false negative conclusions than with false positives, that is, with type II error than with type I error.

21.3.2 Missing data

A second analytic issue relates to missing data for either efficacy or safety evaluations. The set of subjects included in a safety evaluation may differ from those included in the efficacy evaluation. The measurements needed for safety may not be recorded because they never were taken (e.g., no tests of an organ system because there was no suspicion of an effect on that system), because they were considered optional, or for other reasons. Thus, it may not be possible to distinguish those truly missing responses from responses implying no safety concern. Efforts in controlled trials to minimize the amount of missing primary efficacy outcome data frequently cannot be applied to emerging safety concerns. The mechanisms of missingness may be very different for safety outcomes than for efficacy outcomes [Touloumi *et al.* (2002) and Mertens (1993)]. Missing essential information often cannot be anticipated, for example, a spontaneous report of a case of suspected drug-induced pancreatitis that fails to include whether the subject was alcoholic or was examined for gallstones, two of the most common causes of acute pancreatitis. The distinction between characteristics of safety and efficacy outcomes can be minimal, as in the case where the primary efficacy outcomes and major safety outcomes are the same, for example, myocardial infarction. Alternatively, that distinction can be considerable, particularly when the full range of safety outcomes that should optimally be captured is not known at the beginning of the trial and the efficacy outcome is total mortality with potential missingness minimized by input from a national death registry.

Clinical trials of interventions with relatively well-known safety profiles, for example, the third or fourth drug developed in a class, have obvious domains for careful follow-up. For example, studies of antiplatelet agents such as ticlopidine will capture detailed data on hematological response variables, and studies of antiretroviral drugs will evaluate evidence of lipodystrophy. For such a priori treatment group comparisons, the usual testing and estimation approaches apply. However, a new agent without historical background will not have a clear direction for attention to safety outcomes. Analytic assumptions about missingness may not be as viable for missing safety outcomes and for missing values of the primary efficacy outcome and validating missingness assumptions would be difficult at best.

21.3.3 Confounding

Safety and efficacy evaluations are limited by the information available on confounding factors, for example, concomitant medications, intercurrent illnesses, and chronic conditions. Concomitant medications are not easily recorded outside controlled trials, particularly information on over-the-counter (OTC) medications, which are often taken without input from healthcare professionals.

Other confounding factors, such as access to care, may differentially affect safety and efficacy evaluations.

21.3.4 Bias

Biases can both over- and underestimate the relative risk of AEs after exposure to an intervention or product, and can be a particular problem in unblinded trials. Unlike the primary efficacy outcome, adverse event data are often captured passively, in an open-ended fashion, without structured and timely procedures (e.g., diagnostic work-up), and without clear, uniformly applied, and objective definitions. Information bias or diagnostic suspicion bias could occur if the treatment groups were differentially monitored or ascertained with respect to completeness of safety outcome data. Safety responses are often based on subject recall, or on the depth of the interviewers' prompting. Information obtained from computerized records, or queries prompted equally from all treatment groups could ameliorate potential information biases. Lastly, publication bias may affect safety evaluations even more than efficacy evaluations.

21.3.5 Misclassification

Individuals not familiar with the specific definition of an outcome might provide inaccurate information and might confuse the outcome in the information reported. For example, anaphylaxis might be recorded as syncope. Thus, an uncritical review and analysis of the reported outcomes might ignore some outcomes due to misclassification. Even in a well-designed clinical trial such misclassification can lead to biased estimates [O'Neill (1995)].

21.3.6 Multiplicity

Evaluations of either efficacy or safety involve large numbers of comparisons that may then identify either real differences, or chance findings. There are multiple dimensions of concern, multiple outcomes, and possibly multiple comparison groups. A single study may simultaneously evaluate multiple outcomes, for example, EKG and clinical lab data, or liver enzymes, nausea, and jaundice. Occasionally, there is the need for a "no treatment" (or placebo) comparison as well as an active comparator, in order to provide estimates addressing different risk:benefit questions. Multiple comparisons also occur in assessing drug–drug interactions where either efficacy or safety evaluations may differ by drug–drug combinations. Adverse reactions to an intervention may not be distinguishable from events in the natural course of the disease under study, or the target study population may have extensive comorbidities so that the cause of the event is unclear. A variety of comparisons may help distinguish the causal from the coincidental effects, but the strongest experimental design, the randomized controlled trial, provides the context in which adverse event rates elevated over background rates could be detected.

21.4   Analytic Approaches

The analyses of missing data, and particularly the assumptions about the mechanism of missingness, have been extensively addressed in the statistical literature [Little and Rubin (1987) and Laird (1988)]. Designations such as missing completely at random (MCAR), missing at random (MAR), and missing not at random (MNAR) may apply differently to efficacy outcomes than to safety outcomes even for the same subject. Some analytic approaches utilize covariates related to missing (e.g., distance from residence to clinic) or to reasons for discontinuation of therapy (tolerance, toxicity, drug–drug interactions, etc.). Analytic approaches can contribute to and advance the identification of potential safety problems that might not rapidly come to light with less sensitive methods. In evaluating either efficacy or safety, the sensitivity of estimates and hypothesis tests to assumptions and to methods of estimation should be examined.

A common analytic approach is to compare the incidence of each medical/clinical outcome or to compare the mean changes from baseline values [Peace (1987)]. Hypothesis testing and confidence interval estimation for treatment group differences or for evaluating prespecified adverse events of specific concern are frequent analyses; however, safety issues often emerge during the course of a study or a series of studies. The characterization of the available safety data for purposes of regulatory decisions can be called an integrated summary of safety (ISS) [FDA Reviewer Guidance (2005)]. In addition to the guidance offered by regulatory agencies, a variety of statistical approaches to summarizing the safety data has been published [Enas and Goldstein (1995) and Chuang-Stein and Le (2001)]. Various approaches to modeling should be explored for the potential to contribute to both safety and efficacy evaluations, for example, pattern-mixture models [Fitzmaurice, Laird, and Shneyer (2001)], and latent dropout class models [Roy (2003)].

One measure that clinicians may find more immediately useful than relative or absolute risk estimates are the estimates of the number of patients need to treat (NNT), which is the reciprocal of the absolute risk reduction for the treatment. With respect to safety concerns, the metric is the number needed to harm (NNH). These may provide clinicians and patients with information for making therapeutic choices. These measures do have limitations, as they may have wide confidence intervals, apply only to the limited conditions or eligibility of the source trial, depend on the subject's risk at baseline, and be based on the specific period of observations of the source trial [Altman (1998)].

Meta-analyses are often employed to evaluate either efficacy or safety. The difficulties and limitations of meta-analyses to evaluate safety are well demonstrated in Shekelle *et al.* (2003). They summarized adverse events (psychiatric symptoms, autonomic symptoms, upper-gastrointestinal symptoms, and heart palpitations) in 52 controlled trials, and concluded that subjects receiving ephedra or ephedrine for either weight loss or athletic performance, compared to controls, were at two to three times the risk of those adverse events. Given the size of the trials, they could not exclude that more serious adverse events may have occurred at rates less than one per thousand. They reported heterogeneity among the athletic performance trials, but did not observe heterogeneity among the weight loss trials. In another example of meta-analyses of a safety outcome, Freeman, Zehenbauer, and Buchman (2003) reported a meta-analysis of the risk of clinically significant bleeding with anticoagulant therapies. Publication bias, restrictive enrollment, and duration of observation within the trials were all discussed as limitations to both of these meta-analyses.

21.5   Inferences

Analytic results are used to make a range of inferences for personal decisions, and for public health policy and regulatory actions. Recognition of the differences between efficacy and safety evaluations (summarized in Table 21.1) should be part of each of these decisions or actions. Two limits on inferences particularly affect safety evaluations, and have been extensively addressed in both the statistical and the clinical literatures. These are, first, distinguishing causal from coincidental events, and interpreting zero safety events, that is, an absence of evidence [Altman and Bland (1995)].

21.6   Conclusions

Evaluation of efficacy and safety may be based on the same data sources, the same study designs, the same subjects, and sometimes even similar outcome definitions. The careful evaluation of efficacy and safety, however, requires an understanding of the data to inform the respective analytic assumptions and inferences. Recognizing the limits in the available safety information can provide insights into the additional investigations needed to further characterize a safety profile, highlight inadequately assessed areas of concern, and specific safety outcome definitions, and can also suggest improvements in study designs, conduct, and analytic approaches that serve each of the goals of efficacy and safety evaluation.

Table 21.1: Differences that affect the assessments of safety and efficacy throughout product/intervention development

	Safety	**Efficacy**
Design		
A priori defined outcomes	Few	All critical outcomes
Primary outcome parameter	Rarely	Almost always
Scheduled or spontaneous observations	Scheduled evaluations, e.g., toxicity, others spontaneous	According to design schedule
Experimental design	Observational/randomized, controlled	Randomized, controlled
Long-term observation	Rarely	Duration by design
Elicitation of outcome	Uncertain quality of data, often insufficient detail	As designed, and staff trained
Power	Often not addressed	To detect a specified difference
Adequate sample size	Limited	By design
Preferably assessed in population	More broadly defined, possibly healthier population	More narrowly defined, possibly more serious disease patients, e.g., trial eligibility
Comparison group	Occasionally	Often by design
Analytic Issues		
Adjudication of events	Unusual, unless a specific safety outcome is the primary outcome	Often adjudication of primary efficacy outcome
Benefit:risk considerations	Minimize risk	Maximize benefits
Multiplicity	Often ignored	More clearly recognized and addressed in analytic plans
Interim monitoring plan	Rarely	Often
Mechanism of action	Little known; in any body system; often at low incidence	Usually well characterized
Completeness of follow-up	Not often known	Quantifiable
Analytic Approaches		
Mechanisms of missingness	Often unclear	Often unclear, analytic assumptions include MCAR, MAR, or MNAR
Clinical summary measures	Number needed to harm (NNH)	Number needed to treat (NNT)
Summaries	Often descriptive	Inferential

References

1. Altman, D. G. (1998). Confidence intervals for the number needed to treat, *British Medical Journal.* **317**, 1309–1312.

2. Altman, D. G., and Bland, J. M. (1995). Statistics notes: Absence of evidence is not evidence of absence, *British Medical Journal,* **311**, 485.

3. Bender, S., Grohmann, R., Engel, R. R., Degner, D., Dittmann-Balcar, A., and Ruther, E. (2004). Severe adverse drug reactions in psychiatric inpatients treated with neuroleptics, *Pharmacopsychiatry,* **37**, S46–S53.

4. Bombardier, C., Laine, L., Reicin, A., Shapiro, D., Burgos-Vargas, R., Davis, B., Day, R., Ferraz, M. B., Hawkey, C. J., and Hochberg, M. C. (2000). Comparison of upper gastrointestinal toxicity of Rofecoxib and Naproxen in patients with rheumatoid arthritis, *New England Journal of Medicine,* **343**, 1520–1528.

5. Chuang-Stein, C., and Le, V. (2001). Recent advancements in the analysis and presentation of safety data, *Drug Information Journal,* **35**, 377–397.

6. Chuang-Stein, C., Mohberg, N. R., and Musselman, D. M. (1992). Organization and analysis of safety data using a multivariate approach, *Statistics in Medicine,* **11**, 1075–1089.

7. Couzin, J. (2003). Clinical trials: New rule triggers debate over best way to test drugs, *Science,* **299**, 1651–1653.

8. Ellenberg, S. S., Foulkes, M. A., Midthun, K., and Goldenthal, K. L. (2004). Evaluation of new vaccines: How much safety data? In press.

9. Enas, G. G., and Goldstein, D. J. (1995). Defining, monitoring and combining safety information in clinical trials, *Statistics in Medicine,* **14**, 1099–1111.

10. Fauci, A. S. (2003). *Bioterrorism: A Clear and Present Danger*, Rand, Santa Monica, California.

11. FDA Reviewer Guidance (2005). Conducting a clinical safety review of a new product application and preparing a report on the review, `http://www.fda.gov/CDER/GUIDANCE/3580fnl.pdf`.

12. Fitzmaurice, G. M., Laird, N. M., and Shneyer, L. (2001). An alternative parameterization of the general linear mixture model for longitudinal data with non-ignorable drop-outs, *Statistics in Medicine,* **20**, 1009–1021.

13. Freeman, B. D., Zehnbauer, B. A., and Buchman, T. G. (2003). A meta-analysis of controlled trials of anticoagulant therapies in patients with sepsis, *Shock*, **20**, 5–9.

14. Institute of Medicine Committee on Data Standards for Patient Safety (2003). In *Patient Safety: Achieving a New Standard of Care*, National Academic, Washington, DC.

15. Jovanovic, D. R., Algra, A., and van Gijn, J. (2004). Classification of outcomes events in Dutch TIA trial: prognostic value of accepted and rejected events, *Current Medical Research Opinion*, **20**, 255–258.

16. Laird, N. M. (1988). Missing data in longitudinal studies, *Statistics in Medicine*, **7**, 305–315.

17. Little, R. J. A., and Rubin, D. B. (1987). *Statistical Analysis with Missing Data*, John Wiley & Sons, New York.

18. Mertens, T. E. (1993). Estimating the effects of misclassification, *Lancet*, **342**, 418–421.

19. O'Neill, R. T. (1995). Statistical concepts in the planning and evaluation of drug safety from clinical trials in drug development: Issues of international harmonization, *Statistics in Medicine*, **14**, 117–127.

20. Peace, K. E. (1987). Design, monitoring, and analysis issues relative to adverse events, *Drug Informatics Journal*, **21**, 21–28.

21. Roy, J. (2003). Modeling longitudinal data with nonignorable dropouts using a latent dropout class model, *Biometrics*, **59**, 829–836.

22. Shekelle, P. G., Hardy, M. L., Morton, S. C., Maglione, M., Mojica, W. A., Suttorp, M. J., Rhodes, S. L., Jungvig, L., and Gagne, J. (2003). Efficacy and safety of Ephedra and Ephedrine for weight loss and athletic performance: A meta-analysis, *Journal of the American Medical Association*, **289**, 1537–1545.

23. Touloumi, G., Pocock, S. J., Babiker, A. G., and Darbyshire, J. H. (2002). Impact of missing data due to selective dropouts in cohort studies and clinical trials, *Epidemiology*, **13**, 347–355.

24. Walter, S. D., Cook, D. J., Guyatt, G. H., and King, D. (1997). Outcome assessment for clinical trials: How many adjudicators do we need? *Controlled Clinical Trials*, **18**, 27–42.

25. Wingard, J. R., White, M. H., Anaissie, E., Raffalli, J., Goodman, J., and Arrieta, A. (2000). A double-blind comparative trial evaluating the safety of liposomal amphotericin B versus amphotericin B lipid complex in the empirical treatment of febrile neutropenia. L Amph/ABLC Collaborative Study Group, *Clinical Infectious Diseases*, **31**, 1155–1163.

22

Cancer Clinical Trials with Efficacy and Toxicity Endpoints: A Simulation Study to Compare Two Nonparametric Methods

Alexia Letierce and Pascale Tubert-Bitter

Hôptial Bicêtre, Le Kremlin-Bicêtre, France INSERM, Villejuif, France

Abstract: Few methods for cancer clinical trials have been proposed in the past decade to evaluate treatments on the basis of joint efficacy and toxicity endpoints. The primary goal of a new cancer treatment is to improve efficacy. Because of the antagonist relationship between efficacy and toxicity, a critical question is to achieve this improvement without increasing unacceptably the risk of a severe toxicity. In this paper, two methods due to Letierce *et al.* (2003) and Tubert-Bitter *et al.* (2005) are compared in a simulation study. They are both nonparametric and, besides the joint approach of efficacy and toxicity, they consider the cumulative doses at which efficacy and toxicity occur, with the idea that it is better for the patient to attain efficacy at a small dose and to experience toxicity, if it happens, at the highest dose possible. These methods are detailed in the same framework. For the simulation study, the two true correlated doses at which efficacy and toxicity occur are generated from a Clayton model with Weibull marginal distributions. A fixed censoring value is considered, corresponding to the total dose of drug received at the end of the trial by the patients. Treatment groups of size 50 and 100 patients were simulated with 50%, 65%, and 80% of efficacy and 20%, 35%, and 50% of toxicity. Two values for the correlation of the variables were considered. One thousand simulations were run to estimate the type I error rate and the power of the tests. A few features were observed depending on the sample size, the correlation of the variables, and whether the difference between the two simulated treatments concerned efficacy, toxicity, or both.

Keywords and phrases: Cancer, clinical trials, efficacy, toxicity, nonparametrics, Clayton model

22.1   Introduction

In cancer treatment, physicians seek complete remission or at least the reduction of the tumour mass by a significant amount. To this end, they need to employ efficacious drugs in large dosage. Improvements in the control of the toxic effects of the cancer therapies have been realized, such as the introduction of haematopoietic growth factors in chemotherapy to reduce haematological toxicity or the better control of radiation administration in radiotherapy. Yet, the use of larger doses of therapeutics can cause damage to many organs, sometimes very serious and even lethal. In addition, these toxicities can affect the course of the treatment and as a result prevent efficacy. In this context, the question of a global evaluation of treatments, taking into account both of these antagonist effects, efficacy and toxicity, becomes critical.

In the past decade, few methods have been proposed for phase III clinical trials to address the question of a joint analysis of the treatments. Several approaches can be found, and they correspond to different testing hypotheses defining the superiority of a treatment in a multidimensional space. Some methods for one-sided comparisons are based on the derivation of reasonable trade-offs between efficacy and toxicity. Jennison and Turnbull (1993) have developed a parametric method based on the definition of an "indifference region" to analyse one treatment. Two continuous variables measuring efficacy and toxicity are assumed to have a bivariate normal distribution with mean $\mu = (\mu_1, \mu_2)$. Assuming that high values of μ_1 and μ_2 are preferable, two parameters ε_j and Δ_j ($\varepsilon_j < \Delta_j$, $j = 1, 2$) are a priori defined for each variable, to divide the axis into three parts: $\mu_j > \Delta_j$, where the treatment is acceptable, $\mu_j < \varepsilon_j$, where the treatment is unacceptable, and between ε_j and Δ_j, a region of indifference. The intersection of the two axes forms nine parts from which several acceptance or rejection regions can be derived to obtain more or less demanding decision rules, depending on the context of the treatment. Bloch, Lai, and Tubert-Bitter (2001) have proposed a test for the comparison of two treatments A and B, derived from the difference of the vector means of the considered variables, removing the normality assumption. A is preferable to B if one of the univariate differences is strictly positive and the other one is larger than a prespecified quantity, to ensure that the benefit on one endpoint is not obtained at the detriment of the other one. The test is derived with a bootstrap procedure [Efron and Tibshirani (1993)]. Thall and Cheng (1999) have derived a method specifically for the comparison of cancer treatments. It is based on the definition of "target-points" that constitute clinically meaningful improvements over the null hypothesis of "no difference between the two treatments." These points are elicited by the physicians and are expressed in terms of either binary endpoints or continuous measures, possibly censored. The rejection region is obtained by a numerical procedure, assuming that some proper transformation of the two-dimensional difference follows a normal bivariate distribution. All these methods are either parametric, based on the normality of some variables, or they require some parameters to be fixed a priori. These parameters are a threshold of efficacy to attain or a threshold of toxicity not to exceed, or target points.

Two recent methods, by Letierce *et al.* (2003, denoted below by MULTIN) and by Tubert-Bitter *et al.* (2005, denoted below by DISCR), are the focus of attention here. These methods derive nonparametric tests to compare two treatments with both efficacy and toxicity binary endpoints. They additionally take into account the cumulative doses of treatment received by the patient, that respectively achieve efficacy and toxicity, with the idea that it is preferable that the patient experiences efficacy at a small dose of treatment and suffers from toxicity at the largest possible dose, and at best, not at all. If toxicity occurs near the end of the treatment, one can hope the patient will avoid a too serious damage and will be able to continue the treatment till the end, which increases the chance of response. Parametric bivariate models on the doses, with the possibility of censoring, could be fitted but they do not solve the crucial issue of formulating the alternative hypothesis of the superiority of one treatment over another one in a clinical trial. Concerning this matter, only the nonparametric methods MULTIN and DISCR have been proposed in the literature. The other common point of these two latter methods is that they are not based on the specification of any trade-off between the antagonist effects, and consequently, they do not require the definition of any parameter before the analysis. A simulation study is reported in this chapter to compare them. The two approaches are presented in the same framework in Section 22.2, followed by the description of the simulation method in Section 22.3. Then the results are reported in Section 22.4 and some concluding remarks are given in Section 22.5.

22.2 Setting

The two methods MULTIN and DISCR deal with binary endpoints, one for efficacy and one for toxicity. They both add another consideration, that is, which one of the antagonist effects occurs first. Let us introduce the common framework. Consider a patient involved in a clinical trial; he is followed for a certain period of time, planned by the protocol, and receives either the new treatment A or the standard treatment B. Define for each patient two positive random variables X^* and Y^*, respectively, corresponding to the cumulative doses of treatment required to achieve toxicity and efficacy (usually expressed in mg/m^2). Time-to-event variables can be used as well. The variables X^* and Y^* are censored at the total dose of treatment if the corresponding effects are not attained at the end of the treatment. Denoting by Q ($Q > 0$) the total dose of treatment received by the patient at the end of the trial, the observations are $X = \min(X^*, Q)$ and $Y = \min(Y^*, Q)$. Two binary variables T and E are also defined to denote if toxicity and efficacy are attained (respectively, $T = 1$, $E = 1$) or not (respectively, $T = 0$, $E = 0$). Notice that $T = 1$ and $E = 1$ are, respectively, equivalent to $X = X^* \leq Q$ and to $Y = Y^* \leq Q$.

Considering the plane (X^*, Y^*) with the origin $O(0,0)$, the dose Q delimits a square in the first quadrant (OX^*, OY^*). Different situations are possible for the couple (X^*, Y^*) depending on whether X^* and/or Y^* are lower than Q, and on their sequence: (i) $X^* > Q$ and $Y^* > Q$: the necessary doses of treatment to attain toxicity and efficacy are not reached; (ii) $X = X^* \leq Q$ and $Y^* > Q$: only the dose causing toxicity is attained; (iii) $X^* > Q$ and $Y = Y^* \leq Q$: the dose achieving efficacy is attained without causing toxicity; (iv) $X^* \leq Y^* \leq Q$: the doses achieving efficacy and toxicity are both attained, the dose up to toxicity being smaller than the dose up to efficacy; (v) $Y^* < X^* \leq Q$: the doses achieving efficacy and toxicity are attained, with the efficacy obtained at first. In terms of observed values (X, Y, T, E), as plotted in Figure 22.1, the corresponding five parts are: (i') $X = Y = Q$, $T = 0$, $E = 0$; (ii') $X \leq Q$, $Y = Q$, $T = 1$, $E = 0$; (iii') $X = Q$, $Y \leq Q$, $T = 0$, $E = 1$; (iv') $X \leq Y \leq Q$, $T = 1$, $E = 1$; (v') $Y < X \leq Q$, $T = 1$, $E = 1$. The best outcome is the situation (iii') when efficacy is attained without toxicity. Between (iv') and (v') for which the patient experiences both efficacy and toxicity, (v') is preferable because efficacy is attained at a lower dose than toxicity. For (i') and (ii'), efficacy is not reached and the worst outcome is the situation (ii') where the patient experiences toxicity.

The methods compared in this paper share a common approach in the sense that they are based on the division of the plane into these five parts. In MULTIN, by Letierce et al. (2003), two tests on the multinomial repartition of the patients into the five parts are applied. An order of the parts has to be defined first, from the worst outcome, to the best. This is done in the following way: (ii') $\prec$ (i') $\prec$ (iv') $\prec$ (v') $\prec$ (iii'). Let us now renumber these ordered parts from category 1 to category 5. The authors justify the position of category 2, for which $E = 0$ and $T = 0$ by the fact that efficacy is the main aim in cancer trials. The two multinomial parameters $p_A = (p_{A1}, p_{A2}, \ldots, p_{A5})$ and $p_B = (p_{B1}, p_{B2}, \ldots, p_{B5})$ of the probabilities of the five categories for treatments A and B (with $\sum_{i=1}^{5} p_{A_i} = \sum_{i=1}^{5} p_{B_i} = 1$) are compared with likelihood ratio tests that were derived by Dykstra, Kochar, and Robertson (1995). The null hypothesis is $H_0 : p_A = p_B$ and two alternative one-sided hypotheses corresponding to two stochastic orderings are considered. The first alternative hypothesis is the likelihood ratio ordering [Dykstra, Kochar, and Robertson

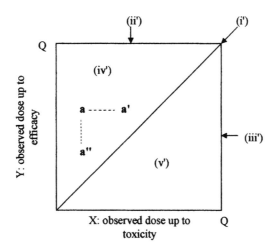

Figure 22.1: The five sets of points (X, Y) on the $Q \times Q$ square. Points $\mathbf{a}(X, Y)$, $\mathbf{a}'(X', Y)$, and $\mathbf{a}''(X, Y')$ illustrate the DISCR method. They satisfy $X' > X$ and $Y' < Y$

(1995)], denoted by LR, and the second is the stochastic ordering [Lehmann (1955)], denoted by ST. The superiority of p_A over p_B for the LR ordering is defined as the ratio p_{Ai}/p_{Bi} is nondecreasing in i, for i in $\{1, 2, \ldots, 5\}$. The superiority of p_A over p_B for the ST ordering is defined as follows: for all j in $\{1, \ldots, 4\}$, $\sum_{i=1}^{j} p_{A_i} \leq \sum_{i=1}^{j} p_{B_i}$ with $\sum_{i=1}^{5} p_{A_i} = \sum_{i=1}^{5} p_{B_i} = 1$. The computation of these tests requires the estimation of isotonic regressions and the calculation of coefficients involved in the asymptotic distribution of the test statistic under the null hypothesis. Indeed, the asymptotic distribution under H_0 is a mixture of chi-squared distributions, called a chi-bar squared distribution [Robertson, Wright, and Dykstra (1988)]. The authors performed a simulation study [Letierce *et al.* (2003)] to estimate the type I error rate and the power of the two tests, in comparison with the usual tests used to compare multinomial distributions (the Wilcoxon test and a scored t-test).

The method DISCR by Tubert-Bitter *et al.* (2005) consists of the construction of an "effectiveness region" in the plane of the observed values (X, Y) for each treatment A and B. This region is determined by a discrimination algorithm that allows us to separate points of two types with a monotone step function [Bloch and Silvermann (1997)]. The authors propose a statistic S that is a sum of two components. The first term is the proportion of efficacious outcomes for which there is no toxicity or for which toxicity occurs at a greater dose than efficacy, that is, points falling in parts (iii′) and (v′) (Figure 22.1). The second term of S concerns the other outcomes, belonging to parts (i′), (ii′), and (iv′) that form a set denoted D. For these points, there may be efficacy, but at a larger dose than toxicity. The algorithm is run on them to discriminate between outcomes for which $E = 1$ and outcomes for which $E = 0$ with an increasing function, with points $E = 1$ supposed to lie under the discriminant function, and points $E = 0$ supposed to lie above it. The monotonicity of the discrimination procedure is required to follow certain constraints: if a given point $\mathbf{a} = (X, Y)$, such as the one plotted in Figure 22.1, is included in the effectiveness region, any point $\mathbf{a}' = (X', Y)$ with $X' > X$ should also be included because it reflects a better outcome (the dose up to toxicity is larger for $\mathbf{a}'$ than for $\mathbf{a}$; i.e., the patient tolerates the treatment better). Similarly, any point $\mathbf{a}'' = (X, Y')$ with $Y' < Y$ should be included in the effectiveness region because efficacy occurs at a lower dose for $\mathbf{a}''$ than for $\mathbf{a}$. The second term of the statistic S is the proportion of efficacious outcomes in the set D, weighted by the area between the diagonal of the square and the discriminant function. The statistic S lies between 0 and 1, $S = 0$ if there is no efficacy, $S = 1$ if efficacy is attained for every patient, and it increases with the number of efficacious outcomes. The computations of the difference between the two groups A and B, S_A–S_B, and of the P-values of the test require us to compute the step monotone discrimination function and to run a bootstrap testing procedure [Efron and Tibshirani (1993)]. The authors showed in their simulation study that the type I error rate of their test was well controlled and that its power was greater than the power of the usual normal test used to compare proportions of efficacious outcomes.

22.3   Method for the Simulation Study

Couples (X^*, Y^*) of random variables were generated from a Clayton copula model with marginal Weibull distributions according to an algorithm based on the one proposed by Marshall and Olkin (1988). Copula models [Genest and Mac Kay (1986)] allow us to handle multivariate distributions by considering the marginal variables. Denoting by S_{X^*, Y^*} the bivariate survival function of X^* and Y^*, and by S_{X^*} and S_{Y^*} the marginal survival functions, a copula C satisfies:

$$S_{X^*, Y^*}(x, y) = C\left(S_{X^*}(x), S_{Y^*}(y)\right).$$

Some copulas C_α, called Archimedean copulas, are generated by a function φ_α satisfying some properties [Genest and Mac Kay (1986)] so that $C_\alpha(u, v) = \varphi_\alpha^{-1}(\varphi_\alpha(u) + \varphi_\alpha(v))$ for (u, v) in $[0, 1]$. α is an association parameter: the greater α is, the stronger is the association between X^* and Y^*. The Clayton copula is an Archimedean copula, for which $\varphi_\alpha(t) = t^{1-\alpha} - 1$ $(\alpha > 1)$ and $C_\alpha(u, v) = \left(u^{1-\alpha} + v^{1-\alpha} - 1\right)^{1/(1-\alpha)}$.

The algorithm by Marshall and Olkin was turned out to handle survival functions instead of distribution functions. It uses the relation

$$S_{X^*,Y^*}(x,y) = \int S_{X^*}(x)^w S_{Y^*}(y)^w dW(w); \qquad (22.1)$$

that is, S_{X^*,Y^*} is the Laplace transform $L(s) = E_W(\exp(-sw))$ of a variable W taken at the point $s = -\log(S_{X^*}) - \log(S_{Y^*})$.

In a Clayton model, the inverse function of φ_α, $\varphi_\alpha^{-1}(s) = (1+s)^{1/(1-\alpha)}$, is the Laplace transform L of a Gamma distribution with parameter $A = 1/(\alpha-1)$. Then, the procedure to generate a random couple (X^*, Y^*) involves the three following stages.

- Firstly, a variable W is generated from a $\Gamma(A,1)$ distribution, whose density function is defined by $f(w) = [1/\Gamma(A)]e^{-w}w^{A-1}$ for $w > 0$;

- Secondly, two independent random variables U and V are generated from the uniform distribution on $[0;1]$;

- And thirdly, U and V are transformed using W and the inverse functions $S_{X^*}^{-1}$ and $S_{Y^*}^{-1}$ of S_{X^*} and S_{Y^*}, to obtain the random variables X^* and Y^*.

Two-parameter Weibull variables $(\gamma_j, \beta_j)_{j=1,2}$, where γ_j is the scale and β_j is the shape of the distribution, were chosen for the marginal distributions because the Weibull model is flexible enough to describe different situations.

To obtain variables X and Y, a constant Q was fixed, representing the total dose of treatment received by the patient and planned in the protocol, assuming that it is the same for every patient. The observations were then $X = \min(X^*, Q)$, $Y = \min(Y^*, Q)$, and the binary variables $T = 0/1$ and $E = 0/1$ defined as previously. Independent realizations were generated and gathered to form two samples of equal size $n = 50$ and $n = 100$ figuring the treatment groups. Observations were classified into categories 1 to 5 to run the tests for the LR ordering and the ST ordering in MULTIN. The test statistic S in DISCR was calculated directly from the observations (X, Y, E, T).

Two values for α were explored: $\alpha = 2$ and $\alpha = 5$. The total dose Q was fixed at 0.8. Both β_1 and β_2 were fixed at 6; γ_1 and γ_2 were made variable so as to obtain different marginal percentages of efficacy and toxicity. Configurations with 80%, 65%, and 50% of efficacy and 20%, 35%, and 50% of toxicity were considered. Nine treatments were labelled by juxtaposing the percentage of efficacy "Exx" and the percentage of toxicity "Eyy" in the following: "$Exx\,Tyy$." Each configuration was generated 1000 times. The two tests of MULTIN were computed in SPlus and DISCR was computed in FORTRAN.

Tests were run for one-sided alternative hypotheses and with a nominal type I error equal to 0.05. Each treatment was compared to itself in order to estimate the type I error rate, and it was compared to each treatment having less or equal efficacy and more or equal toxicity (not equal at the same time). Another configuration in which there is a gain of at least 15% in efficacy and a loss in safety of 15% between treatments A and B was considered: the six following comparisons were performed, between $A = E80T35$ and $B = E65T20$ or $B = E50T20$, $A = E80T50$ and $B = E65T35$ or $B = E50T35$, $A = E65T35$, and $B = E50T20$ and $A = E65T50$ and $B = E50T35$ with the one-sided alternative hypothesis "A is better than B."

22.4 Results

The type I error estimates are reported in Table 22.1 for the two sizes of treatment group. For 1000 simulations, the 95% probability interval of the type I error rate is $[0.036; 0.064]$. Estimates for S are always in this interval, whatever the sample size and the value of the association parameter α. Estimates for the tests of MULTIN are less satisfactory, as LR has sometimes too high a type I error rate and ST is sometimes conservative.

Results for the power estimates are reported in Tables 22.2 and 22.3, respectively, for $n = 50$ and $n = 100$ patients in each group. As expected, a higher power is always observed for the greater sample size for all the tests. The power of the three tests is generally greater for $\alpha = 5$ than for $\alpha = 2$; there are only a few exceptions among the 33 comparisons run for each sample size, that rather happens for ST. When the difference between the two compared treatments only concerns toxicity, the power of DISCR is less than the power of MULTIN, and this is much more marked for a difference of 30% in toxicity, as the power estimates of the MULTIN tests are near 100%. This situation is caused by the fact that DISCR was constructed to compare efficacies, with a penalty for too-toxic treatments. When the difference between the two compared treatments only concerns efficacy, ST has a lower power than the other two tests, which have almost similar powers, for both sample sizes. For a given treatment Exx Tyy, the power for the comparison with treatments $Exx' Tyy'$ (in the list of compared treatments) always increases with the percentage of toxicity Tyy', for a given percentage of efficacy Exx'. For the extreme comparisons, that is, between treatments with very different percentages of efficacy and toxicity, the powers are excellent, near to 100%, even if the powers of the MULTIN tests rise more rapidly when the difference becomes more pronounced. Concerning the comparisons between a treatment $Exx Tyy$ and treatments $Exx' Tyy'$ with $xx' < xx$ and $yy' = yy - 15$, the powers are comparable for the three tests for each sample size and each value of α, but there is a slight superiority of the power of DISCR.

These results are consistent with what the authors found in their respective papers even though the simulations were not conducted in the same way. For

Table 22.1: Type I error rate estimates for $n = 50$ and $n = 100$ patients in each group, for the association parameter $\alpha = 2$ and $\alpha = 5$, obtained from 1000 simulations. LR and ST refer to the MULTIN tests for the likelihood ratio ordering and the stochastic ordering

	$\alpha = 2$			$\alpha = 5$		
	DISCR	LR	ST	DISCR	LR	ST
$n = 50$						
E80 T20	0.055	0.052	0.036	0.052	0.055	0.035
E80 T35	0.041	0.049	0.021	0.042	0.044	0.045
E80 T50	0.052	0.060	0.039	0.046	0.051	0.053
E65 T20	0.054	0.063	0.020	0.055	0.053	0.036
E65 T35	0.037	0.051	0.028	0.054	0.048	0.041
E65 T50	0.047	0.064	0.049	0.052	0.053	0.038
E50 T20	0.062	0.059	0.036	0.059	0.053	0.032
E50 T35	0.052	0.066	0.065	0.053	0.048	0.030
E50 T50	0.063	0.050	0.056	0.049	0.054	0.042
$n = 100$						
E80 T20	0.049	0.051	0.040	0.055	0.056	0.048
E80 T35	0.050	0.060	0.056	0.048	0.060	0.061
E80 T50	0.053	0.049	0.043	0.047	0.047	0.048
E65 T20	0.038	0.066	0.060	0.047	0.054	0.038
E65 T35	0.053	0.054	0.047	0.048	0.041	0.033
E65 T50	0.041	0.044	0.048	0.055	0.079	0.038
E50 T20	0.062	0.044	0.028	0.053	0.060	0.034
E50 T35	0.056	0.058	0.036	0.044	0.065	0.039
E50 T50	0.049	0.075	0.031	0.053	0.059	0.052

Table 22.2: Power estimates for the one-sided comparison of treatment A versus treatment B, with $n = 50$ patients in each group, based on 1000 simulations. See Table 22.1 for the column names

A	B	$\alpha = 2$			$\alpha = 5$		
		DISCR	LR	ST	DISCR	LR	ST
E80 T20	E80 T35	0.118	0.302	0.246	0.099	0.342	0.301
	E80 T50	0.153	0.801	0.794	0.121	0.849	0.875
	E65 T20	0.537	0.536	0.311	0.565	0.555	0.387
	E65 T35	0.696	0.844	0.621	0.717	0.894	0.764
	E65 T50	0.797	0.980	0.944	0.848	0.998	0.995
	E50 T20	0.941	0.939	0.805	0.968	0.971	0.885
	E50 T35	0.980	0.992	0.943	0.995	1	0.992
	E50 T50	0.986	0.999	0.994	0.999	1	1
E80 T35	E80 T50	0.076	0.283	0.238	0.077	0.329	0.343
	E65 T20	0.380	0.361	0.387	0.437	0.403	0.415
	E65 T35	0.553	0.541	0.326	0.600	0.603	0.431
	E65 T50	0.668	0.832	0.634	0.752	0.943	0.879
	E50 T20	0.885	0.890	0.850	0.930	0.914	0.847
	E50 T35	0.946	0.946	0.832	0.977	0.987	0.929
	E50 T50	0.970	0.994	0.959	0.996	1	0.997
E80 T50	E65 T35	0.451	0.392	0.396	0.496	0.441	0.412
	E65 T50	0.580	0.569	0.382	0.682	0.731	0.559
	E50 T35	0.923	0.910	0.864	0.967	0.956	0.880
	E50 T50	0.964	0.951	0.879	0.993	0.998	0.970
E65 T20	E65 T35	0.102	0.304	0.273	0.100	0.340	0.305
	E65 T50	0.182	0.725	0.812	0.201	0.876	0.905
	E50 T20	0.443	0.464	0.242	0.504	0.504	0.304
	E50 T35	0.605	0.784	0.590	0.700	0.898	0.785
	E50 T50	0.729	0.968	0.945	0.844	1	0.999
E65 T35	E65 T50	0.102	0.294	0.274	0.120	0.417	0.399
	E50 T20	0.304	0.290	0.397	0.386	0.342	0.331
	E50 T35	0.458	0.461	0.314	0.574	0.602	0.389
	E50 T50	0.586	0.774	0.636	0.759	0.969	0.891
E65 T50	E50 T35	0.333	0.295	0.366	0.387	0.344	0.301
	E50 T50	0.474	0.466	0.350	0.609	0.708	0.478
E50 T20	E50 T35	0.114	0.309	0.323	0.137	0.397	0.334
	E50 T50	0.204	0.741	0.862	0.295	0.936	0.933
E50 T35	E50 T50	0.107	0.281	0.307	0.137	0.463	0.407

Table 22.3: Power estimates for the one-sided comparison of treatment A versus treatment B, with $n = 100$ patients in each group, based on 1000 simulations. See Table 22.1 for the column names

A	B	$\alpha = 2$			$\alpha = 5$		
		DISCR	LR	ST	DISCR	LR	ST
E80 T20	E80 T35	0.125	0.520	0.525	0.121	0.508	0.574
	E80 T50	0.187	0.973	0.988	0.211	0.997	0.997
	E65 T20	0.806	0.774	0.581	0.817	0.809	0.649
	E65 T35	0.916	0.992	0.945	0.918	0.995	0.985
	E65 T50	0.971	1	1	0.980	1	1
	E50 T20	1	1	0.994	1	1	0.995
	E50 T35	0.999	1	1	1	1	1
	E50 T50	1	1	1	1	1	1
E80 T35	E80 T50	0.094	0.495	0.468	0.126	0.593	0.608
	E65 T20	0.627	0.645	0.748	0.681	0.674	0.738
	E65 T35	0.810	0.786	0.612	0.861	0.869	0.718
	E65 T50	0.902	0.984	0.954	0.951	0.996	0.996
	E50 T20	0.993	0.996	0.996	1	0.997	0.990
	E50 T35	0.999	0.998	0.991	1	1	0.999
	E50 T50	0.999	1	1	1	1	1
E80 T50	E65 T35	0.694	0.620	0.688	0.724	0.677	0.639
	E65 T50	0.837	0.816	0.712	0.882	0.923	0.802
	E50 T35	0.997	0.994	0.991	0.998	0.999	0.995
	E50 T50	0.999	0.999	0.996	1	1	1
E65 T20	E65 T35	0.126	0.467	0.576	0.120	0.576	0.639
	E65 T50	0.251	0.950	0.985	0.307	0.994	0.996
	E50 T20	0.683	0.669	0.506	0.759	0.759	0.557
	E50 T35	0.869	0.966	0.919	0.922	0.997	0.981
	E50 T50	0.945	1	0.999	0.982	1	1
E65 T35	E65 T50	0.112	0.425	0.481	0.146	0.668	0.649
	E50 T20	0.488	0.491	0.697	0.565	0.575	0.641
	E50 T35	0.707	0.697	0.546	0.829	0.883	0.655
	E50 T50	0.838	0.970	0.929	0.948	1	0.998
E65 T50	E50 T35	0.519	0.506	0.633	0.639	0.578	0.563
	E50 T50	0.711	0.697	0.571	0.833	0.925	0.853
E50 T20	E50 T35	0.134	0.486	0.571	0.169	0.622	0.654
	E50 T50	0.281	0.959	0.993	0.413	0.999	0.999
E50 T35	E50 T50	0.136	0.439	0.494	0.200	0.724	0.770

MULTIN, the authors generated directly random multinomial variables for the frequencies of the categories, without considering any underlying distributions for the doses. For DISCR, the model for the random generation of the variables was a trivariate logistic distribution, as the total dose received by the patient was also considered as a random variable, instead of a fixed censoring as simulated in this paper.

22.5 Conclusion

The two compared methods MULTIN and DISCR both take into account the cumulative doses of treatment at which efficacy and toxicity occur. They are both completely nonparametric and they do not need to fix a priori thresholds for the differences of efficacy and toxicity as it is necessary for the other methods [Bloch, Lai, and Tubert-Bitter (2001) and Thall and Cheng (1999)]. They have been developed in the context of cancer trials where efficacy is the primary goal, as it is reflected in MULTIN by the order of category 2, and in DISCR by the definition of the statistic S itself. The simulation study shows different behaviours of these methods depending on whether the simulated difference between the two treatments concerns efficacy, toxicity, or both. It is caused by the definition of the statistic S that rather focuses on efficacy and treats toxicity as a nuisance effect (what it is exactly). Nevertheless, they have excellent powers to detect differences in all the clear-cut cases. In addition, these methods proved to perform better than the other classical methods used in their respective domains, that is, comparison of multinomial distributions for MULTIN and comparison of proportions for DISCR, so that the computational work they require, identical for both, seems to be worth the while. In conclusion, DISCR is not appropriate to compare treatments for which the difference only concerns toxicity but in other cases, the two methods are comparable to analyse treatments with binary endpoints and dose-related effects.

Concerning the two approaches, some points are worth mentioning. With MULTIN, it is possible to deal with more than one toxicity by creating one or more further categories. If one considers two toxicities T_1 and T_2 in a cancer trial, defined by binary variables, and one does not want to give more importance to one or another, the worst category would be $T_1 = 1$, $T_2 = 1$, $E = 0$, and additional categories would be defined from the occurrence of T_1, or T_2, or both, and eventually their sequence. With DISCR, it does not seem possible to handle two toxicities without choosing one or both to define the variable X^*. A reasonable choice of X^* could be the dose up to the first toxicity, whatever the type. The same problem arises when many efficacious assessments have to be taken into account. Thanks to the great adaptability of the definition of the categories in MULTIN, the tests LR and ST can be applied whatever the binary variables, not necessarily antagonist outcomes, whereas for DISCR, variables X^* and Y^* have to reflect antagonist effects (X^* not desirable, Y^* highly desirable). For the two methods, when the two compared treatments do not involve the same drug, X^* and Y^* can be defined in a rank scale as opposed to a dose scale. Otherwise, an appropriate alternative is to express them in terms of duration of the treatment that makes it possible to apply the methods to treatments composed of several drugs.

References

1. Bloch, D. A., Lai, T. L., and Tubert-Bitter, P. (2001). One-sided tests in clinical trials with multiple endpoints, *Biometrics*, **57**, 1039–1047.

2. Bloch, D. A., and Silverman, B. W. (1997). Monotone discriminant functions and their applications in rhumatology, *Journal of the American Statistical Association*, **92**, 144–153.

3. Dykstra, R., Kochar, S., and Robertson, T. (1995). Inference for likelihood ratio ordering in the two-sample problem, *Journal of the American Statistical Association*, **90**, 1034–1040.

4. Efron, B., and Tibshirani, R. J. (1993). *An Introduction to the Bootstrap*, Chapman & Hall, San Francisco.

5. Genest, C., and Mac Kay, J. (1986). The joy of copulas: Bivariate distributions with uniform marginals, *The American Statistician*, **40**, 280–283.

6. Jennison, C., and Turnbull, B. W. (1993). Group sequential tests for bivariate response: Interim analyses of clinical trials with both efficacy and safety endpoints, *Biometrics*, **49**, 741–752.

7. Lehmann, E. (1955). Ordered families of distributions, *Annals of Mathematical Statistics*, **26**, 399–404.

8. Letierce, A., Tubert-Bitter, P., Maccario, J., and Kramar, A. (2003). Two treatment comparison based on joint toxicity and efficacy ordered alternatives in cancer trials, *Statistics in Medicine*, **22**, 859–868.

9. Marshall, A. W., and Olkin, I. (1988). Families of multivariate distributions, *Journal of the American Statistical Association*, **83**, 834–841.

10. Robertson, T., Wright, F. T., and Dykstra, R. L. (1988). *Order-Restricted Statistical Inferences*, John Wiley & Sons, New York.

11. Thall, P., and Cheng, S.-C. (1999). Treatment comparisons based on two-dimensional safety and efficacy alternatives in oncology trials, *Biometrics*, **55**, 746–753.

12. Tubert-Bitter, P., Bloch, D. A., Letierce, A., and Kramar, A. (2005). A nonparametric comparison of the effectiveness of treatments: A multivariate toxicity-penalized approach, *Journal of Biopharmaceutical Statistics*, **15**, 129-142.

23

Safety Assessment in Pilot Studies When Zero Events Are Observed

Rickey E. Carter and Robert F. Woolson

Medical University of South Carolina, Charleston, SC, USA

Abstract: Pilot studies in clinical research settings frequently focus on estimating the frequency of occurrence of certain adverse events. When zero such events are observed, the question of legitimate inference on the true event rate arises. The relationship between binomial and geometric distributions' confidence intervals yields two useful graphical displays and interpretations for the event rate inference in this circumstance. The interval is also closely related to the Bayesian credible interval when the prior distribution for the event rate is uniform. In addition, the simple algebraic expression for the confidence bound is seen to be useful in the context of planning studies.

Keywords and phrases: Bayesian credible interval, binomial distribution, geometric distribution, confidence interval, pilot study

23.1 Introduction

Statisticians collaborating in clinical research settings often assist in the planning and analysis of pilot studies. Although pilot studies may vary in the fundamental objectives, many are designed to explore the safety profile of a drug or a procedure [Spilker (1991) and Friedman, Furberg, and DeMets (1998)]. Often before applying a new therapy to large groups of patients, a small non-comparative study is used to estimate the safety profile of the therapy using relatively few patients. This type of investigation is typically encountered in the authors' experiences as collaborating biostatisticians at our General Clinical Research Center, and to a more limited extent, through our NIDA Clinical Trial Network Regional Research Training Center.

In these settings, a relatively common interest is in deriving knowledge from a pilot investigation in which there are no occurrences of the adverse event under study. This is often the case because initial pilot studies will typically focus on rather major categories of adverse events such as death, respiratory failure, major hemorrhage, and so forth. For example, if a synthetic heparin-like product is under investigation for its ability to prevent occlusion of the arteries, then a major adverse event to be monitored would be major hemorrhage. If initial studies fail to rule out a high probability of major hemorrhagic events, then the product, at that dose regimen, likely will not proceed further to more intensive study. On the other hand, if no hemorrhages are observed in the pilot, how optimistic can one be about the true hemorrhage rate?

Louis (1981) describes a similar clinical setting in the context of diagnostic testing. He notes that many diagnostic tests have relatively small false negative rates (i.e., the likelihood a diseased person will test negative for the disease), and when studying the test among only a few diseased persons, the study may yield zero negative test results. He cautions that this sample result may generate a false sense of optimism for the actual false negative rate. Accordingly, confidence intervals should be reported to reflect the uncertainty accompanying the findings. Of course, a major ingredient in the calculations is the sample size, n, upon which the observation of zero false negatives is made.

In this chapter, we focus on a somewhat different, but related, context. In particular, we utilize the pilot clinical study as our motivation, and examine the inferences (primarily via confidence intervals) that one can make in the setting when no events are observed. We consider three apparently distinct approaches, but as it turns out, all three approaches are mathematically related under the realization of zero events. Interesting reminders of relationships between some basic distributions emerge. The development includes graphical representation of one-sided confidence intervals, which may be useful to clinical researchers and to biostatisticians collaborating in such clinical research settings. Finally, it is noted that one rather simple algebraic expression underlies the resulting inference, and this expression arises from several different viewpoints.

23.2   Clinical Setting

When a novel therapeutic intervention is in development, a pilot clinical study in humans is typically undertaken. In many settings, these pilot studies may be in the formal clinical trial context of phase I and phase II trials, and in others, it may be to explore the intervention in a more limited way [Spilker (1991)].

For many such circumstances there is a specific adverse event that is defined to be critical in determining whether the treatment regimen moves forward for additional testing. If the treatment regimen results in an unacceptably high adverse event rate, then the treatment regimen might not be considered for additional testing. One of the major goals of an initial pilot study would be to estimate the adverse event rate that may result from the therapy.

To narrow the setting further, there are numerous clinical instances wherein the initial expectation is that the therapy has an extremely low chance of eliciting the particular adverse event, and the aim of the pilot study is to attempt to rule out the levels of adverse event rates that do not seem tenable on the basis of the resulting observations in the pilot study.

The situation of particular interest is then one in which no adverse events are realized in a pilot study, and inferences are to be made using this finding. As will be seen in the following sections, there are several statistical approaches applicable when a pilot study yields the finding of zero events, and in the context of confidence intervals, it will be seen that these findings have interpretations with important clinical points of view.

23.3   Notation

For ease of presentation, assume the pilot study will involve n independent patients for which the probability of the adverse event of interest is π, where $0 < \pi < 1$. In the next two sections, two designs are considered. The first is the typical binomial setting in which the number of patients is fixed in advance. The second is one in which the number of participants increases until the first adverse event of interest is observed. The second setting is, of course, the typical geometric distribution setting. In each case, a $100(1 - \alpha)\%$ confidence interval is to be generated for π.

23.4   Binomial Setting

One design common in pilot studies is to select n patients and observe the number of adverse events in this sample. Denote X as the number of patients sampled who experience the adverse event of interest. Then,

$$P(X = x) = \binom{n}{x} \pi^x (1 - \pi)^{n-x} , \qquad x = 0, 1, \ldots, n .$$

Denote π_u as the upper limit of the exact one-sided $100(1 - \alpha)\%$ confidence interval for the unknown proportion, π [Clopper and Pearson (1934)]. Then π_u is the value such that

$$\sum_{j=0}^{x} \binom{n}{j} \pi_u^j (1 - \pi_u)^{n-j} = \alpha . \tag{23.1}$$

When zero events are realized, Eq. (23.1) reduces to

$$(1 - \pi_u)^n = \alpha \ .$$

Accordingly, the upper limit of a one-sided $100(1 - \alpha)\%$ confidence interval for π is

$$\pi_u = 1 - \alpha^{1/n}. \tag{23.2}$$

The resulting $100(1 - \alpha)\%$ one-sided confidence interval is $(0, 1 - \alpha^{1/n})$. Graphically, one can represent this interval on a plot of π against n as illustrated in Figure 23.1 for $\alpha = 0.05, 0.10$, and 0.25. Values of π below $1 - \alpha^{1/n}$ represent the values of π consistent (at the $1 - \alpha$ level of confidence) with observing zero events. This display makes evident the point of clinical concern, viz., with smaller sample sizes a realization of no adverse events is consistent with many potential rates. Some rates may be high enough to be of concern before proceeding to the next stages of clinical investigation.

In a similar manner, one can look at the values of π above $1 - \alpha^{1/n}$ in the graph. Schoenfeld (1980) discussed statistical inference for pilot studies and argued that many clinical researchers design pilot studies asking, "What values of π have at least a $(1 - \alpha)$ chance of generating at least one adverse event?" By reflecting on this question a moment and on the preceding confidence interval development, it can be seen that the area in the graph above $1 - \alpha^{1/n}$ would correspond to the values of π with the chance less than or equal to α of generating zero events; therefore, they are the values of π with probability of $1 - \alpha$ or more of seeing at least one adverse event. Hence, this single graph has an important clinical interpretation from both perspectives.

23.5   Geometric Setting

Another reasonable approach to designing a pilot study in this environment is to sample patients until the first adverse event is realized, and in this way it is the number of patients studied that is the random variable. Denoting Y as the number of patients studied until the first adverse event, then following the usual geometric distribution, we have

$$P(Y = y) = \pi(1 - \pi)^{y-1} \ ; \qquad y = 1, 2, \ldots \ .$$

Now in the context of observing no adverse events, suppose n trials were conducted sequentially and no adverse events were observed. Hence, if one abruptly stopped at this point, one can conclude that $n + 1$ or more trials are required to observe the first adverse event. Accordingly, what values of π correspond to a $100(1 - \alpha)\%$ confidence interval?

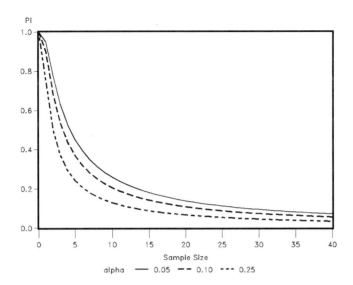

Figure 23.1: Upper limit of the $100(1 - \alpha)\%$ one-sided confidence interval for the true underlying adverse event rate, π, for increasing sample sizes when zero events of interests are observed

In this situation, the $100(1-\alpha)\%$ confidence interval will be the set of values of π that have greater than or equal to α chance of requiring $n + 1$ or more trials to get to the first adverse event. Putting this in probability terms, one has

$$P(Y \geq n+1) = \sum_{y=n+1}^{\infty} \pi(1 - \pi)^{y-1} ,$$

or, in terms of α

$$\sum_{y=n+1}^{\infty} \pi(1 - \pi)^{y-1} \geq \alpha . \qquad (23.3)$$

The preceding expression can be evaluated for each n; however, some algebraic work on the left-hand side of (23.3) yields

$$\begin{aligned}
\sum_{y=n+1}^{\infty} \pi(1 - \pi)^{y-1} &= (1 - \pi)^n \left[\sum_{j=1}^{\infty} \pi(1 - \pi)^{j-1} \right] \\
&= (1 - \pi)^n \cdot 1 \\
&= (1 - \pi)^n .
\end{aligned}$$

Accordingly, following (23.3) the upper limit of the $100(1 - \alpha)\%$ confidence interval for π is

$$\sum_{y=n+1}^{\infty} \pi_u (1 - \pi_u)^y = (1 - \pi_u)^n = \alpha ,$$

which yields

$$\pi_u = 1 - \alpha^{1/n} .$$

This is identical to (23.2); hence, the $100(1 - \alpha)\%$ confidence interval is the same with either formulation when zero adverse events are observed in the n trials.

23.6   Bayesian Credible Interval

A Bayesian approach to the statistical inference with zero events is particularly useful, even with a noninformative (i.e., uniform) prior is considered. One immediate advantage of considering a Bayesian approach is the incorporation of prior information into the estimation of π_u. In particular, the beta distribution describing the posterior distribution is

$$f(\pi|x) = \frac{\Gamma(n + a + b)}{\Gamma(x + a)\Gamma(n - x + b)}\pi^{x+a-1}(1 - \pi)^{n-x+b-1} . \qquad (23.4)$$

When zero events are observed, the $100(1 - \alpha)\%$ Bayesian credible interval for π using an uniform prior $(a = b = 1)$ is $(0, \pi_u)$, where π_u such that

$$1 - \alpha = \int_0^{\pi_u} \frac{\Gamma(n + 2)}{\Gamma(1)\Gamma(n + 1)}(1 - \pi)^n d\pi ,$$

or simply in terms of π_u,

$$\pi_u = 1 - \alpha^{1/(n+1)} .$$

Thus, utilizing a Bayesian approach to estimating the upper limit of the $100(1 - \alpha)\%$ confidence (or credible) interval reduces the upper limit by a factor of $(1 - \alpha^{1/(n+1)})/(1 - \alpha^{1/n})$. Louis (1981) presents this interval as $\pi_u = 1 - \alpha^{1/n}$, a result consistent with the Clopper–Pearson upper limit derived above; however, our calculations show the credible interval to be slightly different. In some pilot studies, reasonable estimates of the adverse event rate may be available, and incorporating this information in terms of a and b in Eq. (23.4) yields increased precision for estimating π, the unknown adverse event in the population under study.

Winkler, Smith, and Fryback (2002) and Thall and Simon (1994) have considered various prior distributions when utilizing Bayesian approaches to related problems. Indeed, one could argue that other values of a and b besides 1 would form a more appropriate prior distribution for π. When zero events are realized and terms are regrouped, Eq. (23.4) reduces to

$$f(\pi|x = 0) = \frac{\Gamma(a + (n + b))}{\Gamma(a)\Gamma(n + b)}\pi^{a-1}(1 - \pi)^{n+b-1} , \qquad (23.5)$$

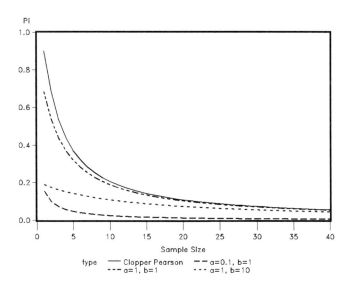

Figure 23.2: Comparisons of upper limit of a 90% Bayesian credible interval for values of a and b

which is beta$(a, n + b)$. Therefore, the upper limit, π_u, of the $(1 - \alpha)\%$ credible interval satisfying

$$1 - \alpha = \int_0^{\pi_u} \frac{\Gamma(a + (n + b))}{\Gamma(a)\Gamma(n + b)} \pi^{a-1} (1 - \pi)^{n+b-1}$$

can be easily obtained from the cumulative distribution of the beta distribution. Figure 23.2 illustrates the effect the selection of a and b have on the upper limit of the 90% Bayesian credible interval in relationship to the Clopper–Pearson interval. For small sample sizes, the effect of a and b is more dramatic. In particular, if $a = 1$ and $b = 10$, 90% of the prior beta distribution is concentrated below $p = .206$. Thus, a result of observing zero adverse events is highly consistent with this prior information and would lead to great efficiency in trial design. However, we caution that more conservative values of a and b, such as $a = b = 1$, should be considered in early phase testing in which limited prior information may be available.

23.7   Clinical Setting: Revisited

One of the major items prompting this work was interest in summarizing safety findings from noncomparative pilot studies in which no adverse events (of a specific type) are observed. As Louis (1981) observed, the clinical observation of zero false negatives in the context of diagnostic testing may generate unreasonable optimism regarding the rate, particularly for smaller sample sizes.

A similar situation does arise in pilot studies, wherein the number of patients studied is typically small and zero observed events may not be an uncommon result. From the perspective of the collaborating biostatistician, it is critical to be able to reflect the uncertainty in the findings, and in most instances offer guidance regarding the interpretation. As seen in the preceding sections, a unifying expression that emerges from the zero adverse events setting is

$$\pi = 1 - \alpha^{1/n} \, , \qquad (23.6)$$

and in this setting, this expression is interpretable as follows.

1. The upper limit of the $100(1 - \alpha)\%$ one-sided confidence interval for π
2. The lower limit for π such that all values of π above it have at least $(1-\alpha)$ probability of yielding 1 or more adverse events in n trials
3. The approximate upper limit of the $100(1-\alpha)\%$ one-sided Bayesian credible interval for π under a uniform $(0,1)$ prior distribution for π

Furthermore, one can consider using (23.6) in other clinically important manners. For instance, an investigator may be planning a pilot study and want to know how large it would need to be to infer with $100(1-\alpha)\%$ confidence that the true rate did not exceed a prespecified π, say π_0, given that zero adverse events were observed. Using (23.6), it follows that

$$n = \frac{\ln \alpha}{\ln(1 - \pi_0)}. \qquad (23.7)$$

Hence, the expression $1 - \alpha^{1/n}$ has a pivotal place in the statistical interpretation of clinical pilot studies in which zero adverse events are observed. It is an upper limit of a confidence interval, a Bayesian prediction interval, and can be easily inverted to address questions of sample size. To illustrate the expression's utility, consider the following example that originated as a part of routine collaboration.

Our Neonatal Intensive Care Unit often treats premature infant births with surfactant to stimulate lung tissue and prevent respiratory failure that could result in death. Once a vial of surfactant is opened, it must be stored in controlled conditions and discharged after 12 hours. Because regular administration of surfactant is delivered on 12 hour intervals, it would be desirable to extend the viability period beyond 12 hours. The question of interest is, "How long is a safe period for storage?" In this setting, in vitro examination of the drug could be used to identify drug samples that have become contaminated as a surrogate endpoint for infection in the premature infant, a likely adverse experience resulting from prolonged storage of the drug. It is desirable to rule out storage conditions not consistent with the general risk of infection, say $\pi_0 = 0.05$, before considering more conclusive testing or treatment of human subjects. Therefore, using Eq. (23.7), we would calculate that 45 vials would need to be contaminant free after a period of prolonged storage to be confident, at the $\alpha = 0.10$ level, that the prolonged storage conditions would be consistent with a contamination risk less than or equal to 0.05. This screening procedure could be replicated at more stringent significance levels to arrive at one or two viable storage conditions that would undergo additional study.

23.8 Summary

In clinical pilot studies, it is common to explore the adverse event profile of a new regimen. In this note, we illustrate how a simple expression has multiple useful clinical interpretations for the generation of confidence intervals when zero events are observed. Settings of fixed and variable sample sizes yield equivalent confidence interval inference in this specialized scenario. This has implications as a practical finding for the interpretation of clinical trial safety data, and offering clinicians advice on the range of adverse event rates that can be thought to be consistent with the observation of zero events. The presented formula offers more flexibility than the "rule of 3" approximation [Lewis (1981)] because it allows for the specification of significance levels other than $\alpha = 0.05$. The ability to choose the significance level might be important when designing or interpreting preliminary data obtained from a pilot study.

Acknowledgements. This work was partially supported by the National Institute of Health grants DA013727 and RR01070.

References

1. Clopper, C. J., and Pearson, E. S. (1934). The use of confidence or fiducial limits illustrated in the case of the binomial, *Biometrika*, **26**, 406–413.

2. Friedman, L. M., Furberg, C., and DeMets, D. L. (1998). *Fundamentals of Clinical Trials*, Springer-Verlag, New York.

3. Lewis, J. A. (1981). Cost-marketing surveillance – How many patients?, *Trends in Pharmacological Sciences*, **2**, 93–94.

4. Louis, T. A. (1981). Confidence intervals for a binomial parameter after observing no successes, *The American Statistician*, **35**, 154.

5. Schoenfeld, D. (1980). Statistical considerations for pilot studies, *International Journal of Radiation Oncology, Biology, Physics*, **6**, 371–374.

6. Spilker, B. (1991). *Guide to Clinical Trials*, Raven, New York.

7. Thall, P. F., and Simon, R. M. (1994). Practical Bayesian guidelines for phase IIB clinical trials, *Biometrics*, **50**, 337–349.

8. Winkler, R. L., Smith, J. E., and Fryback, D. G. (2002). The role of informative priors in zero-numerator problems: Being conservative versus being candid, *The American Statistician*, **56**, 1–4.

PART VII
Clinical Designs

An Assessment of Up-and-Down Designs and Associated Estimators in Phase I Trials

H. K. T. Ng,[1] **S. G. Mohanty,**[2] **and N. Balakrishnan**[2]

[1]*Southern Methodist University, Dallas, TX, USA*
[2]*McMaster University, Hamilton, ON, Canada*

Abstract: In this article, we consider some up-and-down designs that are discussed in Ivanova *et al.* (2003) for estimating the maximum tolerated dose (MTD) in phase I trials: the biased coin design, k-in-a-row rule, Narayana rule, and continual reassessment method (CRM). A large-scale Monte Carlo simulation study, which is substantially more extensive than Ivanova *et al.* (2003), is conducted to examine the performance of these five designs for different sample sizes and underlying dose–response curves. For the estimation of MTD, we propose a modified maximum likelihood estimator (MMLE) in addition to those in Ivanova *et al.* (2003). The selection of different dose–response curves and their parameters allows us to evaluate the robustness features of the designs as well as the performance of the estimators. The results obtained, in addition to revealing that the new estimator performs better than others in many situations, enable us to make recommendations on designs.

Keywords and phrases: Clinical trials, sequential adaptive designs, maximum tolerated dose, isotonic regression estimators, maximum likelihood estimator, robustness, Monte Carlo simulations

24.1 Introduction

In a phase I clinical trial, researchers study a new drug or treatment to determine a safe dose level for humans and also the highest dose that can be tolerated. The standard phase I design is a dose escalation trial in which successive patients are given successively higher doses of the treatment until some of the patients experience unacceptable side effects. In most phase I trials, the patients in the trial are assigned sequentially to various dose levels of a drug one at a time, starting at the lowest dose. If unacceptable side effects are not seen in the first patient, the next patient gets a higher dose. This continues until a dose level is reached that is too toxic, then the next patient gets a lower dose. The goal here is to estimate a dose, usually referred to as the maximum tolerated dose (MTD), which has a prescribed probability, Γ, of toxicity.

For ethical consideration so as to avoid patients being assigned to higher toxic dose levels and for possible improvement of efficiency in estimation by allowing more patients to be assigned to dose levels closer to MTD, it has been seen that up-and-down designs, being sequential and adaptive, are quite suitable.

Based on simulation results, Ivanova *et al.* (2003) have compared four up-and-down designs, viz., the biased coin design, k-in-a-row rule, Narayana rule, and continual reassessment method (CRM), by considering three estimators, viz., the empirical mean, isotonic regression estimator, and maximum likelihood estimator. For the purpose of simulation, they have used only logistic response models with different sets of parameters. In all three scenarios, the MTD is within the selected dose levels. In this chapter, we have carried out a very extensive examination of the same problem, by inclusion of a proposed modified maximum likelihood estimator (MMLE), by adding to the list of norms for comparison the mean squared error of the estimates of the probability at target dose (T-MSE) which is same as MTD [Stylianou *et al.* (2003)] and two more to the list of target doses (viz., $\Gamma = 0.15$ and 0.5), and by considering more response models, particularly ones such that the target dose is outside the selected dose levels for checking the robustness of a design. The MMLE proposed here is a modification of the MLE by means of isotonization and hence is expected to be an improvement over MLE; the simulation results do support this. In Section 24.2, we define the notation and the start-up rule that is used prior to the primary design and describe all designs. Section 24.3 is devoted to putting forth all estimators. The formulation for Monte Carlo simulation is dealt with in Section 24.4. The comparisons of estimators and the designs including conclusions are presented in Sections 24.5 and 24.6, respectively.

24.2 Notation and Designs

The following notation will be used throughout this paper.

K	Number of dose levels
N	Total number of subjects
μ	The maximum tolerated dose (MTD), the target dose
Y	1, 0 depending on whether the outcome is toxic
Γ	$\Pr(Y = 1\|\mu)$
$d_j, \; j = 1, 2, \ldots, K$	The set of ordered dose levels
$Y(n), \; n = 1, 2, \ldots, N$	Outcome for the nth subject (1 or 0)
$D(n), \; n = 1, 2, \ldots, N$	Dose assignment for the nth subject
$Q(d_j), \; j = 1, 2, \ldots, K$	$\Pr(Y = 1\|d_j)$, assumed to be a nondecreasing function of doses
$X_j(n)$	Number of toxic response at dose d_j including the nth patient
$N_j(n)$	Number of assignments to dose d_j including the nth patient
h	The maximum index such that $N_h(n) > 0$ $(h \le k)$

Let $\hat{Q}(d_j, n)$ denote $X_j(n)/N_j(n)$, which is an estimate of $Q(d_j)$ for $j = 1, \ldots, h$ in which the nth subject is included.

A start-up rule is used before the primary design to bring the starting point of the primary design closer to the target. The start-up rule proposed by Storer (1989), and modified by Korn *et al.* (1994), which is employed in Ivanova *et al.* (2003), is described below.

Start-up rule: Given Γ, let k be the closest integer solution of $\Gamma = 1 - 0.5^{1/k}$. Beginning at the lowest dose level, treat k subjects and go to the next higher dose level if no toxicity in the group is observed. Stop as soon as the first toxicity is observed, go to the next lower level and start the primary design. We note that $k = 1, 2, 3, 4$ for $\Gamma = 0.5, 0.2, 0.2, 0.15$, respectively, are the choices we have used.

In this study, the primary design is taken as one of the following five up-and-down designs. To describe the designs, let us assume that the nth subject is assigned to dose level $d_j, \; j = 1, \ldots, K$.

24.2.1   The biased coin design (BCD)

The biased coin design is a randomized design introduced by Durham and Flournoy (1994). For $\Gamma \le 0.5$, the biased coin design assigns the next subject to

(i) Dose level $\max(d_1, d_{j-1})$ if $Y(n) = 1$; that is, toxicity is observed in the previous subject;

(ii) Dose level $\min(d_K, d_{j+1})$ with probability $\Gamma/(1-\Gamma)$ and dose level d_j with probability $1 - [\Gamma/(1-\Gamma)]$, if $Y(n) = 0$.

24.2.2 The k-in-a-row rule (KROW)

The k-in-a-row design was introduced by Gezmu (1996) which can target any $\Gamma = 1 - (0.5)^{1/k}$, where k is a positive integer. The k-in-a-row rule assigns the next subject to

(i) Dose level $\max(d_1, d_{j-1})$ if $Y(n) = 1$;

(ii) Dose level $\min(d_K, d_{j+1})$ if $Y(n) = Y(n-1) = \cdots = Y(n-k+1) = 0$; that is, no toxicity is observed in the k most recent subjects receiving dose d_j;

(iii) Dose level d_j otherwise.

Note that selection of Γ is dependent on positive integer k.

24.2.3 The Narayana rule (NAR)

The Narayana rule was introduced by Narayana (1953) for $\Gamma = 0.5$. This has been modified in Ivanova *et al.* (2003) in order to consider any Γ. The Narayana rule assigns the next subject to

(i) Dose level $\max(d_1, d_{j-1})$ if $\hat{Q}(d_j, n) > \Gamma$ and if there is at least one toxicity among the k most recent responses on the current dose level;

(ii) Dose level $\min(d_K, d_{j+1})$ if $\hat{Q}(d_j, n) < \Gamma$ and if there are no toxicities among the k most recent responses on the current dose level;

(iii) Dose level d_j otherwise.

Note that the rule uses the information on Q through its estimate at every stage.

24.2.4 Continual reassessment method (CRM)

A Bayesian design for a phase I clinical trial, the continual reassessment method, was proposed by O'Quigley, Pepe, and Fisher (1990). The restricted CRM suggested by Faries (1994) and Korn *et al.* (1994) is to avoid a rapid escalation of the dose by prohibiting any skipping of a dose level. For a more comprehensive review on CRM, one may refer to Crowley (2001).

We choose a simple one-parameter dose–response model as the working model for the CRM

$$\Pr(Y = 1 | d_j, a) = \alpha_{d_j}^a,$$

where $(\alpha_1, \alpha_2, \alpha_3, \ldots, \alpha_{11}) = (0.05, 0.1, 0.15, 0.2, 0.25, 0.3, 0.35, 0.4, 0.45, 0.55, 0.7)$. This is the same as given in Ivanova *et al.* (2003).

The prior distribution of a is set to be $g(a) = \exp(-a)$, and is updated using the Bayes theorem as data become available. Assume that n patients have been assigned so far and the nth subject was allocated to level d_j, $j = 1, 2, \ldots, K$. After observing the response of the nth patient, we have the data $\Omega_n = \{(D(1), Y(1)), \ldots, (D(n), Y(n))\}$ and the likelihood function is

$$L_{\Omega_n}(a) = \prod_{j=1}^{n} [\Pr(Y = 1 | D(j), a)]^{Y(j)} [1 - \Pr(Y = 1 | D(j), a)]^{1-Y(j)}.$$

The posterior density of a given $L_{\Omega_n}(a)$ can be computed as

$$f(a | L_{\Omega_n}) = \frac{L_{\Omega_n}(a) g(a)}{\int_0^\infty L_{\Omega_n}(u) g(u) du},$$

and the posterior mean is

$$\hat{a}_n = E(a | \Omega_n) = \int_0^\infty a f(a | \Omega_n) da.$$

The dose–response probabilities can be updated as $\Pr(Y = 1 | d_j, \hat{a}_n)$. According to the restricted CRM, the $(n+1)$th patient is assigned to one of the dose levels d_i such that $|\Pr(Y = 1 | d_i, \hat{a}_n) - \Gamma|$, $i = j - 1, j, j + 1$, is minimized.

24.3 Estimation of Maximum Tolerated Dose

Several estimators of the MTD have been studied by Stylianou and Flournoy (2002) which are also considered in Ivanova *et al.* (2003). In this section, a review of these estimators will be given and a modified maximum likelihood estimator will be proposed. Note that if all the subjects are assigned to the start-up stage, then we will estimate μ by the highest dose without toxicity. This will be so for each estimator described below.

- The Empirical Mean Estimator (EME):
  A simple nonparametric estimator of μ is the mean of the dose assignments distribution, called the empirical mean estimator. It is given by [see, for example, Stylianou and Flournoy (2002)]

$$\hat{\mu}_1 = \frac{1}{N - r + 2} \sum_{i=r}^{N+1} D(i),$$

where r is the first subject in the design stage. Note that the $(N+1)$th dose assignment is included in the estimate.

- The Isotonic Regression Estimator (IS):
  Estimate $Q(d_j)$ by $\hat{Q}(d_j) = \hat{Q}(d_j, N) = X_j(N)/N_j(N)$ for $j = 1, \ldots, h$.

  Estimators based on isotonic regression [see Robertson *et al.* (1988)] can be used here. Because $\hat{Q}(d_1), \hat{Q}(d_2), \ldots, \hat{Q}(d_h)$ may not be isotonic, therefore, the pool adjacent violators algorithm (PAVA) [see Barlow *et al.* (1972)] is used to adjust $\hat{Q}$s to obtain $\hat{Q}^*(d_1) \le \hat{Q}^*(d_2) \le \cdots \le \hat{Q}^*(d_h)$. We can use linear interpolation to get the estimator

  $$\hat{\mu}_{2(linear)} = d_m + \frac{\Gamma - \hat{Q}^*(d_m)}{\hat{Q}^*(d_{m+1}) - \hat{Q}^*(d_m)}(d_{m+1} - d_m),$$

  or use logistic type interpolation to get the estimator

  $$\hat{\mu}_{2(logit)} = d_m + \frac{logit(\Gamma) - logit[\hat{Q}^*(d_m)]}{logit[\hat{Q}^*(d_{m+1})] - logit[\hat{Q}^*(d_m)]}(d_{m+1} - d_m),$$

  where $\hat{Q}^*(d_m) < \Gamma \le \hat{Q}^*(d_{m+1})$ and $logit(Z) = \log[Z/(1 - Z)]$.

  Based on linear interpolation, we propose the estimator (ISLIN) :

  $$\hat{\mu}_{2a} = \begin{cases} d_1, & \text{if } \Gamma < \hat{Q}^*(d_1), \\ d_h, & \text{if } \Gamma > \hat{Q}^*(d_h), \\ \hat{\mu}_{2(linear)}, & \text{otherwise.} \end{cases}$$

  Note that $\hat{\mu}_{2a}$ is equivalent to the modified isotonic estimator (MIE) discussed in Stylianou and Flournoy (2002).

  As the *logit* function is undefined when $\hat{Q}^*(d_m) = 0$ or $\hat{Q}^*(d_{m+1}) = 1$, we will use the following estimator (ISLOG):

  $$\hat{\mu}_{2b} = \begin{cases} d_1, & \text{if } \Gamma < \hat{Q}^*(d_1), \\ d_h, & \text{if } \Gamma > \hat{Q}^*(d_h), \\ \hat{\mu}_{2(linear)}, & \text{if } \hat{Q}^*(d_m) < \Gamma \le \hat{Q}^*(d_{m+1}), \ \hat{Q}^*(d_m) = 0 \\ & \quad \text{or } \hat{Q}^*(d_{m+1}) = 1, \\ \hat{\mu}_{2(logit)}, & \text{otherwise.} \end{cases}$$

- Maximum Likelihood Estimator (MLE):
  Consider the two-parameter logistic model for dose-toxicity function

  $$Q(d_j, a, b) = \frac{\exp(a + bd_j)}{1 + \exp(a + bd_j)}, \qquad j = 1, 2, \ldots, K.$$

  The data are augmented by adding two observations so that the fitted probability shrinks towards Γ by Clogg's correction [Clogg *et al.* (1991)].

The Clogg's correction ensures the existence of the MLE of a and b. We denote the resulting $\hat{Q}$s after Clogg's correction by $\hat{Q}_c(d_1), \hat{Q}_c(d_2), \ldots,$ $\hat{Q}_c(d_h)$. In other words, the MLEs of a and b are computed based on $\hat{Q}_c(d_1), \hat{Q}_c(d_2), \ldots, \hat{Q}_c(d_h)$. Then the MLE of μ is given by

$$\hat{\mu}_3 = \begin{cases} d_1 & \text{if } \hat{\mu}_3' < d_1, \\ d_K & \text{if } \hat{\mu}_3' > d_K, \\ \hat{\mu}_3' & \text{otherwise,} \end{cases}$$

where $\hat{\mu}_3' = \left(\log\left(\frac{\Gamma}{1-\Gamma}\right) - \hat{a}\right)\Big/ \hat{b}$.

- Modified Maximum Likelihood Estimator (MMLE):
  Here, because $\hat{Q}_c(d_1), \hat{Q}_c(d_2), \ldots, \hat{Q}_c(d_h)$ may not be isotonic, we suggest applying the PAVA before computing the MLE of a and b, that is, compute the MLE based on $\hat{Q}_c^*(d_1) \le \hat{Q}_c^*(d_2) \le \cdots \le \hat{Q}_c^*(d_h)$. The resulting MLEs are, say $\hat{a}^*$ and $\hat{b}^*$:

$$\hat{\mu}_4 = \begin{cases} d_1, & \text{if } \hat{\mu}_4' < d_1, \\ d_K, & \text{if } \hat{\mu}_4' > d_K, \\ \hat{\mu}_4', & \text{otherwise,} \end{cases}$$

where $\hat{\mu}_4' = \left(\log\left(\frac{\Gamma}{1-\Gamma}\right) - \hat{a}^*\right)\Big/ \hat{b}^*$.

24.4 Simulation Setting

For the simulation study, we consider the following dose–response curves by assuming the probability of toxicity at dose d_j is given by the relationship:

$$Q(d_j, a, b) = H(a + bd_j), \qquad j = 1, 2, \ldots, K,$$

where $H(\cdot)$ is a monotone function that is twice differentiable. The following models are used in the simulation study.

- Logistic:
$$H(x) = \frac{\exp(x)}{1 + \exp(x)}.$$

- Extreme-value:
$$H(x) = 1 - \exp\left[\exp(x)\right].$$

- Probit:
$$H(x) = \frac{1}{\sqrt{2\pi}} \int_{-\infty}^{x} \exp\left(-\frac{u^2}{2}\right) du.$$

- Generalized Logistic:

$$H(x) = \left[\frac{\exp(x)}{1 + \exp(x)}\right]^{\alpha}, \qquad \alpha > 0.$$

In the simulation study, we use [1] $a = -6.0, b = 1.0$, [2] $a = -4.5, b = 0.5$, [3] $a = -3.0, b = 0.5$, [4] $a = -6.0, b = 0.5$, [5] $a = -1.5, b = 0.25$, and $\alpha = 2.0$ for the generalized logistic curves. The choice of parameters in [1], [2], and [3] will place the target dose level within the selected range of dose levels, and those in [4] and [5] will, respectively, tend to shift them to the right and left within the selected range.

We consider the situation with $K = 11$ dose levels with $d_j = j$, $j = 1, 2, \ldots, 11$ and target toxicity $\Gamma = 0.15, 0.2, 0.3, 0.5$, giving rise to $k = 4, 3, 2, 1$, respectively. Different sample sizes ($N = 15, 25, 35$, and 50) are considered in the simulation study. In each scenario (crossover of dose–response curve, sample size, and target toxicity), we simulated $M = 10000$ samples in order to obtain the estimates for comparison.

It is important to mention here that for each configuration of the parameter (a, b), the four dose–response curves listed above provide a reasonable degree of variation (see Figures 24.1 to 24.5) thus allowing us to evaluate the performance of the designs and estimators under a more flexible response setting. Moreover, our selection of the three groups of the parameter (a, b) as described above help us to examine the robustness features.

24.5   Comparison of Estimators

We use the following criteria for comparison.

- Bias (BIAS) and Mean Squared Error (MSE):
  We compare the five estimators based on the bias and mean squared error which are computed as

$$\text{Bias} = \frac{1}{M}\sum_{i=1}^{M} \hat{\mu}^{(i)} - \mu, \qquad \text{MSE} = \frac{1}{M}\sum_{i=1}^{M}(\hat{\mu}^{(i)} - \mu)^2,$$

  where $\hat{\mu}_i, i = 1, \ldots, M$, are the resulting estimates of μ in each simulation.

- Bias (T-BIAS) and Mean Squared Error (T-MSE) of Probability of Toxicity at Target Dose:
  In a phase I trial, it is important to estimate the probability of toxicity at the target dose which is an estimate of Γ and see how close it is to Γ [see

Stylianou *et al.* (2003)]. Therefore, in addition to the previous criterion, we may use the following bias and mean squared error as measures,

$$\text{T-Bias} = \frac{1}{M} \sum_{i=1}^{M} \left[Q(\hat{\mu}^{(i)}, a, b) - \Gamma \right],$$

$$\text{T-MSE} = \frac{1}{M} \sum_{i=1}^{M} \left[Q(\hat{\mu}^{(i)}, a, b) - \Gamma \right]^2,$$

where $Q(\hat{\mu}^{(i)}, a, b)$ is the probability of toxicity at $\hat{\mu}^{(i)}$ based on the dose–response curve (assume that we know the underlying dose–response curve) in each simulation.

The average BIAS and MSE and the average T-Bias and T-MSE (averaged over the four dose–response curves given earlier) of each estimator for the five parameter configurations [1] to [5] are presented in Tables 24.1 to 24.8, respectively. These results are based on the BCD only. However, we are not presenting results for other designs, because they manifest similar patterns as far as the comparison of estimators is concerned.

From these results, we observe that the isotonic regression estimator based on the logistic interpolation is, in most cases, better than the one based on the linear interpolation. It is also observed that the MMLE is consistently better than the MLE. Moreover, in most cases, the MMLE has better performance than the other estimators in terms of MSE and T-MSE, whereas ISLOG performs better than the MMLE in some scenarios. In addition, our simulation results (not presented here) have revealed that the superiority of MMLE is maintained even when the underlying model is not logistic. Because of these observations, we will use ISLOG and MMLE for comparison of designs.

24.6   Comparison of Designs

We compare the five designs based on the measures described below.

- Mean Squared Error (MSE):
  Because of our observation in Section 24.5 that among the five estimators ISLOG and MMLE have better performance in general, we will use MSE of ISLOG and MMLE for comparison.

- Mean Squared Error of Probability of toxicity at target dose (T-MSE):
  Another natural measure by which the designs can be compared is T-MSE as it measures the closeness of Γ to the probability of toxicity evaluated from the dose–response curve. Hence, it is appropriate to consider T-MSE of ISLOG and MMLE.

- Average Squared Targeting Error (TE):
  The main aim of these designs is to assign most subjects to dose levels
  close to the target level. A measure for the closeness is the average squared
  targeting error as given by

$$\frac{1}{N-r+1}\sum_{i=r}^{N}[D(i)-\mu]^2,$$

  where r is the first subject in the design stage. We then take the average
  of these values over the simulation runs. If we do not go into the design
  stage (all subjects are in the start-up stage), this quantity will be set to
  0 and, therefore, will not be taken into account.

- Average Proportion of Toxic Responses (TOX):
  For ethical reasons, it is important to have as few toxic responses as
  possible. Thus, for comparison of designs, one may calculate average
  proportion of toxic responses as given by

$$\frac{1}{N-r+1}\sum_{i=r}^{N}Y(i),$$

  where r is the first subject in the design stage. We then take the average
  of these values over the simulation runs. If we do not go into the design
  stage (all subjects are in the start-up stage), this quantity will be set to
  0 and, therefore, will not be taken into account.

For the purpose of comparison, we divided the dose–response curves considered in the simulation study into three groups by the location of the true MTD:
(1) within the selected dose levels ([1] $a = -6.0, b = 1.0$; [2] $a = -4.5, b = 0.5$;
[3] $a = -3.0, b = 0.5$); (2) shifted to the right within the selected dose levels ([4]
$a = -6.0, b = 0.5$); and (3) shifted to the left within the selected dose levels ([5]
$a = -1.5, b = 0.25$). Because the BCD is the design most commonly referred to
in the literature, we calculate the ratio of a comparison measure of the BCD to
that of every other design, and use the average value of this ratio as an overall
measure. These values are presented in Tables 24.9 to 24.14. A value less than
1 means the BCD is a better design.

From Tables 24.9 to 24.12, we can see that for the group of dose–response
curves wherein the true MTD are within the selected dose levels, NAR is a
better design in terms of MSE and BCD is a better design in terms of T-MSE.
This additional information, which was not observed earlier, will be of interest
if T-MSE is of primary concern.

KROW performs better in most scenarios for the group of dose–response
curves wherein the true MTD are to the right of the selected dose levels and

BCD is better in most scenarios for the group of dose–response curves wherein the true MTD are on the left of the selected dose levels.

The purpose of an up-and-down design is to have trials close to μ. From this point of view, the efficacy of a design is reflected by comparison of TE (Table 24.13). We can see that CRM targets Γ better than the others, for $\Gamma = 0.15, 0.2$, and 0.3 except when $\Gamma = 0.3$ and the true MTD is shifted to the left within the selected dose levels. For $\Gamma = 0.5$, NAR performs better in most cases but CRM is comparable.

It is well known that the KROW and CRM tend to overdose patients. This can be seen from the measure TOX in Table 24.14. In terms of TOX, it is clear that BCD gives the lowest average proportion of toxic responses and the average proportion of toxic responses of NAR are higher than those of BCD but lower than those of KROW and CRM. In situations where avoiding overdose is the primary concern of the experimenter, for example, when patients who are treated at a dose level above the MTD are expected to have serious health problems or side effects, BCD will be the best choice for phase I trials even though it will suffer from a loss in efficiency in the estimation of MTD. But if avoiding overdose is not a predominant concern, we suggest the use of NAR because it performs well (based on the criteria considered) and has a relatively lower average proportion of toxic responses compared to other designs.

Overall, if we compare the designs from the estimation point of view, CRM outperforms the other designs in general for small values of Γ ($\Gamma = 0.15$ and 0.2). However, its performance becomes worse for larger values of Γ ($\Gamma = 0.3$ and 0.5) even though it has comparatively a higher average proportion of toxic responses in these cases. In these cases when $\Gamma = 0.3$ and 0.5, NAR is observed to be a better design to use. Thus, when one is particularly interested in the case of $\Gamma = 0.5$ (ED50, for example), it is observed that the CRM is undesirable on two counts: one, that the performance is poor in general under the different criteria considered and second, that it has a higher average proportion of toxic responses. In this case, NAR seems to be the best design to use on both grounds.

Finally, Γ and N will usually be known in advance and so the tables presented here can serve as a guideline for selecting a suitable design. For example, if $\Gamma = 0.15$ and $N = 35$, CRM should be used; if its toxicity measure is considered to be too high, NAR should be selected.

Our observation that CRM performs better but rapidly escalates assignment of subjects to highly toxic doses is in agreement with Ivanova *et al.* (2003). However, differing from their conclusion, we find KROW to be not as efficient as CRM or NAR.

An important point to keep in mind is that although the conclusions of Ivanova *et al.* (2003) are based only on the logistic model, our study is not model specific. In addition, we have included MMLE as an estimator and

T-MSE as a criterion for comparison of designs, and therefore have added strength to our conclusions for practical applications.

Acknowledgements. We would like to thank the two referees for their comments and suggestions which resulted in a much improved version of the manuscript.

Table 24.1: Bias and MSE of the estimators under biased-coin design with $N = 15$

	Estimator	$\Gamma = 0.15$		$\Gamma = 0.2$		$\Gamma = 0.3$		$\Gamma = 0.5$	
		Bias	MSE	Bias	MSE	Bias	MSE	Bias	MSE
[1]	EME	-1.148	1.807	-0.858	1.356	-0.528	0.988	-0.219	0.362
	ISLIN	-1.087	1.570	-0.576	0.786	-0.185	0.632	0.004	0.418
	ISLOG	-1.087	1.569	-0.575	0.783	-0.179	0.625	0.005	0.417
	MLE	-1.094	1.604	-0.584	0.902	-0.273	0.819	-0.101	0.393
	MMLE	-1.077	1.536	-0.546	0.747	-0.232	0.639	-0.119	0.380
[2]	EME	-2.907	9.550	-2.652	8.124	-1.686	4.712	-1.014	2.125
	ISLIN	-2.826	9.039	-2.460	7.082	-1.322	3.162	-0.366	1.272
	ISLOG	-2.825	9.032	-2.459	7.073	-1.319	3.146	-0.364	1.270
	MLE	-2.860	9.258	-2.534	7.630	-1.511	4.541	-0.318	1.619
	MMLE	-2.825	9.023	-2.458	7.098	-1.348	3.297	-0.348	1.365
[3]	EME	-0.841	1.667	-0.940	1.900	-0.381	0.552	-0.647	1.299
	ISLIN	-0.675	1.386	-0.593	1.391	-0.033	0.578	-0.098	1.190
	ISLOG	-0.668	1.377	-0.583	1.373	0.002	0.571	-0.097	1.189
	MLE	-0.718	1.430	-0.705	1.675	-0.101	0.451	-0.242	1.369
	MMLE	-0.648	1.320	-0.573	1.344	-0.082	0.407	-0.281	1.198
[4]	EME	-5.586	32.405	-5.198	28.095	-3.399	12.900	-2.336	6.543
	ISLIN	-5.562	32.122	-5.163	27.674	-3.292	11.899	-1.761	4.333
	ISLOG	-5.562	32.122	-5.163	27.673	-3.292	11.896	-1.760	4.332
	MLE	-5.575	32.282	-5.188	28.006	-3.350	12.763	-1.758	5.048
	MMLE	-5.563	32.128	-5.167	27.728	-3.278	11.837	-1.693	4.154
[5]	EME	0.960	1.914	-0.960	1.732	-0.684	1.410	-0.198	0.538
	ISLIN	0.931	1.705	-0.623	1.081	-0.275	0.914	0.068	0.955
	ISLOG	0.943	1.720	-0.620	1.073	-0.265	0.901	0.069	0.954
	MLE	0.983	1.866	-0.660	1.274	-0.401	1.256	-0.127	0.834
	MMLE	0.999	1.847	-0.588	1.030	-0.320	0.929	-0.106	0.731

EME: Empirical Mean Estimator, ISLIN: Isotonic Regression Estimator with Linear Interpolation, ISLIN: Isotonic Regression Estimator with Logistic Interpolation, MLE: Maximum Likelihood Estimator, MMLE: Modified Maximum Likelihood Estimator.

[1] $a = -6.0$, $b = 1.0$, [2] $a = -4.5$, $b = 0.5$, [3] $a = -3.0$, $b = 0.5$, [4] $a = -6.0$, $b = 0.5$, [5] $a = -1.5$, $b = 0.25$.

Table 24.2: Bias and MSE of the estimators under biased-coin design with $N = 25$

	Estimator	$\Gamma = 0.15$ Bias	MSE	$\Gamma = 0.2$ Bias	MSE	$\Gamma = 0.3$ Bias	MSE	$\Gamma = 0.5$ Bias	MSE
[1]	EME	-0.536	1.059	-0.477	0.815	-0.365	0.508	-0.123	0.182
	ISLIN	-0.196	0.657	-0.155	0.495	-0.064	0.343	0.010	0.249
	ISLOG	-0.188	0.647	-0.132	0.485	-0.032	0.338	0.011	0.247
	MLE	-0.182	0.742	-0.184	0.550	-0.158	0.322	-0.095	0.196
	MMLE	-0.139	0.597	-0.149	0.429	-0.152	0.293	-0.104	0.195
[2]	EME	-1.321	3.531	-1.193	3.353	-1.014	2.444	-0.649	0.964
	ISLIN	-1.002	2.415	-0.691	2.034	-0.339	1.336	-0.103	0.735
	ISLOG	-0.995	2.391	-0.677	2.001	-0.313	1.313	-0.102	0.734
	MLE	-1.095	3.029	-0.848	2.977	-0.515	2.016	-0.123	0.724
	MMLE	-0.978	2.387	-0.692	2.045	-0.445	1.440	-0.183	0.707
[3]	EME	-0.511	1.259	-0.606	1.294	-0.483	0.826	-0.380	0.661
	ISLIN	-0.192	1.076	-0.202	1.047	-0.041	0.780	0.047	0.876
	ISLOG	-0.165	1.063	-0.166	1.030	-0.005	0.772	0.047	0.874
	MLE	-0.255	1.216	-0.308	1.233	-0.155	0.681	-0.139	0.722
	MMLE	-0.135	1.002	-0.186	0.946	-0.129	0.592	-0.179	0.670
[4]	EME	-3.050	10.845	-2.155	6.602	-1.808	4.750	-1.953	4.519
	ISLIN	-2.924	9.835	-1.920	5.096	-1.186	2.636	-1.414	2.872
	ISLOG	-2.924	9.830	-1.918	5.084	-1.175	2.608	-1.413	2.870
	MLE	-2.969	10.383	-1.994	6.132	-1.268	3.942	-1.359	2.906
	MMLE	-2.917	9.820	-1.888	5.025	-1.152	2.675	-1.353	2.746
[5]	EME	1.009	1.918	-0.561	1.081	-0.457	0.753	-0.076	0.339
	ISLIN	0.896	1.549	-0.186	0.716	-0.073	0.545	0.085	0.746
	ISLOG	0.918	1.571	-0.157	0.701	-0.040	0.539	0.085	0.743
	MLE	0.967	1.793	-0.230	0.827	-0.167	0.533	-0.080	0.525
	MMLE	0.958	1.656	-0.164	0.632	-0.152	0.461	-0.066	0.481

EME: Empirical Mean Estimator, ISLIN: Isotonic Regression Estimator with Linear Interpolation, ISLIN: Isotonic Regression Estimator with Logistic Interpolation, MLE: Maximum Likelihood Estimator, MMLE: Modified Maximum Likelihood Estimator.

[1] $a = -6.0$, $b = 1.0$, [2] $a = -4.5$, $b = 0.5$, [3] $a = -3.0$, $b = 0.5$, [4] $a = -6.0$, $b = 0.5$, [5] $a = -1.5$, $b = 0.25$.

Table 24.3: Bias and MSE of the estimators under biased-coin design with $N = 35$

	Estimator	$\Gamma = 0.15$		$\Gamma = 0.2$		$\Gamma = 0.3$		$\Gamma = 0.5$	
		Bias	MSE	Bias	MSE	Bias	MSE	Bias	MSE
[1]	EME	-0.475	0.737	-0.414	0.555	-0.308	0.337	-0.089	0.121
	ISLIN	-0.161	0.429	-0.108	0.328	-0.059	0.234	0.005	0.170
	ISLOG	-0.124	0.419	-0.059	0.322	-0.016	0.230	0.006	0.167
	MLE	-0.131	0.455	-0.108	0.302	-0.118	0.197	-0.079	0.139
	MMLE	-0.095	0.350	-0.092	0.254	-0.115	0.188	-0.085	0.139
[2]	EME	-1.046	2.708	-0.931	2.279	-0.750	1.490	-0.515	0.624
	ISLIN	-0.547	1.641	-0.339	1.334	-0.088	0.908	-0.068	0.527
	ISLOG	-0.523	1.603	-0.300	1.303	-0.088	0.895	-0.067	0.524
	MLE	-0.657	2.344	-0.464	1.846	-0.264	1.041	-0.089	0.478
	MMLE	-0.508	1.581	-0.366	1.278	-0.255	0.864	-0.141	0.457
[3]	EME	-0.421	0.938	-0.486	0.945	-0.620	1.199	-0.264	0.429
	ISLIN	-0.106	0.854	-0.107	0.842	-0.113	0.977	0.046	0.660
	ISLOG	-0.059	0.846	-0.058	0.832	-0.081	0.966	0.046	0.656
	MLE	-0.143	0.899	-0.163	0.833	-0.265	1.049	-0.112	0.482
	MMLE	-0.044	0.742	-0.088	0.687	-0.209	0.839	-0.138	0.459
[4]	EME	-1.898	5.443	-1.531	4.093	-1.424	2.977	-1.852	4.019
	ISLIN	-1.604	3.926	-0.981	2.297	-0.704	1.293	-1.345	2.613
	ISLOG	-1.599	3.901	-0.965	2.259	-0.681	1.264	-1.344	2.611
	MLE	-1.706	5.057	-1.070	3.548	-0.691	1.666	-1.309	2.652
	MMLE	-1.578	3.872	-0.942	2.293	-0.681	1.345	-1.307	2.537
[5]	EME	1.030	1.899	-0.482	0.768	-0.375	0.504	-0.022	0.242
	ISLIN	0.868	1.446	-0.120	0.516	-0.052	0.394	0.069	0.566
	ISLOG	0.892	1.465	-0.071	0.506	-0.012	0.389	0.069	0.562
	MLE	0.949	1.710	-0.127	0.504	-0.116	0.328	-0.063	0.370
	MMLE	0.936	1.559	-0.092	0.413	-0.109	0.302	-0.049	0.348

EME: Empirical Mean Estimator, ISLIN: Isotonic Regression Estimator with Linear Interpolation, ISLIN: Isotonic Regression Estimator with Logistic Interpolation, MLE: Maximum Likelihood Estimator, MMLE: Modified Maximum Likelihood Estimator.

[1] $a = -6.0$, $b = 1.0$, [2] $a = -4.5$, $b = 0.5$, [3] $a = -3.0$, $b = 0.5$, [4] $a = -6.0$, $b = 0.5$, [5] $a = -1.5$, $b = 0.25$.

Table 24.4: Bias and MSE of the estimators under biased-coin design with $N = 50$

	Estimator	$\Gamma = 0.15$ Bias	$\Gamma = 0.15$ MSE	$\Gamma = 0.2$ Bias	$\Gamma = 0.2$ MSE	$\Gamma = 0.3$ Bias	$\Gamma = 0.3$ MSE	$\Gamma = 0.5$ Bias	$\Gamma = 0.5$ MSE
[1]	EME	-0.431	0.516	-0.374	0.383	-0.272	0.228	-0.064	0.081
	ISLIN	-0.130	0.285	-0.093	0.225	-0.058	0.154	0.002	0.115
	ISLOG	-0.068	0.276	-0.030	0.218	-0.010	0.150	0.003	0.111
	MLE	-0.068	0.253	-0.062	0.174	-0.084	0.126	-0.063	0.101
	MMLE	-0.048	0.209	-0.054	0.161	-0.080	0.122	-0.067	0.101
[2]	EME	-0.820	1.849	-0.733	1.477	-0.568	0.897	-0.429	0.430
	ISLIN	-0.280	1.104	-0.175	0.893	-0.065	0.635	-0.059	0.373
	ISLOG	-0.227	1.074	-0.123	0.875	-0.030	0.626	-0.059	0.369
	MLE	-0.338	1.425	-0.238	0.942	-0.162	0.570	-0.076	0.316
	MMLE	-0.245	0.978	-0.201	0.747	-0.168	0.526	-0.120	0.304
[3]	EME	-0.341	0.676	-0.409	0.665	-0.927	2.099	-0.190	0.286
	ISLIN	-0.070	0.679	-0.083	0.656	-0.448	1.434	0.023	0.479
	ISLOG	-0.011	0.675	-0.030	0.647	-0.433	1.412	0.022	0.475
	MLE	-0.063	0.623	-0.091	0.546	-0.654	2.043	-0.091	0.357
	MMLE	0.008	0.540	-0.044	0.481	-0.502	1.466	-0.109	0.344
[4]	EME	-1.264	3.269	-1.167	2.480	-1.216	2.059	-1.798	3.783
	ISLIN	-0.647	1.668	-0.474	1.073	-0.553	0.913	-1.309	2.508
	ISLOG	-0.616	1.625	-0.434	1.035	-0.529	0.892	-1.308	2.507
	MLE	-0.723	2.646	-0.498	1.495	-0.491	0.915	-1.289	2.547
	MMLE	-0.610	1.636	-0.463	1.055	-0.521	0.892	-1.289	2.476
[5]	EME	1.047	1.883	-0.416	0.521	-0.317	0.345	0.017	0.175
	ISLIN	0.840	1.364	-0.090	0.369	-0.054	0.276	0.045	0.431
	ISLOG	0.865	1.377	-0.031	0.360	-0.012	0.271	0.045	0.427
	MLE	0.926	1.610	-0.065	0.301	-0.078	0.216	-0.050	0.275
	MMLE	0.905	1.438	-0.045	0.267	-0.072	0.205	-0.038	0.264

EME: Empirical Mean Estimator, ISLIN: Isotonic Regression Estimator with Linear Interpolation, ISLIN: Isotonic Regression Estimator with Logistic Interpolation, MLE: Maximum Likelihood Estimator, MMLE: Modified Maximum Likelihood Estimator.

[1] $a = -6.0$, $b = 1.0$, [2] $a = -4.5$, $b = 0.5$, [3] $a = -3.0$, $b = 0.5$, [4] $a = -6.0$, $b = 0.5$, [5] $a = -1.5$, $b = 0.25$.

Table 24.5: T-Bias and T-MSE of the estimators under biased-coin design with $N = 15$

	Estimator	$\Gamma = 0.15$		$\Gamma = 0.2$		$\Gamma = 0.3$		$\Gamma = 0.5$	
		T-Bias	T-MSE	T-Bias	T-MSE	T-Bias	T-MSE	T-Bias	T-MSE
[1]	EME	-0.102	0.012	-0.099	0.016	-0.078	0.032	-0.060	0.027
	ISLIN	-0.100	0.012	-0.074	0.012	-0.013	0.030	0.000	0.030
	ISLOG	-0.100	0.012	-0.074	0.012	-0.012	0.030	0.001	0.030
	MLE	-0.101	0.012	-0.072	0.012	-0.027	0.030	-0.030	0.029
	MMLE	-0.100	0.012	-0.071	0.012	-0.025	0.029	-0.035	0.029
[2]	EME	-0.118	0.015	-0.150	0.024	-0.144	0.031	-0.137	0.038
	ISLIN	-0.117	0.015	-0.145	0.023	-0.122	0.025	-0.048	0.026
	ISLOG	-0.117	0.015	-0.145	0.023	-0.122	0.025	-0.047	0.026
	MLE	-0.118	0.015	-0.146	0.023	-0.129	0.027	-0.037	0.028
	MMLE	-0.117	0.015	-0.145	0.023	-0.124	0.025	-0.044	0.027
[3]	EME	-0.048	0.006	-0.066	0.010	-0.041	0.007	-0.091	0.026
	ISLIN	-0.039	0.006	-0.039	0.009	0.003	0.009	-0.012	0.024
	ISLOG	-0.039	0.006	-0.038	0.009	0.008	0.009	-0.012	0.024
	MLE	-0.042	0.005	-0.045	0.009	-0.006	0.007	-0.033	0.026
	MMLE	-0.038	0.005	-0.037	0.009	-0.004	0.006	-0.040	0.024
[4]	EME	-0.142	0.020	-0.187	0.035	-0.245	0.062	-0.299	0.099
	ISLIN	-0.141	0.020	-0.186	0.035	-0.243	0.061	-0.235	0.070
	ISLOG	-0.141	0.020	-0.186	0.035	-0.243	0.061	-0.235	0.070
	MLE	-0.141	0.020	-0.186	0.035	-0.243	0.061	-0.228	0.068
	MMLE	-0.141	0.020	-0.186	0.035	-0.243	0.061	-0.227	0.067
[5]	EME	0.098	0.018	-0.089	0.014	-0.083	0.027	-0.029	0.012
	ISLIN	0.094	0.017	-0.059	0.011	-0.023	0.025	0.010	0.020
	ISLOG	0.095	0.017	-0.059	0.011	-0.021	0.025	0.010	0.020
	MLE	0.100	0.019	-0.060	0.011	-0.037	0.026	-0.019	0.017
	MMLE	0.102	0.019	-0.056	0.011	-0.031	0.024	-0.016	0.016

EME: Empirical Mean Estimator, ISLIN: Isotonic Regression Estimator with Linear Interpolation, ISLIN: Isotonic Regression Estimator with Logistic Interpolation, MLE: Maximum Likelihood Estimator, MMLE: Modified Maximum Likelihood Estimator.

[1] $a = -6.0$, $b = 1.0$, [2] $a = -4.5$, $b = 0.5$, [3] $a = -3.0$, $b = 0.5$, [4] $a = -6.0$, $b = 0.5$, [5] $a = -1.5$, $b = 0.25$.

T-Bias: Bias of probability of toxicity at target dose; T-MSE: MSE of probability of toxicity at target dose.

Table 24.6: T-Bias and T-MSE of the estimators under biased-coin design with $N = 25$

	Estimator	$\Gamma = 0.15$		$\Gamma = 0.2$		$\Gamma = 0.3$		$\Gamma = 0.5$	
		T-Bias	T-MSE	T-Bias	T-MSE	T-Bias	T-MSE	T-Bias	T-MSE
[1]	EME	-0.033	0.014	-0.048	0.015	-0.063	0.019	-0.036	0.015
	ISLIN	0.005	0.015	-0.001	0.016	0.001	0.019	0.002	0.019
	ISLOG	0.006	0.015	0.003	0.016	0.009	0.020	0.002	0.019
	MLE	0.010	0.015	-0.006	0.014	-0.024	0.016	-0.029	0.016
	MMLE	0.012	0.015	-0.004	0.014	-0.024	0.015	-0.024	0.016
[2]	EME	-0.061	0.008	-0.068	0.014	-0.091	0.021	-0.092	0.019
	ISLIN	-0.050	0.007	-0.036	0.012	-0.023	0.017	-0.013	0.016
	ISLOG	-0.050	0.007	-0.035	0.012	-0.020	0.017	-0.013	0.016
	MLE	-0.051	0.007	-0.041	0.013	-0.037	0.018	-0.018	0.015
	MMLE	-0.049	0.007	-0.036	0.012	-0.035	0.017	-0.026	0.015
[3]	EME	-0.024	0.007	-0.041	0.009	-0.050	0.010	-0.055	0.014
	ISLIN	0.000	0.008	-0.003	0.010	0.005	0.013	0.006	0.018
	ISLOG	0.002	0.008	0.000	0.010	0.010	0.013	0.006	0.018
	MLE	-0.002	0.007	-0.011	0.010	-0.010	0.010	-0.021	0.015
	MMLE	0.004	0.007	-0.003	0.009	-0.008	0.009	-0.027	0.014
[4]	EME	-0.120	0.015	-0.128	0.019	-0.162	0.033	-0.265	0.078
	ISLIN	-0.118	0.015	-0.122	0.018	-0.114	0.023	-0.199	0.052
	ISLOG	-0.118	0.015	-0.122	0.018	-0.113	0.023	-0.198	0.052
	MLE	-0.118	0.015	-0.122	0.018	-0.111	0.024	-0.189	0.049
	MMLE	-0.118	0.015	-0.120	0.018	-0.109	0.023	-0.190	0.049
[5]	EME	0.102	0.018	-0.047	0.013	-0.062	0.017	-0.011	0.008
	ISLIN	0.088	0.014	-0.002	0.014	0.002	0.018	0.011	0.015
	ISLOG	0.090	0.015	0.002	0.014	0.008	0.018	0.011	0.015
	MLE	0.097	0.018	-0.006	0.013	-0.016	0.015	-0.013	0.011
	MMLE	0.095	0.016	-0.002	0.012	-0.015	0.014	-0.011	0.010

EME: Empirical Mean Estimator, ISLIN: Isotonic Regression Estimator with Linear Interpolation, ISLIN: Isotonic Regression Estimator with Logistic Interpolation, MLE: Maximum Likelihood Estimator, MMLE: Modified Maximum Likelihood Estimator.

[1] $a = -6.0$, $b = 1.0$, [2] $a = -4.5$, $b = 0.5$, [3] $a = -3.0$, $b = 0.5$, [4] $a = -6.0$, $b = 0.5$, [5] $a = -1.5, b = 0.25$.

T-Bias: Bias of probability of toxicity at target dose; T-MSE: MSE of probability of toxicity at target dose.

Table 24.7: T-Bias and T-MSE of the estimators under biased-coin design with $N = 35$

	Estimator	$\Gamma = 0.15$		$\Gamma = 0.2$		$\Gamma = 0.3$		$\Gamma = 0.5$	
		T-Bias	T-MSE	T-Bias	T-MSE	T-Bias	T-MSE	T-Bias	T-MSE
[1]	EME	-0.038	0.009	-0.049	0.011	-0.059	0.014	-0.026	0.010
	ISLIN	-0.001	0.010	-0.002	0.011	-0.003	0.014	0.001	0.014
	ISLOG	0.004	0.010	0.008	0.012	0.008	0.014	0.001	0.013
	MLE	0.003	0.009	-0.004	0.009	-0.020	0.011	-0.025	0.012
	MMLE	0.005	0.008	-0.003	0.009	-0.019	0.010	-0.027	0.012
[2]	EME	-0.047	0.008	-0.057	0.011	-0.072	0.015	-0.075	0.013
	ISLIN	-0.020	0.007	-0.012	0.011	-0.002	0.014	-0.009	0.012
	ISLOG	-0.019	0.007	-0.008	0.011	0.002	0.014	-0.009	0.012
	MLE	-0.022	0.007	-0.019	0.010	-0.019	0.013	-0.013	0.011
	MMLE	-0.018	0.007	-0.016	0.010	-0.020	0.012	-0.021	0.010
[3]	EME	-0.022	0.005	-0.034	0.007	-0.062	0.014	-0.039	0.009
	ISLIN	0.004	0.007	0.003	0.009	-0.001	0.015	0.006	0.014
	ISLOG	0.008	0.007	0.008	0.009	0.003	0.015	0.006	0.014
	MLE	0.002	0.006	-0.002	0.007	-0.018	0.013	-0.017	0.010
	MMLE	0.008	0.006	0.003	0.007	-0.015	0.012	-0.021	0.010
[4]	EME	-0.090	0.010	-0.096	0.014	-0.139	0.025	-0.256	0.073
	ISLIN	-0.082	0.009	-0.065	0.011	-0.073	0.014	-0.191	0.049
	ISLOG	-0.082	0.009	-0.064	0.011	-0.071	0.014	-0.191	0.048
	MLE	-0.083	0.009	-0.063	0.011	-0.066	0.015	-0.185	0.047
	MMLE	-0.081	0.009	-0.061	0.011	-0.068	0.014	-0.186	0.047
[5]	EME	0.103	0.018	-0.045	0.010	-0.055	0.012	-0.003	0.006
	ISLIN	0.083	0.013	0.001	0.011	0.002	0.014	0.009	0.012
	ISLOG	0.086	0.013	0.008	0.011	0.010	0.014	0.009	0.012
	MLE	0.094	0.017	-0.001	0.009	-0.012	0.010	-0.010	0.008
	MMLE	0.091	0.014	0.002	0.009	-0.011	0.010	-0.008	0.008

EME: Empirical Mean Estimator, ISLIN: Isotonic Regression Estimator with Linear Interpolation, ISLIN: Isotonic Regression Estimator with Logistic Interpolation, MLE: Maximum Likelihood Estimator, MMLE: Modified Maximum Likelihood Estimator.

[1] $a = -6.0$, $b = 1.0$, [2] $a = -4.5$, $b = 0.5$, [3] $a = -3.0$, $b = 0.5$, [4] $a = -6.0$, $b = 0.5$, [5] $a = -1.5, b = 0.25$.

T-Bias: Bias of probability of toxicity at target dose; T-MSE: MSE of probability of toxicity at target dose.

Table 24.8: T-Bias and T-MSE of the estimators under biased-coin design with $N = 50$

	Estimator	$\Gamma = 0.15$		$\Gamma = 0.2$		$\Gamma = 0.3$		$\Gamma = 0.5$	
		T-Bias	T-MSE	T-Bias	T-MSE	T-Bias	T-MSE	T-Bias	T-MSE
[1]	EME	-0.042	0.006	-0.051	0.008	-0.056	0.010	-0.020	0.007
	ISLIN	-0.005	0.006	-0.005	0.008	-0.007	0.009	0.000	0.010
	ISLOG	0.006	0.007	0.008	0.008	0.006	0.009	0.001	0.009
	MLE	0.003	0.005	-0.001	0.006	-0.014	0.007	-0.020	0.009
	MMLE	0.005	0.005	0.000	0.006	-0.014	0.007	-0.021	0.009
[2]	EME	-0.040	0.006	-0.049	0.008	-0.058	0.010	-0.063	0.009
	ISLIN	-0.005	0.006	-0.003	0.008	0.001	0.010	-0.008	0.009
	ISLOG	-0.001	0.006	0.003	0.008	0.005	0.010	-0.008	0.008
	MLE	-0.007	0.006	-0.009	0.007	-0.012	0.008	-0.012	0.007
	MMLE	-0.004	0.005	-0.007	0.006	-0.014	0.008	-0.018	0.007
[3]	EME	-0.019	0.004	-0.031	0.005	-0.087	0.021	-0.028	0.006
	ISLIN	0.004	0.005	0.002	0.007	-0.036	0.018	0.003	0.010
	ISLOG	0.009	0.006	0.008	0.007	-0.034	0.018	0.003	0.010
	MLE	0.005	0.004	0.001	0.005	-0.052	0.020	-0.014	0.008
	MMLE	0.010	0.004	0.004	0.005	-0.042	0.018	-0.017	0.007
[4]	EME	-0.061	0.007	-0.081	0.010	-0.127	0.021	-0.251	0.070
	ISLIN	-0.030	0.006	-0.031	0.007	-0.060	0.011	-0.187	0.047
	ISLOG	-0.028	0.006	-0.028	0.007	-0.057	0.011	-0.186	0.047
	MLE	-0.028	0.006	-0.029	0.007	-0.051	0.011	-0.183	0.046
	MMLE	-0.027	0.006	-0.030	0.007	-0.055	0.011	-0.184	0.046
[5]	EME	0.105	0.018	-0.044	0.007	-0.049	0.009	0.003	0.004
	ISLIN	0.079	0.012	0.000	0.008	-0.002	0.009	0.006	0.009
	ISLOG	0.082	0.012	0.008	0.008	0.006	0.010	0.006	0.009
	MLE	0.090	0.015	0.002	0.006	-0.008	0.007	-0.008	0.006
	MMLE	0.087	0.013	0.004	0.006	-0.007	0.007	-0.007	0.006

EME: Empirical Mean Estimator, ISLIN: Isotonic Regression Estimator with Linear Interpolation, ISLIN: Isotonic Regression Estimator with Logistic Interpolation, MLE: Maximum Likelihood Estimator, MMLE: Modified Maximum Likelihood Estimator.

[1] $a = -6.0$, $b = 1.0$, [2] $a = -4.5$, $b = 0.5$, [3] $a = -3.0$, $b = 0.5$, [4] $a = -6.0$, $b = 0.5$, [5] $a = -1.5, b = 0.25$.

T-Bias: Bias of probability of toxicity at target dose; T-MSE: MSE of probability of toxicity at target dose.

Table 24.9: Ratio of MSE for ISLOG to Biased coin design

Γ	Designs	Within Selected Dose Levels				Right of Selected Dose Levels				Left of Selected Dose Levels			
		N = 15	N = 25	N = 35	N = 50	N = 15	N = 25	N = 35	N = 50	N = 15	N = 25	N = 35	N = 50
0.15	KROW	1.15	0.88	0.81	0.98	1.03	1.44	1.95	1.78	0.54	0.61	0.72	0.80
	NAR	1.67	1.32	1.17	1.16	1.02	1.29	1.63	1.65	0.78	0.82	0.89	0.90
	CRM	1.03	1.18	1.37	1.46	0.97	0.80	1.85	1.87	0.80	1.00	1.06	1.06
0.2	KROW	1.32	0.96	1.03	1.17	1.06	1.97	2.04	1.57	0.53	0.63	0.78	0.87
	NAR	1.23	1.08	1.06	1.18	1.04	1.53	1.69	1.47	0.79	0.86	0.95	1.00
	CRM	1.28	1.25	1.37	1.42	1.18	1.26	1.91	1.47	1.02	1.11	1.26	1.41
0.3	KROW	1.33	0.96	1.03	1.10	1.17	2.11	1.55	1.28	0.65	0.75	0.89	0.93
	NAR	1.21	1.10	1.18	1.25	1.10	1.53	1.33	1.28	0.95	1.05	1.10	1.09
	CRM	1.18	1.10	1.17	1.16	0.78	1.70	1.01	0.86	0.99	1.15	1.35	1.55
0.5	KROW	1.01	1.00	1.00	1.02	1.01	0.98	1.00	0.99	0.99	0.99	0.99	1.00
	NAR	1.05	1.18	1.22	1.24	0.86	0.98	1.04	1.04	1.19	1.27	1.27	1.28
	CRM	0.72	0.73	0.72	0.67	1.15	0.78	0.72	0.69	0.89	0.99	1.04	0.94

KROW: k-in-a-row rule, NAR: Narayana rule, CRM: Continual Reassessment Model.

Table 24.10: Ratio of T-MSE for ISLOG to biased coin design

Γ	Designs	Within Selected Dose Levels				Right of Selected Dose Levels				Left of Selected Dose Levels			
		N = 15	N = 25	N = 35	N = 50	N = 15	N = 25	N = 35	N = 50	N = 15	N = 25	N = 35	N = 50
0.15	KROW	0.80	0.32	0.40	0.70	1.01	1.03	0.84	0.96	0.44	0.54	0.67	0.76
	NAR	0.68	0.81	0.74	0.87	1.01	1.05	0.91	1.00	0.72	0.78	0.86	0.87
	CRM	1.03	0.89	1.07	1.45	0.99	0.93	1.40	1.45	1.02	1.00	1.09	1.27
0.2	KROW	0.88	0.52	0.63	0.83	1.02	1.22	1.08	1.12	0.46	0.57	0.73	0.85
	NAR	0.95	0.70	0.80	1.01	1.01	1.17	1.10	1.13	0.74	0.82	0.92	0.99
	CRM	1.05	0.90	1.28	1.52	1.05	1.09	1.51	1.42	0.96	1.06	1.31	1.52
0.3	KROW	0.98	0.78	0.94	1.07	1.06	1.59	1.33	1.21	0.61	0.73	0.88	0.94
	NAR	1.02	0.97	1.11	1.19	1.03	1.31	1.22	1.21	0.94	1.04	1.09	1.08
	CRM	0.91	1.05	1.28	1.34	0.93	1.52	1.11	0.99	0.90	1.14	1.40	1.67
0.5	KROW	1.00	1.00	1.00	1.01	1.01	0.99	1.00	0.99	0.99	1.00	1.00	1.00
	NAR	1.05	1.15	1.19	1.21	0.87	0.99	1.04	1.04	1.16	1.22	1.23	1.24
	CRM	0.77	0.78	0.79	0.76	1.12	0.84	0.78	0.75	0.89	1.00	1.06	0.97

KROW: k-in-a-row rule, NAR: Narayana rule, CRM: Continual Reassessment Model.

Table 24.11: Ratio of MSE for MMLE to biased coin design

Γ	Designs	Within Selected Dose Levels				Right of Selected Dose Levels				Left of Selected Dose Levels			
		N = 15	N = 25	N = 35	N = 50	N = 15	N = 25	N = 35	N = 50	N = 15	N = 25	N = 35	N = 50
0.15	KROW	1.20	1.23	1.16	1.10	1.03	1.46	2.21	2.16	0.66	0.68	0.75	0.77
	NAR	2.31	1.69	1.42	1.26	1.01	1.30	1.74	1.84	0.87	0.88	0.93	0.92
	CRM	1.02	1.19	1.37	1.31	0.97	0.73	1.63	1.72	1.01	1.03	1.04	1.04
0.2	KROW	1.39	1.33	1.36	1.30	1.06	1.96	2.02	1.93	0.68	0.69	0.75	0.78
	NAR	1.29	1.28	1.24	1.24	1.03	1.54	1.71	1.57	0.88	0.90	0.95	0.97
	CRM	1.21	1.34	1.41	1.24	1.17	1.05	1.91	1.53	1.03	1.04	1.10	1.13
0.3	KROW	1.44	1.29	1.32	1.24	1.17	1.87	1.91	1.80	0.75	0.79	0.82	0.79
	NAR	1.26	1.21	1.22	1.17	1.11	1.53	1.47	1.36	0.95	0.98	0.99	0.95
	CRM	1.32	1.27	1.27	1.08	0.79	2.06	1.37	1.07	0.98	1.05	1.02	0.96
0.5	KROW	1.01	1.00	1.00	1.01	1.02	0.99	1.00	1.00	0.99	1.04	0.99	0.99
	NAR	1.00	0.99	1.02	1.05	0.86	0.94	1.03	1.07	0.93	0.91	0.90	0.90
	CRM	1.01	0.93	0.85	0.76	1.51	0.89	0.80	0.77	1.19	1.10	1.02	0.88

KROW: *k*-in-a-row rule, NAR: Narayana rule, CRM: Continual Reassessment Model.

Table 24.12: Ratio of T-MSE for MMLE to biased coin design

Γ	Designs	Within Selected Dose Levels				Right of Selected Dose Levels				Left of Selected Dose Levels			
		N = 15	N = 25	N = 35	N = 50	N = 15	N = 25	N = 35	N = 50	N = 15	N = 25	N = 35	N = 50
0.15	KROW	0.90	0.50	0.60	0.72	1.01	1.06	0.93	1.11	0.58	0.63	0.71	0.74
	NAR	0.93	1.15	0.90	0.91	1.00	1.06	0.98	1.09	0.83	0.86	0.93	0.91
	CRM	1.02	1.01	1.08	1.23	0.99	0.92	1.27	1.38	1.00	1.01	1.03	1.07
0.2	KROW	0.98	0.76	0.81	0.86	1.02	1.21	1.08	1.23	0.61	0.64	0.70	0.74
	NAR	1.02	0.89	0.95	1.04	1.01	1.16	1.12	1.14	0.84	0.88	0.93	0.95
	CRM	1.02	1.03	1.24	1.21	1.05	1.03	1.49	1.34	0.97	0.98	1.10	1.15
0.3	KROW	1.09	1.03	1.13	1.10	1.06	1.44	1.56	1.55	0.71	0.76	0.79	0.76
	NAR	1.06	1.05	1.10	1.08	1.03	1.28	1.30	1.24	0.93	0.96	0.98	0.94
	CRM	1.03	1.12	1.20	1.06	0.94	1.70	1.28	1.07	0.90	1.00	1.01	0.98
0.5	KROW	1.00	1.00	0.99	1.00	1.01	1.00	1.00	1.00	0.99	1.04	0.99	1.00
	NAR	1.01	0.98	1.00	1.03	0.89	0.95	1.03	1.07	0.93	0.91	0.90	0.89
	CRM	1.01	0.92	0.85	0.77	1.39	0.90	0.83	0.80	1.17	1.10	1.01	0.88

KROW: *k*-in-a-row rule, NAR: Narayana rule, CRM: Continual Reassessment Model.

Table 24.13: Ratio of TE to biased coin design

Γ	Designs	Within Selected Dose Levels				Right of Selected Dose Levels				Left of Selected Dose Levels			
		$N=15$	$N=25$	$N=35$	$N=50$	$N=15$	$N=25$	$N=35$	$N=50$	$N=15$	$N=25$	$N=35$	$N=50$
0.15	KROW	1.19	1.11	0.96	0.89	1.14	1.17	1.41	1.43	0.74	0.71	0.71	0.72
	NAR	1.07	1.09	1.06	1.10	1.07	1.09	1.21	1.29	0.93	0.95	1.00	1.06
	CRM	1.24	1.20	1.23	1.32	1.13	1.17	1.50	1.62	1.04	1.05	1.07	1.16
0.2	KROW	1.24	1.10	1.01	0.98	1.15	1.22	1.44	1.47	0.75	0.72	0.73	0.74
	NAR	1.11	1.12	1.14	1.20	1.06	1.11	1.24	1.33	0.97	1.02	1.08	1.15
	CRM	1.31	1.17	1.24	1.35	1.17	1.25	1.58	1.66	1.02	1.05	1.12	1.24
0.3	KROW	1.17	1.11	1.09	1.08	1.08	1.28	1.34	1.37	0.83	0.82	0.83	0.84
	NAR	1.10	1.14	1.19	1.26	1.04	1.15	1.21	1.29	1.01	1.09	1.16	1.24
	CRM	1.16	1.11	1.22	1.33	1.11	1.41	1.56	1.69	0.98	1.01	1.08	1.20
0.5	KROW	1.00	1.00	1.00	1.00	1.00	1.00	1.00	1.00	1.00	1.00	1.00	1.00
	NAR	1.04	1.11	1.19	1.27	0.97	1.05	1.11	1.18	1.07	1.16	1.22	1.29
	CRM	0.85	0.95	1.06	1.17	1.11	1.21	1.31	1.36	1.05	1.10	1.14	1.22

KROW: k-in-a-row rule, NAR: Narayana rule, CRM: Continual Reassessment Model.

Table 24.14: Ratio of TOX to biased coin design

Γ	Designs	Within Selected Dose Levels				Right of Selected Dose Levels				Left of Selected Dose Levels			
		$N=15$	$N=25$	$N=35$	$N=50$	$N=15$	$N=25$	$N=35$	$N=50$	$N=15$	$N=25$	$N=35$	$N=50$
0.15	KROW	0.32	0.52	0.46	0.47	0.34	0.29	0.32	0.51	0.79	0.76	0.76	0.76
	NAR	0.50	0.73	0.66	0.70	0.50	0.59	0.53	0.67	0.93	0.96	0.98	1.01
	CRM	0.46	0.61	0.66	0.77	0.65	0.49	0.41	0.74	0.93	0.94	0.96	1.01
0.2	KROW	0.43	0.57	0.55	0.55	0.41	0.50	0.59	0.62	0.79	0.77	0.77	0.78
	NAR	0.70	0.75	0.75	0.79	0.63	0.68	0.72	0.75	0.95	0.97	1.00	1.02
	CRM	0.45	0.60	0.69	0.79	0.53	0.52	0.68	0.76	0.86	0.89	0.94	0.99
0.3	KROW	0.76	0.71	0.72	0.73	0.80	0.75	0.78	0.81	0.83	0.83	0.84	0.84
	NAR	0.88	0.86	0.88	0.90	1.09	0.87	0.85	0.85	0.96	0.99	1.01	1.03
	CRM	0.64	0.64	0.74	0.81	1.11	0.75	0.76	0.79	0.82	0.85	0.89	0.94
0.5	KROW	1.00	1.00	1.00	1.00	0.99	1.00	1.00	1.00	1.00	1.00	1.00	1.00
	NAR	1.03	1.02	1.00	1.00	1.02	0.94	0.92	0.90	1.04	1.04	1.03	1.03
	CRM	0.68	0.76	0.81	0.86	0.89	0.86	0.86	0.86	0.81	0.85	0.88	0.91

KROW: k-in-a-row rule, NAR: Narayana rule, CRM: Continual Reassessment Model.

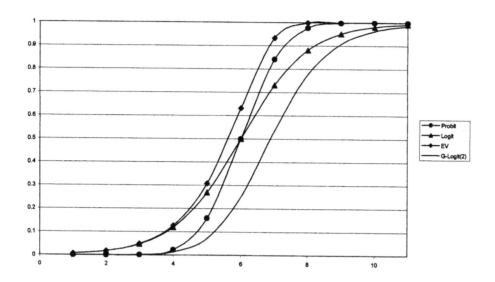

Figure 24.1: Dose–response curves with parameters $a = -6.0$, $b = 1.0$

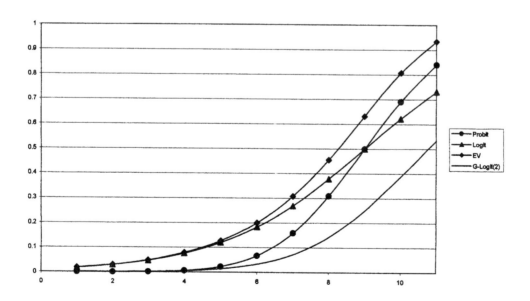

Figure 24.2: Dose–response curves with parameters $a = -4.5$, $b = 0.5$

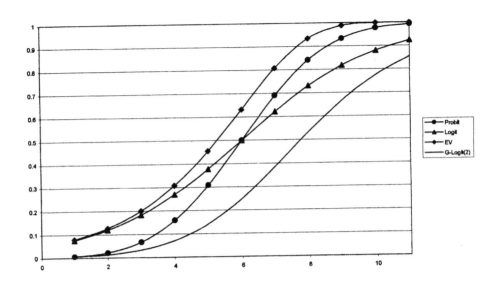

Figure 24.3: Dose–response curves with parameters $a = -3.0$, $b = 0.5$

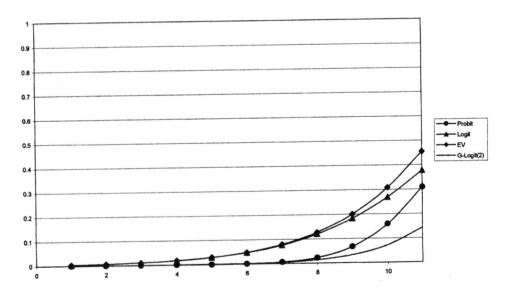

Figure 24.4: Dose–response curves with parameters $a = -6.0$, $b = 0.5$

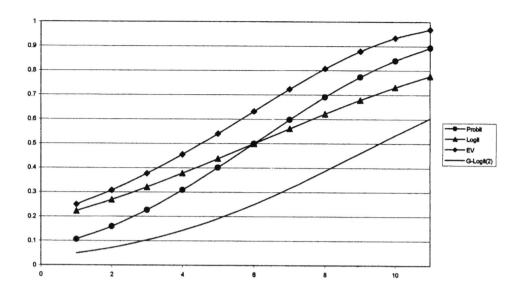

Figure 24.5: Dose–response curves with parameters $a = -1.5$, $b = 0.25$

References

1. Barlow, R. E., Bartholomew, D. J., Bremner, J. M., and Brunk, H. D. (1972). *Statistical Inference under Order Restrictions*, John Wiley & Sons, New York.

2. Clogg, C. C., Rubin, D. B., Schenker, N., Schultz, B., and Weidman, L. (1991). Multiple imputation of industry and occupation codes in census public-use samples using Bayesian logistic regression, *Journal of the American Statistical Association*, **86**, 68–78.

3. Crowley, J. (2001). *Handbook of Statistics in Clinical Oncology*, Marcel Dekker, New York.

4. Durham, S. D., and Flournoy, N. (1994). Random walks for quantile estimation, In *Statistical Decision Theory and Related Topics V* (Eds., S. S. Gupta and J. O. Berger), pp. 467–476, Springer-Verlag, New York.

5. Durham, S. D., and Flournoy, N. (1995). Up-and-down designs I. Stationary treatment distributions, In *Adaptive Designs* (Eds., N. Flournoy and W. F. Rosenberger), pp. 139–157, Institute of Mathematical Statistics, Hayward, California.

6. Durham, S. D., Flournoy, N., and Rosenberger, W. F. (1997). A random walk rule for phase I clinical trials, *Biometrics*, **53**, 745–760.

7. Faries, D. (1994). Practical modifications of the continual reassessment method for phase I cancer clinical trials. *Journal of Biopharmaceutical Statistics*, **4**, 147–164.

8. Gezmu, M. (1996). The geometric up-and-down design for allocating dosage levels, *Ph.D. Dissertation*, American University, Washington, DC.

9. Ivanova, A., Montazer-Haghighi, A., Mohanty, S. G., and Durham, S. D. (2003). Improved up-and-down designs for phase I trails, *Statistics in Medicine*, **22**, 69–82.

10. Korn, E. L., Midthune, D., Chen, T. T., Rubinstein, L. V., Christian, M. C., and Simon, R. M. (1994). A comparison of two phase I trial designs, *Statistics in Medicine*, **13**, 1799–1806.

11. Narayana, T. V. (1953). Sequential procedures in the probit analysis, *Ph.D. Dissertation*, University of North Carolina, Chapel Hill, NC.

12. O'Quigley, J., Pepe, M., and Fisher, L. (1990). Continual reassessment method: a practical design for phase I clinical trials in cancer, *Biometrics*, **46**, 33–48.

13. Robertson, T., Wright, F. T., and Dykstra, R. L. (1988). *Order Restricted Statistical Inference*, John Wiley & Sons, New York.

14. Storer, B. E. (1989). Design and analysis of phase I clinical trials, *Biometrics*, **45**, 925–937.

15. Stylianou, M., and Flournoy, N. (2002). Dose finding using the biased coin up-and-down design and isotonic regression, *Biometrics*, **58**, 171–177.

16. Stylianou, M., Proschan, M., and Flournoy, N. (2003). Estimating the probability of toxicity at the target dose following an up-and-down design, *Statistics in Medicine*, **22**, 535–543.

25

Design of Multicentre Clinical Trials with Random Enrolment

Vladimir V. Anisimov and Valerii V. Fedorov

GlaxoSmithKline, New Frontiers Science Park (South), Harlow, Essex, UK
GlaxoSmithKline, Upper Providence R&D Laboratory, RI, USA

Abstract: This chapter is devoted to the investigation of multicentre clinical trials with random enrolment, where the patients enter the centres at random according to doubly stochastic Poisson processes. We consider two-arm trials and use a random-effects model to describe treatment responses. The time needed to complete the trial (recruitment time) and the variance of the estimator of the Expected Combined Response to Treatment (ECRT) are investigated for different enrolment scenarios, and closed-form expressions and asymptotic formulae are derived. Possible delays in initiating centres and dropouts of patients are also taken into account. The developed results lead to rather simple approximate formulae which can be used to design a trial.

Keywords and phrases: Multicentre clinical trial, combined response to treatment, random enrolment, recruitment time, optimization

25.1 Introduction

A large clinical trial usually involves multiple centres. The analysis of multicentre clinical trials includes several key variables such as the recruitment time, the variance of the estimated ECRT, and the risk function, which includes possible costs for treatments, cost of enrolment, centre initiation, advertisement expenses, and so on, and potential revenue loss due to delay of the trial.

For the sake of simplicity, we consider the case with only two treatments. When treatments and centres are fixed effects, a combined response to treatment as the measure of the treatment effect difference was introduced in Dragalin *et al.* (2002). In Fedorov, Jones, and Rockhold (2002), this definition was extended to the case of the random-effects model for the treatment effects with a fixed number of patients per centre. Because at the design stage the number of patients that actually will be enrolled at each centre is not known and can be viewed as a random variable, these results were extended by Anisimov, Fedorov, and Jones (2003) to the case where the patients arrive at centres according to Poisson processes with fixed rates. However, with many centres (several hundred) and a large number of descriptors for these centres, it is expedient to model enrolment rates as a sample from some population. In this chapter, we extend the results of Anisimov, Fedorov, and Jones (2003) to the case when the patients arrive at different centres according to doubly stochastic Poisson processes with gamma or arbitrary distributed rates.

One problem in designing a multicentre trial can be formulated as follows: find the optimal numbers of centres and patients minimizing a risk function given the restrictions on the variance of the estimator of ECRT.

Assume that we plan to recruit in total n patients at N medical centres. Consider the following costs: C_i, the cost of initiating and running the ith centre; c_k, the cost of treating the kth patient; and R, the potential revenue loss per time unit due to the late market entering. Here, C_i and c_k are random variables with known expectations $C = E[C_i]$ and $c = E[c_k]$. Denote by $T_e(n, N)$ the recruitment time (the time needed to enrol all n patients at N centres) under some enrolment strategy e. The linear loss function can be defined as follows,

$$\mathcal{L}(n, N) = \sum_{i=1}^{N} C_i + \sum_{k=1}^{n} c_k + RT_e(n, N).$$

The risk function is

$$L(n, N) = \mathbf{E}[\mathcal{L}(n, N)] = CN + cn + R\,\mathbf{E}[T_e(n, N)]. \qquad (25.1)$$

If n_{ij} is the number of patients actually recruited in centre i on treatment j, then $n = \sum_{i,j} n_{ij}$. Let $\zeta^2(\{n_{ij}\})$ be the variance of the estimator of ECRT for the enrolment $\{n_{ij}\}$. At the design stage, we do not know the values n_{ij}. Assume that they are random and consider the averaged by distribution of $\{n_{ij}\}$ variance $\zeta^2(n, N) = \mathbf{E}[\zeta^2(\{n_{ij}\})]$ given n and N.

The simplest design optimization problem is: find the values n^* and N^* such that

$$\{n^*, N^*\} = \arg\min_{n,N} L(n, N) \quad \text{given that} \quad \zeta^2(n, N) \le v^2, \qquad (25.2)$$

where v is some specified small value.

Alternatively, we can consider the minimization of the risk function given the condition $\mathbf{P}(\zeta^2(\{n_{ij}\}) \le v^2)$, or the minimization of a certain quantile of a loss function $\mathbf{P}(\mathcal{L}(n, N) > L_*)$ given the restrictions on the variance of the estimator of the ECRT.

The solution of the optimization problem includes several stages. Firstly, we analyze the recruitment time which is one of the key decision variables at the planning stage of a multicentre trial. Secondly, we analyze the variance of the estimator of the ECRT under different enrolment scenarios and derive the first-order approximation formulae which are simple and intuitively transparent. Finally, we solve the optimization problem.

25.2   Recruitment Time Analysis

We assume that the patients arrive at centre i according to a doubly stochastic Poisson process [or Cox process; see Kovalenko, Kuznetsov, and Shurenkov (1996, p. 141)], with random rate λ_i, where λ_i are sampled from a population with a gamma or arbitrary distribution. In addition, there can be dropouts of patients and random delays in initiating the centres. At this stage, we study only the recruitment time and do not investigate different schemes for how the patients at each centre can be allocated to the treatments.

Consider the following three enrolment policies.

(1) A competitive policy means stopping when the total number of enrolled patients reaches a prescribed level n. In this case, the recruitment time $T_1(n, N)$ is called a *competitive* time.

(2) A balanced enrolment policy means waiting until the number of patients in every centre reaches some fixed value $n_0 = n/N$. The recruitment time $T_2(n, N)$ is called a *balanced* time.

(3) A restricted enrolment policy means that every centre has to enrol at least n_* patients and cannot enrol more than n^* patients, where n_* and n^* are given threshold levels. The recruitment time $T_3(n, N)$ in this case is called a *restricted* time.

Note that the balanced policy leads to trials with minimal variance of the estimator of the ECRT [Fedorov, Jones, and Rockhold (2002)], but the recruitment time in this case can be too large.

Let $n_i(t)$ be the number of recruited patients at centre i at time t and $n(t) = \sum_{i=1}^{N} n_i(t)$ be the total number of patients recruited at time t at all N centres.

If the rates λ_i are fixed, then $n_i(t)$ is a Poisson process with rate λ_i and $n(t)$ is a Poisson process with rate $\hat{\lambda} N$, where $\hat{\lambda} = \sum_{i=1}^{N} \lambda_i / N$. Denote by $Ga(\alpha, \beta)$ a random variable which has a gamma distribution with p.d.f. $p(x, \alpha, \beta) = e^{-\beta x} \beta^\alpha x^{\alpha-1} / \Gamma(\alpha)$, where α and β are the shape and rate parameters, respectively, and $\Gamma(\alpha)$ is a gamma function. $T_1(n, N)$ is the time of the nth event for the Poisson process $n(t)$ and it has a gamma distribution with parameters $\alpha = n$ and $\beta = \sum_i \lambda_i = \hat{\lambda} N$. Thus,

$$\bar{T}_1 = \mathbf{E}[T_1(n, N)] = n/\hat{\lambda} N, \quad S_1^2 = \mathbf{Var}[T_1(n, N)] = n/(\hat{\lambda} N)^2.$$

The result [Johnson, Kotz, and Balakrishnan (1994, p. 340)] on the normal approximation of a standardized gamma distribution implies that for any fixed N as $n \to \infty$, the variable $(T_1(n, N) - \bar{T}_1)/S_1$ converges in distribution to the standard normal random variable $\mathcal{N}(0, 1)$.

Consider now the case when the rates λ_i are sampled from a gamma distribution with parameters $(\alpha_\lambda, \beta_\lambda)$, and denote by $T_1 = T_1(n, N)$ a competitive time. Recalling that for a given collection $\{\lambda_i\}$ the time T_1 has a gamma distribution with parameters $\alpha = n$ and $\beta = \sum_i \lambda_i$, one may conclude that T_1 is gamma distributed with parameters $\alpha = n$ and $\beta = Ga(\alpha_\lambda N, \beta_\lambda)$, where the rate parameter is random. Integrating by the distribution of β, one may verify that T_1 has a Pearson Type VI distribution with p.d.f. [Johnson, Kotz, and Balakrishnan (1994, p. 381)]

$$p(x \mid n, N, \alpha_\lambda, \beta_\lambda) = \frac{1}{\boldsymbol{B}(n, \alpha_\lambda N)} \frac{x^{n-1} \beta_\lambda^{\alpha_\lambda N}}{(x + \beta_\lambda)^{n + \alpha_\lambda N}}, \quad x \geq 0, \qquad (25.3)$$

where $\boldsymbol{B}(i, a)$ is a beta function. From (25.3), we can conclude that for $\alpha_\lambda N > 2$,

$$\bar{T}_1 = \mathbf{E}[T_1] = \frac{\beta_\lambda n}{\alpha_\lambda N - 1}, \quad S_1^2 = \mathbf{Var}[T_1] = \frac{\beta_\lambda^2 n(n + \alpha_\lambda N - 1)}{(\alpha_\lambda N - 1)^2 (\alpha_\lambda N - 2)}. \qquad (25.4)$$

Consider the asymptotic properties of T_1. Denote convergence in probability by the symbol $\overset{\text{P}}{\longrightarrow}$. It is known [Johnson, Kotz, and Balakrishnan (1994, p. 17)] that the normal distribution is the limiting distribution for all Pearson types. Using the asymptotic properties of a gamma distribution, one can prove that as $n \to \infty$ and $N \to \infty$, $T_1/\bar{T}_1 \overset{\text{P}}{\longrightarrow} 1$, and the variable $(T_1 - \bar{T}_1)/S_1$ converges in distribution to $\mathcal{N}(0, 1)$.

The condition that both $N \to \infty$ and $n \to \infty$ is necessary and sufficient. Note that in the case of deterministic rates, we need only the condition $n \to \infty$; see Anisimov, Fedorov, and Jones (2003).

Limit theorems for doubly stochastic Poisson processes are studied by Snyder and Miller (1991). Note that our result does not follow from Theorem 7.2.2. of Snyder and Miller (1991) because, in our case, the value $\beta_\lambda n/\alpha_\lambda N$, which plays the role of t of Snyder and Miller (1991), may not tend to infinity.

Consider now a general case when the rates λ_i are sampled from a population with arbitrary distribution. In this case, the moment and distribution functions of T_1 in general cannot be calculated in closed form. Thus, we provide an asymptotic analysis. Assume that λ_i have finite second moments and denote $\mathbf{E}[\lambda_i] = \bar{\lambda}$, $\mathbf{Var}[\lambda_i] = \sigma^2$. Suppose that $\bar{\lambda} > 0$, $\sigma^2 \geq 0$.

Theorem 25.2.1 *If* $n \to \infty$ *and* $N \to \infty$, *then* $\bar{\lambda}NT_1/n \xrightarrow{P} 1$, *and the variable* $\alpha_{n,N}(T_1 - n/\bar{\lambda}N)$ *converges in distribution to* $\mathcal{N}(0,1)$, *where* $\alpha_{n,N} = \bar{\lambda}^2 N n^{-1}(\bar{\lambda}^2/n + \sigma^2/N)^{-1/2}$.

The proof is given in Appendix A.1. Note that this result includes in particular the cases when $\sigma^2 = 0$ (the rates are fixed) and when the rates have a gamma distribution.

The results of Theorem 25.2.1 can be extended to a practical case where there are r groups of centres of different types (quick or slow recruitment, for example). Assume that the kth group contains N_k centres and the recruitment rates for this group are sampled from a population with arbitrary distribution with mean $a_k \geq 0$ and variance $\sigma_k^2 \geq 0$. Let $N \to \infty$, $N_k/N \to g_k \geq 0$, $k = 1, \ldots, r$. Denote $\bar{\lambda} = \sum_{k=1}^{r} g_k a_k$, $\sigma^2 = \sum_{k=1}^{r} g_k \sigma_k^2$, $A_N = \sum_{k=1}^{r} a_k N_k$, and assume that $\bar{\lambda} > 0$, $\sigma^2 > 0$.

Theorem 25.2.2 *As* $n \to \infty$ *and* $N \to \infty$, $\bar{\lambda}NT_1/n \xrightarrow{P} 1$, *and the variable* $\alpha_{n,N}(T_1 - n/A_N)$ *converges in distribution to* $\mathcal{N}(0,1)$,

The proof follows along the same lines and is therefore omitted.

Consider now trials with delays and dropouts. Assume that λ_i satisfy conditions of Theorem 25.2.1. Suppose that each patient stays in the trial only with probability $p > 0$, and with probability $1 - p$ the patient leaves the trial. In addition, allow for a random delay τ_i in initiating centre i, where the variables τ_i are sampled from a population with mean $m \geq 0$ and variance $b^2 \geq 0$. For simplicity, let τ_i be bounded by some constant C_τ. Denote a competitive time as above by T_1. Set

$$M_{n,N} = m + n/(p\bar{\lambda}N), \qquad \beta_{n,N} = p\bar{\lambda}^2 N\sqrt{N}\Big/\sqrt{\sigma^2 n^2 + \bar{\lambda}^2 p^2 b^2 N^2 + \bar{\lambda}^2 nN}.$$

Theorem 25.2.3 *If* $n \to \infty$, $N \to \infty$, *and* $\lim M_{n,N} > C_\tau$, *then* $T_1/M_{n,N} \xrightarrow{P} 1$ *and* $\beta_{n,N}(T_1 - M_{n,N})$ *converges in distribution to* $\mathcal{N}(0,1)$.

The proof is given in Appendix A.2.

These results can be also extended to the case where there are different groups of centres.

The analysis of other enrolment characteristics such as the cumulative arrival process, the total cost of enrolment, and so on, can be provided as well. Consider, as an example, $n(t)$, the total number of patients enrolled at all centres up to time t. Suppose that the conditions of Theorem 25.2.1 (or Theorem 25.2.2) are satisfied. Assume for simplicity that there are no delays ($m = 0$) and dropouts appear with probability $1 - p$. Consider the normalized process $\gamma_N(t) = (n(t) - p\bar{\lambda}tN)/\sqrt{N}$, $t > 0$.

Lemma 25.2.1 *As $N \to \infty$, the process $\gamma_N(t)$ converges (in the sense of weak convergence in Skorokhod space) to the process $\gamma_0(t) = p\sigma\xi t + \sqrt{\bar{\lambda}p}\,w(t)$, where $w(t)$ is a standard Wiener process, $\mathbf{E}[w(t)] = 0$, $\mathbf{Var}[w(t)] = t$, ξ is independent of $w(t)$, and has a normal distribution with parameters $(0,1)$.*

The proof is given in Appendix A.3.

This implies that for modelling $n(t)$, we can use the approximation $n(t) \approx p\bar{\lambda}tN + \sqrt{N}\left(p\sigma t\,\xi + \sqrt{p\bar{\lambda}}\,w(t)\right)$.

Consider now a balanced time $T_2(n, N)$. Suppose first that the rates λ_i are fixed and $\lambda_i \equiv \lambda$. Let $t_k^{(i)}$ be the time of arrival of the kth patient at the ith centre. Then $t_k^{(i)}$ has a gamma distribution with parameters (k, λ), and for any $x > 0$,

$$\mathbf{P}(T_2(n, N) \le x) = \mathbf{P}(\max_{i=1,\dots,N} t_{n_0}^{(i)} \le x) = \mathbf{P}(Ga(n_0, \lambda) \le x)^N.$$

Consider the case when the rates λ_i are random and sampled from a gamma population with parameters $(\alpha_\lambda, \beta_\lambda)$. In this case, $t_k^{(i)}$ is a doubly stochastic random variable of the form $t_k^{(i)} = Ga(k, Ga(\alpha_\lambda, \beta_\lambda))$. Denote $\gamma(k, \alpha_\lambda, \beta_\lambda) = Ga(k, Ga(\alpha_\lambda, \beta_\lambda))$. Then for any $x > 0$,

$$\mathbf{P}(T_2(n, N) \le x) = \mathbf{P}(\max_{i=1,\dots,N} t_{n_0}^{(i)} \le x) = \mathbf{P}(\gamma(n_0, \alpha_\lambda, \beta_\lambda) \le x)^N, \qquad (25.5)$$

where $\gamma(n_0, \alpha_\lambda, \beta_\lambda)$ according to (25.3) has a Pearson Type VI distribution with p.d.f. $p(x) = x^{n_0-1}\beta_\lambda^{\alpha_\lambda}\boldsymbol{B}(n_0, \alpha_\lambda)^{-1}(x + \beta_\lambda)^{-(n+\alpha_\lambda)}$, $x \ge 0$.

Equation (25.5) can be written in a convenient form suitable for computation

$$\mathbf{P}(T_2(n, N) \le x) = \boldsymbol{I}\left(n_0, \alpha_\lambda, \frac{x}{\beta_\lambda + x}\right)^N, \qquad x > 0, \qquad (25.6)$$

where $\boldsymbol{I}(i, \alpha_\lambda, x) = \boldsymbol{B}(i, \alpha_\lambda, x)/\boldsymbol{B}(i, \alpha_\lambda)$, and $\boldsymbol{B}(i, \alpha_\lambda, x)$ is the incomplete beta function:

$$\boldsymbol{B}(i, \alpha_\lambda, x) = \int_0^x t^{i-1}(1 - t)^{\alpha_\lambda-1}dt, \qquad 0 \le x \le 1.$$

In fact, by definition, $\boldsymbol{I}(i, \alpha_\lambda, x)$ is a distribution function of a beta random variable $beta(i, \alpha_\lambda)$ with parameters (i, α_λ). Now we can use a representation [Johnson, Kotz, and Balakrishnan (1995, p. 248)]: $\gamma(i, \alpha_\lambda, \beta_\lambda) = \beta_\lambda beta(i, \alpha_\lambda)(1 - beta(i, \alpha_\lambda))^{-1}$, which implies (25.6).

Let us compare enrolment policies. Assume that $n_0 = n/N$ and $n_* < n_0 < n^*$. Then stochastically $T_1(n, N) < T_3(n, N) < T_2(n, N)$, which means, for any $t > 0$,

$$\mathbf{P}(T_1(n, N) > t) < \mathbf{P}(T_3(n, N) > t) < \mathbf{P}(T_2(n, N) > t), \qquad (25.7)$$

and $\mathbf{E}[T_1(n, N)] < \mathbf{E}[T_3(n, N)] < \mathbf{E}[T_2(n, N)]$, respectively. Numerical calculations show that a balanced time is essentially larger than a competitive time

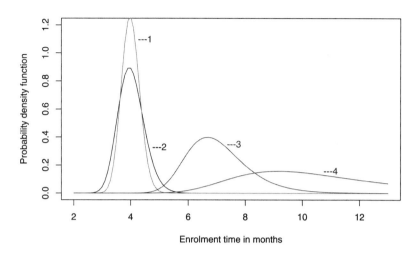

Figure 25.1: Comparison of recruitment times. $n = 160, N = 20$. Competitive time: **1** – fixed rates with $\lambda = 2$; **2** – gamma rates, $\mathbf{E}[\lambda] = 2, \mathbf{Var}[\lambda] = 0.5$. Balanced time: **3** – fixed rates with $\lambda = 2$; **4** – gamma rates, $\mathbf{E}[\lambda] = 2, \mathbf{Var}[\lambda] = 0.5$

and the variation in rates essentially inflates the recruitment time (see Figure 25.1).

For restricted recruitment time, we cannot write a closed-form solution, but it follows from (25.7) that in some sense the restricted time is somewhere between competitive and balanced times and it essentially depends on the threshold levels n_* and n^*.

25.3   Analysis of Variance of the Estimated ECRT

Consider a clinical trial in which n patients are enrolled at N centres. Denote by n_{ij} the number of patients on treatment j in centre i, $i = 1, 2, \ldots, N$; $j = 1, 2$. Let $n_i = n_{i1} + n_{i2}$ be the total number of patients in centre i. The problem is how to combine the treatment responses at different centres to a combined response to treatment. Different approaches are considered in Dragalin *et al.* (2002), Fedorov, Jones, and Rockhold (2002), Gallo (2000), and Senn (1997, 2000), for example. Following Fedorov, Jones, and Rockhold (2002), we use a random-effects model: a response given by patient k on treatment j in centre i is

$$y_{ijk} = \mu_{ij} + \varepsilon_{ijk}, \tag{25.8}$$

where often $\{\varepsilon_{ijk}\}$ are assumed to be independent and normally distributed, $\mathbf{E}[\varepsilon_{ijk}] = 0$ and $\mathbf{Var}[\varepsilon_{ijk}] \equiv \sigma^2$. The variables ε_{ijk} describe the within-centre variability. The centre mean vector $\boldsymbol{\mu}_i = [\mu_{i1}, \mu_{i2}]^\top$ is assumed to be sampled from the bivariate normal distribution $\mathcal{N}(\boldsymbol{\mu}, \boldsymbol{V})$, where $\boldsymbol{\mu} = [\mu_1, \mu_2]^\top$ and $\boldsymbol{V}$ for convenience is presented in the form $\boldsymbol{V} = \sigma^2 \boldsymbol{\Lambda}$. The treatment effect difference at centre i is $\delta_i = \mu_{i1} - \mu_{i2}$, and the ECRT is defined as follows: $\delta = \mathrm{ECRT} = \sum_{i=1}^N E[\delta_i]/N = \mu_1 - \mu_2$.

Let $\bar{y}_{ij.} = \sum_{k=1}^{n_{ij}} y_{ijk}/n_{ij}$ if $n_{ij} > 0$, and 0 otherwise, $i = 1, \ldots, N$, $j = 1, 2$, and $\bar{\boldsymbol{y}}_i = [\bar{y}_{i1.}, \bar{y}_{i2.}]^\top$. Given N and $\{n_{ij}\}$, the best linear unbiased estimator of $\boldsymbol{\mu}$ [see Fedorov, Jones, and Rockhold (2002)] is

$$\hat{\boldsymbol{\mu}} = \left\{ \sum_{i=1}^N \mathbf{W}_i \right\}^{-1} \sum_{i=1}^N \mathbf{W}_i \bar{\boldsymbol{y}}_i, \qquad (25.9)$$

where, if all $n_{ij} > 0$, $\mathbf{W}_i = (\boldsymbol{\Lambda} + \mathbf{M}_i^{-1})^{-1}$, and $\mathbf{M}_i$ is a diagonal matrix with entries $\{n_{i1}, n_{i2}\}$. If in the ith centre there are no patients on treatment j' (i.e., $n_{ij'} = 0$), where $j' = 1$ or 2, then formula (25.9) still applies, but now for $j \neq j'$ the (j, j)th entry of the matrix $\mathbf{W}_i$ is $(\Lambda_{jj} + 1/n_{ij})^{-1}$ and all other entries are zeros.

The estimator of the ECRT is $\hat{\delta} = \boldsymbol{\ell}^\top \hat{\boldsymbol{\mu}} \boldsymbol{\ell} = \hat{\mu}_1 - \hat{\mu}_2$, where $\boldsymbol{\ell}^\top = [1, -1]$.

In Fedorov, Jones, and Rockhold (2002), the following formula for the variance of $\hat{\delta}$ is derived: for given n_{ij},

$$\zeta^2[\{n_{ij}\}] = \mathbf{Var}[\hat{\delta} \mid n_{ij}] = \sigma^2 \boldsymbol{\ell}^\top \left\{ \sum_{i=1}^N \mathbf{W}_i \right\}^{-1} \boldsymbol{\ell}. \qquad (25.10)$$

As n_{ij} are random values due to random enrolment, then the averaged variance [Anisimov, Fedorov, and Jones (2003)] is

$$\zeta^2(n, N) = \mathbf{Var}[\hat{\delta}] = \sigma^2 \boldsymbol{\ell}^\top \mathbf{E}\left[\left\{ \sum_{i=1}^N \mathbf{W}_i \right\}^{-1} \right] \boldsymbol{\ell}. \qquad (25.11)$$

In particular, if the trial is completely balanced (in each centre $n_{ij} = n/2N$), then

$$\zeta^2(n, N) = \frac{4\sigma^2}{n} + \frac{s^2}{N}, \qquad (25.12)$$

where $\sigma^2 = \mathbf{Var}[\varepsilon_{ijk}]$ (within-centre variability) and $s^2 = \boldsymbol{\ell}^\top \boldsymbol{V} \boldsymbol{\ell}$ (between-centre variability).

25.4   Inflation of the Variance Due to Random Enrolment

The expressions in (25.10) and (25.11) have quite a complicated form. We give simpler approximate formulae which can be used at the design stage and for solving the optimization problem. The results of simulation show that these formulae work very well for a very wide range of parameters.

The type of approximation essentially depends on the relationship between σ^2 and s^2. Let us consider the case when s^2 is relatively small compared to σ^2, as is often seen in practical situations. If the patients are equally allocated between treatments, it was shown by Anisimov, Fedorov, and Jones (2003) that the first-order approximation of the variance in (25.10) is

$$\zeta^2[\{n_{ij}\}] \approx \frac{4\sigma^2}{n} + \frac{s^2}{n^2}\sum_{i=1}^{N} n_i^2 = \frac{4\sigma^2}{n} + \frac{s^2}{N}(1+\omega_n^2), \qquad (25.13)$$

where $\omega_n^2 = \left[\sum_{i=1}^{N}(n_i-\bar{n})^2\right]/(\bar{n}^2 N)$, $\bar{n} = \sum_{i=1}^{N} n_i/N = n/N$. The averaged variance is

$$\zeta^2(n,N) \approx \frac{4\sigma^2}{n} + \frac{s^2}{n^2}\sum_{i=1}^{N} \mathbf{E}[n_i^2] = \frac{4\sigma^2}{n} + \frac{s^2}{N}(1+\mathbf{E}[\omega_n^2]). \qquad (25.14)$$

The computation of the right-hand side of (25.14) depends on the type of enrolment model we study. Consider the competitive enrolment policy. Assume first that the rates λ_i are fixed. Denote $p_i = \lambda_i/\Lambda_N$, $i = 1,2,\ldots,N$, where $\Lambda_N = \sum_{i=1}^{N}\lambda_i$. Given n, the vector $\{n_i, \ i = 1,\ldots,N\}$ has a multinomial distribution with parameters $(n, p_1, \ldots, p_N)$, and n_i has a binomial distribution with parameters (n, p_i), Thus, $\mathbf{E}[n_i^2] = n(n-1)p_i^2 + np_i$ and we can represent (25.14) up to the terms of order $O(1/nN)$ in the form

$$\zeta^2(n,N) \approx \frac{4\sigma^2}{n} + \frac{s^2}{N}\left(\frac{N}{n} + N\sum_{i=1}^{N} p_i^2\right) = \frac{4\sigma^2}{n} + \frac{s^2}{N}\left(1 + \frac{N}{n} + \omega_\lambda^2\right), \quad (25.15)$$

where $\omega_\lambda^2 = \left[\sum_{i=1}^{N}(\lambda_i - \bar{\lambda})^2\right]/(\bar{\lambda}^2 N)$. In particular, if $\lambda_i \equiv \lambda$ (stochastically balanced case), then $\omega_\lambda^2 = 0$.

If the rates λ_i are random, then in (25.15) we need to take $\mathbf{E}[\omega_\lambda^2]$. Thus, if λ_i are sampled from some population with arbitrary distribution, then at large N, $\mathbf{E}[\omega_\lambda^2] \approx \bar{\omega}_\lambda^2 = \mathbf{Var}[\lambda]/(\mathbf{E}[\lambda])^2$, and at large n and N,

$$\zeta^2(n,N) \approx \frac{4\sigma^2}{n} + \frac{s^2}{N}\left(1 + \frac{N}{n} + \bar{\omega}_\lambda^2\right). \qquad (25.16)$$

If λ_i are sampled from a gamma distribution with parameters $(\alpha_\lambda, \beta_\lambda)$, we can calculate exactly the expectation on the right-hand side in (25.15). In this case $p_i = Ga(\alpha_\lambda, \beta_\lambda)^{-1}(Ga(\alpha_\lambda, \beta_\lambda) + Ga((N-1)\alpha_\lambda, \beta_\lambda))$, where $Ga(\alpha_\lambda, \beta_\lambda)$ and $Ga((N-1)\alpha_\lambda, \beta_\lambda)$ are independent. Thus, p_i has a standard beta distribution with parameters $(\alpha_\lambda, (N-1)\alpha_\lambda)$. As $\mathbf{E}[p_i^2] = (\alpha_\lambda + 1)/(N(\alpha_\lambda N + 1))$ [Johnson, Kotz, and Balakrishnan (1995, p. 217)], we get

$$\bar{\omega}_\lambda^2 = (N-1)/(\alpha_\lambda N + 1). \tag{25.17}$$

Therefore, if the rates vary (which is always true in practical situations), the variance is larger compared to the stochastically balanced case where $\lambda_i \equiv \lambda$. The following table summarizes the results on the inflation of the variance.

Model	Enrolment	Variance
Fixed effects	Deterministic, balanced	$\frac{4\sigma^2}{n}$
Random effects	Deterministic, balanced	$\frac{4\sigma^2}{n} + \frac{s^2}{N}$
Random effects	Poisson, equal rates	$\frac{4\sigma^2}{n} + \frac{s^2}{N}\left(1 + \frac{N}{n}\right)$
Random effects	Varying rates	$\frac{4\sigma^2}{n} + \frac{s^2}{N}\left(1 + \frac{N}{n} + \mathbf{E}[\omega_\lambda^2]\right)$

These results show that the additional sources of variability add extra terms and increase the variance of the estimator of ECRT. Thus, using the traditional approach may lead to underpowered studies.

These results are supported by a simulation study showing that for a very wide range of scenarios at large enough $n \geq 200$ and $N \geq 20$, the first-order approximation (25.12) is a very close lower boundary for the variance of the estimator of the ECRT. The models with varying and gamma rates have a larger variance and the expansions (25.15) and (25.17) improve the approximations.

25.5   Solution of the Optimization Problem

Consider only the case when s^2 is smaller than σ^2 as this is often seen in practical situations. Let us study a competitive enrolment policy which is the most common one. Assume first that λ_i are sampled from a gamma distribution with parameters $(\alpha_\lambda, \beta_\lambda)$. According to (25.4), $\mathbf{E}[T_1(n, N)] = \beta_\lambda n/(\alpha_\lambda N - 1)$ and the risk function (25.1) can be written in the form $L(n, N) = CN + cn + \beta_\lambda Rn/(\alpha_\lambda N - 1)$. To find an approximate solution, we use (25.16) with $\bar{\omega}_\lambda^2$ in the form (25.17). Thus, the optimization problem (25.2) can be written in the following form. Find

$$\{n^*, N^*\} = \arg\min_{n,N} L(n, N) \text{ given that } \frac{4\sigma^2 + s^2}{n} + \frac{(\alpha_\lambda + 1)s^2}{\alpha_\lambda N + 1} \leq v^2. \tag{25.18}$$

To solve the problem (25.18) in closed form, we replace $L(n, N)$ by the expression $L^*(n, N) = CN + cn + \beta_\lambda Rn/(\alpha_\lambda N + 1)$, which is asymptotically equivalent at large N. Now the optimization problem up to some constants is equivalent to problem (27) of Fedorov, Jones, and Rockhold (2002) [see also problems (6.2) and (6.3) of Anisimov, Fedorov, and Jones (2003)]. Solving it in the same way, we get

$$N^* = \frac{(\alpha_\lambda + 1)s^2}{\alpha_\lambda v^2} + \frac{1}{v^2}\sqrt{\frac{4\sigma^2 + s^2}{C\alpha_\lambda}}\sqrt{c(\alpha_\lambda + 1)s^2 + \beta_\lambda Rv^2},$$

$$n^* = \frac{4\sigma^2 + s^2}{v^2 - \frac{(\alpha_\lambda+1)s^2}{\alpha_\lambda N^* + 1}}. \qquad (25.19)$$

Using these formulae we can calculate the variance $\zeta^2(n^*, N^*)$ and the power of the optimal trial, respectively.

If λ_i are sampled from a population with a general distribution and N is large enough, then according to Theorem 25.2.1 we can use the approximation $\mathbf{E}[T_1(n, N)] \approx n/\bar\lambda N$ and the expression (25.16) for the variance. In this case the optimization problem has the form: find

$$\{n^*, N^*\} = \arg\min_{n,N}\left\{CN + cn + \frac{Rn}{\bar\lambda N}\right\}$$

$$\text{given that} \quad \frac{4\sigma^2 + s^2}{n} + \frac{(1 + \bar\omega_\lambda^2)s^2}{N} \leq v^2. \qquad (25.20)$$

According to Fedorov, Jones, and Rockhold (2002) and Anisimov, Fedorov, and Jones (2003), a solution of (25.20) has the form

$$N^* = \frac{(1 + \bar\omega_\lambda^2)s^2}{v^2} + \frac{1}{v^2}\sqrt{\frac{4\sigma^2 + s^2}{C}}\sqrt{(1 + \bar\omega_\lambda^2)cs^2 + Rv^2/\bar\lambda}, \quad n^* = \frac{4\sigma^2 + s^2}{v^2 - \frac{(1+\bar\omega_\lambda^2)s^2}{N^*}}.$$

Consider now a problem of minimization of a certain quantile $\mathbf{P}(\mathcal{L}(n, N) > L_*)$ of the loss function $\mathcal{L}(n, N)$ given that $\zeta^2(n, N) \leq v^2$.

According to Theorems 25.2.1–25.2.3, we can use a normal approximation for $T_1(n, N)$ in the form $T_1(n, N) \approx A_{n,N} + B_{n,N}\mathcal{N}(0, 1)$ for a very wide range of enrolment models, where the values $A_{n,N}$ and $A_{n,N}$ are calculated in closed form. For the sake of simplicity, assume that all other costs are nonrandom and $C_i \equiv C$, $c_i \equiv c$. Then the problem of minimization of $\mathbf{P}(\mathcal{L}(n, N) > L_*)$, where for $T_1(n, N)$ we use a normal approximation, is equivalent to the problem of minimization of the expression $(CN + cn + RA_{n,N} - L_*)/RB_{n,N}$.

For example, under the conditions of Theorem 25.2.3, $A_{n,N} = M_{n,N}$, $B_{n,N} = \beta_{n,N}^{-1}$, and the optimization problem has the form: find

$$\{n^*, N^*\} = \arg\min_{n,N}\beta_{n,N}(CN + cn + RM_{n,N} - L_*)$$

$$\text{given that} \quad \frac{4\sigma^2 + s^2}{n} + \frac{(1 + \bar\omega_\lambda^2)s^2}{N} \leq v^2. \qquad (25.21)$$

This problem can be easily solved numerically for any given values of the parameters.

25.6   Conclusions

We consider a multicentre trial under quite general and practical assumptions taking into account random enrolment. The developed results lead to simple approximate formulae which can be used at the design and planning stages of multicentre clinical trials. These results prove that random enrolment increases the mean and the variance of the recruitment time and the variance of the estimated ECRT and decreases the power of the trial. To achieve the necessary power, we need to increase the number of centres N, as well as the number of patients n.

These facts should be taken into account at the design and planning stages of multicentre clinical trials because the use of the traditional approach may lead to underpowered studies.

Appendix

A.1   Proof of Theorem 25.2.1

We use the following representation (in the sense of the equality of distributions): $T_1 = Ga(n, \Lambda_N) = Ga(n, 1)/\Lambda_N$, where $\Lambda_N = \sum_i \lambda_i$. As λ_i are independent, we can apply the Law of Large Numbers: as $N \to \infty$, $\Lambda_N/\bar{\lambda}N \xrightarrow{P} 1$. Thus, as $n \to \infty, N \to \infty$, $\bar{\lambda}NT_1(n,N)/n = (Ga(n,1)/n) \times (\Lambda_N/\bar{\lambda}N)^{-1} \xrightarrow{P} 1$. Furthermore, if $\sigma > 0$,

$$\alpha_{n,N}(T_1(n,N) - n/\bar{\lambda}N) = \left(c_{n1} \frac{Ga(n,1) - n}{\sqrt{n}} + c_{n2} \frac{\Lambda_N - \bar{\lambda}N}{\sigma\sqrt{N}} \right) \frac{\bar{\lambda}N}{\Lambda_N}, \quad (A.1)$$

where $c_{n1} = \alpha_{n,N}\sqrt{n}/\bar{\lambda}N$, $c_{n2} = \alpha_{n,N}\, n\sigma N^{-3/2}/\bar{\lambda}^2$, and $c_{n1}^2 + c_{n2}^2 = 1$. Noting that the variables $(Ga(n,1)-n)/\sqrt{n}$ and $(\Lambda_N - \alpha N)/(\sigma\sqrt{N})$ are independent and, for large n and N, are both asymptotically standard normally distributed, we prove that the right-hand side of (A.1) is asymptotically standard normally distributed.

A.2   Proof of Theorem 25.2.3

Denote by $\Pi_\lambda(t)$ a Poisson process with parameter λ. Let $\chi_i = \chi(\tau_i \leq t)$ be the indicator of the event $\{\tau_i \leq t\}$; that is, $\chi_i = 1$ if $\tau_i \leq t$, and $\chi_i = 0$ otherwise. Denote $Q_N(t) = p\sum_{i=1}^{N} \lambda_i(t - \tau_i)\chi_i$, $\Lambda_N = \sum_i \lambda_i$. We can write representations

$$n(t) = \sum_{i=1}^{N} \Pi_{p\lambda_i}((t - \tau_i)\chi_i) = \Pi_1(Q_N(t)),$$

$$\mathbf{P}(T_1(n, N) \leq t) = \mathbf{P}(Ga(n, 1) \leq Q_N(t)). \tag{A.2}$$

If $t > C_\tau$, then for all i, $\chi_i = 1$ and $Q_N(t) = p\sum_{i=1}^{N} \lambda_i(t - \tau_i)$. Therefore,

$$\mathbf{P}(T_1(n, N) \leq t) = \mathbf{P}\left(\frac{Ga(n, 1) + p\sum_{i=1}^{N} \lambda_i \tau_i}{p\Lambda_N} \leq t\right). \tag{A.3}$$

Under the conditions of Theorem 25.2.3 we can apply the Law of Large Numbers: as $n \to \infty, N \to \infty$,

$$\Lambda_N \Big/ N\bar{\lambda} \xrightarrow{\mathrm{P}} 1, \quad \left(Ga(n, 1) + p\sum_{i=1}^{N} \lambda_i \tau_i\right) \Big/ (n + p\bar{\lambda}mN) \xrightarrow{\mathrm{P}} 1.$$

These relationships imply that $T_1(n, N)/M_{n,N} \xrightarrow{\mathrm{P}} 1$. Furthermore, using (A.2) we can write a relationship $\mathbf{P}(\beta_{n,N}(T_1(n, N) - M_{n,N}) \leq z) = \mathbf{P}(\zeta_{n,N}q_N \leq z)$, where

$$\zeta_{n,N} = \beta_{n,N}\left(Ga(n, 1) + p\sum_{i=1}^{N} \lambda_i(\tau_i - M_{n,N})\right) \Big/ (p\bar{\lambda}N), \quad q_N = \bar{\lambda}N \Big/ \Lambda_N. \tag{A.4}$$

One can calculate that $\mathbf{E}[\zeta_{n,N}] = 0$, $\mathbf{Var}[\zeta_{n,N}] = 1$ and under conditions of Theorem 25.2.3, as $n \to \infty, N \to \infty$, the variable $\zeta_{n,N}$ converges in distribution to $\mathcal{N}(0, 1)$. As $q_N \xrightarrow{\mathrm{P}} 1$, this implies the statement of Theorem 25.2.3.

A.3   Proof of Lemma 25.2.1

Using the property that as $N \to \infty$, the random variable $(\Lambda_N - \bar{\lambda}N)\big/\sqrt{N}$ converges in distribution to $\mathcal{N}(0, \sigma^2)$, we can write for any $t > 0$ the following relationship for the characteristic function of the process $\zeta_N(t)$: as $N \to \infty$,

$$\begin{aligned}
\mathbf{E}\left[\exp\{i\theta\zeta_N(t)\}\right] &= \mathbf{E}\left[\exp\left\{p\Lambda_N t(e^{i\theta/\sqrt{N}} - 1) - i\theta p\bar{\lambda}t\sqrt{N}\right\}\right] \\
&\approx \mathbf{E}\left[\exp\left\{i\theta pt(\Lambda_N - \bar{\lambda}N)/\sqrt{N} - pt\theta^2\Lambda_N/2N\right\}\right] \\
&\to \mathbf{E}\left[\exp\{-(p^2\sigma^2t^2 + \bar{p}\lambda t)\theta^2/2\}\right],
\end{aligned}$$

where $\mathbf{i} = +\sqrt{-1}$. Thus, for any $t > 0$, $\zeta_N(t)$ converges in distribution to the variable $\zeta_0(t) = p\sigma\xi t + \sqrt{p\bar{\lambda}}\, w(t)$. As the process $\zeta_N(t)$ has conditionally independent increments, we can prove in the same way that the increments of $\zeta_N(t)$ weakly converge to the increments of $\zeta_0(t)$ and also check the weak compactness in Skorokhod space.

References

1. Anisimov, V., Fedorov, V., and Jones, B. (2003). Optimization of clinical trials with random enrollment, *GSK BDS Technical Report, 2003–03*.

2. Dragalin, V., Fedorov, V., Jones, B., and Rockhold, F. (2002). Estimation of the combined response to treatment in multicentre trials, *Journal of Biopharmaceutical Statistics*, **11**, 275–295.

3. Fedorov, V., Jones, B., and Rockhold, F. (2002). The design and analysis of multicentre trials in the random effects setting, *GSK BDS Technical Report, 2002–03*.

4. Gallo, P. P. (2000). Center-weighting issues in multicenter clinical trials, *Journal of Biopharmaceutical Statistics*, **10**, 145-163.

5. Johnson, N. L., Kotz, S., and Balakrishnan, N. (1994). *Continuous Univariate Distributions*, Vol. 1, Second edition, John Wiley & Sons, New York.

6. Johnson, N. L., Kotz, S., and Balakrishnan, N. (1995). *Continuous Univariate Distributions*, Vol. 2, Second edition, John Wiley & Sons, New York.

7. Kovalenko, I. N., Kuznetsov, N. Yu., and Shurenkov, V. M. (1996). Models of random processes, In *A Handbook for Mathematicians and Engineers*, CRC Press, Boca Raton, Florida.

8. Senn, S. (1997). *Statistical Issues in Drug Development*, John Wiley & Sons, Chichester, U.K.

9. Senn, S. (2000). The many modes of meta, *Drug Information Journal*, **34**, 535-549.

10. Snyder, D., and Miller, M. (1991). *Random Point Processes in Time and Space*, Second edition, Springer-Verlag, New York.

26

Statistical Methods for Combining Clinical Trial Phases II And III

Nigel Stallard and Susan Todd

The University of Warwick, Coventry, UK
The University of Reading, Reading, UK

Abstract: This chapter reviews recently developed methodology for designs that combine clinical trial phases II and III in a single trial. The designs enable both selection of the best of a number of experimental treatments and comparison of this treatment with a control treatment, and allow the trial to be stopped early if the best experimental treatment is insufficiently promising or is clearly superior to the control. The stopping rules are constructed to preserve the overall type I error rate for the trial. Two-stage designs are reviewed briefly and two multistage methods based, respectively, on the adaptive and group-sequential approaches are described in detail. The latter are illustrated by a trial to compare three doses of a new drug for the treatment of Alzheimer's disease.

Keywords and phrases: Adaptive designs, phase II/III trials, select and test designs, sequential clinical trials, treatment selection

26.1 Introduction

In the statistical design of clinical trials to evaluate new drugs, an area of considerable interest is the combination of clinical trial phases II and III into a single trial, because this allows the drug development process to be accelerated. Trial design methods with this aim have been proposed by Thall *et al.* (1988, 1989), Schaid *et al.* (1990), Bauer and Kieser (1999), Stallard and Todd (2003), Royston *et al.* (2003), and Inoue *et al.* (2002). Their approaches extend the sequential design of clinical trials where two or more interim analyses are conducted as data accumulate through the course of the trial. In essence, the new methods use one or more of the earlier interim analyses to replace the phase II trial. A single trial is thus conducted which allows selection of one or more of the experimental treatments, as would usually take place in a phase II trial, as well as the comparison of the selected treatment(s) with the control treatment as in a phase III trial. With the exception of Royston et al. (2003) and Inoue et al. (2002), all of the cited papers focus on the construction of frequentist designs in which the overall type I error rate allowing for the treatment selection is controlled. These two papers, however, address a slightly different problem in the combination of phases II and III: that of the use of a definitive endpoint in the final 'phase III' analysis and a surrogate endpoint in the interim 'phase II' analysis. Royston et al. (2003) propose a frequentist solution to this problem, whereas Inoue et al. (2002) adopt a Bayesian method. Although the use of surrogate endpoints is considered briefly in the Discussion section, most of this chapter is concerned with frequentist methods that allow for treatment selection based on the use of the same endpoint throughout. The chapter provides a review of such methods, illustrating the advantages that their use might bring and highlighting when they are most appropriate. An example of a clinical trial to compare several dose levels of galantamine for the treatment of Alzheimer's disease is used to illustrate and compare the newer methods and future directions and challenges in this field are discussed.

Following this introductory section, we give an overview of the clinical testing process for a new drug in Section 26.2, explaining the roles played by phase II and phase III clinical trials. The advantages and limitations associated with the combination of phases II and III are then discussed. As several of the methods described rely on statistical methodology for sequential clinical trials comparing a single experimental treatment with a control treatment, a brief summary of this area is given in Section 26.2. The main description of the methods combining phases II and III is given in Section 26.3, together with the illustrative example. We end with a discussion of the methodology and remaining challenges in Section 26.4.

26.2 Background

26.2.1 The clinical evaluation programme for new drugs

The programme of clinical evaluation of a new drug prior to application to regulatory authorities for registration can be divided into three phases. Phase I clinical trials are small-scale trials in which the first exposure to humans of the new drug is carefully assessed. The focus is on the safety of the drug, and the subjects will often be healthy volunteers. A control group may be included to maintain blindness, but formal comparison between treated and control groups is unusual. A number of doses of the new drug are generally used, with the aim of determining the maximum tolerated dose; the highest dose that can be administered without causing an unacceptably high level of side effects.

Phase II clinical trials are both the first trials conducted in the target patient population and the first in which treatment efficacy is assessed. They are usually conducted using a control group and double-blind randomization. Although a maximum tolerated dose will have been determined by phase I trials, phase II may include a number of doses, dosing patterns, or formulations. The main purpose of these trials is to act as screens to decide which new drugs are worthy of further evaluation in phase III trials. The trials are relatively small-scale, with sample sizes of a few hundred or less, to avoid large commitment of resources. In order to minimize trial duration, a short-term or surrogate endpoint can be primarily considered.

The aim of phase III trials is to provide definitive evidence of the efficacy and safety of a drug for regulatory approval. These are large-scale trials conducted in the target patient population, requiring several hundred or more patients. The large sample size, and hence the high cost and long duration of such trials means that a single dose level is compared with a control treatment, which may be a placebo or a standard therapy in a double-blind randomised trial. The primary endpoint is chosen to reflect the clinical setting. This is often an endpoint, such as survival, obtained after long-term follow-up. To provide confirmatory evidence of treatment efficacy, regulatory authorities generally require two phase III trials.

26.2.2 Combining clinical trial phases II and III

Approaches that allow the clinical testing programme to be completed more quickly or with fewer patients without any compromise in the level of evidence provided are appealing to companies acting in the competitive field of drug development. Such approaches are also of benefit to society if effective drugs can be made available more quickly as indicated in Section 112 of the US FDA Modernization Act of 1997 on Expediting Study and Approval of Fast Track Drugs. One movement towards accelerated drug development that has been very successful over the last few decades is the application of sequential methods in phase III clinical trials comparing a single experimental treatment with a control. This approach allows analysis of accumulating data to be conducted during the course of a trial, with the trial being stopped as soon as sufficient evidence has been observed to conclude that the experimental treatment is superior to the control, or that the experimental treatment is insufficiently superior to make continuation of the trial worthwhile. Overviews of sequential clinical trial methods are given by Whitehead (1997) and Jennison and Turnbull (2000).

Of more recent interest, with the same aim of accelerating the drug testing process, has been the possibility of designs that combine the usually distinct phases of development. The range of methods for combining phases II and

III that have been proposed are described in detail and compared in Section 26.3 below. We first consider the situations in which combination of the two phases is and is not possible and desirable. We may consider three distinct cases. The first is that in which phases II and III involve efficacy evaluation in different patient populations. This is common in cancer trials, for example, when patients are often enrolled in phase II trials only after the failure of first-line therapy. In this case, it seems reasonable to consider phases II and III separately, and there is very little scope for combining them. The second case is that in which the patient populations for phases II and III are the same, but a different primary endpoint is used in the two phases. For example, it is common to use a rapidly observable endpoint in a phase II trial, with long-term survival considered in phase III. In this case, there might be some scope for combining phases II and III, but existing methods would have to be extended. This extension is an area of current research. In the third case, in which the same patient population and endpoint are used for phases II and III, a combined trial seems both suitable and desirable. For the remainder of the chapter, it will be this case that is considered.

If two separate phase III trials are required, we suggest that the first could be conducted using a combined phase II/III approach as discussed here and the second conducted comparing the chosen experimental treatment with the control treatment using a more conventional phase III design.

26.2.3   Background to sequential clinical trials

Several of the methods for clinical trials that combine phases II and III are based on extensions of sequential methods for trials that compare a single experimental treatment group with a control group. This section describes two such methods, the group-sequential method and the adaptive design approach, introducing the key underlying concepts and some notation and terminology that will be used in the description of the combined phase II/phase III designs, in Section 26.3.

In a sequential trial to compare a single experimental group with a control group, a test statistic giving some measure of treatment difference is compared with a stopping boundary at a series of interim analyses. The trial stops as soon as the stopping boundary is reached, or after some maximum number, n, of interim analyses. Let θ be a measure of the treatment difference, with $\theta > 0$, $\theta = 0$, and $\theta < 0$ corresponding, respectively, to superiority, equality, and inferiority of the experimental treatment to the control. The aim of the trial is to test the null hypothesis $H_0 : \theta = 0$ in favour of the one-sided alternative hypothesis $\theta > 0$. Whitehead (1997) proposes use of the efficient score for θ as a test statistic, which may be compared with stopping limits that depend on the observed Fisher's information at the interim analysis. The efficient score and observed information at the jth interim analysis will be denoted by Z_j and V_j, respectively.

Forms for θ and the corresponding Z_j and V_j for a number of settings are given by Whitehead (1997). In the case of normal data, for example, he takes θ to be the standardised difference in means. If the experimental and control groups have, respectively, n_E and n_C observations and observed means $\bar{x}_E$ and $\bar{x}_C$, and the sum of the squares of all observations (taken over both groups) is Q, then Z and V are given by

$$Z = n_E n_C (\bar{x}_E - \bar{x}_C)/\{n_E + n_C\}D \tag{26.1}$$

and

$$V = n_E n_C/(n_E + n_C) - Z^2/2\{n_E + n_C\}, \tag{26.2}$$

where $D = \{Q/(n_E + n_C) - (n_E \bar{x}_E + n_C \bar{x}_C)^2/(n_E + n_C)^2\}^{1/2}$. In this case, under H_0, when the expected value of Z is zero, if $n_E = n_C$, V is approximately equal to $n_C/2$.

It can be shown that in a wide range of settings, asymptotically, for large sample sizes and small θ, $Z_1 \sim N(\theta V_1, V_1)$, and the increment in efficient score at the jth interim analysis, $Z_j - Z_{j-1}$, is independent of Z_{j-1}, with $Z_j - Z_{j-1} \sim N(\theta(V_j - V_{j-1}), (V_j - V_{j-1}))$ [Scharfstein *et al.* (1987)]. In the group sequential method at the jth interim analysis, $j = 1, \ldots, n$, Z_j are compared with stopping limits, l_j and u_j. If $Z_j \geq u_j$, the trial will be stopped with H_0 rejected in favour of the one-sided alternative, $\theta > 0$. If $Z_j \leq l_j$, the trial will be stopped without rejection of H_0. If $l_j < Z_j < u_j$, the trial continues to the $(j+1)$th interim analysis, with $l_n = u_n$ so that the trial must stop at the nth interim analysis if not before.

The values of l_j and u_j, $j = 1, \ldots, n$, may be chosen so as to satisfy some specified α-spending function as introduced by Lan and DeMets (1983). Using the approach proposed by Stallard and Facey (1995) for asymmetric tests that may stop for futility with overall one-sided type I error rate $\alpha/2$, two increasing functions, $\alpha_U^* : [0, 1] \to [0, \alpha/2]$, with $\alpha_U^*(0) = 0$ and $\alpha_U^*(1) = \alpha/2$, and $\alpha_L^* : [0, 1] \to [0, 1-\alpha/2]$, with $\alpha_L^*(0) = 0$ and $\alpha_L^*(1) = 1-\alpha/2$, are specified. Stopping limits are then constructed so as to satisfy

$$\text{Pr}(\text{stop and reject } H_0 \text{ at or before look } j \mid H_0) = \alpha_U^*(t_j) \tag{26.3}$$

and

$$\text{Pr}(\text{stop and do not reject } H_0 \text{ at or before look } j \mid H_0) = \alpha_L^*(t_j), \tag{26.4}$$

with $t_j = V_j/V_{\max}$, where $V_{\max}$ is the planned value of V_n.

The values of l_j and u_j, to give a test to satisfy (26.3) and (26.4), can be obtained via a recursive numerical integration technique based on the asymptotic distribution of Z first described by Armitage *et al.* (1969). Further details are given by Jennison and Turnbull (2000). A numerical search may be used to find $V_{\max}$ so that the procedure has the required power under some specified alternative hypothesis.

Bauer and Köhne (1994) present the adaptive design approach that allows for more design modification than the group-sequential method. Considering a two-stage sequential trial, they propose that the evidence of a treatment difference at the jth stage of the trial for $j = 1, 2$, is summarised by a one-sided p-value, p_j, for the test of the null hypothesis, $H_0 : \theta = 0$, where, as above, θ is some measure of treatment difference. The evidence from the two stages is then combined via the product of the p-values, $p_1 p_2$. Suppose that the trial stops at the first interim analysis with rejection of H_0 if $p_1 \leq \alpha_1$ and without rejection of H_0 if $p_1 \geq \alpha_0$, for some α_1 and α_0. Bauer and Köhne show that in order to achieve overall one-sided type I error rate $\alpha/2$, a critical value of $c_{\alpha/2} = (\alpha/2 - \alpha_1)/(\log \alpha_0 - \log \alpha_1)$ must then be used for the product of p-values at the second stage. The only assumption is that p_1 and p_2 are independent and have a $U[0, 1]$ distribution under H_0. This is generally satisfied by the fact that the p-values are based on observations from different groups of patients. In contrast to the group-sequential approach, this means that considerable flexibility in the modification of the sequential design can be allowed without affecting the type I error rate.

Wassmer (1999) describes how the Bauer and Köhne procedure can be extended to allow more than two stages. Suppose that at the jth stage for $j = 1, \ldots, n$, the product of p-values $p_1 \times \cdots \times p_j$ is calculated and compared with a critical value $c_{\alpha(j)}$, with the trial being stopped and H_0 rejected if $p_1 \times \cdots \times p_j \leq c_{\alpha(j)}$, and being stopped for futility if $p_j \geq \alpha_0^{(j)}$, for some choice of $c_{\alpha(j)}$, $j = 1, \ldots, n$, and $\alpha_0^{(j)}$, $j = 1, \ldots, n - 1$. Wassmer shows that the probability of stopping and rejecting the null hypothesis at the jth interim analysis is equal to P_j, given recursively by

$$P_j = c_{\alpha(j)} \sum_{k=1}^{j} \left(\prod_{i=1}^{k-1} \log(\alpha_0^{(j-i)}) \right) (Y_k - X_k), \qquad (26.5)$$

where $X_k = \sum_{i=1}^{j-k-1} (1/(j-k+1-i)!) \log^{j-k+1-i} \left((c_{\alpha(i)} \prod_{l=i+1}^{j-k-1} \alpha_0^{(l)})/c_{\alpha(j-k)} \right)$ $\times (P_i/c_{\alpha(i)})$ and $Y_k = \log^{j-k} \left((\prod_{i=1}^{j-k-1} \alpha_0^{(i)})/c_{\alpha(j-k)} \right)/(j-k)!$ with $\log^i(x)$ denoting $(\log(x))^i$, $c_{\alpha(0)} = 1$ and $\sum_{i=a}^{b} x_i = 0$ and $\prod_{i=a}^{b} x_i = 1$ if $a > b$.

Values of $\alpha_0^{(j)}$ and $c_{\alpha(j)}$, $j = 1, \ldots, n$, may be constructed so that the test satisfies (26.3) and (26.4) for some specified spending function, provided these are such that the $c_{\alpha(j)}$ values are decreasing. At the first interim analysis, the probabilities under the null hypothesis of stopping and rejecting or not rejecting H_0 are, respectively, $P_1 = c_{\alpha(1)}$ and $1 - \alpha_0^{(1)}$, so that these can be set equal to $\alpha_U^*(t_1)$ and $\alpha_L^*(t_1)$, respectively. At the jth interim analysis, the probability under H_0 of stopping for futility given that the trial has not stopped earlier is

$1 - \alpha_0^{(j)}$. If the values of $c_{\alpha^{(h)}}$ and $\alpha_0^{(h)}$, for $h = 1, \ldots, j-1$, have been obtained so that the test satisfies (26.3) and (26.4) for earlier looks, the probability of not having stopped before the jth look is $1 - \alpha_U^*(t_{j-1}) - \alpha_L^*(t_{j-1})$. The probability of stopping at the jth look and not rejecting H_0 is thus equal to $(1 - \alpha_0^{(j)})(1 - \alpha_U^*(t_{j-1}) - \alpha_L^*(t_{j-1}))$. To satisfy (26.3) and (26.4), this must be equal to $\alpha_L^*(t_j) - \alpha_L^*(t_{j-1})$, so that $\alpha_0^{(j)} = (1 - \alpha_U^*(t_{j-1}) - \alpha_L^*(t_j))/(1 - \alpha_U^*(t_{j-1}) - \alpha_L^*(t_{j-1}))$. It is also desired that the probability of stopping at the jth interim analysis and rejecting H_0 is equal to $\alpha_U^*(t_j) - \alpha_U^*(t_{j-1})$. A value of $c_{\alpha^{(j)}}$ to achieve this can be found from (26.5) with P_j set equal to $\alpha_U^*(t_j) - \alpha_U^*(t_{j-1})$.

As in the two-stage design, the only requirement for (26.3) and (26.4) to be satisfied, and hence for the preservation of the overall type I error rate, is that $p_1, \ldots, p_n$ follow independent uniform distributions under H_0. This allows considerable design flexibility. Indeed, in principle at least, H_0 may be changed from one interim analysis to the next to provide a final test of the intersection of the null hypotheses considered, though the practical value of such a strategy might be questioned.

26.3 Methods for Combining Phases II and III

As indicated in Section 26.1 above, one of the aims of a phase II clinical trial is to compare competing treatments, which may be the same drug administered at different doses or with different treatment regimens, or different drugs, in terms of their efficacy to choose the most effective. The aim of a phase III clinical trial is to compare a single treatment with a control treatment with the hope of obtaining definitive evidence of a treatment effect. An approach to combining phases II and III into a single trial must thus focus on both selecting the best of a number of treatments and comparing this with the control treatment. In view of this dual nature, the designs for combining phases II and III are sometimes known as 'select and test' designs.

In detail, we suppose k competing experimental treatments, which we will denote by $T_1, \ldots, T_k$, are to be compared with each other and with a control treatment, T_0. Let θ_i be a measure of the superiority of treatment T_i relative to T_0, with $\theta_i > 0$, $\theta_i = 0$, and $\theta_i < 0$ corresponding, respectively, to superiority, equality, and inferiority of T_i. The aims of the combined phase II/III trial are to both select the best experimental treatment and to test the global null hypothesis $H_0 : \theta_1 = \cdots = \theta_k = 0$, with controlled type I error rate.

26.3.1   Two-stage methods

Methods for combining phases II and III were proposed by Thall *et al.* (1988) and Schaid *et al.* (1990). Both papers propose trials conducted in two stages, with a single interim analysis at the end of the first stage, at which the trial will be stopped if results are insufficiently promising. In the first stage, patients are randomized between a number of experimental treatments and a control treatment, with the aim of selecting the best treatment or treatments for continuation to the second stage. The final analysis is performed at the end of the second stage, and uses data from both the second and the first stages for those treatments continuing to the end of the trial.

Thall *et al.* (1988, 1989) proposed a method for trials with a binary endpoint in which, providing the trial has not been stopped, only the best treatment from the first look continues with the control treatment to the second stage. The overall type I error rate, given the critical values at the two analyses may be obtained through the use of a normal approximation if a control group is included in the first stage [Thall *et al.* (1988)] or by binomial calculations if there is no control group [Thall *et al.* (1989)]. A numerical search can thus be used to obtain the critical value at the final analysis given that at the first stage, and the latter can be chosen to minimize the required sample size subject to a specification of the power of the trial.

Schaid *et al.* (1990) propose a method for trials with a survival endpoint. Their method allows any number of the experimental treatments to continue to the second stage along with the control. The overall type I error rate is maintained by imposing a Bonferroni correction as if no experimental arms could be dropped, leading to a design that is more flexible than that suggested by Thall *et al.* (1988), but is generally conservative.

26.3.2   A multistage group-sequential method

More recently proposed methods for combining phase II and phase III clinical trials build on sequential clinical trial methodology to allow trials that may be conducted in more than two stages. The frequentist properties of the test can be specified via spending functions as in (26.3) and (26.4), where now the test is of the global null hypothesis, with rejection of this in the one-sided direction that some experimental treatment is superior to the control.

Stallard and Todd (2003) proposed a method based on the group-sequential approach described in Section 26.2. It is assumed that randomization is initially to the k experimental treatments and the control. At the first interim analysis the best of the experimental treatments is selected, and, if the trial does not stop at this point, further randomization is between the control and this treatment only. The trial then proceeds with a series of interim analyses comparing this treatment with the control. The combination of evidence from the different stages in the trial is achieved through the calculation of efficient score statistics for $\theta_1, \ldots, \theta_k$.

Suppose that at the first interim analysis, the efficient score and observed Fisher's information for θ_i are, respectively, $Z_{i,1}$ and $V_{i,1}$, $i = 1, \ldots, k$. If the sample size for each treatment arm is the same, it is often reasonable to assume that $V_{1,1} = \cdots = V_{k,1}$. Because an approximate maximum likelihood estimate of θ_i is given by $Z_{i,1}/V_{i,1}$, the best treatment is the one with the largest value of $Z_{i,1}$. Let $S = \arg\max\{Z_{i,1}\}$, that is, the value of i for which $Z_{i,1}$ is largest, so that the selected treatment is T_S. A test of the global null hypothesis can be based on the observed value of $Z_{S,1}$. Based on the assumption that $V_{1,1} = \cdots = V_{k,1}$, Stallard and Todd (2003) derive the density of $Z_{S,1}$. As only T_S and T_0 continue beyond the first stage of the trial, data from subsequent stages can be summarized by the statistics $Z_{S,j}$ and $V_{S,j}$. As in the case of a trial with a single experimental treatment, the increment $Z_{S,j} - Z_{S,j-1}$ is asymptotically $N(\theta_S(V_{S,j} - V_{S,j-1}), (V_{S,j} - V_{S,j-1}))$ and independent of $Z_{S,j-1}$. The joint density of $Z_{S,1}, \ldots, Z_{S,k}$ can thus be obtained from the density of $Z_{S,1}$ using recursive numerical integration in a similar way to that described by Armitage *et al.* (1969) and Jennison and Turnbull (2000) to give a stopping boundary that satisfies (26.3) and (26.4) for specified spending functions.

26.3.3   A multistage adaptive design method

An alternative approach to the design of a trial combining phases II and III has been proposed by Bauer and Kieser (1999). They use the adaptive design approach described in Section 26.2 above. Although they describe a two-stage method, the approach of Wassmer can be used to extend their approach to a multistage setting. In general, at the jth stage, patients are randomized between the control treatment and some subset τ_j of $\{T_1, \ldots, T_k\}$. Although the flexibility of the adaptive design approach allows τ_j to be chosen in any way, typically τ_1 would be taken to be $\{T_1, \ldots, T_k\}$ and $\tau_j \subseteq \tau_{j-1}$ for $j > 1$, so that randomization is initially to all treatments, with ineffective treatments dropped through the course of the trial and no dropped treatment reinstated. At the jth stage a p-value, p_j, is calculated as a test of the global null hypothesis based on the new data from that stage and the product of p-values up to and including that stage is compared with appropriate critical values to decide whether the trial should be stopped. To preserve the overall type I error rate, the p-value must allow for the multiple comparison of several experimental treatments with a control. Bauer and Kieser (1999) give a brief discussion of alternative methods including a simple Bonferroni correction. Using this approach, at the jth stage, one-sided p-values would be obtained for the comparison of each of the treatments in τ_j with the control. The smallest of these p-values, corresponding to the treatment most superior to the control, would then be multiplied by the number of treatments, that is, $|\tau_j|$, to correct for the multiple comparisons, to give p_j. The product $p_1 \times \cdots \times p_j$ is then compared with $c_{\alpha(j)}$, and p_j is compared with $\alpha_0^{(j)}$ as described above to give a test with overall error rates as specified by the spending functions (26.3) and (26.4).

26.3.4   Example—a multistage trial comparing three doses of a new drug for the treatment of Alzheimer's disease

Stallard and Todd (2003) illustrate their method with the example of a clinical trial to assess the effectiveness of galantamine for the treatment of Alzheimer's disease. Patients were randomized to receive the placebo or galantamine at a dose of 18 mg/day, 24 mg/day, or 36 mg/day.

The original trial was conducted as three simultaneous group-sequential triangular tests [see Whitehead (1997, Section 3.7) for details of the triangular test], each one comparing a single dose of galantamine with the placebo control. Comparison was in terms of the cognitive portion of the Alzheimer's disease assessment scale (ADAS) score, which was assumed to be normally distributed. Sample size calculations indicated that a maximum of 100 patients on each treatment arm would be needed, and it was planned to conduct interim analyses when results were available from groups of 20 patients on each arm, so that a maximum of five interim analyses was anticipated. Using the result that the observed Fisher's information, V, is approximately equal to half of the number of patients per group, this corresponds to V increasing by 10 each look.

As an alternative to the three simultaneous triangular tests that take no account of the multiple comparisons, the selection of the best galantamine dose and comparison of this with the control treatment could be conducted using either of the methods described in Section 26.3 above, as illustrated in the remainder of this section. To give a test with similar properties to that actually used, the combined phase II/III test may be designed to satisfy (26.3) and (26.4) with spending functions corresponding to the triangular test. The form of the spending functions is given by Whitehead (1997). For a test with overall one-sided type I error rate of 0.025 and five equally spaced interim analyses planned, we get $(\alpha_U^*(0.2), \alpha_U^*(0.4), \alpha_U^*(0.6), \alpha_U^*(0.8), \alpha_U^*(1)) = (0.001, 0.010, 0.019, 0.024, 0.025)$ and $(\alpha_L^*(0.2), \alpha_L^*(0.4), \alpha_L^*(0.6), \alpha_L^*(0.8), \alpha_L^*(1)) = (0.185, 0.733, 0.933, 0.973, 0.975)$. The critical values for the product of p-values, $c_{\alpha(j)}$, $j = 1, \ldots, 5$, obtained from Eq. (26.5) with these spending function values are not decreasing, so that critical values satisfying these spending functions cannot be found using (26.5). In particular, because $c_{\alpha(1)} = \alpha_U^*(0.2)$, the small value of the spending function for the upper boundary at this first look results in $c_{\alpha(1)} < c_{\alpha(2)}$. Stopping boundaries were instead obtained using a slight modification of the triangular test spending function, with the values given in the second and third columns of Table 26.1.

Table 26.1: Critical values for the Stallard and Todd (2003) and Bauer and Kieser (1999) designs for the galantamine trial

Look (j)	Spending Functions $\alpha_L^*(t_j)$	$\alpha_U^*(t_j)$	Stallard and Todd Critical Values l_j	u_j	Bauer and Kieser Critical Values $\alpha_0^{(j)}$	$c_{\alpha^{(j)}}$
1	0.2	0.002	-0.461	10.1	0.800	0.002
2	0.7	0.01	4.01	12.0	0.373	0.00134
3	0.9	0.02	8.32	13.4	0.310	0.000691
4	0.97	0.024	14.2	16.0	0.125	0.000210
5	0.975	0.025	18.1	18.1	.	0.000140

The critical values for $Z_{S,j}$, l_j, and u_j obtained using the approach of Stallard and Todd (2003) are given in Table 26.1. The values are calculated assuming that for each of the three comparisons with control, the observed Fisher's information, V, increases by 10 at each interim analysis. Also given in Table 26.1 are the critical values for the products of p-values, $\alpha_0(j)$ and $c_{\alpha^{(j)}}$, for $j = 1, \ldots, 5$. The boundary values for the Stallard and Todd approach are also plotted against V in Figure 26.1. The figure shows the roughly triangular shape of the continuation region bounded by the stopping boundaries. The continuation region is similar in shape to the triangular tests of Whitehead (1997), but is moved upwards due to the selection of the best treatment at the first interim analysis.

Table 26.2 gives a summary of the comparison of each dose with the placebo at the first two interim analyses. The values of the efficient score, Z, and observed Fisher's information, V, for each comparison are obtained from expressions (26.1) and (26.2), so that Z represents the cumulative evidence of a difference between the dose group and placebo based on all of the data accumulated thus far in the trial. The p-values for the first interim analysis are given by $p_{i,1} = 1 - \Phi(Z_{i,1}/V_{i,1})$, $i = 1, \ldots, 3$, and so correspond to an analysis based on the asymptotic normality of the efficient score statistics $Z_{i,1}$. Because the full data for the trial were unavailable, the p-values that would be obtained from a similar analysis of the data from the new patients at the second interim analysis have been approximated by $p_{i,2} = 1 - \Phi((Z_{i,2} - Z_{i,1})/(V_{i,2} - V_{i,1}))$, $i = 1, \ldots, 3$, because the values of Z_i and V_i for the new patients' data are likely to be similar to the increments $(Z_{i,2} - Z_{i,1})$ and $(V_{i,2} - V_{i,1})$.

It can be seen that the values of observed Fisher's information, V, are close to the expected values of 10 at the first interim analysis and 20 at the second interim analysis. The values of the efficient score, Z, at the first interim analysis are plotted against the values of V in Figure 26.1. At this interim analysis, the 24 mg/day dose appears the best, so that this dose is considered for continuation

Table 26.2: Observed test statistics for the galantamine trial

Comparison	Look 1			Look 2		
	$Z_{i,1}$	$V_{i,1}$	$p_{i,1}$	$Z_{i,2}$	$V_{i,2}$	$p_{i,2}$
18 mg/day vs. placebo	4.28	11.79	0.1063	4.29	20.61	0.4987
24 mg/day vs. placebo	7.89	10.82	0.0082	13.78	19.58	0.0233
36 mg/day vs. placebo	4.64	11.01	0.0810	8.39	20.30	0.1093

along with the control in the Stallard and Todd (2003) design. As the value of Z for the comparison of this dose with the control is between l_1 and u_1 given in Table 26.1, the trial continues to the second interim analysis. At the second look, the value of Z for the comparison of the 24 mg/day dose with the placebo is 13.78. This value is also plotted in Figure 26.1. As it exceeds the value for u_2 given in Table 26.1, using the Stallard and Todd design, the trial would be stopped at this point and it would be concluded that the 24 mg/day dose is superior to the control.

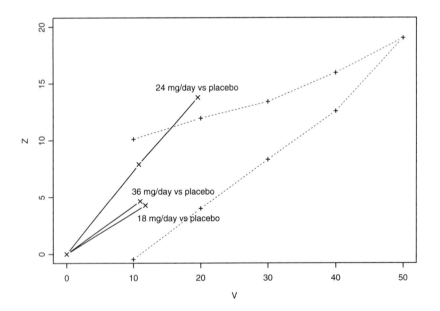

Figure 26.1: Group-sequential stopping boundary and sample paths for the galantamine trial with efficient score, Z, plotted against observed Fisher's information, V

With the Bauer and Kieser (1999) approach, the critical values are obtained exactly as in the case of comparison of a single experimental treatment with control. The correction for the use of multiple doses must be made in calculation of the p-values that are compared with those critical values. At the first stage there are three comparisons with control. A simple Bonferroni correction thus uses, as the p-value for the test of the global null hypothesis, the smallest of the three p-values observed and multiplies this by three. This gives a p_1 of $3 \times 0.0082 = 0.0246$. As this is larger than $c_{\alpha^{(1)}}$ and smaller than $\alpha_0^{(1)}$ from Table 26.1, the trial continues. With the Bauer and Kieser (1999) approach, any number of doses may continue to the second stage. We therefore illustrate how the trial would proceed in two different cases. In the first, as in the Stallard and Todd design, only the 24 mg/day dose proceeds to the second stage along with the placebo. In the second case, both the 18 and 24 mg/day doses continue to the second stage. This case might correspond to a situation in which the lowest effective dose is sought and it was considered that there was insufficient evidence from the first stage alone to reject the 18 mg/day dose.

In the first case, the p-value for comparison of the 24 mg/day dose with the control at the second stage does not need correcting for multiple comparisons as only one comparison is conducted at this interim analysis. The product of p-values is thus equal to $0.0246 \times 0.0233 = 0.000573$. In the second case, again applying a Bonferroni correction, now to allow for the two comparisons conducted at the second interim analysis, the product of p-values is equal to $0.0246 \times 2 \times 0.0233 = 0.001146$. In both cases, the product of p-values is smaller than $c_{\alpha^{(2)}}$ from Table 26.1, so that, as in the Stallard and Todd design, the trial would be stopped at this point.

26.4 Discussion and Future Directions

This chapter has provided a review of recent research work on designs for clinical trials that combine phases II and III, focusing in particular on the multistage approach of Stallard and Todd (2003) and the approach of Bauer and Kieser (1999) that may be extended to a multistage method using the technique proposed by Wassmer (1999). Although both the Stallard and Todd and the Bauer and Kieser methods achieve similar aims and may lead to the same conclusion, the underlying statistical methodology is different. The Stallard and Todd method is based on the group-sequential approach. This means that the number of experimental treatments that will be compared with the control treatment at each stage must be specified in advance. As formulated by Stallard and Todd, only a single experimental treatment is allowed to continue beyond the first interim analysis. This is in contrast to the Bauer and Kieser approach, which is based on the adaptive design approach of Bauer and Köhne (1994) and allows a great amount of flexibility in the design, including the possibility to continue with any number of experimental treatments at any stage. Although the adaptive designs have been criticized for a lack of power compared with the group-sequential approach due to the fact that the product of p-values used as a test statistic is not a sufficient statistic for the parameter of interest [see Jennison and Turnbull (2003) and Tsiatis and Mehta (2003)], the difference in power may be very small in practice [Kelly *et al.* (2005)]. A more severe practical problem may be the fact that for the adaptive design approach, the p-values are based on the separate data sets observed at each interim analysis. When the test used to construct the p-values is based on an asymptotic result, this may hold poorly in these small samples, leading to inaccurate type I error rates.

A feature of both multistage methods described above is that they formally test the global null hypothesis that all experimental treatments are of identical efficacy as the control. Rejection of the null hypothesis thus indicates that some experimental treatment is superior to the control, but does not give information on individual treatment comparisons. As an example, suppose that two experimental treatments are compared with a control using the Bauer and Kieser design, and that at the first interim analysis T_1 is superior to T_0 and T_2 is inferior. Suppose that the trial continues with both treatments and that at the second interim analysis, based on the new data, T_2 is superior to T_0 and T_1 is inferior. The corrected p-values from the two stages may be such that the global null hypothesis can be rejected based on the p-value product without rejection of either $H_{01} : \theta_1 = 0$ or $H_{02} : \theta_2 = 0$. The restriction in the Stallard and Todd approach that only the best experimental treatment from the first stage continues to subsequent stages means that the evidence against the null hypothesis from the different stages arises from comparison of the same experimental treatment with the control, so that this problem does not arise. In the Stallard and Todd design, the need to specify in advance the rule for deciding which treatments are to be used in the different stages might also be seen as an advantage by the regulatory authorities, who do not always look favourably on unplanned design modification.

Although, as reported above, great advances have been made recently in the methodology available for combined phase II/III clinical trials, this remains an area of active research. One outstanding challenge is the question of analysis after such a trial. Another is the use of information on a surrogate endpoint early in the trial as discussed by, for example, D'Agostino (2000), Zhang *et al.* (1997), and Shih *et al.* (2003). Whilst some work on the use of surrogate endpoints in the setting of combined phase II/phase III clinical trials has been undertaken [see, for example, Todd and Stallard (2005) and Stallard and Todd (2005)], some difficulties remain. The optimal design of trials of this sort, particularly the division of resources between assessment of several experimental treatments early in the trial and the more detailed comparison of a single experimental treatment with a control later in the trial, is also an area in which more work is needed.

Acknowledgements. The authors are grateful to Gernot Wassmer for assistance with implementation of the multistage adaptive design approach, to an anonymous referee for helpful comments on the chapter, and to Professor Auget and the organising committee of the International Conference on Statistics in Health Sciences for the opportunity to present this work. Some of the work reported here was developed at a workshop organised by the authors in Reading in March 2004. The authors are grateful to the UK Engineering and Physical Sciences Research Council for funding the workshop and to participants for their input.

References

1. Armitage, P., McPherson, C. K., and Rowe, B. C. (1969). Repeated significance tests on accumulating data, *Journal of the Royal Statistical Society, Series A*, **132**, 235–244.

2. Bauer P., and Kieser M. (1999). Combining different phases in the development of medical treatments within a single trial, *Statistics in Medicine*, **18**, 1833–1848.

3. Bauer, P., and Köhne, K. (1994). Evaluation of experiments with adaptive interim analyses, *Biometrics*, **51**, 1315–1324.

4. D'Agostino, R. B. (2000). Controlling alpha in a clinical trial: the case for secondary endpoints, *Statistics in Medicine*, **19**, 763–766.

5. Inoue, L. Y. T., Thall, P. F., and Berry, D. A. (2002). Seamlessly expanding a randomized phase II trial to phase III, *Biometrics*, **58**, 823–831.

6. Jennison, C., and Turnbull, B. W. (2000). *Group Sequential Methods with Applications to Clinical Trials*, Chapman & Hall, London.

7. Jennison, C., and Turnbull, B. W. (2003). Mid-course sample size modification in clinical trials based on the observed treatment effect, *Statistics in Medicine*, **22**, 971–993.

8. Kelly, P. J., Sooriyarachchi, M. R., Stallard, N., and Todd, S. (2005). A practical comparison of group-sequential and adaptive designs, *Journal of Biopharmaceutical Statistics*, **15**, 719–738.

9. Lan, K. K. G., and DeMets, D. L. (1983). Discrete sequential boundaries for clinical trials, *Biometrika*, **70**, 659–663.

10. Royston, P., Parmar, M. K. B., and Qian, W. (2003). Novel designs for multi-arm clinical trials with survival outcomes with an application in ovarian cancer, *Statistics in Medicine*, **22**, 2239–2256.

11. Schaid, D. J., Wieand, S., and Therneau, T. M. (1990). Optimal two-stage screening designs for survival comparisons, *Biometrika*, **77**, 507–513.

12. Scharfstein, D. O., Tsiatis, A. A., and Robins, J. M. (1987) Semiparametric efficiency and its implication on the design and analysis of group-sequential studies. *Journal of the American Statistical Association*, **92**, 1342-1350.

13. Shih, W. J., Ouyang, P., Quan, H., Lin, Y., Michiels, B., and Bijnens, L. (2003). Controlling type I error rate for fast track drug development programmes, *Statistics in Medicine*, **22**, 665–675.

14. Stallard, N., and Facey, K. M. (1996). Comparison of the spending function method and the Christmas tree correction for group sequential trials, *Journal of Biopharmaceutical Statistics*, **6**, 361–373.

15. Stallard, N., and Todd, S. (2003). Sequential designs for phase III clinical trials incorporating treatment selection, *Statistics in Medicine*, **22**, 689–703.

16. Stallard, N., and Todd, S. (2005). Point estimates and confidence regions for sequential trials involving selection, *Journal of Statistical Planning and Inference*, **135**, 402–419.

17. Thall, P. F., Simon, R., and Ellenberg, S. S. (1988). A two-stage design for choosing among several experimental treatments and a control in clinical trials, *Biometrics*, **45**, 537–547.

18. Thall, P. F., Simon, R., and Ellenberg, S. S. (1989). Two-stage selection and testing designs for comparative clinical trials, *Biometrika*, **75**, 303–310.

19. Todd, S., and Stallard, N. (2005). A new clinical trial design combining phases II and III: Sequential designs with treatment selection and a change of endpoint, *Drug Information Journal*, **39**, 109–118.

20. Tsiatis, A. A., and Mehta, C. (2003). On the inefficiency of the adaptive design for monitoring clinical trials, *Biometrika*, **90**, 367–378.

21. Wassmer, G. (1999). Multistage adaptive test procedures based on Fisher's product criterion, *Biometrical Journal*, **41**, 279–293.

22. Whitehead, J. (1997). *The Design and Analysis of Sequential Clinical Trials*, John Wiley & Sons, Chichester, UK.

23. Zhang, J., Quan, H., Ng, J., and Stepanavage, M. E. (1997). Some statistical methods for multiple endpoints in clinical trials, *Controlled Clinical Trials*, **18**, 204–221.

27

SCPRT: A Sequential Procedure That Gives Another Reason to Stop Clinical Trials Early

Xiaoping Xiong,[1] **Ming Tan,**[2] **and James Boyett**[1]

[1] *St. Jude Children's Research Hospital, Memphis, TN, USA*
[2] *University of Maryland, Baltimore, MD, USA*

Abstract: A sequential clinical trial is designed with given significance level and power to detect a certain difference in the parameter of interest and the trial will be stopped early when data collected at an early stage of the trial have produced enough, in one sense or another, evidence for the conclusion of the hypotheses. Different sequential test designs are available for a same requirement of significance level and power. On the other hand, a same set of observed data can be interpreted as outcomes of different sequential designs with the same significance level and power. Therefore for same observed data, the conclusion of a test may be significant by one sequential design but insignificant by another sequential test design. This phenomenon may lead to the question of whether applying sequential test design to clinical trials is rational. Withstanding this challenge, the sequential conditional probability ratio test (SCPRT) offers a special feature such that a conclusion made at an early stopping is unlikely to be reversed if the trial were not stopped but continued to the planned end. The SCPRT gives a sound reason to stop a trial early; that is, if the trial were not stopped as it should, then adding more data and continuing the trial by the planned end would not change the conclusion. With an SCPRT procedure, a sequential clinical trial is designed not only with given significance level and power, but also with a given probability of discordance which controls the chance that conclusion at an early stage would differ from that at the final stage of the trial. In particular, the SCPRT procedure based on Brownian motion on information time is simple to use and can be applied to clinical trials with different endpoints and different distributions.

Keywords and phrases: Sequential analysis, hypothesis testing

27.1   Introduction

Whether we realize it or not, clinical trials are experiments with human subjects and hence there is a conflict between the scientific merits of clinical trials and the ethical concerns on the trials in terms of sample sizes. The scientific merits of clinical trials require larger sample sizes for more reliable results, whereas the ethical concerns in clinical trials demand that fewer patients should be exposed to the inferior treatment. In addition, the scientific merits also conflict with the efficiency of clinical trials in light of the many potential research initiatives competing for clinical trials, whereas the number of patients and resources available for clinical trials is very limited. The sequential clinical trials provide a better solution to balance these conflicts, by which fewer patients will be exposed to the inferior treatment, the test is more efficient with smaller expected sample sizes, and investigators can monitor data at early stages of a trial. Motivated by improving the efficiency of sampling for inspection of ammunition production in World War II, Wald (1947) proposed the first sequential procedure as the sequential probability ratio test (SPRT) in the United States in 1943, and independently in the same year, Bernard (1946) proposed a similar sequential procedure as the problem of gambler's ruin in the United Kingdom. Since then, the sequential test procedures have been widely applied in industry, economics, business, and other fields. The application of sequential designs to clinical trials, although started in early 1950, did not sail smoothly through the clinical trial community. This is because some properties of sequential procedures are unappealing to clinical investigators. The past decades witnessed many authors' efforts to improve sequential designs to make them more suitable for clinical trials: for example, the sequential medical plans by Bross (1952) and Armitage (1957), the truncated SPRT by Anderson (1960), the uniformly most powerful (UMP) sequential test by Alling (1966), the direct method by Aroian (1968), the repeated significance tests by Armitage *et al.* (1969), the modified UMP sequential test by Breslow (1970), the Pocock boundaries by Pocock (1977), the O & F boundaries by O'Brien and Fleming (1979), the stochastic curtailing by Lan *et al.* (1982), the triangular sequential design by Whitehead and Stratton (1983), the spending function by Lan and DeMets (1983), and the repeated confidence interval approach by Jennison and Turnbull (1989). A recent book by Jennison and Turnbull (2000) summarizes various group-sequential methods and applications to clinical trials. The sequential procedure offers an advantage with smaller sample size on average as compared with the fixed sample test. However, the enthusiasm for sequential procedures by clinical trial investigators could have been discouraged by concerns such as, "Is the conclusion reliable?" when the trial was stopped early and the conclusion was drawn from a smaller sample, or, "Would the conclusion be reversed if the trial were not stopped and had got more samples?" On the other hand, although the sequential trial is expected to stop with a smaller sample size, it may end up with a substantially larger sample size than that of the fixed sample size test. The bottom line is that medical investigators are conservative and would be hesitant to use the sequential procedure if they do not feel confident about it. Consequently, the question is, what should be the ideal sequential test procedures for clinical trials? In our opinion, at least, an ideal sequential test procedure should be consistent in conclusions at different interim and final looks, and for which the efficiency of the test should be judged not only by the expected sample size but also by the maximum sample size.

27.2 The SCPRT Procedure

The Sequential Conditional Probability Ratio Test (SCPRT) procedure was proposed by Xiong (1993, 1995), based on one of the results in Xiong (1991). The special properties of SCPRT are that the (maximum) sample size of the sequential test is not larger than that of the (reference) fixed sample size test, and that the probability of discordance as a design parameter can be controlled to any small level, where the discordance is the disagreement between the conclusion reached by the sequential test and that by the fixed sample test at the final stage or the planned end. The SCPRT is derived using the ratio of maximum conditional likelihoods which are conditioned on the future value of the test statistic at the final stage. The likelihood ratio is the ratio of maximum likelihood that the test statistic at the final stage will end at the rejection region to the maximum likelihood that this test statistic will end at the acceptance region. The SCPRT procedures have been developed so far for several distributions such as binomial, normal, exponential, Poisson, Gamma, and Brownian motion in a technical report [Xiong (1993)] and published papers [Xiong (1995) and Xiong *et al.* (2003)]. In this paper, we sketch the basic concepts of SCPRT using the example of SCPRT for Brownian motion on information time for those who are mainly interested in clinical trial applications, and details of this procedure can be found in Xiong *et al.* (2003). For Brownian motion $S_t \sim N(\delta t, t)$ on information time $[0,1]$ to test hypotheses $H_0 : \delta \leq 0$ versus $H_a : \delta > 0$ with significance level α, the ratio of maximum conditional likelihoods is defined as

$$LR(t, S_t|z_\alpha) = \frac{\max_{\{s>z_\alpha\}} f(S_t|S_1 = s)}{\max_{\{s\leq z_\alpha\}} f(S_t|S_1 = s)}, \qquad (27.1)$$

where S_t is the test statistic at current information time t; S_1 is the S_t at future information time $t = 1$; $f(S_t|S_1)$ is the likelihood of S_t given S_1; z_α (upper α-quantile of standard normal distribution) is the cutoff value for S_1.

By taking the log of LR in (27.1), the stopping rule is defined as

$$\log(LR(t_k, S_{t_k}|z_\alpha)) > a \quad \text{or} \quad \log(LR(t_k, S_{t_k}|z_\alpha)) < -b, \qquad (27.2)$$

where a and b are positive numbers. Applications can be greatly simplified by letting $a = b$ which produces symmetric sequential boundaries. Derived from equations in (27.2) with $a = b$, the upper and lower boundaries for S_{t_k} are, respectively,

$$a_k = z_\alpha t_k + \sqrt{2at_k(1 - t_k)} \quad \text{and} \quad b_k = z_\alpha t_k - \sqrt{2at_k(1 - t_k)}, \qquad (27.3)$$

where $(t_1, \ldots, t_K)$ are the information times specified by investigators for the interim and final analyses. If the hypotheses are $H_0 : \delta \geq 0$ versus $H_a : \delta < 0$, then the upper and lower boundaries should be

$$a_k = -z_\alpha t_k + \sqrt{2at_k(1 - t_k)} \quad \text{and} \quad b_k = -z_\alpha t_k - \sqrt{2at_k(1 - t_k)}. \qquad (27.4)$$

The a in the above equations is called the boundary coefficient, and can be determined through the probability of discordance using Table 27.1. If investigators of a clinical trial are interested in only one side of the boundaries (e.g., the upper boundaries), then the other side of the boundaries (e.g., the lower boundaries) can be deleted. For the design after deletion, the power function (including its two special values, the significance level, and the power for detecting the given alternative) change very little if a small $\rho_{\max}$ was chosen for the design before deletion (e.g., $\rho_{\max} = 0.0054$). The $\rho_{\max}$ for the design after deletion is about half of that for the design before deletion.

Table 27.1: Boundary coefficient a for given K and ρ

For any K		Boundary Coefficient a				
ρ	ρ_{max}	$K = 2$	$K = 3$	$K = 4$	$K = 5$	$K = 6$
0.005	0.0012	3.315	3.895	4.227	4.459	4.636
0.01	0.0025	2.699	3.271	3.595	3.819	3.987
0.02	0.0054	2.109	2.645	2.953	3.166	3.327
0.03	0.0084	1.769	2.285	2.583	2.789	2.945
0.04	0.0116	1.532	2.031	2.320	2.521	2.672
0.05	0.0149	1.353	1.835	2.118	2.313	2.460
0.06	0.0183	1.209	1.678	1.951	2.142	2.287
0.08	0.0256	0.987	1.431	1.693	1.876	2.015
0.10	0.0331	0.821	1.243	1.494	1.669	1.803

27.2.1 Controlling the boundary

The only undetermined parameter in Eqs. (27.3) and (27.4) is the boundary coefficient a which controls the width of the continuation region between the upper and lower boundaries: the smaller the a, the narrower the region is. For a sequential design, it is critical to choose an appropriate a, which can be determined intuitively through using the probability of discordance defined as follows. Let D be the event that the sequential test and the non-sequential test at the final stage reach different conclusions on sequentially collected data. The probability of discordance $P_\delta(D)$ depends on δ, and is maximized at $\delta = z_\alpha$. The maximum probability of discordance is defined as $\rho_{\max} = \max_\delta P_\delta(D)$, and the maximum conditional probability of discordance is defined as $\rho = \max_s P(D|S_1 = s)$. The relationships among a and $\rho_{\max}$ and ρ are given in Table 27.1, in which K is the total number of interim looks and the final look. The principle for choosing an appropriate a is that the design should be as efficient as possible, while keeping the significance level and power of the sequential test about the same as that of the fixed sample size test at the final stage. The smaller the a, the larger are ρ and $\rho_{\max}$, and the smaller is the expected sample size. Because a smaller $\rho_{\max}$ is desirable and a larger expected sample size is undesirable, one has to choose the a by balancing the two opposite desirabilities in accordance with the very utility in the clinical trial. In general, we recommend to choose an a that produces $\rho = 0.02$ or $\rho_{\max} = 0.0054$, which implies that on average there are 5.4 cases of reversing conclusion in 1000 trials using this design under the most unfavorable scenario ($\delta = z_\alpha$).

27.2.2 Boundaries in terms of *P*-values

For practical convenience, users may prefer sequential boundaries in terms of the (nominal) critical P-values, and accordingly the sequential test statistic in terms of the (nominal) observed P-value. At information time t_k, the variance of test statistic S_t is $\mathrm{Var}(S_{t_k}) = t_k$; then the upper and lower boundaries can be standardized by $a_k, b_k / \sqrt{\mathrm{Var}(S_{t_k})} = z_\alpha \sqrt{t_k} \pm \sqrt{2a(1-t_k)}$. For testing hypotheses $H_0 : \delta \leq 0$ versus $H_a : \delta > 0$, the (nominal) critical P-values (critical significance levels) are

$$P_{a_k} = 1 - \Phi\left(z_\alpha\sqrt{t_k} + \sqrt{2a(1-t_k)}\right) \quad \text{and} \quad P_{b_k} = 1 - \Phi\left(z_\alpha\sqrt{t_k} - \sqrt{2a(1-t_k)}\right)$$

$$(27.5)$$

for the upper and lower boundaries, respectively. The test statistic S_k can be standardized as $S_{t_k} / \sqrt{\mathrm{Var}(S_{t_k})} = S_{t_k} / \sqrt{t_k}$. Hence, the (nominal) observed P-value at stage k is

$$P_{S_k} = 1 - \Phi\left(S_{t_k} / \sqrt{t_k}\right). \qquad (27.6)$$

The trial should be stopped if the observed P-value $\leq$ critical P-value on the upper boundary, or $\geq$ critical P-value on the lower boundary. If the hypotheses are $H_0 : \delta \geq 0$ versus $H_a : \delta < 0$, then the critical P-values are

$$P_{a_k} = \Phi\left(-z_\alpha\sqrt{t_k} + \sqrt{2a(1-t_k)}\right) \quad \text{and} \quad P_{b_k} = \Phi\left(-z_\alpha\sqrt{t_k} - \sqrt{2a(1-t_k)}\right)$$

$$(27.7)$$

for the upper and lower boundaries, respectively; and the observed P-value at stage k is

$$P_{S_k} \quad = \quad \Phi\left(S_{t_k}/\sqrt{t_k}\right). \tag{27.8}$$

The trial should be stopped if the observed P-value $\geq$ critical P-value on the upper boundary, or $\leq$ critical P-value on the lower boundary. The observed P-value in (27.6) or (27.8) at stage k is actually same as the P-value (of one-sided test) for the regular nonsequential test applied to the data up to stage k, which is available from regular analysis of updated data using SAS, SPlus, or other statistical packages.

27.3   An Example

Assume the X_is are normally distributed with mean μ_x and variance $\sigma_x^2 = 1$, and the Y_is are normally distributed with mean μ_y and variance $\sigma_y^2 = 1.5^2$. To test $H_0 : \mu_x \leq \mu_y$ versus $H_a : \mu_x > \mu_y$, with significance level $\alpha = 0.05$ and power $1 - \beta = 0.8$ for detecting an alternative $\delta = \mu_x - \mu_y = 0.3$, the sample sizes for a nonsequential test are calculated as $m = m_x = m_y = 224$. For the sequential test, assume the interim and final looks are planned when 25%, 50%, 75%, and 100% of the data are collected; hence the information times are $(0.25, 0.5, 0.75, 1)$ and sample sizes are $(56, 112, 168, 224)$ for those looks. The test statistic is

$$S_{t_k} \quad = \quad n_k(\bar{X}_{n_k} - \bar{Y}_{n_k})/\sqrt{m(\sigma_x^2 + \sigma_y^2)}, \tag{27.9}$$

where $t_k = n_k/m$ for $k = 1,\ldots,4$. Assume $\rho = 0.02$; then $a = 2.953$ and $\rho_{\max} = 0.0054$ from Table 27.1. The SCPRT upper and lower boundaries are $(1.4635, 2.0375, 2.2860, 1.6449)$ and $(-0.6411, -0.3927, 0.1813, 1.6449)$ by Eq. (27.3). The critical P-values are $(0.0017, 0.002, 0.0042, 0.05)$ for the upper boundary and $(0.9001, 0.7107, 0.4171, 0.05)$ for the lower boundary by Eq. (27.5).

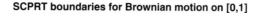

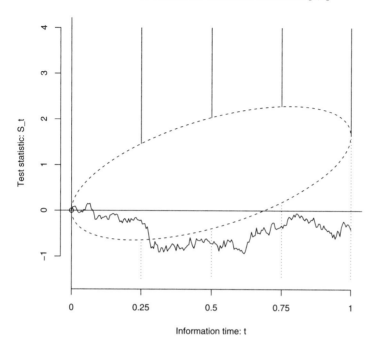

Figure 27.1: Sequential test statistic S_t simulated under H_0: $\mu_x - \mu_y = 0$

Under H_0 assuming $\mu_x = \mu_y = 0$, we simulated 224 X_is and 224 Y_is, from which the test statistic S_t was a process on information time interval $[0,1]$ emulating a Brownian motion, as shown in Figure 27.1. On the four interim and final looks, $(S_{t_1}, \ldots, S_{t_4}) = (-0.2083, -0.7161, -0.3262, -0.4142)$ and the observed P-values $= (0.6615, 0.8444, 0.6468, 0.6606)$. The observed P-value is greater than the critical P-value of the lower boundary at $k = 2$ (i.e., $0.8444 > 0.7107$) and hence the trial should be stopped with sample size $n_2 = 112$ and a conclusion of not significant. As shown in Figure 27.1, the test statistic S_t exited the lower boundary at $t_2 = 0.5$, and if the trial did not stop as it should at $t_2 = 0.5$ but continued to the planned end, then the test statistic at $t_4 = 1$ would fall in the acceptance region and the conclusion would still be the same as not significant.

Under H_a assuming $\mu_x = 0.4$ and $\mu_y = 0$, a simulation similar to the above leads to a process of test statistic S_t as plotted in Figure 27.2. On the four looks $(S_{t_1}, \ldots, S_{t_4}) = (0.8004, 2.3843, 2.6519, 3.3241)$ and the observed P-values $= (0.0547, 0.0004, 0.0011, 0.0004)$. The observed P-value is smaller than the critical P-value of the upper boundary at $k = 2$ (i.e., $0.0004 < 0.002$) and

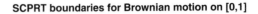

SCPRT boundaries for Brownian motion on [0,1]

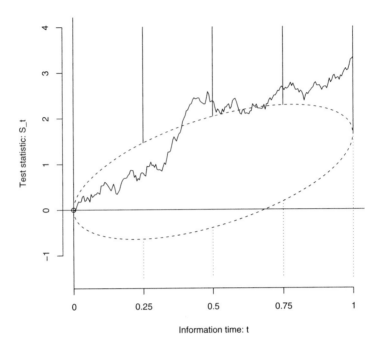

Figure 27.2: Sequential test statistic S_t simulated under H_a: $\mu_x - \mu_y = 0.3$

hence the trial should be stopped with sample size $n_2 = 112$ and conclusion of significant. As shown in Figure 27.2, the test statistic S_t exited the upper boundary at $t_2 = 0.5$, and if the trial did not stop as it should at $t_2 = 0.5$ but continued to the planned end, then the test statistic at $t_4 = 1$ would fall in the rejection region and the conclusion would still be the same as significant.

27.4   SCPRT with Unknown Variance

In the statistical design of clinical trials, the variance σ^2 has to be assumed known for calculating the sample size and the test statistic. However, in reality, the variance is usually unknown and its estimate $\hat{\sigma}^2$ is used for the sample size calculation, which leads to a loss of power. In the table below, for a nonsequential test designed with significance level $\alpha = 0.05$ and power $1 - \beta = 0.8$, the actual (overall) power is calculated for different n which is the sample size for $\hat{\sigma}^2$. For example, the actual power is 0.74 instead of 0.8 when $n = 10$.

Sample size for $\hat{\sigma}^2$: n	10	20	30	40	80	100
Overall power: $E(1-\hat{\beta})$	0.74	0.772	0.781	0.786	0.793	0.795

For a clinical trial design in which $\hat{\sigma}^2$ instead of σ^2 was used for calculating sample size, in order to reach a targeted overall power $1-\beta$, the loss of power can be compensated by using a nominal power $1-\beta^*$ which is a solution of the equation,

$$1 - \beta = (1 - \beta^*) - \frac{\phi(z_{\beta*})}{4(n-1)}\left\{(z_\alpha + z_{\beta*}) + (z_\alpha + z_{\beta*})^2 z_{\beta*}\right\}.$$

For significance level $\alpha = 0.05$ and the targeted power $1-\beta = 0.80$, the nominal power $1-\beta^*$ is calculated for different n in the table below. For example, for $n = 10$, $1-\beta^* = 0.867$ which is substantially larger than the targeted power $1-\beta = 0.8$.

n for $\hat{\sigma}^2$	10	20	30	40	80	100
Nominal power $1-\beta^*$	0.867	0.831	0.82	0.815	0.807	0.806

We now give a nonsequential test procedure that guarantees significance level and power for any unknown true σ^2. Assume σ^2 is estimated by $\hat{\sigma}^2$ with sample size $n = 20$ and then this $\hat{\sigma}^2$ is used to calculate the sample size $\hat{m}^*$ (an estimate of m^*) for a design of a test with significance level $\alpha = 0.05$ and targeted power $1-\beta^* = 0.831$ (corresponding to $n = 20$ in the table above). The conditional power for this test given $\hat{\sigma}^2$ is $1-\hat{\beta}^*$ which is random and unknown (because it depends on the random $\hat{\sigma}^2$ and the unknown σ^2). However, the overall power for this procedure (that includes estimating σ^2, calculating the sample size of the test using $\hat{\sigma}^2$, and carrying out a test with sample size $\hat{m}^*$) is $E(1-\hat{\beta}^*) = 0.80(= 1-\beta)$ for any unknown true σ^2.

Based on the nonsequential test procedure above, we then develop an adaptive SCPRT procedure for which the significance level and power of a sequential test procedure can be retained for any true variance. This procedure was built on the property that the SCPRT is a sequential test in accordance with conclusions of the nonsequential test with the same significance and power. At each look k, σ^2 is reestimated as $\hat{\sigma}^2_k$, and by which the final sample size (unknown m) is reestimated as $\hat{m}_k$. Then the SCPRT boundaries are recalculated using the updated estimate of final sample size $\hat{m}_k$. The upper quantile of t distribution, $t_\alpha(n-1)$, is used (instead of z_α for the standard normal distribution) for calculating the boundaries. Ultimately, the adaptive SCPRT design keeps the power of the test for any unknown true σ^2. For example, to test hypotheses of $\mu_0 = 0$ versus $\mu_a = 0.5$ with significance level $\alpha = 0.05$ and power $1-\beta = 0.8$, the operating characteristics (OC) for the adaptive SCPRT (t-test) are given in Table 27.2, in which different scenarios are assumed for the unknown true variance σ^2 $(= 1, 16, 64)$ and the maximum conditional probability of discordance ρ $(= 0.005, 0.02)$.

Table 27.2: OC for the adaptive SCPRT with unknown variance

True σ^2	Fixed Sample Size Test with Known σ^2 Sample Size m	Adaptive SPCRT with Unknown σ^2 t-Test; Nominal $\alpha = 0.04$				
		ρ	α	$1 - \beta$	$E_{\mu_0} N$	$E_{\mu_a} N$
1	25	0.005	0.051	0.802	22.2	24.6
		0.02	0.053	0.802	20.8	23.5
16	396	0.005	0.045	0.797	353	391
		0.02	0.050	0.790	323	367
64	1583	0.005	0.047	0.796	1416	1570
		0.02	0.053	0.790	1296	1470

27.5 Clinical Trials with Survival Data

In this section, we apply SCPRT procedures to clinical trials for comparing two survival curves (treatment and control). There are two scenarios for this type of sequential procedures. The first scenario is for regular clinical trials in which enrollments for the treatment group and control group are both prospective, and synchronize in proportion of total enrollments at each stage. The second scenario is for the clinical trials with historical controls, in which the enrollment of the control group had been completed before the start of the clinical trial, whereas the treatment group is prospectively and sequentially enrolled. For this scenario, the comparison at each stage is between the partially enrolled treatment group and the whole control group.

Assume observations for the treatment group are X_is with hazard rate λ_x, and observations for control group are Y_is with hazard rate λ_y. The hypotheses of interest are $H_0 : r \leq 1$ versus $H_a : r > 1$, where $r = \lambda_y/\lambda_x$. Let m_x and m_y be sample sizes for the treatment and control groups, respectively. Let $\pi = m_x/(m_x + m_y)$ and $1 - \pi = m_y/(m_x + m_y)$ be proportions of pooled patients for the two groups. Let a be the length of the enrollment period and f be the length of the followup period in the clinical trial, and a and f are the same for both groups. Assume $G_x(t)$ and $G_y(t)$ are survival functions for X_i and Y_i, respectively. Let $A = (1/6)\{G_x(f) + 4G_x(0.5a + f) + G_x(a + f)\}$ and $B = (1/6)\{G_y(f) + 4G_y(0.5a + f) + G_y(a + f)\}$, as in Collett (2003). Suppose we want to test the hypothesis with significance level α and power $1 - \beta$ for detecting alternative r_a. For the first scenario of sequential design, the proportion π should have been given, by which the (maximum) sample size of the control group is

$$m_y = \frac{(z_\alpha + z_\beta)^2}{\pi[1 - B - \pi(A - B)](\log r_a)^2}, \qquad (27.10)$$

and the sample size of the treatment group is $m_x = m_y\pi/(1-\pi)$. For the second scenario of sequential design, the sample size of control group m_y should have been given; then the proportion π is calculated as the solution of Eq. (27.10), and by which the sample size of the treatment group is $m_x = m_y\pi/(1 - \pi)$.

In a uniform way, we describe how to calculate the sequential test statistic for the two scenarios of sequential designs. Assume distinct event times $\tau_1 < \tau_2 < \cdots < \tau_j < \cdots$ across two groups, where the event time is defined as the length of time from the accrual to the event for a patient. At time τ_j, let d_j^x be the number of events in the treatment group and d_j^y the number of events in the control group. Let n_j^x and n_j^y be the numbers of patients at risk just before time τ_j for the two groups. Consequently, $d_j = d_j^x + d_j^y$ is the total number of events at time τ_j among a total of $n_j = n_j^x + n_j^y$ patients just before τ_j. At the kth look of the sequential clinical trial, let $\tau^*(k)$ be the calendar time, and by which a log-rank score is defined as $U_k = \sum_j(d_{j\tau^*(k)}^x - e_{j\tau^*(k)}^x)$, where $d_{j\tau^*(k)}^x$, $e_{j\tau^*(k)}^x$, $n_{j\tau^*(k)}^x$, $d_{j\tau^*(k)}$, and $n_{j\tau^*(k)}$ are those as d_j^x, e_j^x, n_j^x, d_j, and n_j but calculated from the data up to calendar time $\tau^*(k)$. The variance of U_k is $V_k = \sum_j v_{j\tau^*(k)}^x$, where $v_{j\tau^*(k)}^x = n_{j\tau^*(k)}^x n_j^y d_{j\tau^*(k)}(n_{j\tau^*(k)} - d_{j\tau^*(k)})/n_{j\tau^*(k)}^2(n_{j\tau^*(k)} - 1)$. We define the sequential test statistic as $S_{t_k} = U_k/V_K^{*1/2}$ for $k = 1, \ldots, K - 1$, where $V_K^* = \{(z_\alpha + z_\beta)/\{\ln(r_a)\}^2$ is the projected final variance; $t_k = V_k/V_K^*$ is the projected information time. At the final stage K, the true variance V_K is used instead of V_K^*, and so $t_K = 1$ and $S_{t_K} = U_K/V_K^{1/2}$. For sequential procedures with survival data, the information time t_k cannot be specified in advance, but can be calculated from V_k with data up to the stage k, where the kth look is designed according to the calendar time or the number of patients enrolled since the start of the clinical trial. At stage k, the SCPRT boundaries for S_{t_k} can be calculated by (27.3) with information time t_k and boundary coefficient a which was determined from the prespecified probability of discordance ρ and the total number of looks K. For practical convenience, one does not need to calculate S_{t_k}s. The observed P-value P_{S_k} is available as the P-value from regular survival (nonsequential) test applying to the data up to stage k, for which the critical P-values P_{a_k} and P_{b_k} are available by (27.5) or (27.7) with $t_k = V_k/V_K^*$. If at some stage k for the first time, P_{S_k} is less than or equal to P_{a_k}, or greater than or equal to P_{b_k}, then the trial will be stopped. We illustrate here the SCPRT procedure for the design and analysis of clinical trials with survival data using a simulation example below.

Example: Assume X_is are distributed with Exponential(μ_x) with hazard $\lambda_x = 1/\mu_x$ for the treatment group, and assume Y_is are distributed with Exponential(μ_y) with hazard $\lambda_y = 1/\mu_y$ for the control group. Suppose hypotheses $H_0 : r \leq 1$ versus $H_a : r > 1$ are to be tested with $\alpha = 0.05$ and power $1 - \beta = 0.8$ for detecting $r_a = 1.6$ for r $(= \lambda_y/\lambda_x = \mu_x/\mu_y)$. Assume the length of the accrual period in clinical trial is $a = 4$ years, and assume the length of the follow-up period is $f = 1$ year. Assume interim and final looks are planned at calendar time $(2, 3, 4, 5)$ years from the start of the clinical trial. For sample size calculation, assume $\mu_y = 5$ years and thus under H_a we have $\mu_x = 8$ years. Hence $G_y(t) = e^{-0.2t}$ and $G_x(t) = e^{-0.125t}$, by which $A = 0.6945$ and $B = 0.5636$ are calculated. For the first scenario of sequential design (i.e., for regular clinical trials with prospective enrollment for both treatment and control groups), assume $\pi = 0.5$ (sample sizes of two groups are equal), then $m_y = m_x = 151$ by Eq. (27.10). For the second scenario of sequential design (for the clinical trials with historical controls), assume the sample size for controls is $m_y = 170$, then the proportion for treatment group $\pi = 0.5843$ is calculated by (27.10), and hence $m_x = 140$.

We now simulate data for the second sequential design scenario, for which sample sizes $m_x = 140$ and $m_y = 170$. With interim and final looks at 2, 3, 4, and 5 years, the information times $(t_1, \ldots, t_4) = (0.3889, 0.6264, 0.8725, 1)$ are calculated from simulated data. The SCPRT upper boundary $(a_1, \ldots, a_4) = (0.5451, 0.1453, -0.6244, -1.6449)$ and lower boundary $(b_1, \ldots, b_4) = (-1.8243, -2.2060, -2.2457, -1.6449)$ by Eq. (27.4), for which the boundary coefficient $a = 2.953$ from Table 27.1 for a specified $\rho = 0.02$ ($\rho_{\max} = 0.0054$) and $K = 4$. The sequential test statistic at the four stages is $(S_{t_1}, \ldots, S_{t_4}) = (-1.0476, -2.2299, -2.6425, -3.0113)$. The clinical trial should stop at the second stage because the test statistic crosses the boundaries for the first time at $(S_{t_2} = -2.2299 \leq -2.2060 = b_2)$. The decision made at the second stage is in accordance with that made at the planned end if the study were not stopped, that is, both rejecting H_0. In terms of nominal P-values for practical convenience, the critical P-values are $(P_{a_1}, \ldots, P_{a_4}) = (0.809, 0.573, 0.252, 0.05)$ for upper boundaries (for acceptance of H_0), and are $(P_{b_1}, \ldots, P_{b_4}) = (0.0017, 0.0027, 0.0081, 0.05)$ for lower boundaries (for rejection of H_0), calculated by (27.7). The observed P-values are $(P_{S_1}, \ldots, P_{S_4}) = (0.0465, 0.0024, 0.0023, 0.0013)$, calculated by (27.8).

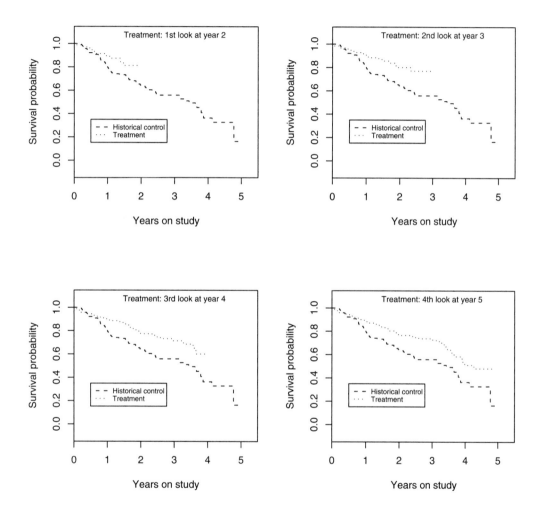

Figure 27.3: Clinical trial with historical control: survival curves at different looks

27.6   Conclusion

Ethical consideration and availability of patients are major concerns for statistical designs of clinical trials. Sequential procedures lessen the conflict between the scientific merits and the ethical concerns of clinical trials in terms of sample sizes, and improve the efficiency of clinical trials by having smaller expected sample sizes. However, medical investigators are hesitant to apply sequential procedures for designing studies because some properties of sequential procedures are not suitable for this application. SCPRT procedures meet the challenge by providing properties useful in clinical trials, especially one that provides a sound reason (from a scientific point of view) to stop a trial early: *if the trial were not stopped as it should, then adding more data and continuing the trial until the planned end would not change the conclusion.* A sequential clinical trial by SCPRT is designed not only with given significance level and power, but also with a given probability of discordance. The SCPRT procedure based on Brownian motion on information time is simple to use, and in particular is appropriate for clinical trials that compare two populations for which distributions are not normal. The distribution of the observed difference between two groups usually approximates the normal distribution well even when sample sizes are small, and thus meets the application condition for the SCPRT procedure based on Brownian motion on information time. Computer software for implementing the designs described in this paper is available from the Web site www.stjuderesearch.org/depts/biostats.

Acknowledgements. The research work was supported in part by CA 21765 and by the American Lebanese Syrian Associated Charities, the fund raising arm of St. Jude Children's Research Hospital, both in Memphis, Tennessee, USA.

References

1. Anderson, T. W. (1960). A modification of the sequential probability ratio test to reduce the sample size, *Annals of Mathematical Statistics*, **31**, 165–197.

2. Alling, D. M. (1966). Closed sequential tests for binomial probabilities, *Biometrika*, **53**, 73–84.

3. Armitage, P. (1957). Restricted sequential procedure, *Biometrika*, **44**, 9–26.

4. Armitage, P., McPherson, C. K., and Rowe, B. C. (1969). Repeated significance tests on accumulating data, *Journal of the Royal Statistical Society, Series A*, **132**, 235–244.

5. Aroian, L. A. (1968). Sequential analysis, direct method, *Technometrics*, **10**, 125–132.

6. Bernard, G. A. (1946). Sequential tests in industrial statistics, *Journal of the Royal Statistical Society*, **8** (1), *Suppl.* 1–21.

7. Breslow, N. (1970). Sequential modification of the UMP test for binomial probabilities, *Journal of the American Statistical Association*, **65**, 639–648.

8. Bross, I. (1952). Sequential medical plans, *Biometrics*, **8**, 188–205.

9. Collett, D. (2003). *Modeling Survival Data in Medical Research*, 2nd edition, Chapman & Hall/CRC, London.

10. Jennison, C., and Turnbull, B. W. (1989). Interim analyses: The repeated confidence interval approach (with discussion), *Journal of the Royal Statistical Society, Series B*, **51**, 305–361.

11. Jennison, C., and Turnbull, B. W. (2000). *Group Sequential Methods with Applications to Clinical Trials*, Chapman & Hall/CRC, New York.

12. Lan, K. K. G., Simon, R., and Halperin, M. (1982). Stochastically curtailed tests in long-term clinical trials, *Sequential Analysis*, **1**, 207–219.

13. Lan, K. K. G., and DeMets, D. L. (1983). Discrete sequential boundaries for clinical trials, *Biometrika*, **70**, 659-663.

14. O'Brien, P. C., and Fleming, T. R. (1979). A multiple testing procedure for clinical trials, *Biometrics*, **35**, 549–556.

15. Pocock, S. J. (1977). Group sequential methods in the design and analysis of clinical trials, *Biometrika*, **64**, 191–199.

16. Wald, A. (1947). *Sequential Analysis*, John Wiley & Sons, New York.

17. Whitehead, J., and Stratton, I. (1983). Group sequential clinical trials with triangular continuation regions, *Biometrics*, **39**, 227–236.

18. Xiong, X. (1991). Sequential analysis for hypergeometric distribution, *Ph.D. Dissertation*, Department of Statistics, Purdue University, W. Lafayette, Indiana.

19. Xiong, X. (1993). Principle of generalized conditional PLR sequential test and its applications, *Technical Report 93-15*, Department of Statistics, Purdue University, W. Lafayette, Indiana.

20. Xiong, X. (1995). A class of sequential conditional probability ratio tests, *Journal of the American Statistical Association*, **90**, 1463–1473.

21. Xiong, X., Tan, M., and Boyett, J. (2003). Sequential conditional probability ratio tests for normalized test statistic on information time, *Biometrics*, **59**, 624–631.

PART VIII
MODELS FOR THE ENVIRONMENT

Seasonality Assessment for Biosurveillance Systems

Elena N. Naumova and Ian B. MacNeill

Tufts University School of Medicine, Boston, MA, USA
University of Western Ontario, London, ON, Canada

Abstract: Biosurveillance systems for infectious diseases typically deal with nonlinear time series. This nonlinearity is due to the non-Gaussian and non-stationary nature of an outcome process. Infectious diseases (ID), waterborne and foodborne enteric infections in particular, are typically characterized by a sequence of sudden outbreaks, which are often followed by long low endemic levels. Multiple outbreaks occurring within a relatively short time interval form a seasonal pattern typical for a specific pathogen in a given population. Seasonal variability in the probability of exposure combined with a partial immunity to a pathogen adds to the complexity of seasonal patterns. Although seasonal variation is a well-known phenomenon in the epidemiology of enteric infections, simple analytical tools for examination, evaluation, and comparison of seasonal patterns are limited. This obstacle also limits analysis of factors associated with seasonal variations. The objectives of this paper are to outline the notion of seasonality, to define characteristics of seasonality, and to demonstrate tools for assessing seasonal patterns and the effects of environmental factors on such patterns. To demonstrate these techniques, we conducted a comparative study of seasonality in *Salmonella* cases as reported by the state surveillance system in relation to seasonality in ambient temperature, and found that the incidence in *Salmonella* infection peaked two weeks after a peak in temperature. The results suggest that ambient temperature can be a potential predictor of *Salmonella* infections at a seasonal scale.

Keywords and phrases: Seasonality, δ-method, ambient temperature, *Salmonella* infection, biosurveillance

28.1   Introduction

We define "disease seasonality" as systematic periodic fluctuations within the course of a year that can be characterized by the magnitude, timing, and duration of a seasonal increase. Variations in seasonal characteristics in temporal, spatial, or demographic contexts provide important clues to factors influencing disease occurrence. We consider stability in seasonality, expressed by some measure of variation in the above-mentioned characteristics of a seasonal pattern, as an indicator of synchronization in disease incidence by environmental and/or social processes. Meteorological factors, and ambient temperature in particular, appear to be critically linked to seasonal patterns of disease. Recent studies indicate that meteorological disturbances may influence the emergence and proliferation of water- or foodborne pathogens. It is quite plausible that seasonal fluctuation in ambient temperature might affect the timing and intensity of infectious outbreaks. Therefore, we examined seasonal patterns in both infections and temperature time series and then compared characteristics of seasonality.

28.1.1   Conceptual framework for seasonality assessment

This synchronization in disease incidence and environmental factors can be viewed as a special case when multiple time series exhibit common periodicities [MacNeill (1977)]. The conceptual format for measuring the temporal relation between seasonal patterns in environmental temperatures and disease incidence is shown in Figure 28.1. Considering two characteristics of seasonality: the magnitude and the timing of a seasonal peak, we define a set of measures. The measures related to timing are (1) the position of the maximum point on the seasonal curve of exposure (i.e., temperature) or disease incidence, (2) the position of the minimum point on the seasonal curve of exposure or disease incidence, and (3) the lag, which is the difference between time of exposure maximum and time of disease incidence maximum. The magnitude related measures are (1) maximum value on the seasonal curve of exposure or incidence of disease, (2) minimum value on the seasonal curve of exposure or incidence of disease, (3) the amplitude, which is the difference between maximum and minimum values on the seasonal curve for exposure or incidence of disease, and (4) the relative intensity, which is the ratio of maximum value and minimum value on the seasonal curve. Thus, the task of measuring the temporal relation between seasonal patterns is translated to the problem of estimating the lag and associations among measures of timing and intensity.

This concept is easy to express via Model 1 as follows.

$$Y(t) = \gamma \cos(2\pi\omega t + \psi) + e(t), \tag{28.1}$$

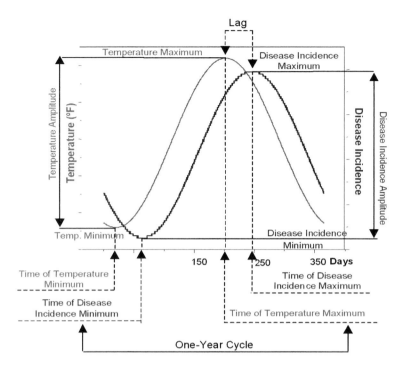

Figure 28.1: Characteristics of seasonality: Graphical depiction and definition for daily time series of exposure (ambient temperature) and outcome (disease incidence) variables

where $Y(t)$ is a time series, the periodic component has a frequency of ω, an amplitude of γ, and a phase angle of ψ, and $\{e(t),\ t = 1, 2, \ldots, n\}$ is an i.i.d. sequence of random variables with $E[e(t)] = 0$ and $\text{Var}[e(t)] = \sigma^2$. From a user standpoint, this model offers the highly desirable property of being easy to interpret. The model describes a seasonal curve by a cosine function with symmetric rise and fall over a period of a full year. The locations of two points at which this seasonal curve peaks and has the lowest value can be determined using a shift, or phase angle parameter, ψ. This parameter reflects the timing of the peak relative to the origin. For convenience, an origin can be set at the beginning of a calendar year, January 1. So, if $\psi = 0$, there is no shift of a peak relative to the origin. If $\psi = \pi$, the peak shifts to the summer, that is, to the 182nd day. If $\pi < \psi < 2\pi$, there is a shift toward fall; or if $\psi < \pi$, there is a shift toward spring. The parameter can be used for seasonality comparison and can be expressed in days. The amplitude of fluctuations between two extreme points is controlled via a parameter γ; if $\gamma = 0$, there is no seasonal increase.

This Model 1 is equivalent to Model 2:

$$Y(t) = \beta_1 \sin(2\pi\omega t) + \beta_2 \cos(2\pi\omega t) + e(t), \tag{28.2}$$

which is more convenient to fit by least squares, a procedure available in much commercial statistical software. Below we demonstrate an approach that allows us to combine the ease of fitting Model 2 and the simplicity and elegance of interpretation of Model 1, by using the δ-method.

28.2 δ-Method in Application to a Seasonality Model

This methodology, whose origin is remote, enables one to obtain a workable approximation to the mean, variances, and covariances of a function of random variables whose means and variances are either known or for which there exist consistent estimators.

28.2.1   Single-variable case

Let X be a random variable with $E(X) = \mu$ and $\text{Var}(X) = \sigma^2$. Also let $X_1, X_2, \ldots, X_n$, be a sequence of i.i.d. random variables each with the same distribution as X. If $\overline{X}_n = n^{-1} \sum_{i=1}^{n} X_i$, then $E(\overline{X}_n) = \mu$ and $\sigma^2_{\overline{X}_n} = \sigma^2/n$. Hence, $\overline{X}_n \to \mu$ as $n \to \infty$, where convergence is in each of: probability, a.e., and mean square. Now let $f()$ be a function of one variable that may be expanded in Taylor's series; that is,

$$f(x) = f(x_0) + (x - x_0)f'(x_0) + \frac{(x - x_0)^2}{2!} f''(x_0) + \cdots \quad .$$

In consequence of the above,

$$Y_n = f\left(\overline{X}_n\right) = f(\mu) + \left(\overline{X}_n - \mu\right) f'(\mu) + O\left(\frac{1}{n}\right).$$

Because $\overline{X}_n \to \mu$, $f\left(\overline{X}_n\right) \to f(\mu)$, and $f'\left(\overline{X}_n\right) \to f'(\mu)$,

$$
\begin{aligned}
&f\left(\overline{X}_n\right) - f(\mu) \\
&= \left(\overline{X}_n - \mu\right) \left[f'(\overline{X}_n) - \left\{ f'(\overline{X}_n) - f'(\mu) \right\} \right] + O\left(\frac{1}{n}\right) \\
&= \left(\overline{X}_n - \mu\right) f'(\overline{X}_n) - \left(\overline{X}_n - \mu\right) \left\{ f'(\overline{X}_n) - f'(\mu) \right\} + O\left(\frac{1}{n}\right) \\
&= \left(\overline{X}_n - \mu\right) f'(\overline{X}_n) + O\left(\frac{1}{n}\right).
\end{aligned}
$$

Therefore, $E\left[Y_n - f(\mu)\right]^2 = E\left[\overline{X}_n - \mu\right]^2 \left\{ f'\left(\overline{X}_n\right) \right\}^2 + O\left(\frac{1}{n^{1/2}}\right)$. That is

$$\sigma^2_{Y_n} = \sigma^2_{\overline{X}_n} \left\{ f'\left(\overline{X}_n\right) \right\}^2 + O\left(\frac{1}{n^{1/2}}\right),$$

where σ^2 may be estimated consistently by $\hat{\sigma}^2 = n^{-1} \sum_{i=1}^{n} \left(X_i - \hat{X}_n \right)^2$. Thus, for large samples: $E[Y_n] \cong f' \left(\overline{X}_n \right)$ and $\sigma_{Y_n}^2 \cong \left\{ f' \left(\overline{X}_n \right) \right\}^2 (\hat{\sigma}_{Xn}^2 / n)$.

28.2.2 Two-variables case

Let $f(\cdot, \cdot)$ be a function of two random variables X and Y, whose means (μ_x and μ_y), variances (σ_x^2 and σ_y^2), and covariance (σ_{xy}) are known. Consider the first few terms in the Taylor's series expansion of $f(\cdot, \cdot)$:

$$
\begin{aligned}
f(X, Y) &= f(\mu_x, \mu_y) + (X - \mu_x) \left. \frac{\partial f}{\partial X} \right|_{\mu_x, \mu_y} + (Y - \mu_y) \left. \frac{\partial f}{\partial Y} \right|_{\mu_x, \mu_y} \\
&\quad + \frac{1}{2}(X - \mu_x)^2 \left. \frac{\partial^2 f}{\partial X^2} \right|_{\mu_x, \mu_y} + \frac{1}{2}(Y - \mu_y)^2 \left. \frac{\partial^2 f}{\partial Y^2} \right|_{\mu_x, \mu_y} \\
&\quad + (X - \mu_x)(Y - \mu_y) \left. \frac{\partial^2 f}{\partial X \partial Y} \right|_{\mu_x, \mu_y} + \cdots .
\end{aligned}
$$

Then, by neglecting higher-order terms in the expansion, one can obtain a large sample approximation to $E[f(X, Y)]$ as follows.

$$
E[f(X, Y)] \cong f(\mu_x, \mu_y) + \frac{\sigma_x^2}{2} \left. \frac{\partial^2 f}{\partial X^2} \right|_{\mu_x, \mu_y} + \frac{\sigma_y^2}{2} \left. \frac{\partial^2 f}{\partial Y^2} \right|_{\mu_x, \mu_y} + \sigma_{xy} \left. \frac{\partial^2 f}{\partial X \partial Y} \right|_{\mu_x, \mu_y} .
$$

Similarly, a large sample approximation to the variance of $f(X, Y)$ can be obtained as follows.

$$
\mathrm{Var}[f(X, Y)] \cong \sigma_x^2 \left(\left. \frac{\partial f}{\partial X} \right|_{\mu_x, \mu_y} \right)^2 + \sigma_y^2 \left(\left. \frac{\partial f}{\partial Y} \right|_{\mu_x, \mu_y} \right)^2 + 2\sigma_{xy} \left(\left. \frac{\partial f}{\partial X} \frac{\partial f}{\partial Y} \right|_{\mu_x, \mu_y} \right) .
$$

Now we consider large sample results. Let X_{1n} and X_{2n} be two sequences of random variables with $\mathrm{Var}(X_{1n}) = n^{-1}\sigma_{11}$, $\mathrm{Var}(X_{2n}) = n^{-1}\sigma_{22}$, and $\mathrm{Cov}(X_{1n}, X_{2n}) = n^{-1}\sigma_{12}$. The estimators for the parameters are denoted by $\hat{\mu}_{jn}$ and $\hat{\sigma}_{jkn}$, $j, k = 1, 2$. These estimators are assumed to be consistent. Then

$$
\begin{aligned}
Y_n &= f(\hat{\mu}_{1n}, \hat{\mu}_{2n}) + (\hat{\mu}_{1n} - \mu_1) \left. \frac{\partial f}{\partial \mu_1} \right|_{\hat{\mu}_{1n}, \hat{\mu}_{2n}} + (\hat{\mu}_{2n} - \mu_2) \left. \frac{\partial f}{\partial \mu_2} \right|_{\hat{\mu}_{1n}, \hat{\mu}_{2n}} \\
&\quad + \frac{1}{2}(\hat{\mu}_{1n} - \mu_1)^2 \left. \frac{\partial^2 f}{\partial \mu_1^2} \right|_{\hat{\mu}_{1n}, \hat{\mu}_{2n}} + \frac{1}{2}(\hat{\mu}_{2n} - \mu_2)^2 \left. \frac{\partial^2 f}{\partial \mu_2^2} \right|_{\hat{\mu}_{1n}, \hat{\mu}_{2n}} \\
&\quad + (\hat{\mu}_{1n} - \mu_1)(\hat{\mu}_{2n} - \mu_2) \left. \frac{\partial^2 f}{\partial \mu_1 \partial \mu_2} \right|_{\hat{\mu}_{1n}, \hat{\mu}_{2n}} + \cdots .
\end{aligned}
$$

Because $E(\hat{\mu}_{jn} - \mu_j) \to 0$, $j = 1, 2$, and $\hat{\sigma}_{jkn} = (1/n)\hat{\sigma}_{jk}$ $j, k = 1, 2$, $E[Y_n] \cong f(\hat{\mu}_{1n}, \hat{\mu}_{2n})$, then

$$\sigma_{Y_n}^2 \cong \hat{\sigma}_{11n}\left(\frac{\partial f}{\partial \mu_1}\Big|_{\hat{\mu}_{1n}, \hat{\mu}_{2n}}\right)^2 + \hat{\sigma}_{22n}\left(\frac{\partial f}{\partial \mu_2}\Big|_{\hat{\mu}_{1n}, \hat{\mu}_{2n}}\right)^2$$

$$+ 2\hat{\sigma}_{12n}\left(\frac{\partial f}{\partial \mu_1}\Big|_{\hat{\mu}_{1n}, \hat{\mu}_{2n}}\right)\left(\frac{\partial f}{\partial \mu_2}\Big|_{\hat{\mu}_{1n}, \hat{\mu}_{2n}}\right).$$

More generally, it can be shown that

$$E[f(X_1, X_2, \ldots, X_k)]$$

$$\cong f(\mu_{x_1}, \mu_{x_2}, \ldots, \mu_{x_k}) + \frac{1}{2}\sum_{i=1}^{k}\sum_{j=1}^{k}\sigma_{x_i x_j}\frac{\partial^2 f}{\partial X_i \partial X_j}\Big|_{\mu_{x_1}, \mu_{x_2}, \ldots, \mu_{x_k}}$$

and

$$\text{Var}[f(X_1, X_2, \ldots, X_k)] \cong \sum_{i=1}^{k}\sum_{j=1}^{k}\sigma_{x_i x_j}\left(\frac{\partial f}{\partial X_i}\frac{\partial f}{\partial X_j}\Big|_{\mu_{x_1}, \mu_{x_2}, \ldots, \mu_{x_k}}\right).$$

28.2.3   Application to a seasonality model

Now by using the δ-method we demonstrate how we can relate parameters of two models: Model 1 and Model 2. Consider a time series $\{Y(t), t = 1, 2, \ldots, n\}$ and the traditional model for seasonality, Model 2:

$$Y(t) = \beta_1 \sin(2\pi\omega t) + \beta_2 \cos(2\pi\omega t) + e(t),$$

where $\{e(t), t = 1, 2, \ldots, n\}$ is an i.i.d. sequence of random variables with $E[e(t)] = 0$ and $\text{Var}[e(t)] = \sigma^2$. Note that $\cos(2\pi\omega t + \psi) = \cos(2\pi\omega t)\cos(\psi) - \sin(2\pi\omega t)\sin(\psi)$.

If $\beta_1 = -\gamma\sin\psi$ and $\beta_2 = \gamma\cos\psi$, then $\gamma\cos(2\pi\omega t + \psi) = \beta_1\sin(2\pi\omega t) + \beta_1\cos(2\pi\omega t)$.

Also, $\beta_1/\beta_2 = -\sin(\psi)/\cos(\psi) = -\tan(\psi)$ and $\gamma^2 = \beta_1^2 + \beta_2^2$. Therefore, $\gamma = a(\beta_1^2 + \beta_2^2)^{1/2}$, where $a = -1$ when $\beta_2 < 0$ and $a = 1$ otherwise; and $\psi = -\arctan(\beta_1/\beta_2)$ with $\frac{\pi}{2} < \psi < \frac{\pi}{2}$. It may be noted that a change of sign of gamma results in a phase shift of $\pm\pi$. Also,

$$\frac{\partial\gamma}{\partial\beta_1} = a\beta_1/(\beta_1^2 + \beta_2^2)^{1/2}, \qquad \frac{\partial\gamma}{\partial\beta_2} = a\beta_2/(\beta_1^2 + \beta_2^2)^{1/2},$$

$$\frac{\partial\psi}{\partial\beta_1} = -\beta_2/(\beta_1^2 + \beta_2^2), \qquad \frac{\partial\psi}{\partial\beta_2} = \beta_1/(\beta_1^2 + \beta_2^2).$$

To fit the Model 2 by OLS, we let $Y' = \{Y(1), Y(2), \ldots, Y(n)\}$ be the vector of observations; $e' = \{e(1), e(2), \ldots, e(n)\}$ be the vector of noise variables; $\beta' =$

$\{\beta_1, \beta_2\}$ be the vector of parameters; and X be the design matrix where $X_{k1} = \sin(\omega k)$ and $X_{k2} = \cos(\omega k)$, $k = 1, 2, \ldots, n$. Then for $Y = X\beta + e$, the least squares estimators are $\hat{\beta} = (X'X)^{-1}X'Y$, and the variance–covariance matrix is $\mathrm{Cov}(\hat{\beta}) = \sigma^2(X'X)^{-1}$. If $\hat{Y} = X\hat{\beta}$, then we denote the vector of residuals by $\hat{e} = Y - \hat{Y}$. The unknown variance may be consistently estimated by $\hat{\sigma}^2 = n^{-1}e'e$. Because OLS estimators of the parameters of Model 2 are consistent, we have consistent estimators for β_1, β_2, and σ^2.

Models 1 and 2 are equivalent, therefore we can fit Model 2 to obtain the estimates for the amplitude and phase parameters by applying the δ-method. Thus, we have $E[\hat{\beta}'] = E[(\hat{\beta}_1, \hat{\beta}_2)] \to (\beta_1, \beta_2) = \beta'$ and

$$\mathrm{Cov}(\hat{\beta}) = \sigma^2(X'X)^{-1} = \begin{pmatrix} \hat{\sigma}^2_{\beta_1} & \hat{\sigma}_{\beta_1\beta_2} \\ \hat{\sigma}_{\beta_1\beta_2} & \hat{\sigma}^2_{\beta_1} \end{pmatrix} \approx \sigma^2(X'X)^{-1}.$$

For the amplitude $\gamma = f(\beta_1, \beta_2) = (\beta_1^2 + \beta_2^2)^{1/2}$, the estimates are

$$\hat{\gamma} = f(\hat{\beta}_1, \hat{\beta}_2) = (\hat{\beta}_1^2 + \hat{\beta}_2^2)^{1/2}$$

and

$$\mathrm{Var}(\hat{\gamma}) = (\hat{\sigma}^2_{\beta_1}\hat{\beta}_1^2 + \hat{\sigma}^2_{\beta_2}\hat{\beta}_2^2 + 2\hat{\sigma}_{\beta_1\beta_2}\hat{\beta}_1\hat{\beta}_2)/(\hat{\beta}_1^2 + \hat{\beta}_2^2).$$

The phase angle estimate is $\hat{\psi} = -\arctan(\hat{\beta}_1/\hat{\beta}_2)$ and corresponding variance estimate is

$$\mathrm{Var}(\hat{\psi}) = (\hat{\sigma}^2_{\beta_1}\hat{\beta}_2^2 + \hat{\sigma}^2_{\beta_2}\hat{\beta}_1^2 - 2\hat{\sigma}_{\beta_1\beta_2}\hat{\beta}_1\hat{\beta}_2)/(\hat{\beta}_1^2 + \hat{\beta}_2^2)^2.$$

28.2.4 Potential model extension

Model 2 can be extended to a more general Model 3 for seasonality as

$$Y(t) = \beta_0 + \beta_1\sin(2\pi\omega t) + \beta_2\cos(2\pi\omega t) + \beta_3\sin(4\pi\omega t) + \beta_2\cos(4\pi\omega t) + e(t), \tag{28.3}$$

where ω is the frequency of the seasonal component and 2ω is its first harmonic. The vector form of the model uses the following notation.

$$Y' = \{Y(1), Y(2), \ldots, Y(n)\};$$

$$e' = \{e(1), e(2), \ldots, e(n)\};$$

$$\beta' = \{\beta_0, \beta_1, \beta_2, \beta_3, \beta_4\};$$

and the $(n \times 5)$ design matrix X has as kth row

$$\{1, \sin(2\pi\omega t), \cos(2\pi\omega t), \sin(4\pi\omega t), \cos(4\pi\omega t)\}.$$

Model 3 can now be rewritten as described above with an alternative Model 4 as

$$Y(t) = \beta_0 + \gamma_1 \cos(2\pi\omega t + \psi_1) + \gamma_2 \cos(4\pi\omega t + \psi_2) + e(t). \qquad (28.4)$$

The relations between the parameters of Models 3 and 4 are as follows: $\gamma_1^2 = \beta_1^2 + \beta_2^2$; $\psi_1 = -\arctan(\beta_1/\beta_2)$; $\gamma_2^2 = \beta_3^2 + \beta_4^2$; $\psi_2 = -\arctan(\beta_3/\beta_4)$ and $\beta_1 = -\gamma_1 \sin(\psi_1)$; $\beta_2 = \gamma_1 \cos(\psi_1)$; $\beta_3 = -\gamma_2 \sin(\psi_2)$; $\beta_4 = \gamma_2 \cos(\psi_2)$. The estimation for β_0 is the same for each of Models 3 and 4. The partial derivatives are those given in Models 1 and 2, but it should be noted that many of the derivatives are zero; that is,

$$\frac{\partial \gamma_1}{\partial \beta_0} = \frac{\partial \gamma_1}{\partial \beta_3} = \frac{\partial \gamma_1}{\partial \beta_4} = \frac{\partial \gamma_2}{\partial \beta_0} = \frac{\partial \gamma_2}{\partial \beta_3} = \frac{\partial \gamma_2}{\partial \beta_4} = 0,$$

$$\frac{\partial \psi_1}{\partial \beta_0} = \frac{\partial \psi_1}{\partial \beta_3} = \frac{\partial \psi_1}{\partial \beta_4} = \frac{\partial \psi_2}{\partial \beta_0} = \frac{\partial \psi_2}{\partial \beta_3} = \frac{\partial \psi_2}{\partial \beta_4} = 0,$$

and

$$\frac{\partial \beta_0}{\partial \beta_i} = 0, \qquad i = 1, \ldots, 4; \qquad \text{also} \qquad \frac{\partial \beta_0}{\partial \beta_0} = 1.$$

This simplifies the computation of the standard error estimates for $(\beta_0, \gamma_1, \psi_1, \gamma_2, \psi_2)$. Thus, we have the following estimates for Model 4 based on the fit for Model 3:

$$\hat{\beta}_0 = \hat{\beta}_0; \qquad \hat{\gamma}_1 = (\hat{\beta}_1^2 + \hat{\beta}_2^2)^{1/2}; \qquad \hat{\gamma}_2 = (\hat{\beta}_3^2 + \hat{\beta}_4^2)^{1/2};$$
$$\hat{\psi}_1 = -\arctan(\hat{\beta}_1/\hat{\beta}_2); \qquad \hat{\psi}_2 = -\arctan(\hat{\beta}_3/\hat{\beta}_4).$$

To obtain the estimates of the standard errors of the parameters $\Omega = (\beta_0, \gamma_1, \psi_1, \gamma_2, \psi_2)$, we denote the matrix of partial derivatives of the Model 4 parameters with respect to Model 3 by $\left.\frac{\partial \Omega}{\partial \beta}\right|_\beta$. Then

$$\text{Cov}(\hat{\Omega}) \cong \left(\left.\frac{\partial \Omega}{\partial \beta}\right|_\beta\right)' (\hat{\sigma}^2 (X'X)^{-1}) \left(\left.\frac{\partial \Omega}{\partial \beta}\right|_\beta\right).$$

28.2.5   Additional considerations

Here we intend to apply the proposed method for assessing seasonality in infectious diseases that typically have one annual peak and are measured by counting cases occurring over prespecified time periods (e.g., days, weeks, months). Therefore, two main aspects of the method of implementation should be discussed: the underlying distribution of the case counting process and the orthogonality of the design matrix.

It is plausible to assume a Poisson process for a rare event such as a case of infection in a large closed population that satisfies a requirement of non-negativity in a time series of counts. Suppose the mean-value function for a Poisson process follows Model 2 or 3. Then the process will have as its tth component a Poisson variate with parameter $\lambda(t)$. Unless $\lambda(t) = \lambda$ for all t, the process will not have constant variance. In a case of nonconstant variance, the OLS parameters will be biased. To reduce this bias, we will use an iterative weighted least squares approach implemented via standard statistical software for a generalized Poisson regression.

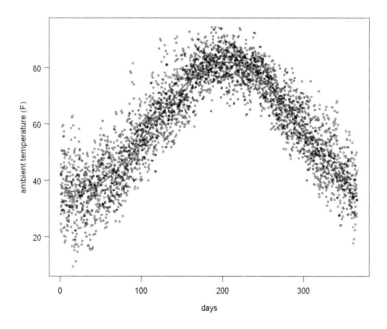

Figure 28.2: Seasonal curve for ambient temperature in temperate climate of Massachusetts, USA. Solid line is the fitted mean-value function

When fitting a trigonometric polynomial to a set of data, it is helpful if the columns of the design matrix X are orthogonal. Suppose that a time period consists of n equal subintervals of length $1/n$, and the data are collected at the end of each time subinterval. For a one-year study period, a year is a time period of one unit in length divided into 365 subunits, that is, days, each of $1/365$th of the unit. For the proposed Model 1, the frequency ω equals 1, meaning that in one full cycle per unit of time (year) the first harmonic has twice this frequency, or there are two full cycles per year. Then the design matrix X will have columns that are orthogonal and $X'X$ will be a diagonal matrix.

28.3   Application to Temperature and Infection Incidence Analysis

To examine the relations between seasonal patterns in ambient temperature and disease incidence, we study time series of daily mean temperature and counts of *Salmonella* that have been established over the last decade in Massachusetts, USA. Ten years of temperature daily observations and *Salmonella* counts, superimposed for ease of seasonality visualization are shown in Figures 28.2 and 28.3. Figure 28.4 demonstrates daily counts of *Salmonella* with respect to the corresponding temperature values. As we can see, there are apparent increases in *Salmonella* cases in warm summer months, as well as respective increases in variability in these time periods. A daily rate of *Salmonella* is 0.78 cases per 1,000,000 population.

Our first step was to describe the seasonal pattern in temperature and infections over the last decade. We used a generalized linear model (GLM) with a

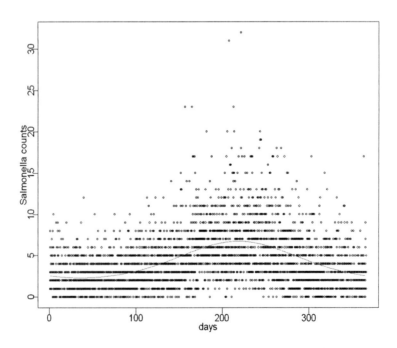

Figure 28.3: Seasonal curve for salmonella cases in Massachusetts, USA. Solid line is the fitted mean-value function

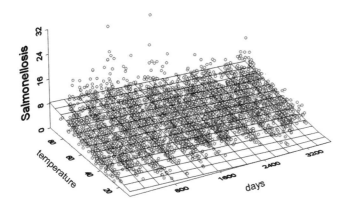

Figure 28.4: Temporal pattern in daily *Salmonella* cases (*Z*-axis) with respect to ambient temperature values in C° (*Y*-axis) over time (*X*-axis)

Gaussian distribution for the outcome when the variable of interest is ambient temperature,

$$Y(t) = \beta_0 + \beta_1 \sin(2\pi\omega t) + \beta_2 \cos(2\pi\omega t) + e(t), \qquad (28.5)$$

and a Poisson distribution if the studied outcome is daily disease counts,

$$\log(E[Y(t)]) = \beta_0 + \beta_1 \sin(2\pi\omega t) + \beta_2 \cos(2\pi\omega t) + e(t). \qquad (28.6)$$

In both cases, β_0 is an intercept that estimates a baseline of a seasonal pattern. With t as time, expressed in days for a time series of length N ($t = 1, 2, \ldots, N$, where N is the number of days in a time series), we set $\omega = 1/365$ to properly express the annual cycle. The $\exp\{\beta_0\}$ for the Poisson regression reflects a mean daily disease count over a study period. We estimated the mean-value function using Models 5 and 6, as well as using the estimates of the amplitude and phase angle, and obtained the exact same plot (Figures 28.2 and 28.4).

Now, using the estimates of the amplitude and the phase angle, the proposed characteristics of seasonality can be expressed as follows.

1. The average maximum value on the seasonal curve of exposure, $\max\{Y(t)\}$ $= \beta_0 + \gamma$, or incidence of disease, $\max\{Y(t)\} = \exp\{\beta_0 + \gamma\}$;

2. The average minimum value on the seasonal curve of exposure, $\min\{Y(t)\}$ $= \beta_0 - \gamma$, or incidence of disease, $\min\{Y(t)\} = \exp\{\beta_0 - \gamma\}$;

3. The average intensity, the difference between maximum and minimum values on the seasonal curve for exposure, $I = 2\gamma$, or incidence of disease, $I = \exp\{\beta_0 + \gamma\} - \exp\{\beta_0 - \gamma\}$;

4. The average relative intensity, the ratio of maximum value and minimum value on the seasonal curve, for exposure, $I_R = (\beta_0^2 - \gamma^2)/(\beta_0 - \gamma)^2$, or incidence of disease, $I_R = \exp\{2\gamma\}$;

5. The average peak timing (in days), a position of the maximum point on the seasonal curve of exposure or disease incidence, $P = 365(1 - \psi/\pi)/2$;

6. The average lag, $P_E - P_D$, the difference between peak timing of exposure, P_E, and peak timing of disease incidence, P_E.

The results of fitting Model 2, as well as the estimated amplitude and phase angle parameters are shown in Table 28.1. We used S-Plus glm-function to fit the models. S-Plus codes for estimation of seasonality parameters are available on request. Suggested models demonstrate that a seasonal component explained 83% of variability in daily temperature and 23% in counts of *Salmonella* infections. The *Salmonella* infections peaked two weeks after a peak in temperature.

Table 28.1: Characteristics of seasonal curves for ambient temperature and *Salmonella* cases

	Temperature Parameters Value (Std.error)	Disease Parameters Value (Std.error)
Intercept—β_0	58.971 (0.1213)	1.377 (0.0086)
sin(2*π*time/365)—β_1	−9.187 (0.1716)	−0.3111 (0.0117)
cos(2*π*time/365)—β_2	−21.093 (0.1715)	−0.4331 (0.0118)
Null variance (df = 3652)	1163591	8967
Residual variance (df = 3650)	196222	6871
% variance explained	83%	23%
Amplitude—γ	22.9698	0.5412
Phase angle—ψ	−0.4071	−0.6489
Relative intensity—I_R	2.2760	2.9519
Peak timing—P	206.1	220.2

Next, we hypothesized that temporality in ambient temperature will determine, in part, the timing and magnitude of peaks and we explored associations between seasonal characteristics in disease and temperature. Specifically, we asked the question, "Do the timing and/or intensity of a seasonal peak in ambient temperature predict the timing and/or intensity of the seasonal peak for an enteric infection?" In order to answer this question, we examined seasonal characteristics in ambient temperature and *Salmonella* infections in the manner described above for each year separately and then examined the synchronization of seasonal patterns in temperature and *Salmonella* counts. A few interesting observations are: moderate association exists between relative intensities for temperature and *Salmonella* cases ($\rho = 0.648$), and negative correlation exists between average minimum values for temperature and average maximum values for *Salmonella* infections ($\rho = -0.806$). These results suggest that ambient temperature can be a potential predictor of *Salmonella* infections at a seasonal scale.

28.4 Conclusion

An ability to provide estimates for seasonality characteristics as a set of parameters was the main objective in developing the presented models. The presented set of analytical tools allows for comprehensive, systematic, and detailed examination of a seasonal pattern in daily time series of continuous and discrete outcomes. The application indicates the promise of these techniques to produce sensible and intuitively appearing functional relationships. The suggested conceptual structure permits the description of seasonal patterns and their comparison. In fitting a GLM with a cosine function for a seasonal curve we assumed that a pattern described by a cosine curve has a symmetric rise and fall, and a cosine curve with a period of a full year has a point at which it peaks and a point with the lowest value. We demonstrated an approach, in which we combine the ease of fitting one model with the simplicity and elegance of interpretation of another one, by using the δ-method. We also demonstrated that the proposed technique could be extended to a more general case, for example, when two seasonal peaks can be identified. Clearly, further experience in using these techniques and some theoretical work are required. It is important to compare the performance of models with well-documented statistical techniques for seasonality evaluation, to expand visual presentation of modeling results, and to provide step-by-step instructions for implementing these statistical procedures in practical settings for public health professionals. The presented models and parameter estimation procedures allow for a straightforward interpretation, are easy to perform using commercial statistical software, and are valuable tools for investigating seasonal patterns in biosurveillance.

One methodological aspect of this exercise deserves special comment. The vast majority of epidemiological studies that have examined the seasonality of diseases used crude quarterly or monthly aggregate data which prevent a fully detailed, accurate, or comprehensive analysis of a seasonal pattern and may even be misleading [da Silva Lopes (1999)]. Examination of weekly rates substantially improves the evaluation of seasonal curves when compared to monthly data, but a systematic approach to the issue of week standardization has often been lacking. The use of daily time series enabled us to detect significant differences in the seasonal peaks of infections, which would have been lost in a study that used monthly cumulative information. The effective use of the presented methods requires data collected over a long period with sufficient frequency. An efficient surveillance system has similar requirements. The vast majority of continuously monitored surveillance systems collect data on a daily basis and focus on the use of daily time series.

Acknowledgements. We wish to thank Drs. Jeffrey Griffiths and Andrey Egorov for their thoughtful suggestions, and Drs. Alfred DeMaria and Bela Matyas and the Massachusetts Department of Public Health for providing us with surveillance data. We would also like to thank the USA EPA, the National Institute of Allergy and Infectious Diseases, and the National Institute of Environmental Health Sciences that provided funding through the Subcontract Agreement, AI43415, and ES013171 grants, respectively.

References

1. MacNeill, I. B. (1977). A test of whether several time series share common periodicities, *Biometrika*, **64**, 495–508.

2. da Silva Lopes, A. C. B. (1999). Spurious deterministic seasonality and autocorrelation corrections with quarterly data: Further Monte Carlo results, *Empir Econ.*, **24**, 341–359.

29

Comparison of Three Convolution Prior Spatial Models for Cancer Incidence

Erik-A. Sauleau,[1] **Monica Musio,**[2] **Arnaud Etienne,**[1] **and Antoine Buemi**[1]

[1] *Cancer Registry of Haut-Rhin, Mulhouse, France*
[2] *University of Cagliari, Cagliari, Italy*

Abstract: Generalized linear models with a Poisson distribution are often used to model cancer registry data stratified by sex, age, year, and little geographical units. We compare three different approaches which take into account possible spatial correlation among neighbouring units, using lung cancer incidence data. Inference is fully Bayesian and uses Markov chain Monte Carlo techniques. Comparison between models is based on the Deviance Information Criterion (DIC).

Keywords: Bayesian hierarchical spatial model, conditional autoregressive model, distance model, P-splines, cancer registry, incidence, lung cancer

29.1 Introduction

The cancer registries collect data for calculation of incidence and survival of different sites of cancer. Among influential factors, age and sex are collected. Environmental factors are also important but they are not gathered by the registries. To take into account the cumulative effect of such unobserved covariates, a spatial effect is added in the models: each case in the cancer registry is geographically located by his address, reported to the geographical unit it belongs to, and eventually located by the geographical coordinates of its centroid, that is, the centre of the geographical unit, derived mathematically and weighted to approximate a sort of 'centre of gravity.' This location is used as a proxy for environmental exposure. During the last ten years, spatial modelling has become a topic of great interest. Many atlases of diseases or publications before the year 1990 have represented by some geographical unit the maximum likelihood estimate of relative risks under Poisson assumption. If O is the number of observed cases and E the expected cases (both are cases for incidence or deaths for mortality), these estimates are O/E, which correspond to the standardized incidence ratio (SIR) or to the standardized mortality ratio. Such a model ignores the correlation between geographical units: the outcome in a unit is more similar to the outcome of a proximate unit than the outcome of an arbitrary unit. Different kinds of methods have been developed for taking into account this correlation. Non-Gaussian spatial data are frequently modelled using generalized linear mixed models, with location-specific random effect. The correlation between units can be taken into account in a joint way or in a conditional way. The conditional way uses a singular precision matrix whereas the joint approach models the variance–covariance matrix. The joint modelling can be considered as a first step of kriging modelling [Diggle, Tawn, and Moyeed (1998)]. The spatial effect is normally distributed with mean μ and variance–covariance $\sigma^2 V$. For example, in an exponential model, the element v_{ij} of the V matrix is given by $\exp[-(d_{ij}/\rho)]$, where d_{ij} is the Euclidian distance between two units and ρ is a given random "attenuation" factor. On the other hand, the conditional way yields conditional autoregressive models [Besag, York, and Mollié (1991) and Mollié (1996)] whose expansion is a multivariate normal. A particular form of this model is a pure autocorrelation model, which is named the intrinsic conditional autoregressive (ICAR) model. In this model, the force of the autocorrelation is maximum, measured by a so-called adjacency matrix, an indicator matrix of direct neighbourhood (i.e., geographical units sharing a boundary). The conditional spatial effect ϕ is then a normal with a mean which is the mean of the spatial effect around each unit and the variance is proportional to the number of neighbours n_i of each unit (all neighbours of i constituting the set ∂). This can then be written as

$$\phi_i | \phi_{-i} \sim N \left(\frac{\sum_{j \in \partial} \phi_j}{n_i}, \frac{z}{n_i} \right). \tag{29.1}$$

The only parameter to be estimated is a variance parameter z. A nonspatially structured exchangeable normal distribution $\theta_i \sim N[0, (1/\tau_\theta)]$ is often added to the autocorrelation part and represents an heterogeneity part, which is aimed to distribute spatially some residual variability. A particular model is called the 'convolution prior' [Besag, York, and Mollié (1991)], a sum of this heterogeneity term and an ICAR component.

The goal of all the previous models is to take into account the outcome of neighbours for each geographical unit. Beside these distance and adjacency models, there is an interesting other series of smoothing functions, such as two-dimensional P-splines. The spatial effect is now an unknown surface which can be approximated by the tensor product of two one-dimensional B-splines [Lang and Brezger (2004)]. B-splines provide a useful tool for fitting complicated models with smooth components. In general, if u_+ defines the positive part of a function u (equal to u if u is positive and 0 otherwise), a smoothing B-spline

of degree l for a variable x is a linear combination of $1, x, x^2, \ldots, x_l, (x - \kappa_1)_+^l,$
$\ldots, (x - \kappa_K)_+^l$ [Ruppert, Wand, and Carroll (2003)]. The K points κ are points
equally spaced between the minimal value of x and its maximal and are called
knots. If the centroid of the geographical units has coordinates (x, y), then
the smoothing surface is defined by $f(x, y) = \sum^m \sum^m \pi_{ij} B_i(x) B_j(y)$, where
B_i and B_j are B-splines and π are the coefficients of the linear combinations
of B-splines. In a Bayesian framework, the most commonly used priors on π
are based on the four nearest neighbours [Lang and Brezger (2004)] and are
specified in first-order random walks:

$$\pi_{ij} \sim N\left(\frac{1}{4}\left(\pi_{(i-1)j} + \pi_{(i+1)j} + \pi_{i(j-1)} + \pi_{i(j+1)}\right), \frac{1}{\tau_\pi}\right). \qquad (29.2)$$

These methods of disease mapping are useful for cancer registries only if they
fulfill some conditions. Geographical units highlighted with a particular high
or low risk must have internal plausibility (relation between cancer and known
exposure, relative constancy over time, etc.) and also external (spatial pattern
of contiguous regions). The smoothing proposed by these methods should be
sufficient for a public health utilization which cannot focus on several isolated
geographical units.

Our aim is to compare, using a lung cancer incidence data set from the registry of the Haut-Rhin department in France, three "convolution prior" models: the first with an ICAR model, the second with a joint exponential-distance
model, and the third with two-dimensional P-splines. In all these three models,
an heterogeneity part is added and modelled as an exchangeable normal. Our
approach is fully Bayesian with Markov chains and Monte Carlo inference. The
example of lung cancer is chosen because of the high incidence in the population of this site and its known epidemiology; see, for example, Hill, Millar,
and Connelly (2003) and Janssen-Heijnen and Coebergh (2003). Among its risk
factors, the main one is tobacco habits and of less importance is atmospheric
or occupational exposure (asbestos, nickel, etc.). This cancer is a male one (1
female for 5 males) but the incidence for female grows for 35–44 age categories
because of new smoking habits. A peak of incidence is reached about 70 years
old. This location of cancer is threefold more frequent in cities than in rural
zones.

29.2   Material and Methods

The data are from the cancer registry of the Haut-Rhin. The Haut-Rhin *department* is located in the north-east of France sharing a boundary with Germany
and Switzerland. It has 3525 km^2 and 707,555 inhabitants (in 1999) in a very

dense irregular lattice of 377 municipalities ('communes') which are our geographical units. The largest distance between two geographical units is about 95 kms. We extract the counts of lung cancer by age, sex, year of diagnosis and geographical unit. The age is categorized into nine groups: the interval [0–44 years], the 5-year intervals [45–49], ..., [75–79], and the interval [80 and more]. Our data are available and validated between 1988 and 1999 (renumbered as 1 to 12). The total number of cases is 3415, unequally split between 2903 for males and 513 for females. The temporal evolution of numbers of cases is different between sexes. For males, the number of cases is 218 in 1988 and 230 in 1999 with little variations between 231 and 247 in the interval (except 281 cases in 1996). For females, the number is 20 in 1988 and 62 in 1998 with increasing from 26 to 52 in the interval. The population at risk during these 12 years is 8,240,000 with 4,200,000 females. By geographical unit, this population varies from about 55 to about 110,000 (from 25 to 56,000 for female) by year. Due to covariates, the data set consists of counts of cases distributed in 81,432 cells.

Following Clayton and Kaldor (1987), we assume that the number of observed cases O follows a Poisson distribution: $O|. \sim P(E.e^{\mu .})$, where E denotes the number of cases expected and μ is a linear combination of covariate effects (the symbol '.' stands for all these covariates). Hence, we build the different models with outcome O_{sati} (the counts of cases) and as covariates: sex s (1 or 2), age category a ($a \in [1 - A]$ where $A = 9$), year of diagnosis t ($t \in [1 - T]$ where $T = 12$), and geographical units i ($i \in [1 - N]$ where $N = 377$). Population counts are known by age, sex, and geographical unit for 1990 and 1999 (national census). We use the 1990 population for 1988, 1989, 1990, and 1991. The population of 1999 is used for 1998 and 1999. A linear interpolation on the years 1993 and 1996 is used for 1992 to 1994 and for 1995 to 1997. If we denote by R the population counts, we then get the estimation for R_{sati}. For the calculation of expected counts E, $E_{sati} = \hat{p}R_{sati}$, where $\hat{p}$ estimates a global risk by

$$\hat{p} = \frac{\sum^2 \sum^A \sum^T \sum^N O_{sati}}{\sum^2 \sum^A \sum^T \sum^N R_{sati}}.$$

The modelling of the spatial effect, say Ψ, takes the form of a sort of 'convolution prior' as it associates a factor θ for heterogeneity and a factor ϕ for correlation, and will yield three different hierarchical main models, just differing on the specification of ϕ. The first level of the hierarchy, for all three models, is the Poisson level for observed cases in geographical unit i, for sex s, age a, and time t:

$$O_{sati} \sim P(E_{sati}e^{\mu_{sati}}) \quad \text{where } \mu_{sati} = \alpha + \beta_s + \gamma_a + \delta_t + \Psi_i. \qquad (29.3)$$

exhibit an age effect increasing (in mean from -0.7 to 0.7) with maxima for 60–69 years categories and then decreasing to -0.2 for the oldest age category. The M-SMOOTH model shows about the same range of effect but with a constant low risk for the two youngest categories of age, then a higher steady state in 50–79 years categories (about 0), and then a peak for the oldest category (0.8). The attenuation factor ρ of the M-EXP model exhibits a narrow credible interval but its distribution is very near to the upper bound of the prior uniform distribution. The M-ICAR yields the more precise value for heterogeneity (the strongest of the three different estimates for τ_θ), but with a coefficient of variation more than 1 contrary to the M-EXP. *A contrario*, the M-EXP model gives a poor value for $1/\sigma^2$, compared to the value of λ and the precision τ_ϵ in the P-splines.

Gathering the data over the 12 years, the age categories, and genders, the SIRs are from 0 (in 54 geographical units) to 4.3, without any clear spatial structure (Figure 29.1). Figure 29.2 represents the mapping of the exponential of 'main' spatial effects (Figures 29.2a,b,c) and the exponential of the heterogeneity components (Figures 29.2d,e,f) for the three models. For all three models, the heterogeneity part is the same in terms of spatial position (several dispersed geographical units with high residual heterogeneity) but also in values: the mean is 1.0 for all the geographical units, with a maximum at 1.2 or 1.3 and a minimum at 0.9 (all values in term of exponential effect). The main effect is 1.0 in mean (with a maximum at 1.2 and a minimum at 0.8). The maps for M-EXP and M-SMOOTH seem to be smoother than that for M-ICAR. The M-ICAR exhibits three subregions with high risk but one is along the eastern boundary and the other corresponding to two of the cities in the region. The M-SMOOTH highlights the same two central subregions (more markedly than M-ICAR) but also another one along the western boundary. The M-EXP shows an identical pattern to M-ICAR. At the nominal level of 95%, no geographical unit exhibits a 'significant' spatial effect either with the M-ICAR model or with the M-SMOOTH (all credible intervals include 0). With the M-SMOOTH model and at the level of 80%, the units in a subregion along the eastern boundary have low risk and all the units in the central subregion constitute a contiguous set of units with higher risks. But credible intervals for the effect in the units along the western boundary all include 0.

For the three models, iterations required more memory than we had, so we had to access the disk as virtual memory, a process that dramatically slowed down the computation. This problem was stronger with the M-ICAR and M-EXP models in WinBUGS. Very globally, burn-in phase of 5000 iterations is the norm and estimations on 50,000 further iterations are enough for estimations (little less in WinBUGS). The times for achieving 1000 simulations are 7200 seconds for M-ICAR, 12,000 for M-EXP, and 1500 seconds for M-SMOOTH.

Table 29.1: Estimation of parameters for the three models

Parameter	Model	Mean	Sd	p2.5	Median	p97.5
Fixed Effects						
α	M-ICAR	-5.68	0.199	-6.10	-5.67	-5.31
	M-EXP	-5.59	0.898	-6.61	-6.03	-3.86
	M-SMOOTH	0.182	0.142	-0.0988	0.180	0.472
β_1	M-ICAR	0.0632	0.00469	0.0540	0.0634	0.0726
	M-EXP	0.0633	0.00489	0.0537	0.0634	0.0728
	M-SMOOTH	0.0614	0.00534	0.0521	0.0614	0.0711
β_2	M-ICAR	-0.140	0.00797	-0.156	-0.140	-0.124
	M-EXP	-0.140	0.00812	-0.156	-0.140	-0.125
	M-SMOOTH	-0.156	0.00810	-0.172	-0.156	-0.140
γ_1	M-ICAR	-0.770	0.206	-1.14	-0.780	-0.319
	M-EXP	-0.847	0.223	-1.27	-0.859	-0.385
	M-SMOOTH	-0.386	0.148	-0.657	-0.383	-0.118
γ_2	M-ICAR	-0.514	0.204	-0.874	-0.525	-0.0614
	M-EXP	-0.591	0.220	-1.01	-0.603	-0.129
	M-SMOOTH	-0.378	0.150	-0.686	-0.374	-0.0951
γ_3	M-ICAR	-0.121	0.201	-0.473	-0.132	0.332
	M-EXP	-0.197	0.217	-0.600	-0.212	0.262
	M-SMOOTH	0.0854	0.145	-0.206	0.0870	0.370
γ_4	M-ICAR	0.321	0.199	-0.0237	0.310	0.772
	M-EXP	0.245	0.216	-0.150	0.228	0.702
	M-SMOOTH	-0.0542	0.128	-0.325	-0.0515	0.213
γ_5	M-ICAR	0.750	0.198	0.406	0.731	1.20
	M-EXP	0.668	0.214	0.280	0.649	1.12
	M-SMOOTH	-0.00276	0.125	-0.274	-0.000132	0.265
γ_6	M-ICAR	0.759	0.197	0.421	0.747	1.21
	M-EXP	0.681	0.214	0.294	0.663	1.13
	M-SMOOTH	-0.00965	0.118	-0.281	-0.00702	0.258
γ_7	M-ICAR	0.443	0.198	0.0996	0.431	0.893
	M-EXP	0.366	0.215	-0.0238	0.349	0.823
	M-SMOOTH	-0.00346	0.118	-0.275	-0.000830	0.264
γ_8	M-ICAR	0.00913	0.200	-0.338	-0.00446	0.461
	M-EXP	-0.0670	0.217	-0.463	-0.0823	0.388
	M-SMOOTH	-0.0694	0.128	-0.341	-0.0668	0.198
γ_9	M-ICAR	-0.211	0.202	-0.566	-0.223	0.242
	M-EXP	-0.288	0.218	-0.695	-0.304	0.171
	M-SMOOTH	0.805	0.199	0.465	0.811	1.111
ρ	M-EXP	3.42E-4	9.26E-5	1.54E-4	3.50E-4	4.89E-4
Precisions of the Spatial Effects						
τ_θ	M-ICAR	53.1	70.5	17.1	37.6	184
	M-EXP	46.4	36.2	16.5	36.0	142
	M-SMOOTH	44.7	80.2	18.7	48.7	215
λ	M-ICAR	44.9	57.5	8.00	28.2	199
$\frac{1}{\sigma^2}$	M-EXP	7.05	8.81	0.328	3.04	32.1
τ_ϵ	M-SMOOTH	24.3	31.6	8.73	29.7	276

29.4 Discussion

Comparing with the mapping of the crude SIRs (Figure 29.1), maps of the main effect of the three spatial models are smoother—less with the M-ICAR model— with obvious spatial similarity between neighbouring geographical units (Figure 29.2). All three models exhibit a very global weak heterogeneity component but in some of the geographical units strong values remain. Furthermore, according to our three models there is little main spatial effect also. In fact the main effect in value is clearly the age effect for the M-ICAR and the M-EXP models. The main effect in the M-SMOOTH is the overall risk (constant α), but other effects also play a role (which is quite diffuse). For this model, the age effect does not have a classical form (with an incidence peak about 70 years). For all three models, the sex–time effect are the same and coherent with the published papers; see, for example, Janssen-Heijnen and Coebergh (2003). The models identify two central subregions with high risk. M-ICAR identifies another subregion along the eastern boundary, and M-SMOOTH another subregion along the western boundary and also a subregion along the eastern boundary with low risk. An edge effect cannot be kept off although it seems to be too massive. The lack of difference between M-ICAR and M-EXP is a little surprising as the region has geographical units with very different sizes and shapes, and so differences are expected when the models rely on distance between units rather than on adjacency. This is perhaps due to a very weak spatial effect and some differences will arise if the spatial effect is stronger. Finally, the best model according to the DIC is the M-SMOOTH.

When the disease mapping is for descriptive purposes, the user needs to know first how important is the effect drawn on her maps and if it is accurate to model disease risk with spatial model and autocorrelation. A first step can be made with a simple Potthoff–Whittinghill's test [Potthoff and Whittinghill (1966)] to investigate if risks are homogeneous in the study region. Then in a second step a Moran's I statistic [Moran (1948)] can be used to test if risks are spatially related in the study region. Because distributions of these statistics are difficult to derive, it is possible to use a bootstrap approach for estimating their distributions [Gómez-Rubio, Ferrándiz, and López (2003)].

A main problem occurring with count data with several covariates is that the data have many zero counts. Furthermore, the models contain a large number of parameters with high correlations. The consequences of these facts are unambiguous. MCMC samplers need a large amount of iterations for convergence and the mixing can be very poor. Different solutions can then be found. It is possible to aggregate the data in both time and space to some level that represents an equilibrium between the sparseness of cases and the spatial or temporal information of the data. However, this point is difficult to find without any prior

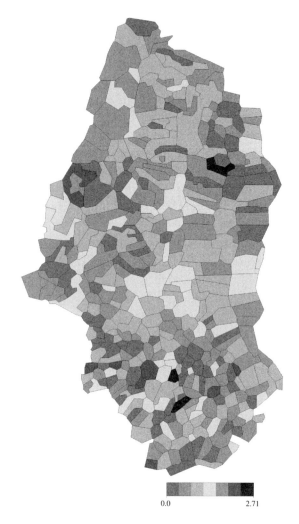

Figure 29.1: Standardized incidence ratios for lung cancer by geographical unit

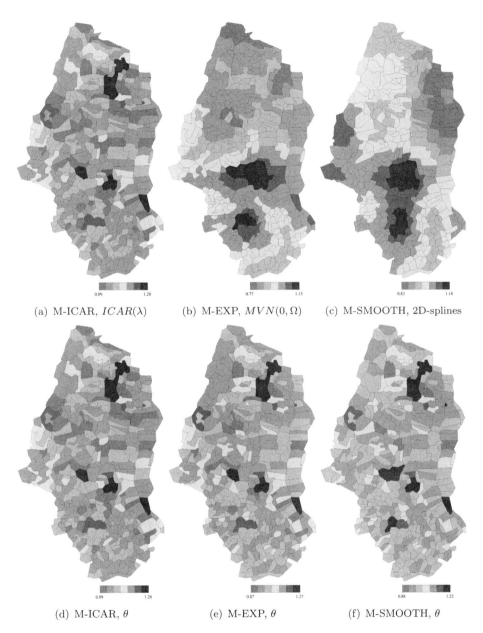

(a) M-ICAR, $ICAR(\lambda)$ (b) M-EXP, $MVN(0, \Omega)$ (c) M-SMOOTH, 2D-splines

(d) M-ICAR, θ (e) M-EXP, θ (f) M-SMOOTH, θ

Figure 29.2: Mapping of spatial effects for lung cancer (exponential of the values)

knowledge. Another solution is the reparametrization of the models: for example, by centering (in the M-EXP model) or by considering no further the spatial effects θ and ϕ but $\theta + \phi$ and ϕ [Waller *et al.* (1997)]. And finally, changing the sampler can improve mixing of parameters. For our three different models, we use two different software: WinBUGS which allows to choose the algorithm in relation to the models and BayesX which implements a block updating algorithm [Rue (2001) and Knorr-Held and Rue (2002)]. In WinBUGS, the most efficient algorithms, among those open to choice, are the rejection sampling for the M-ICAR and the slice sampling for the M-EXP. Considering the time spent by convergence, it seems that the best algorithm is the block-update but it is difficult to compare M-ICAR and M-EXP algorithms because a considerable amount of computation time for M-EXP is spent on the inversion at each step of the variance matrix (the algorithm has N^3 complexity). For M-ICAR, it has been shown [Haran, Hodges, and Carlin (2003)] that a structured MCMC, a class of block-update MCMC algorithms using different size blocks, to which the one of BayesX belongs, with or without reparametrization, improves the mixing and sometimes the number of effective samples generated by a second of time. All these considerations tend to suggest that block-update MCMC is the more accurate algorithm (BayesX can also be used for the M-ICAR model).

In the M-EXP model, the choice of prior on ρ is very subjective and a sensitivity analysis should be conducted on this choice. The convolution prior model, like the M-ICAR model, is highly sensitive to the prior specification [MacNab (2003)] and also needs a sensitivity analysis on the choice of λ and τ_θ. Different values for the parameters of τ_θ, for example, $\Gamma(0.001, 0.001)$ and $\Gamma(1, 1)$, can be used. The precision λ of the ICAR is then adapted with respect to these new values. For priors on all the precisions in our models (which only concern normal distributions), we chose to use proper conjugate priors and our priors are $\Gamma(G, G)$. When $G \to 0$, we get an improper posterior distribution and thus we set G to the 'reasonable' value 0.01. According to Gelman (2004), it could be possible to use other priors for precision or for the standard deviation of normal distribution. For example, we could choose as a noninformative prior an uniform distribution on a wide positive range or, if a more informative prior were desired, a distribution of the positive t-family which has a better behaviour near 0 than inverse-Γ, for example, a positive-Cauchy distribution.

In our models, we take into account the age at the diagnosis and the year at the diagnosis. Nevertheless, there is a growing literature about the cohort of birth effect and so we have to model this effect as well. For example, Schmid, and Held (2004), in a binomial model, use random walks and Gaussian random Markov fields for age, time, cohort with interaction space–time or space–cohort. Lagazio, Dreassi, and Biggeri (2001) use a conditional autoregressive prior for cohort effect (adjacent cohorts of a cohort c are the cohort $c - 1$ and $c + 1$), whereas Lagazio, Biggeri, and Dreassi (2003) use random walks prior for main age, period, and cohort effects and some interactions space–time and space–cohort.

Another way to address the problem of disease mapping is by using partition models. These models stay in the strict definition of mapping whereas they split the region of study in a series of a priori unknown subregions with homogeneous risks as cluster analysis does. But no formal test for clustering is allowed with these methods. For example, Knorr-Held and Rasser (2000) and Giudici, Knorr-Held, and Rasser (2000), for taking into account some categorical covariates, model log-risk in each subregion as a normal distribution. The method used in these two articles is related to that of Schlattmann and Böhning (1993) who use mixture models. Denison and Holmes (2001) make use of Voronoi tessellation for building subregions.

The cancer registries have to produce incidence data for each site of cancer, taking into account (or not) several covariates. The M-SMOOTH model is the fastest one to converge whereas M-EXP can take one day. Furthermore, M-SMOOTH seems to be less sensitive to prior choice than M-EXP and M-ICAR and so sensitivity analysis can be reduced (but not cancelled). Globally, our results agree with those of a recent paper [Best, Richardson, and Thomson (2005)], which includes M-EXP and M-ICAR models but not the M-SMOOTH. This chapter concludes that the exponential model (M-EXP) does not perform well. Its issues are based on simulation study. Beyond these results are some public health consequences, which have to rely on an accurate smoothing. For example, the descriptions of subregions are not so strictly defined for the M-ICAR model as compared to those for the M-SMOOTH model. Finally, the model using a spatial smoothing with Bayesian P-splines seems to be the more accurate model among all those we have tested.

Acknowledgements. The authors are grateful to Avner Bar-Hen and Marc Colonna for valuable comments on a draft of this chapter, and to the reviewers whose comments have improved its clarity.

References

1. Bernardinelli, L., Clayton, D., and Montomoli, C. (1995). Bayesian estimates of disease maps: How important are priors? *Statistics in Medicine*, **14**, 2411–3241.

2. Besag, J., York, J., and Mollié, A. (1991). Bayesian image restoration, with two applications in spatial statistics (with discussion), *Annals of the Institute of Statistical Mathematics*, **43**, 1–59.

3. Best, N., Richardson, S., and Thomson, A. (2005). A comparison of Bayesian spatial models for disease mapping, *Statistical Methods in Medical Research*, **14**, 35–59.

4. Brezger, A., Kneib, T., and Lang, S. (2005). *BayesX*, Version 1.4, Available at http://www.stat.uni-muenchen.de/~lang/bayesx.

5. Clayton, D., and Kaldor, J. (1987). Empirical Bayes estimates of age-standardized relative risks for use of disease mapping, *Biometrics*, **43**, 671–681.

6. Denison, D. G. T., and Holmes. C. C. (2001). Bayesian partitioning for estimating disease risk, *Biometrics*, **57**, 143–149.

7. Diggle, P. J., Tawn, J. A., and Moyeed, R. A. (1998). Model-based geostatistics, *Applied Statistics*, **47**, 299–350.

8. Gelman, A. (2004). Prior distributions for variance parameters in hierarchical models, June 2004, Available at
   http://www.stat.columbia.edu/~gelman/research/unpublished/.

9. Gelman, A., Carlin, J., Stern, H., and Rubin, D. (1995). *Bayesian Data Analysis*, Chapman & Hall, London.

10. Giudici, P., Knorr-Held, L., and Rasser, G. (2000). Modelling categorical covariates in Bayesian disease mapping by partition structures, *Statistics in Medicine*, **19**, 2579–2593.

11. Gómez-Rubio, V., Ferrándiz, J., and López, A. (2003). Detecting clusters of diseases with R, In *Proceedings of the Third International Workshop on Distributed Statistical Computing* (Eds., F. Leisch K. Hornik and A. Zeileis), Vienna, Austria.

12. Haran, M., Hodges, J. S., and Carlin, B. P. (2003). Accelerating computation in Markov random field models for spatial data via structured MCMC, *Journal of Computational and Graphical Statistics*, **12**, 249–264.

13. Hill, G., Millar, W., and Connelly, J. (2003). "The great debate" 1: Smoking, lung cancer, and cancer epidemiology, *Canadian Bulletin of Medical History*, **20**, 367–386.

14. Janssen-Heijnen, M. L. and Coebergh, J. W. (2003). The changing epidemiology of lung cancer in Europe, *Lung Cancer*, **41**, 245–258.

15. Knorr-Held, L., and Besag, J. (1998). Modelling risk from a disease in time and space, *Statistics in Medicine*, **17**, 2045–2060.

16. Knorr-Held, L., and Rasser, G. (2000). Bayesian detection of clusters and discontinuities in disease maps, *Biometrics*, **56**, 13–21.

17. Knorr-Held, L., and Rue, H. (2002). On block updating in Markov random field models for disease mapping, *Scandinavian Journal of Statistics*, **29**, 597–614.

18. Lagazio, C., Biggeri, A., and Dreassi, E. (2003). Age-period-cohort models and disease mapping, *Environmetrics*, **14**, 475–490.

19. Lagazio, C., Dreassi, E., and Biggeri, A. (2001). A hierarchical Bayesian model for space-time variation of disease risk, *Statistical Modelling*, **1**, 17–29.

20. Lang, S. and Brezger, A. (2004). Bayesian P-splines, *Journal of Computational and Graphical Statistics*, **13**, 183–212.

21. MacNab, Y. C. (2003). Hierarchical Bayesian modeling of spatially correlated health service outcome and utilization rates, *Biometrics*, **59**, 305–316.

22. Mollié, A. (1996). Bayesian mapping of disease, In *Markov Chain Monte Carlo in Practice* (Eds., W. R. Gilks, S. Richardson, and J. C. Wakefield), pp. 359–379, Chapman and Hall, New York.

23. Moran, P. A. (1948). The interpretation of statistical maps, *Journal of the Royal Statistical Society, Series B*, **10**, 243–251.

24. Potthoff, R. F., and Whittinghill, M. (1966). Testing for homogeneity: II. The Poisson distribution, *Biometrika*, **53**, 183–190.

25. Rue, H. (2001). Fast sampling of Gaussian Markov random fields with applications, *Journal of the Royal Statistical Society, Series B*, **63**, 325–338.

26. Ruppert, D., Wand, M. P., and Carroll, R. J. (2003). *Semiparametric Regression*, Cambridge University Press, Cambridge, UK.

27. Schlattmann, P., and Böhning, D. (1993). Mixture models and disease mapping, *Statistics in Medicine*, **12**, 1943–1950.

28. Schmid, V., and Held, L. (2004). Bayesian extrapolation of space-time trends in cancer registry data, *Biometrics*, **60**, 1034–1042.

29. Spiegelhalter, D. J., Best, N., Carlin, B. P., and Van der Linde, A. (2002). Bayesian measures of model complexity and fit (with discussion), *Journal of the Royal Statistical Society, Series B*, **64**, 583–639.

30. Spiegelhalter, D. J., Thomas, A., Best, N., and Lunn, D. (2003). *WinBUGS Version 1.4 User Manual*, Institute of Public Health, Cambridge, U.K.

31. Waller, L. A., Carlin, B. P., Xia, H., and Gelfand, A. E. (1997). Hierarchical spatio-temporal mapping of disease rates, *Journal of the American Statistical Association*, **92**, 607–617.

30

Longitudinal Analysis of Short-Term Bronchiolitis Air Pollution Association Using Semiparametric Models

Sylvie Willems,[1] **Claire Segala,**[1] **Manuel Maidenberg,**[2] **and Mounir Mesbah**[3]

[1]*SEPIA-SANTE, Melrand, France*
[2]*RESPIRER, Paris, France*
[3]*LSTA, Université de Pierre et Marie Curie, Paris, France*

Abstract: The first aim of this work is to clearly present a very popular semi-parametric methodology often used to estimate the association between death or hospital counting data and pollution data and to estimate short-term effects of ambient air pollution on infant bronchiolitis hospital consultations. Infant bronchiolitis is a frequent infectious disease caused by a virus, the syncethial respiratory virus (RSV). Normally, contact with this virus is responsible for a cold, but in infant and in some circumstances, especially at the beginning of winter, the virus can be responsible for a severe respiratory disease which can lead to numerous hospital consultations and hospitalizations. A critical comparison of its practical application using S-Plus, R, or SAS Proc Gam is performed. It appears that more work is needed to get a satisfactory implementation of the Schwartz method in SAS with similar results to those in S-Plus or R.

Keywords and phrases: GAM model, air pollution, semiparametric models

30.1 Introduction

Time series studies of air pollution and health estimating associations between day-to-day variations in air pollution concentrations and day-to-day variations in adverse health outcomes have been widely used since the 1980s and have motivated reassessment of air quality standards in the United States and Europe.

In the last ten years, many advances have been made in the statistical modeling of air pollution time series studies. Standard regression methods used initially have been replaced by semiparametric approaches. Use of generalized additive models [GAMs; Hastie and Tibshirani (1990)] became popular in the mid-1990s. In a recent issue of *American Journal of Epidemiology*, Dominici *et al.* (2002) discuss the fact that the gam default convergence criteria defined in S-Plus version 3.4, (and, to a lesser degree in SAS) were not sufficiently rigorous for these analyses; the result was an overestimation of the effect of air pollution on health. More recently, in a issue of *Epidemiology*, Ramsay *et al.* (2003) point out that S-Plus and SAS GAM functions use a computational approximation which, in the presence of a large correlation between the nonlinear functions included in the model (called concurvity), can underestimate the standard errors of the relative rates. The community of air pollution researchers is now faced with the obligation of repeating analyses that have used the GAM function in S-Plus and considering further methodological issues [Health Effect Institute (2003)]. Researchers over the past decade have found other ways to fit GAM. Penalized regression splines (P-Splines) using R software are an example of a technique with similar characteristics to smoothing splines, that requires much less computation for standard errors. From 1997 to 2001, daily means of environmental variables including pollution data and meteorological data were gathered. In order to evaluate the impact of the GAM problems, data are analyzed using different methods:

– GAM using LOESS functions and the default convergence parameters (using S-Plus and SAS software)

– GAM using more stringent convergence parameters than the default setting (in S-Plus) and GAM using P-Splines (in R)

The aim of this work is to estimate short-term effects of PM10 on infant bronchiolitis hospital consultations. Infant bronchiolitis is a frequent infectious disease caused by a virus, the syncethial respiratory virus (RSV). Normally, contact with this virus is responsible for a cold, but in infants and in some circumstances, especially at the beginning of winter, the virus can be responsible for a severe respiratory disease which leads to numerous hospital consultations and hospitalizations. The bronchiolitis and environmental data are first presented in Section 30.2. Secondly, the methods used are detailed. GAMs are described in Section 30.3.1. The particular strategy applied in the case of air pollution time series studies is then expounded (Section 30.3.2). Next, in Section 30.3.3, criticism about the use of standard statistical software to fit GAM is displayed. Results of the bronchiolitis study are finally presented in Section 30.4.

30.2 Data

The study consists of a longitudinal data analysis based on ecological sanitary and environmental data.

30.2.1 Sanitary data

For 43 hospitals of the Paris region, the number of hospital consultations have been provided by the ERBUS ("Epidémiologie et Recueil des Bronchiolites en Urgence pour Surveillance") network for the period between 1997 and 2000, [Thélot *et al.* (1998)], given a standardized definition. Bronchiolitis is defined as respiratory dyspnea and/or sibilants and wheezing for an infant of less than 3 years old during the supervision period. Particularly, the counts are available for the period between the 15th of October and the 15th of January for each year. In 1999–2000, some hospitals momentarily stopped the data collection. To avoid missing values problems, only the 34 hospitals that provided complete data were retained for the study.

30.2.2 Environmental data

From 1997 to 2001, daily means of PM10 (particles with an aerometric diameter less than 10 microg) and meteorological data were gathered. Air pollutants were routinely measured at the stations of the AIRPARIF network. We retained PM10 data from the nine urban background monitoring sites representative of ambient air pollution in the geographical area (greater Paris). The daily average (SE) during the study period was 24.2 (10.4) micro/m^3. Weather data corresponding to Paris and its outer suburbs were provided by Meteo France. Twelve covariates were transmitted for the period beginning 01/01/1996 and finishing 12/31/2000. Five of them were chosen using the results of a previously performed principal components analysis [Tual (2003)]. The idea was to retain the covariates that carry the most information about the principal components. The weather factors retained for this study are the daily minimal temperature, the relative humidity, the daily precipitation, the daily average wind strength, and the pressure at sea level.

470 S. Willems et al.

30.3 Methods

30.3.1 Generalized additive models

GAMs [Hastie and Tibshirani (1990) and Xiang (2002)] assume that the mean of the dependent variable depends on an additive predictor through a nonlinear function. Let Y be a response random variable and $X = (X_1, \ldots, X_p)$ be a set of predictor variables. The standard linear regression model assumes the expected value of Y has a linear form and can be written as

$$E(Y|X) = f(X_1, \ldots, X_p) = \beta_0 + \beta_1 X_1 + \cdots + \beta_p X_p. \qquad (30.1)$$

The additive model generalizes the linear model by modeling the expected value of Y as

$$E(Y|X) = f(X_1, \ldots, X_p) = s_0 + s_1(X_1) + \cdots + s_p(X_p), \qquad (30.2)$$

where $s_i(X)$, $i = 1, \ldots, p$ are smooth functions. These functions are not given a parametric form but instead are estimated in a nonparametric fashion. GAMs extend traditional linear models in another way, viz., by allowing for a link between $f(X_1, \ldots, X_p)$ and the expected value of Y. Hence, GAMs consist of a random component, an additive component, and a link function relating these two components. The response Y, the random component, is assumed to have a density in the exponential family

$$f_Y(y; \theta; \phi) = \exp\left\{ \frac{y\theta - b(\theta)}{a(\phi)} + c(y; \phi) \right\}, \qquad (30.3)$$

where θ is called the natural parameter and ϕ the scale parameter. The additive component is the quantity η defined as

$$\eta = s_0 + s_1(X_1) + \cdots + s_p(X_p), \qquad (30.4)$$

where $s_i(X)$, $i = 1, \ldots, p$, are smooth functions. Finally, the relationship between the mean $E(Y|X)$ of the response variable Y and η is defined by a link function $g(E(Y|X)) = \eta$.

Scatterplot smoothing functions, commonly referred to as smoothers, are central to GAMs. A smoother is a mathematical technique for approximating an observed variable Y by a smooth function of one (or several) independent variables(s). Some examples of commonly used smoothers are smoothing splines, regression splines, LOESS functions (locally estimated polynomial regression), and kernel smoothers. These methods are nonparametric because they make no parametric assumption about the shape of the function being estimated. Each smoother has a parameter that determines how smooth the resulting function will be. For the LOESS function, that parameter is called the *span*. For smoothing splines and natural splines, the degree of smoothing can be specified through the degrees of freedom parameter. In general, the amount of smoothing selected will have more impact than the type of smoother chosen. Further information about smooth functions can be found in Hastie and Tibshirani (1990).

GAMs have the advantage that they allow greater flexibility than the traditional parametric modeling tools. They relax the usual parametric assumption and enable us to uncover hidden structure in the relationship between the independent variables and the dependent variable. The link amounts to allowing for an alternative distribution for the underlying random variation besides just the normal distribution. GAMs can therefore be applied to a much wider range of data analysis problems. In particular, they are widely used for air pollution time series studies.

30.3.2   Air pollution time series studies strategy

A time series analysis of air pollution and health raises distributional and modeling issues. On any given day, only a small portion of the population consults or is hospitalized. This number is a count, which suggests that a Poisson process is the underlying mechanism being modeled.

Analysis of the health effects of air pollution must account for other time-varying factors that may affect health outcomes to avoid taking the effects of such factors for pollution effects. Indeed, the basic issue in modeling is to control properly potential confounding. Many variables show systematic variation in time. Because any two variables that show a long-term trend must be correlated, searches for correlations that are more likely to be causal must exclude these trends. A second common attribute of many variables that evolve over time is seasonality. These variations would be present even if these factors were not causally related, and will induce correlations among them. Again, to focus on possibly causal associations, it is necessary to remove these patterns. A final systematic component that may bias time series regressions involves calendar-specific days such as day of week or holiday effects.

After season and trend, weather terms are the most important covariates to enter the model. The variables will be there to carry information about the effects of short-term variations in weather on health effect. The effects of all the explanatory variables may be immediate, or may occur with some lag.

Repeated measurements are likely to be dependent. In the case where two observations closer together in time are more alike than two randomly chosen observations, this is referred to as serial correlation. If the serial correlation in the outcome is due to omitted covariates or imperfectly controlled for covariates, serial correlation will be observed in the residuals of the model. Autoregressive models represent efficient schemes to take the serial correlation into account.

Consequently, it is essential to take into account time effects and serial correlation to identify and estimate the short-term relation between pollution and health events without bias. The model building is done, in accordance with the methodology developed by Schwartz et al. (1996), including step by step: long-term variations (trend), medium-term variations (seasonality), short-term variations (calendar-specific days, weather factors), short-term relations with the different pollutants, and autoregressive terms if necessary.

Note that, because of the high correlations between the pollutants, multi-pollutant models are seldom considered.

During the model-building process, diagnostics plots are used to evaluate the success of the approach. First, a plot of the residuals versus time can often identify long wavelength patterns that remain. These patterns should disappear as one goes along. Secondly, a plot of the predicted outcome over time can also be quite useful. The comparison of the graph of the predicted series and the graph of the initial series allows us to judge the quality of the model. Finally, a graph of the partial autocorrelation of the residuals of the model is very important. The sum of the autocorrelations should be as near to 0 as possible and, ideally, at the end of the analysis, the autocorrelation function of the residuals should be a white noise. In the case of morbidity, the autocorrelation is also due to intrinsic factors and is more difficult to suppress. Sometimes, an important residual autocorrelation remains on the first lag. It is, however, necessary to obtain a white noise beyond the ten first lags as well as a reduction of the autocorrelation on the first lags.

Let Y be the response variable studied, $date$, the covariate representing the time (in days), and $X_1, \ldots, X_k$, the different weather factors. Note pol is the pollutant considered, $J_1 = I(\text{Sunday})$, $J_6 = I(\text{Friday})$, $\ldots$, $F = I(\text{official holiday})$, $V = I(\text{holidays})$, where I is the indicator function. Let $X = (date, X_1, \ldots, X_k, pol, J_1, \ldots, J_6, F, V)$ be the set of all the covariates. Note $lo_{sp_{date}}(date)$ is the LOESS function for $date$ with a span equal to sp_{date}, and for $1 \leq i \leq k$, $lo_{sp_i}(X_i)$ is the LOESS function for the weather factor i and a span equal to sp_i. Let $lo_{sp_{pol}}(pol)$ be the LOESS function corresponding to the pollutant (with a span equal to sp_{pol}) and verifying

$$lo_{sp_{pol}}(pol) = \beta pol + f(pol), \qquad (30.5)$$

with $f(pol)$, a nonlinear function of the pollutant, and $\beta_0, \beta_{11}, \ldots, \beta_{16}, \beta_2, \beta_3$, and β, the parameters of the model. The model can be written as

$$\log\{E(Y|X)\} = \beta_0 + lo_{sp_{date}}(date) + \beta_{11} J_1 + \cdots + \beta_{16} J_6 + \beta_2 F$$
$$+ \beta_3 V + lo_{sp_{pol}}(pol) + \sum_{1 \leq i \leq k} lo_{sp_i}(X_i) = a. \qquad (30.6)$$

A model differing from the preceding one by the fact that the effect of the pollutant is linear is also interesting. This model has the form

$$
\begin{aligned}
\log\{E(Y|X)\} = {}& \beta_0 + lo_{sp_{date}}(date) + \beta_{11}J_1 + \cdots + \beta_{16}J_6 + \beta_2 F \\
& + \beta_3 V + \beta pol + \sum_{1 \le i \le k} lo_{sp_i}(X_i) = b.
\end{aligned} \tag{30.7}
$$

Because (30.5), models (30.6) and (30.7) are nested and because the distribution used is the Poisson distribution, a χ^2-test can be performed to compare them. Indeed, the deviance corresponding to a Poisson distribution is given by

$$
2 \sum_i \left\{ y_i (\log(\frac{y_i}{\mu_i})) - (y_i - \mu_i) \right\}.
$$

The difference of the deviances in models (30.6) and (30.7) has, therefore, the following form.

$$
S = 2 \sum_i \left\{ y_i f(pol) - (\exp(a) - \exp(b)) \right\}. \tag{30.8}
$$

The statistic S follows a chi-square distribution. If the two models are not significantly different, model (30.7) will be preferred for ease of interpretation.

At this step, some autocorrelation terms can be introduced in the model if it is necessary. Let $AR_1, \ldots, AR_j$, be these terms. The final model then becomes

$$
\begin{aligned}
\log\{E(Y|X)\} = {}& \beta_0 + lo_{sp_{date}}(date) + \beta_{11}J_1 + \cdots + \beta_{16}J_6 + \beta_2 F \\
& + \beta_3 V + \beta pol + \sum_{1 \le i \le k} lo_{sp_i}(X_i) + \sum_{1 \le l \le j} AR_l.
\end{aligned} \tag{30.9}
$$

The pollutant parameter can now be interpreted. Indeed, for $pol = 1$, model (30.9) becomes

$$
\begin{aligned}
\log\{E(Y|X)|pol = 1\} = {}& \beta_0 + lo_{sp_{date}}(date) + \beta_{11}J_1 + \cdots + \beta_{16}J_6 \\
& + \beta_2 F + \beta_3 V + \beta + \sum_{1 \le i \le k} lo_{sp_i}(X_i) + \sum_{1 \le l \le j} AR_l.
\end{aligned} \tag{30.10}
$$

Similarly, for $pol = 0$, model (30.9) can be written as

$$
\begin{aligned}
\log\{E(Y|X)|pol = 0\} = {}& \beta_0 + lo_{sp_{date}}(date) + \beta_{11}J_1 + \cdots + \beta_{16}J_6 \\
& + \beta_2 F + \beta_3 V + \sum_{1 \le i \le k} lo_{sp_i}(X_i) + \sum_{1 \le l \le j} AR_l.
\end{aligned} \tag{30.11}
$$

By subtracting (30.10) and (30.11), the following equation is obtained,

$$
\log\{E(Y|X)|pol = 1\} - \log\{E(Y|X)|pol = 0\} = \beta, \tag{30.12}
$$

which can be rewritten as

$$\log \left\{ \frac{[E(Y|X)|pol = 1]}{[E(Y|X)|pol = 0]} \right\} = \beta. \tag{30.13}$$

The exponential of the parameter β can therefore be interpreted as the relative risk of the variable Y for an increase of one unity of the value of the pollutant.

Note that another strategy could be adopted. The autocorrelation terms could be inserted in the model before comparing the LOESS function of the pollutant to a linear effect of this pollutant. In this work, it was chosen to add the autocorrelation terms at the end. Autocorrelation terms are introduced only for taking the serial correlation into account.

30.3.3 Criticism about the use of standard statistical software to fit GAM to epidemiological time series data

Recently, major concern has been raised about the numerical accuracy of the estimates of pollutant effect obtained by fitting GAM. Ramsay *et al.* (2003) and Dominici *et al.* (2002) identified important critical points in the analysis of epidemiological time series using commercial statistical software that fits GAM by a backfitting algorithm. Two criticisms have been made specifically. First, the default convergence criteria of the backfitting algorithm defined in S-Plus (and, to a lesser degree, in SAS) are too lax to assure convergence and lead to upwards biased estimates of pollutant effect. Secondly, the estimated standard errors obtained by fitting GAM in S-Plus or SAS are biased.

As demonstrated in Section 30.3.1, the GAM is a generalization of linear regression. Most of the familiar diagnosis tests for fitting linear regression models have analogues to fitting GAMs. One important exception to this rule is concurvity, the nonparametric analogue of multicollinearity. Multicollinearity is present in the data if some subset of the regressors is highly correlated. It leads to highly unstable and highly correlated parameter estimates associated with the multicollinear variables. Concurvity is a nonparametric extension of this concept. Concurvity occurs when a function $s(X_i)$ of one of the variables, say X_p, can be approximated by a linear combination of functions $s(X_1), \ldots, s(X_{p-1})$ of the other variables. As is the case for linear regression, the parameter estimates of a fitted GAM are highly unstable if there is concurvity in the data. If data exhibit relevant a degree of concurvity, the convergence of the backfitting algorithm can be very slow [Biggeri *et al.* (2002)]. Dominici *et al.* (2002) showed that when a smooth function for time and a smooth function for weather are included in the model, the greater the degree of concurvity, the greater is the overestimation of the pollutant effect.

At present, S-Plus and SAS provide no diagnostic tools for assessing the impact of concurvity on a fitted GAM. The inability of the GAMs to detect concurvity can lead to misleading statistical inferences, notably an overstatement of the significance of the association between air pollution and health status. Because of the way variances are estimated in the S-Plus and SAS GAM functions, the variance estimates do not reflect the instability of the parameter estimates. The variance estimates produced by the GAM function will be biased downwards in the case of concurvity. Indeed, both statistical softwaresprovide an approximation of the variance–covariance matrix, which takes into account only the linear component of the variable that was fit with a smooth function. That leads to confidence intervals on linear parameters being too narrow and in misleading *P*-values for hypothesis tests based on variance estimates, resulting in an inflated type I error.

Some solutions to these problems have been suggested [Samet *et al.* (2003)]. It was first proposed to replace GAM functions with those using stricter convergence criteria. That was suggested to correct the GAM convergence problem while acknowledging that the problem with standard error estimates was not addressed. Secondly, it could be interesting to use alternative modeling approaches to GAM fitted by A backfitting algorithm. The use of generalized linear models (GLMs) with natural cubic splines, using approximately the same degrees of freedom as were used in the original GAMs or the use of GAM with penalized regression spline fitted by the direct method in R software, which correctly computes the variance–covariance matrix, are two solutions. These solutions were suggested for correcting problems with the standard errors.

In the case of the bronchiolitis study, it was decided to evaluate the sensitivity of the results by fitting: firstly, GAM by the backfitting algorithm using S-Plus with default or stringent convergence criteria and secondly, GAM by the direct method implemented in R 1.6.2 software. A comparison between S-Plus and SAS results has also been performed.

30.4   Results

The different programs used to produce results here can be obtained from the authors on request. An example is presented for S-Plus, and a comparison with R and SAS is discussed.

30.4.1   Series of number of hospital consultations: Results with S-Plus

This section deals with the model-building process of the daily number of hospital consultations for infant bronchiolitis for the period between 1997 and 2000, using the S-Plus method.

For each model tested, a graphical validation step consisting of examination of the graph of the residual, and/or the autocorrelation, and/or the partial autocorrelation of its residuals and the graph of the LOESS function for the new introduced variable is performed. Due to the large number of these models, only a few representative graphs will be presented here.

Long term and seasonal variations

Figure 30.1 displays the daily number of hospital consultations for infant bronchiolitis in the 34 hospitals considered for this study. The series shows clearly some seasonal variations. A peak can be observed each winter.

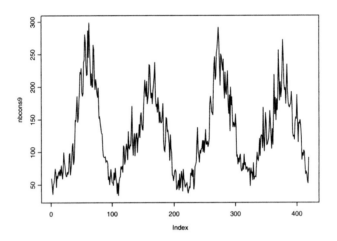

Figure 30.1: Daily number of hospital consultations for bronchiolitis

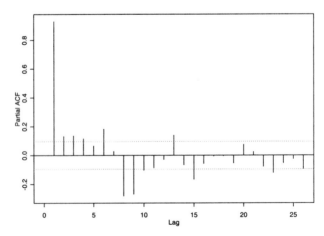

Figure 30.2: Autocorrelations of the daily number of hospital consultations for bronchiolitis

The autocorrelation of the number of hospital consultations is given in Figure 30.2. The interval around 0 represents the 95% confidence interval of the test of the null hypothesis "null autocorrelation." This graph shows that some serial correlation is present in the data. The autocorrelation on the first lag is very high.

Long-term and seasonal variations are first modeled by introducing the time in the model. A LOESS function is used as a smoothing function. By looking at the different validation graphs, a span equal to 0.15 is retained. Figures 30.3 and 30.4 show, respectively, the graph of the residuals of the model and the graph of partial autocorrelation of these residuals. After adjustment for the trend and seasonal variations, the partial autocorrelation of the residuals decreases considerably on the first lag and is low on the last lags. Some lags are, however, still significantly different from 0.

Figure 30.5 displays the LOESS function corresponding to the time. It represents the part of the logarithm of the number of hospital consultations explained by this covariate. The seasonal variations of the daily number of hospital consultations can be clearly observed. Indeed, the four peaks are present on this graph.

At this step, the model can be written as

$$\log\{E(nb|X)\} = \beta_0 + lo_{0.15}(date), \tag{30.14}$$

with nb as the number of hospital consultations in the 34 hospitals retained for the study.

Short-term variations

The next step consists in modeling the short-term variations by introducing the variables corresponding to the days of the week (six binary variables J1,... ,J6, with Sunday as reference), official holidays (binary variable: F), and holidays (binary variable: V). After each introduction, the graphs of partial autocorrelation of the residuals of the model and the part of the logarithm of the number of consultations explained by each covariate were produced and evaluated. The model obtained after this step can then be written as

$$\log\{E(nb|X)\} = \beta_0 + lo_{0.15}(date) + \beta_{11}J_1 + \cdots + \beta_{16}J_6 + \beta_2 F + \beta_3 V. \tag{30.15}$$

After taking these covariates into account, the partial autocorrelation of the residuals becomes null on the last lags.

Introduction of the weather factors

All five weather factors could be introduced in the model. The minimal temperature is the first included in the model. It was decided to choose the lag for

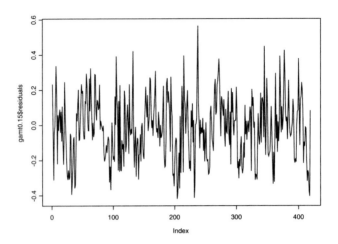

Figure 30.3: Residuals of model (30.14)

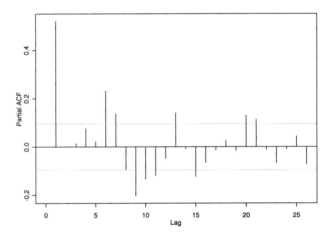

Figure 30.4: Partial autocorrelation of the residuals after introduction of the time

this covariate using the "AIC-criterion" and to keep the same lag for the other weather factors. The minimal temperature at lag 1 is retained. Let $tmin1$ be this variable. As for the covariate representing the time, a LOESS function is used to model the effect of minimal temperature at lag 1. A span equal to 0.8 is retained by looking at the validation graphs. Then, successively, the relative humidity, the daily precipitation, the wind strength, and the atmospheric pressure were taken into consideration. As for the minimal temperature, the examination of the validation graphs allows us to choose the span value. The final

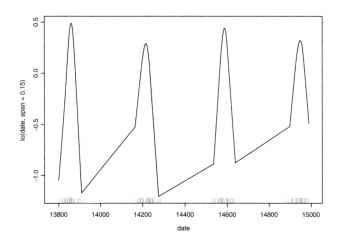

Figure 30.5: LOESS function corresponding to the time

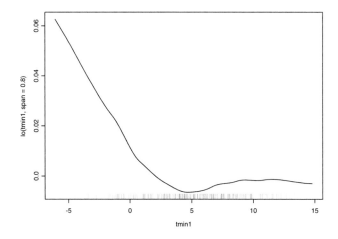

Figure 30.6: LOESS function for the minimal temperature

model at this step is

$$
\begin{aligned}
\log\{E(nb|X)\} = {} & \beta_0 + lo_{0.15}(date) + \beta_{11}J_1 + \cdots + \beta_{16}J_6 + \beta_2 F \\
& + \beta_3 V + lo_{0.8}(tmin1) + lo_{0.6}(humrel1) + lo_{0.7}(precipit1) \\
& + lo_{0.7}(forcvent1) + lo_{0.9}(pressmer1).
\end{aligned}
$$

$$(30.16)$$

Short-term relations with air pollution

For PM10, two indicators were analyzed. Let $pm10A1$ be the average of the pollutant concentration over 2 days (the day considered and the previous day) and $pm10A5$ be the average of the pollutant concentration over 6 days (the day considered and the 5 previous days). Only one of these indicators is included in the model at a time. A LOESS function with a span value equal to 0.7 is used to model the pollutant effect [Le Tertre (2003)]. If the introduction of the pollutant is pertinent, the model is compared, as explained in Section 30.3.2, to a model presenting a linear effect of this pollutant.

Table 30.1 displays summary of the p-values corresponding to the introduction of PM10.

Table 30.1: Summary of the introduction of the different pollutants

Pollutant	$pm10A1$	$pm10A5$
p-value	0.0626	$\mathbf{1.3736 * 10^{-6}}$

The introduction of the average over 6 days is significant and a new model is obtained as

$$\log\{E(nb|X)\} = A + lo_{0.7}pm10A5. \tag{30.17}$$

The model containing a linear trend of the pollutant is equivalent to the one including a LOESS function. Table 30.4.1 displays a summary of the p-values corresponding to the test of the null hypothesis, "Model with linear term is equivalent to model with LOESS function."

Table 30.2: Summary of the test comparing the model including a linear term and the one with a LOESS function

Pollutant	$pm10A5$
p-value	**0.1639**

The pollutant for which the linear term is retained is the particle matter less than 10 μm in aerodynamic diameter. These models can then be written as

$$\log\{E(nb|X)\} = A + \beta pm10A5. \tag{30.18}$$

For the particle matter less than 10 μm in aerodynamic diameter, a comparison between the LOESS function and the linear term is shown in Figure 30.7.

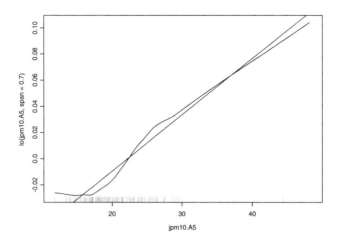

Figure 30.7: Comparison between LOESS function and linear term for $pm10A5$

A lot of serial correlation remains on the first lag. Some autoregressive terms are therefore introduced in the model. After looking at the validation graphs, it was decided to introduce three autoregressive terms in the model. Hence, the final model has the following form.

$$\log\{E(nb|X)\} = A + \beta pm10A5 + \sum_{1 \le l \le 4} AR_l. \tag{30.19}$$

The graph of the partial autocorrelation of the residuals of these final models is produced. A graph of partial autocorrelation very close to a white noise can be observed. A graphical comparison between the series and the predictive values for the final model shows us that this model is good.

It has been shown in Section 30.3.2 that the exponential of the parameter β can be interpreted as the relative risk of the number of hospital consultations for an increase of one unity of the value of the pollutant. Table 30.3 displays the estimate of the parameter β, its standard error, the corresponding t-value, the relative risk for an increase of 10 unities of the pollutant, and its confidence interval.

The model-building process was repeated using more stringent convergence parameters than the default setting. Results obtained were exactly the same.

Table 30.3: Summary of the estimates of the final models

Model	β	Standard Error	t-Value	Relative Risk	CI$(-)$	CI$(+)$
$pm10A5$	0.0083	0.0013	6.2506	1.0863	1.0585	1.1149

30.4.2 Series of number of hospital consultations: Results with R

Models obtained in the previous section are rebuilt using R software. LOESS functions are replaced by penalized splines with a number of knots k and a smoothing parameter λ instead of a span parameter. The model-building process under R is not done from the beginning. Concerning the specific days and the weather factors, for an easier comparison with S-Plus results, the covariates retained in Section 30.4.1 will be used here. Hence, the five weather factors will be used at lag 1. Moreover, only one pollutant, the particle matter less than 10 μm in aerodynamic diameter, for which the relation hospital consultations–pollutant has been expressed in relative risk (in Section 30.4.1) is considered.

A model without any pollutant is built first. Spline functions are used to model the effect of the time and of the weather factors. By looking at the validation graphs, the selected model is

$$
\begin{aligned}
\log&\{E(nb|X)\} \\
&= \beta_0 + s_{40\&5.8*10^4}(date) + \beta_{11}J_1 + \cdots + \beta_{16}J_6 + \beta_2F + \beta_3V \\
&\quad + s_{5\&5.1*10^{11}}(tmin1) + s_{8\&5.6*10^4}(humrel1) + s_{6\&2.3*10^5}(precipit1) \\
&\quad + s_{5\&1*10^6}(forcvent1) + s_{5\&8*10^6}(pressmer1), \quad\quad (30.20)
\end{aligned}
$$

with $s_{40\&5.8*10^4}(date)$ being a penalized spline of the time using a number of knots k equal to 40 and a smoothing parameter λ equal to $5.8*10^4$. The graph of the partial autocorrelation of the residuals of this model was produced and examined. Only for very few lags, is the partial autocorrelation significatively different from 0.

The next step is the introduction of the pollutant. Particle matter less than 10 μm improves the model significantly (p-values are $3.6085*10^{-5}$) .

The penalized splines corresponding to this pollutant were examined. The number of hospital consultations increases with the pollutants. Because this function is almost a perfect line, the model including a linear term for the pollutant is preferred to the one including a nonparametric function of the same pollutant. This new model is

$$\begin{aligned}
\log\{E(nb|X)\} \\
= \quad & \beta_0 + s_{40\&5.8*10^4}(date) + \beta_{11}J_1 + \cdots + \beta_{16}J_6 + \beta_2 F + \beta_3 V \\
& + s_{5\&5.1*10^{11}}(tmin1) + s_{8\&5.6*10^4}(humrel1) + s_{6\&2.3*10^5}(precipit1) \\
& + s_{5\&1*10^6}(forcvent1) + s_{5\&8*10^6}(pressmer1) + \beta pm10A5. \quad (30.21)
\end{aligned}$$

The graph of the partial autocorrelation of the residuals of the final model was produced. Almost a white noise can be observed. Therefore, it was decided not to introduce autoregressive terms in this case.

Again, the exponential of the parameter β can be interpreted as the relative risk of the number of consultations for an increase of one unity of the value of the pollutant. Table 30.4 displays the estimate of the parameter β, its standard error, the t-value, the relative risk for an increase of 10 unities of the pollutant, and its confidence interval.

Table 30.4: Summary of the estimates of the final models

Model	β	Standard Error	t-Value	Relative Risk	CI$(-)$	CI$(+)$
$pm10$ (30.21)	0.0043	0.0010	4.159	1.0441	1.0231	1.0655

Using p-splines with R, the estimate of the increase in consultations dropped to 4.4 percent per 10 mg/m^3 increase in PM10 with a standard error of 0.0010, compared with 8.6 percent (se: 0.0013) using LOESS with S-Plus.

30.4.3   SAS results

As in S-Plus, proc GAM in SAS allows us to fit GAMs using LOESS functions. However, the smoothing parameter differs from S-Plus. Instead of a "span parameter," the LOESS function needs a "*DF* parameter." An option allows us to ask the value of the smoothing parameter to be selected by generalized cross-validation. The default method in SAS uses $DF = 4$ for each smooth function. It is also permitted to choose a particular DF for each function. This last method is equivalent to playing with the spans in S-Plus.

In order to compare S-Plus and SAS software, the models obtained using S-Plus have also been implemented in SAS. They are first programmed using, for each LOESS function, the DF value given in the S-Plus output. The LOESS functions corresponding to the different covariates of the model can be obtained. They appear, more or less, to be the ones obtained using S-Plus.

The use of SAS software to apply this method on the bronchiolitis data has some disadvantages. First, SAS looks for functions with values of DF as close as possible to the values asked. That leads to smooth functions different from those asked. For instance, the obtained graph does not show, as expected, the four peaks corresponding to the seasonal variations of the daily number of hospital consultations. Secondly, it takes longer than S-Plus. Indeed, for the bronchiolitis data, a program runs several hours in SAS whereas it is almost instantaneous in S-Plus. Finally, the validation graphs used to construct the model step by step are not provided in the options of the GAM-procedure in SAS. They can be obtained more easily in S-Plus.

An interesting challenge could be building a SAS macro that allows SAS procedures (GAM and others, such as Arima and Graphs) to perform the Schwartz method.

30.5 Discussion

Numerous time series studies have linked levels of particulate air pollution to daily mortality and cardiorespiratory hospitalizations. However, the study of the specific role of air pollution as a risk factor for specific respiratory disease is not usual. This study, conducted in Paris during four successive winters, found that prevailing levels of PM10 had measurable short-term effects on hospital consultations for an infectious disease in infants, bronchiolitis.

Generalized additive models (GAMs) with smoothing splines were used for this purpose and models are presented in detail in this paper. Because of the critical points identified in the analysis of epidemiological time series using commercial statistical software which fits GAMs by a backfitting algorithm, a sensibility analysis was performed using S-Plus, R, and SAS software.

The model-building process was done in accordance with the method proposed by Schwartz, controlling for weather, season, and other longer-term time-varying factors to minimize confounding the effect estimates for the air pollutant. Models were first constructed using LOESS functions in the GAM function S-Plus. PM10 (particle matter less than 10 μm) present an effect that can be expressed in terms of a relative risk of hospital consultation for an increase of a certain amount of the pollutant concentration. An increase of 10 μg/m^3 of the particle matter less than 10 μm raises the risk of hospital consultation for bronchiolitis of 8.6% [95% CI is (5.9; 11.5)]. Because it was raised that the default convergence criteria of the backfitting algorithm would be too lax to assure convergence, the model-building process was repeated using more stringent convergence parameters than the default setting; results obtained were identical.

The models obtained in S-Plus were then rebuilt using R software. LOESS functions were replaced by penalized splines. An increase of 10 μg/m^3 of the particle matter less than 10 μm raises this risk of only 4.4% [95% CI (2.3; 6.6)]. S-Plus provides no diagnosis tools for assessing the impact of concurvity on a fitted GAM. S-Plus version 3.4 leads to an overstatement of the significance of the association between air pollution and health status. Moreover, S-Plus provides an approximation of the variance–covariance matrix, which takes into account only the linear component of the variable fitted with a smooth function. That would lead to confidence intervals on linear parameters being too narrow. As was expected, the relative risks obtained using S-Plus are higher than the ones obtained with R. However, with this data set, confidence intervals around the estimate are similar (and even a little larger) in S-Plus than in R.

The model-building process is easier to implement in S-Plus than in R. Indeed, using the LOESS function in S-Plus, values must be chosen for the span of each covariate for which the effect is modeled using a smooth function. Using penalized splines in R, values for two parameters (k and λ) have to be selected for each covariate. Therefore, for ease of comparison, we first build the models using S-Plus before working with R.

Using GAM in SAS is more difficult. Indeed, the validation graphs used to construct the model step by step are not provided in the options of the GAM procedure in SAS. Creating SAS macros for an application of the Schwartz method will be of interest. However, in the case of the bronchiolitis data, SAS software does not seem to be very appropriate because of the time necessary to run the different programs. Moreover, implementation in SAS presents more problems than in S-Plus.

The methodological issues in time series analysis of air pollution epidemiology are important as the air pollution effect is small and possibly confounded by varying factors that are correlated with pollution exposures. The potential for incorrect standard errors in GAMs was known [Hastie and Tibshirani (1990)], but the new methods had not been implemented in widely used software, and therefore have not reached epidemiologists. Actually, the S-Plus default convergence parameters have already been revised in the new S-Plus version and revisions of GAM software implementation, to enable "exact" calculations of the standard errors are underway.

Our work has permitted us to show that the pollutants would have a short-term incidence on infant bronchiolitis and to confirm the overestimation of the risks by the implementation of GAMs in S-Plus, version 3.4.

Acknowledgements. This study was supported by Conseil Scientifique de l'ANTADIR. The authors are grateful to Délégation à l'Information Médicale et à L'Epidémiologie, AP-HP, Paris who provided ERBUS data.

References

1. Biggeri, A., Baccini, M., Accetta, G., and Lagazio C. (2002). Estimates of short-term effects of air pollutants in Italy, *Epidemiologia e Prevenzione*, **26**, 203–205 (in Italian).

2. Dominici, F., McDermott, A., Zeger, S. L., and Samet, J. (2002). On the use of generalized additive models in times-series studies of air pollution and health, *American Journal of Epidemiology*, **156**, 193.

3. Hastie, T. J. and Tibshirani, R. J. (1990). *Generalized Additive Models*, Chapman & Hall, London.

4. Health Effects Institute, (2003). *Revised Analyses of Time-Series Studies of Air Pollution and Health*, Boston, Massachusetts.

5. Le Tertre, A. (2003). Personal Communication, INVS, Paris.

6. Ramsay, T. O., Burnett, R. T., and Krewski, D. (2003). The effect of concurvity in generalized additive models linking mortality to ambient particulate matter, *Epidemiology*, **14**, 18–23.

7. Samet, J. M., Dominici, F., McDermott, A., and Zeger, S. L. (2003). New problems for an old design: Time series analyses of air pollution and health, *Epidemiology*, **14**, 11–17.

8. SAS Stat Documentation (2001). Chapter 4: The GAM Procedure Release 8.1.

9. Schwartz, J., Spix, C., Touloumi, G., Bacharova, L., Barumamdzadeh, T., Le Tertre, A., Piekarski, T., Leon, A. P., Pönka, A., Rossi, G., Saez, M., Schouten, J. P. (1996). Methodological issues in studies of air pollution and daily counts of deaths or hospital admissions, *Journal of Epidemiology and Community Health*, **50** (Sup. 1), S3–S11.

10. Thélot, B., Bénichou, J. J., Cheron, G., Chevalier, B., Begué, P., and Bourrillon, A. (1998). Surveillance épidémiologique hospitalière de la bronchiolite du nourisson par le réseau ERBUS, *Revue d'Epidemiologie et de Santé Publique*, **46**, 277–288.

11. Tual, S. (2003). Rapport de stage, Etude de l'impact des facteurs environnementaux extérieurs et des facteurs de susceptibilité individuelle dans la survenue d'affections respiratoires et cardio-vasculaires, Rapport de stage, IUT Statitisque et Informatique de Vannes, Vannes, France.

12. Xiang, D. (2002). Fitting generalized additive models with the GAM procedure, In *Statistics, Data Analysis, and Data Mining*, SUGI Proceeding.

PART IX
GENOMIC ANALYSIS

31

Are There Correlated Genomic Substitutions?

M. Karnoub,[1] **P. K. Sen,**[2] **and F. Seillier-Moiseiwitsch**[3]

[1] *GlaxoSmithKline, Research Triangle Park, NC, USA*
[2] *University of North Carolina at Chapel Hill, Chapel Hill, NC, USA*
[3] *Georgetown University, Washington, DC, USA*

Abstract: Evidence shows that mutations along some genomes do not all occur independently. This paper introduces statistical methodology for testing the assumption of independence of the substitution processes acting at two different positions. We consider specific pairs of sites along a genome of interest. For each pair, we focus on the distribution of double mutations away from the consensus (i.e., the most frequent configuration) conditioning on the total number of sequences and on the consensus pair. The resulting test statistic is applicable to general contingency tables that have an arbitrary number of rows and columns.

Keywords and phrases: Contingency table, genomic sequences, independence, statistical test

31.1 Introduction

For genomic sequences, the probabilistic model underlying analytical methods relies, more often than not, on the assumption that positions undergo independent mutation processes. For example, in phylogenetic reconstruction, many popular models for the substitutions at a single position stem from the reversible continuous-time time-homogeneous Markov chain model by imposing various constraints on the rate parameters [Tavaré (1986) and Rodrígues *et al.* (1990)]. The assumption of independence can be relaxed in a number of ways. For instance, Felsenstein and Churchill (1996) consider a hidden Markov model for the assignment of substitution rates at different positions, which results in correlated rates and implies that, once these rates are fixed, positions undergo independent mutation processes. Violation of the assumption of independence leads to the overestimation of genetic distances and therefore to erroneous phylogenetic reconstructions [Seillier-Moiseiwitsch *et al.* (1998)]. It is, therefore, critical to assess whether this assumption holds. The methodology introduced in this paper can serve to check this assumption. It is suitable for contingency tables with an arbitrary number of rows and columns. A statistical test for 2×2 tables or for the total number of double mutations in a contingency table of arbitrary dimension was published in Karnoub, Seillier-Moiseiwitsch, and Sen (1999).

Here, we are concerned with detecting correlated substitutions. Via the consensus character (either amino acid or nucleotide depending on the nature of the data) at a position we can identify changes at that position. Consequently, to locate the correlated changes at different positions, we need to condition on the joint consensus. Other techniques [Korber *et al.* (1993) and Bickel *et al.* (1996)] do not take this consensus into account and thus test for independence between positions rather than independence of substitutions. In these papers, departures from independence can be caused by correlations between a consensus and a change; this type of correlation is not of interest in our case. Furthermore, these tests are not suitable for situations where a strong consensus is expected [Karnoub (1997)].

The outline of this chapter is as follows. In Section 31.2, we describe the probabilistic model underlying the contingency tables. Parameter estimates are derived in Section 31.3. We present a χ^2-type test in Section 31.4. A power study is described in Section 31.5. In Section 31.6, we summarize the results of some simulations. We close this chapter with a data analysis (Section 31.7) and a brief discussion (Section 31.8).

31.2 The Probabilistic Model

In some contexts, it is justifiable to treat sequences as independent, at least as a first assumption. In the case of sequences from the immunodeficiency virus (HIV), for instance, replication cycles are short (e.g., 1 to 2 days) and each cycle yields a number of substitutions (1 to 10). When sequences are sampled from different individuals, hundreds of rounds of replication are likely to separate any two viruses, with each position having had many opportunities to mutate. Furthermore, functionality of the resulting proteins drives survival/fitness of the organism. Functionality depends on structure, and thus dictates whether a position is allowed to mutate and whether substitutions at one position work in concert with events at other positions. Hence, structural constraints and high turn-over rates overwhelm ancestral relationships.

Consider a specific pair of sites along the sequences of interest, say positions I and J. At position I, over all sequences, the characters (amino acids or nucleotides) are $A_{I1}, A_{I2}, \ldots, A_{Ic}$, whereas at position J they are $A_{J1}, A_{J2}, \ldots,$

Table 31.1: Contingency table summarizing the observed characters (either amino acids or nucleotides) at two generic positions

Position I

		A_{I1}	A_{I2}	$\ldots$	A_{Ic}	Total
	A_{J1}	n_{11}, p_{11}	n_{12}	$\ldots$	n_{1c}	$n_{1.}$
		consensus	p_{12}		p_{1c}	$p_{1.}$
	A_{J2}	n_{21}	n_{22}	$\ldots$	n_{2c}	$n_{2.}$
		p_{21}	p_{22}		p_{2c}	$p_{2.}$
Position J	$\vdots$	$\vdots$	$\vdots$	$\ddots$	$\vdots$	$\vdots$
	A_{Jr}	n_{r1}	n_{r2}	$\ldots$	n_{rc}	$n_{r.}$
		p_{r1}	p_{r2}		p_{rc}	$p_{r.}$
	Total	$n_{.1}$	$n_{.2}$	$\ldots$	$n_{.c}$	n
		$p_{.1}$	$p_{.2}$		$p_{.c}$	

A_{Jr}. The indices c and r run to at most 4 for nucleotides and at most 20 for amino acids. Table 31.1 gives the observed counts for all possible pairs of characters at these positions. By convention, the $(1,1)$-cell contains the number of sequences with the consensus configuration. Observed counts are denoted by n_{ij} and the corresponding random variables by N_{ij}. Let N_{ij} be the number of sequences with A_{Ii} at position I and A_{Jj} at position J, and p_{ij} the probability of having this configuration. Any sequence in the first row or the first column but not in the $(1,1)$-cell sustained a single mutation away from the consensus. All sequences outside the first row and column had two mutations. The total number of observed sequences is represented by N and its realization by n.

The interest here is in investigating whether departures from the consensus characters at two positions are correlated. Clearly, the identification of substitutions relies on the identification of the consensus pair. This is essentially our reasoning behind conditioning on the consensus cell. In addition, there are two statistical arguments in favor of conditioning on N_{11}. First, the data are presented in a usually large $r \times c$ contingency table (with r and c between 2 and 20) with many empty and low-frequency cells. Hence, the exact test conditional on fixed marginals has little power. To gain power, the table needs to be reduced. To this end, we use the consensus cell as it does not contain information on the correlation between mutations. The consensus being data dependent, conditioning on this consensus affects the table structure and the probability model. Second, the size of N_{11} affects the power of the test: its order of magnitude is different from those of other entries (see Tables 31.5 and 31.6). Conditioning on N_{11}, again, improves power.

It is argued [Karnoub (1997)] that the familiar Fisher's exact test based on the hypergeometric law or its large-sample (normal) approximation are not justifiable in the present context. Indeed, conditioning on the marginal totals is not an option because we do not have any knowledge about the total number of mutations with a specific character at any one of the positions. We could, however, remove the conditioning by taking the expected values and variances over all possible marginals. Because the asymptotic distribution of the conditional test statistic does not depend on these, we would still retain the normal distribution as the unconditional distribution of the test statistic. But, we need to deal with the fact that we know the consensus and the number of sequences with this consensus. The maximality of N_{11} and its being fixed to n_{11} are not easily handled in such a setup. We therefore develop a test where we condition on the total sample size and on the fact that we know that the $(1,1)$ cell is maximal and equal to n_{11}.

The standard distributions associated with cell counts in contingency tables are: the Poisson model obtained with a sampling plan that has no restrictions on the total sample size, the multinomial model with a fixed total sample size, and independent multinomial distributions for the rows with fixed row totals or independent multinomial distributions for the columns with fixed column totals [Bishop, Fienberg, and Holland (1975)]. For these sampling models, the marginal totals are sufficient statistics for testing the independence of two factors. Furthermore, under the assumption of independence of the factors, the maximum-likelihood estimates under the above sampling processes exist, are unique, and, if none of the marginals is 0, they are equal. In fact, when the total sample size is fixed, the multinomial and Poisson schemes are equivalent [Bishop, Fienberg, and Holland (1975)]. The Poisson model is usually preferred when the events are rare; that is, the cell counts are small. In view of the nature of our data, we adopt this model here.

The assumptions are:

1. The cell counts N_{ij} are mutually independent and have a Poisson distribution with means λ_{ij},

$$P\left(N_{ij} = n_{ij}\right) = \frac{e^{-\lambda_{ij}} \, \lambda_{ij}^{n_{ij}}}{n_{ij}!} \, , \qquad 1 \leq i \leq r, \qquad 1 \leq j \leq c.$$

2. $\lambda_{11} \gg \lambda_{ij}$ for all $(i,j) \neq (1,1)$ and the λ_{ij}s are all greater than 5, preferably greater than 10.

Let $\lambda = \sum\limits_{(i,j)} \lambda_{ij}$. The two hypotheses of interest are

- The null hypothesis H_0: $\lambda_{ij} = \lambda \, \alpha_i \, \beta_j$ for all (i,j), $\sum\limits_i \alpha_i = 1$, $\sum\limits_j \beta_j = 1$.

- The alternative hypothesis H_1: the cell counts are not restricted in any way.

Let $N_* = N - N_{11}$, $n_* = n - n_{11}$ and let $\lambda_* = \lambda - \lambda_{11}$. We derive the joint distribution of the cell counts, given the fixed $(1,1)$-cell count n_{11} and the fixed total sample size n. First,

$$P\left(N_{11} = n_{11},\ N_{12} = n_{12}, \ldots, N_{rc} = n_{rc}\,|\,N_{11} = n_{11}\right) = e^{-\lambda_*}\,\frac{\displaystyle\prod_{(i,j)\neq(1,1)} \lambda_{ij}^{n_{ij}}}{\displaystyle\prod_{(i,j)\neq(1,1)} n_{ij}!}\,.$$

As for the distribution of N_* given the fixed $(1,1)$-cell count n_{11},

$$P\left(N_* = n_*\,|\,N_{11} = n_{11}\right) = \frac{P\left(N_* = n_*,\ N_{11} = n_{11}\right)}{P\left(N_{11} = n_{11}\right)} = e^{-\lambda_*}\,\frac{\lambda_*^{n_*}}{n_*!}\,.$$

Therefore,

$$P\left(N_{12} = n_{12}, \ldots, N_{rc} = n_{rc}\,|\,N_{11} = n_{11}\,,\ N = n\right)$$
$$= \begin{cases} \dfrac{P\left(N_{12} = n_{12}, \ldots, N_{rc} = n_{rc}\,|\,N_{11} = n_{11}\right)}{P\left(N = n\,|\,N_{11} = n_{11}\right)} & \text{if } n_{11} + \ldots + n_{rc} = n \\ 0 \quad \text{otherwise}\,. \end{cases}$$

Now, $P\left(N = n\,|\,N_{11} = n_{11}\right) = P\left(N_* = n_*\,|\,N_{11} = n_{11}\right)$. If $\lambda_{11} \gg \lambda_{ij}$ for all $(i,j) \neq (1,1)$ and $\lambda_{ij} > 5$ (cf. Appendix 31.1), then

$$P\left(N_{12} = n_{12}, \ldots, N_{rc} = n_{rc}\,,\ N_{11}\ \text{maximum}\,|\,N_{11} = n_{11}\right)$$
$$\approx P\left(N_{12} = n_{12}, \ldots, N_{rc} = n_{rc}\,|\,N_{11} = n_{11}\right)\,,$$

$$P\left(N_* = n_*\,,\ N_{11}\ \text{maximum}\,|\,N_{11} = n_{11}\right) \approx P\left(N_* = n_*\,|\,N_{11} = n_{11}\right)$$

$$P\left(N_{12} = n_{12}, \ldots, N_{rc} = n_{rc}\,|\,N_{11} = n_{11}, N_{11}\ \text{maximum}\,,\ N = n\right)$$
$$\approx \frac{n_*}{n_{12}!\,n_{21}! \ldots n_{rc}!}\left(\frac{\lambda_{12}}{\lambda_*}\right)^{n_{12}}\left(\frac{\lambda_{21}}{\lambda_*}\right)^{n_{21}} \cdots \left(\frac{\lambda_{rc}}{\lambda_*}\right)^{n_{rc}}\,.$$

This is thus an $((r \times c) - 1)$-multinomial distribution with parameters n_* and λ_{ij}/λ_*, $1 \leq i \leq r$, $1 \leq j \leq c$. The expected values, variances, and covariances of the cell counts under this conditional model are

$$E\left(N_{ij}\,|\,N_{11} = n_{11},\ N_{11}\ \text{maximum}\,,\ N_* = n_*\right) \approx n_*\,\frac{\lambda_{ij}}{\lambda_*}$$

$$\text{Var}\left(N_{ij}\,|\,N_{11} = n_{11},\ N_{11}\ \text{maximum}\,,\ N_* = n_*\right) \approx n_*\,\frac{\lambda_{ij}}{\lambda_*}\left(1 - \frac{\lambda_{ij}}{\lambda_*}\right)$$

$$\text{Cov}\left(N_{ij},\ N_{kl}\,|\,N_{11} = n_{11},\ N_{11}\ \text{maximum}\,,\ N_* = n_*\right) \approx -n_*\,\frac{\lambda_{ij}}{\lambda_*}\,\frac{\lambda_{kl}}{\lambda_*}\,.$$

31.3 Parameter Estimation

Under H_0,

$$P\left(N_{11} = n_{11}, \ldots, N_{rc} = n_{rc} \mid N_{11} = n_{11}, N_{11} \text{ maximum}, N = n\right)$$
$$\approx \frac{n_*}{n_{12}! \, n_{21}! \, \ldots \, n_{rc}!} \left(\frac{\alpha_1 \beta_2}{1 - \alpha_1 \beta_1}\right)^{n_{12}} \left(\frac{\alpha_2 \beta_1}{1 - \alpha_1 \beta_1}\right)^{n_{21}} \cdots \left(\frac{\alpha_r \beta_c}{1 - \alpha_1 \beta_1}\right)^{n_{rc}}.$$

This conditional law is a function of the $(r + c - 2)$ parameters α_i and β_j, $1 \leq i \leq r - 1$, $1 \leq j \leq c - 1$. As there are $(r \times c - 2)$ degrees of freedom, non-estimability of the parameters is not a issue. However, to comply with the constraints imposed by fixing $N_{11} = n_{11}$ and $N = n$, we estimate $\Theta = \alpha_1 \beta_1$ from the marginal distribution of N_{11} and utilize $\widehat{\Theta}$ in the log-likelihood for α_i and β_j, $1 \leq i \leq r - 1$, $1 \leq j \leq c - 1$.

The marginal distribution of N_{11} given n is, under H_0,

$$P\left(N_{11} = n_{11} \mid N = n\right) = \frac{n!}{n_{11}! \, (n - n_{11})!} \, (\alpha_1 \beta_1)^{n_{11}} \, (1 - \alpha_1 \beta_1)^{n_*}.$$

Because $(\partial^2 L_0(\Theta))/\partial \Theta^2 = -(n_{11}/\Theta^2) - (n_*/((1 - \Theta)^2)) < 0$, the maximum likelihood estimate of Θ based on this marginal law is $\widehat{\Theta} = n_{11}/n$.

To simplify computations, we keep the log-likelihood as a function of all αs and βs and maximize it with respect to the constraints

$$\alpha_r = 1 - \sum_{1 \leq i \leq r-1} \alpha_i, \quad \beta_c = 1 - \sum_{1 \leq j \leq c-1} \beta_j \quad \text{and} \quad \Theta = \widehat{\Theta}.$$

Maximizing the log-likelihood is the same as minimizing

$$f\left(\alpha_i, \beta_j, 1 \leq i \leq r, 1 \leq j \leq c\right)$$
$$= -\left(n_{1.} - n_{11}\right) \log \alpha_1 - \sum_{i \neq 1} n_{i.} \log \alpha_i - \left(n_{.1} - n_{11}\right) \log \beta_1 - \sum_{j \neq 1} n_{.j} \log \beta_j$$

subject to the constraints

$$g_1\left(\alpha_i, \beta_j, 1 \leq i \leq r, 1 \leq j \leq c\right) = \alpha_1 + \alpha_2 + \cdots + \alpha_r - 1 = 0$$
$$g_2\left(\alpha_i, \beta_j, 1 \leq i \leq r, 1 \leq j \leq c\right) = \beta_1 + \beta_2 + \cdots + \beta_c - 1 = 0$$
$$g_3\left(\alpha_i, \beta_j, 1 \leq i \leq r, 1 \leq j \leq c\right) = \alpha_1 \beta_1 - \widehat{\Theta} = 0.$$

Now represent the gradient of a function h by ∇h and define

$$\mathbf{g}\left(\alpha_i, \beta_j, 1 \leq i \leq r, 1 \leq j \leq c\right) = \begin{bmatrix} g_1\left(\alpha_i, \beta_j\right) \\ g_2\left(\alpha_i, \beta_j\right) \\ g_3\left(\alpha_i, \beta_j\right) \end{bmatrix}.$$

The first-order necessary condition for finding a point at which $f(\alpha_i, \beta_j)$ attains its minimum is that there exists a vector $\mu^\tau = (\mu_1, \mu_2, \mu_3)$ such that

$$\nabla f^\tau + \mu^\tau \nabla g^\tau = 0$$

[Luenberger (1984)]. Because

$$\nabla f^\tau = \left[-\frac{n_{1.} - n_{11}}{\alpha_1} \quad -\frac{n_{2.}}{\alpha_2} \quad \cdots \quad -\frac{n_{r.}}{\alpha_r} \quad -\frac{n_{.1} - n_{11}}{\beta_1} \quad -\frac{n_{.2}}{\beta_2} \quad \cdots \quad -\frac{n_{.c}}{\beta_c} \right]$$

and
$$\nabla g^\tau = \begin{bmatrix} 1 & 1 & \cdots & 1 & 0 & 0 & \cdots & 0 \\ 0 & 0 & \cdots & 0 & 1 & 1 & \cdots & 1 \\ \beta_1 & 0 & \cdots & 0 & \alpha_1 & 0 & \cdots & 0 \end{bmatrix}_{3\times(r+c)},$$

this condition is equivalent to

$$\frac{n_{1.} - n_{11}}{\alpha_1} = \mu_1 + \mu_3 \beta_1 \quad (1) \qquad \frac{n_{2.}}{\alpha_2} = \mu_1 \quad (2) \qquad \cdots \qquad \frac{n_{r.}}{\alpha_r} = \mu_1 \quad (r)$$

$$\frac{n_{.1} - n_{11}}{\beta_1} = \mu_2 + \mu_3 \alpha_1 \quad (r+1) \qquad \frac{n_{.2}}{\beta_2} = \mu_2 \quad (r+2) \qquad \cdots \qquad \frac{n_{.c}}{\beta_c} = \mu_2 \quad (r+c)$$

$$(2)\cdots(r) \Longrightarrow n_{2.} + \cdots + n_{r.} = \mu_1 (\alpha_2 + \cdots + \alpha_r) \iff \mu_1 = \frac{n - n_{1.}}{1 - \alpha_1}$$

$$(r+2)\cdots(r+c) \Longrightarrow n_{.2} + \cdots + n_{.c} = \mu_2 (\beta_2 + \cdots + \beta_r) \iff \mu_2 = \frac{n - n_{.1}}{1 - \beta_1}$$

$$(1) \Longrightarrow \mu_3 = \widehat{\Theta}^{-1} (n_{1.} - n_{11} - \mu_1 \alpha_1)$$

(1) and $(r+1) \Longrightarrow$
$$n_{1.} - n_{.1} = \mu_1 \alpha_1 - \mu_2 \beta_1$$

$$\iff (n - n_{.1}) \alpha_1{}^2 + (n_{.1} - n_{1.}) \alpha_1 - \widehat{\Theta} (n - n_{1.}) = 0$$

$$\Longrightarrow \quad \tilde{\alpha}_1 = \frac{1}{2} \left\{ 1 - \frac{n - n_{1.}}{n - n_{.1}} + \left\{ \left(1 - \frac{n - n_{1.}}{n - n_{.1}} \right)^2 + 4 \widehat{\Theta} \frac{n - n_{1.}}{n - n_{.1}} \right\}^{1/2} \right\},$$

the other solution to the quadratic equation being negative. From Eqs. (2) to $(r + c)$, we obtain

$$\tilde{\alpha}_i = \frac{n_{i.}}{\mu_1} = \frac{n_{i.} (1 - \tilde{\alpha}_1)}{n - n_{1.}} \quad 2 \le i \le r$$

$$\widetilde{\beta}_1 = \frac{\widehat{\Theta}}{\widetilde{\alpha}_1} \quad \text{and} \quad \widetilde{\beta}_j = \frac{n_{.j}}{\mu_2} = \frac{n_{.j} \left(1 - \widetilde{\beta}_1 \right)}{n - n_{.1}} \quad 2 \le j \le c \ .$$

31.4 New Test Statistic

The proposed test statistic focuses on the inner-cell counts, that is, N_{ij} for $2 \le i \le r$ and $2 \le j \le c$. It combines the standardized inner-cell counts N_{ij}.

The component statistics of interest therefore are

$$\widetilde{Z}_{ij} = \frac{1}{n^{1/2}} \left(N_{ij} - n \, \widetilde{\alpha}_i \, \widetilde{\beta}_j \right) \qquad 2 \le i \le r \quad \text{and} \quad 2 \le j \le c \ .$$

In order to study their large sample properties, we consider the classical standardized variables

$$Z_{ij} = \frac{1}{n^{1/2}} \left(N_{ij} - n \frac{\lambda_{ij}}{\lambda} \right) \qquad i = 1, \dots r, \qquad j = 1, \dots c.$$

Under H_0,

$$Z_{ij} = \frac{1}{n^{1/2}} \left(N_{ij} - n \, \alpha_i \, \beta_j \right) \ .$$

Note that

$$
\begin{aligned}
\widetilde{Z}_{ij} &= \frac{1}{n^{1/2}} \left(N_{ij} - n \, \widetilde{\alpha}_i \, \widetilde{\beta}_j - n \, \alpha_i \, \beta_j + n \, \alpha_i \, \beta_j \right) \\
&= \frac{1}{n^{1/2}} \left(N_{ij} - n \, \alpha_i \, \beta_j \right) - n^{1/2} \, \widetilde{\alpha}_i \, \widetilde{\beta}_j + n^{1/2} \, \alpha_i \, \beta_j \\
&= Z_{ij} + n^{1/2} \, \alpha_i \, \beta_j - n^{1/2} \, \frac{n_{i.} \, n_{.j}}{(n - n_{1.}) \, (n - n_{.1})} \left(1 - \widetilde{\alpha}_1 \right) \left(1 - \widetilde{\beta}_1 \right) \ .
\end{aligned}
$$

In Appendix 31.2, we linearize $\widetilde{\alpha}_1$, $\widetilde{\beta}_1$, and $(n_{i.} \, n_{.j})/((n - n_{1.}) \, (n - n_{.1}))$ for $2 \le i \le r$, $2 \le j \le c$. These results lead to

$$
\begin{aligned}
\widetilde{Z}_{ij} &= Z_{ij} + \frac{2 \, \alpha_i \, \beta_j}{\alpha_1 + \beta_1 - 2 \, \alpha_1 \, \beta_1} \, Z_{11} \\
&\quad - \frac{\alpha_i \, \beta_j \, \beta_1}{\alpha_1 + \beta_1 - 2 \, \alpha_1 \, \beta_1} \left(Z_{1.} - \frac{1 - \alpha_1}{1 - \beta_1} \, Z_{.1} \right) \\
&\quad + \frac{\alpha_i \, \beta_j \, \alpha_1 \, (1 - \beta_1)}{(1 - \alpha_1) \, (\alpha_1 + \beta_1 - 2 \, \alpha_1 \, \beta_1)} \left(Z_{1.} - \frac{1 - \alpha_1}{1 - \beta_1} \, Z_{.1} \right) \\
&\quad - \beta_j \, Z_{i.} - \alpha_i \, Z_{.j} - \frac{\alpha_i \, \beta_j}{1 - \alpha_1} \, Z_{1.} - \frac{\alpha_i \, \beta_j}{1 - \beta_1} \, Z_{.1} + O_p \left(n^{-1/2} \right) \\
&= Z_{ij} + \kappa_{11}^{ij} \, Z_{11} + \kappa_{1.}^{ij} \, Z_{1.} + \kappa_{.1}^{ij} \, Z_{.1} + \kappa_{i.}^{ij} \, Z_{i.} + \kappa_{.j}^{ij} \, Z_{.j} + O_p \left(n^{-1/2} \right),
\end{aligned}
$$

where

$$\kappa_{11}^{ij} = \frac{2 \, \alpha_i \, \beta_j}{\alpha_1 + \beta_1 - 2 \, \alpha_1 \, \beta_1} \quad , \quad \kappa_{1.}^{ij} = -\frac{2 \, \alpha_i \, \beta_j \, \beta_1}{\alpha_1 + \beta_1 - 2 \, \alpha_1 \, \beta_1}$$

$$\kappa_{.1}^{ij} = -\frac{2 \, \alpha_i \, \beta_j \, \alpha_1}{\alpha_1 + \beta_1 - 2 \, \alpha_1 \, \beta_1} \quad , \quad \kappa_{i.}^{ij} = -\beta_j \quad \text{and} \quad \kappa_{.j}^{ij} = -\alpha_i \ .$$

With $\mathbf{Z}^\tau = [Z_{11} \ Z_{12} \ \cdots \ Z_{1c} \ Z_{21} \ Z_{22} \ \cdots \ Z_{2c} \ \cdots \ Z_{r1} \ Z_{r2} \ \cdots \ Z_{rc}]_{1 \times rc}$,

$$\widetilde{Z}_{ij} = \mathbf{C}(\mathbf{ij})^\tau \, \mathbf{Z} + o_p(1) \qquad 2 \le i \le r \quad , \quad 2 \le j \le c,$$

where $\mathbf{C(ij)}^\tau = \begin{bmatrix} C_{11}^{ij} & C_{12}^{ij} & \cdots & C_{1c}^{ij} & C_{21}^{ij} & C_{22}^{ij} & \cdots & C_{2c}^{ij} & \cdots & C_{r1}^{ij} & C_{r2}^{ij} & \cdots & C_{rc}^{ij} \end{bmatrix}_{1\times rc}$
with all entries being 0 except

$$C_{11}^{ij} = \frac{2\,\alpha_i\,\beta_j\,(1-\alpha_1-\beta_1)}{\alpha_1+\beta_1-2\,\alpha_1\,\beta_1}\quad, \qquad C_{1k}^{ij} = -\frac{2\,\alpha_i\,\beta_j\,\beta_1}{\alpha_1+\beta_1-2\,\alpha_1\,\beta_1}\qquad k\neq 1,\,j,$$

$$C_{1j}^{ij} = -\frac{2\,\alpha_i\,\beta_j\,\beta_1}{\alpha_1+\beta_1-2\,\alpha_1\,\beta_1}-\alpha_i\quad, \qquad C_{i1}^{ij} = -\frac{2\,\alpha_i\,\beta_j\,\alpha_1}{\alpha_1+\beta_1-2\,\alpha_1\,\beta_1}-\beta_j,$$

$$C_{u1}^{ij} = -\frac{2\,\alpha_i\,\beta_j\,\alpha_1}{\alpha_1+\beta_1-2\,\alpha_1\,\beta_1}\qquad u\neq 1,\,i\quad, \qquad C_{ij}^{ij} = 1-\beta_j-\alpha_i,$$

$$C_{uj}^{ij} = -\alpha_i\quad u\neq 1,\,i, \qquad C_{ik}^{ij} = -\beta_j \qquad k\neq 1,\,j.$$

Let $\mathbf{P}^\tau = \begin{bmatrix} \alpha_1\,\beta_1 & \alpha_1\,\beta_2 & \cdots & \alpha_1\,\beta_c & \cdots & \alpha_r\,\beta_1 & \alpha_r\,\beta_2 & \cdots & \alpha_r\,\beta_c \end{bmatrix}$ and $\mathbf{D_P}$
be the diagonal matrix with the entries of $\mathbf{P}$ as elements. Then $\mathbf{Var_0}(\mathbf{Z}) = \mathbf{D_P} - \mathbf{PP}^\tau$.

Consider $\widetilde{\mathbf{Z}}^\tau = \begin{bmatrix} \widetilde{Z}_{22} & \cdots & \widetilde{Z}_{2c} & \cdots & \widetilde{Z}_{r2} & \cdots & \widetilde{Z}_{rc} \end{bmatrix}_{1\times(r-1)(c-1)}$. The variance–covariance matrix under H_0 of $\widetilde{\mathbf{Z}}$, namely, $\mathbf{Var_0}\left(\widetilde{\mathbf{Z}}\right)$, has diagonal elements $\mathrm{Var_0}\left(\widetilde{Z}_{ij}\right)$ and off-diagonal elements $\mathrm{Cov_0}\left(\widetilde{Z}_{ij},\widetilde{Z}_{kl}\right)$ for $2\leq i,\,k\leq r$, $2\leq j,\,l\leq c$ and $(i,\,j)\neq(k,\,l)$:

$$\mathrm{Var_0}\left(\widetilde{Z}_{ij}\right) \approx \mathbf{C(ij)}^\tau\,\mathbf{Var_0}(\mathbf{Z})\,\mathbf{C(ij)}$$
$$\mathrm{Cov_0}\left(\widetilde{Z}_{ij},\widetilde{Z}_{kl}\right) \approx \mathbf{C(ij)}^\tau\,\mathbf{Var_0}(\mathbf{Z})\,\mathbf{C(kl)}\ .$$

The matrix

$$\mathbf{Var_0}\left(\widetilde{\mathbf{Z}}\right) \approx \begin{bmatrix} \mathbf{C(22)}^\tau \\ \mathbf{C(23)}^\tau \\ \vdots \\ \mathbf{C(rc)}^\tau \end{bmatrix}(\mathbf{D_P}-\mathbf{PP}^\tau)\begin{bmatrix} \mathbf{C(22)} & \mathbf{C(23)} & \cdots & \mathbf{C(rc)} \end{bmatrix}$$

has rank at most $(r-1)\,(c-1)$, which is the number of independent parameters, and has a generalized inverse.

In summary, the new test statistic is

$$\widetilde{\mathbf{Z}}^\tau\left\{\widehat{\mathbf{Var_0}\left(\widetilde{\mathbf{Z}}\right)}\right\}^-\widetilde{\mathbf{Z}},$$

where $\left\{\mathbf{Var_0}\left(\widetilde{\mathbf{Z}}\right)\right\}^-$ stands for the generalized inverse of $\mathbf{Var_0}\left(\widetilde{\mathbf{Z}}\right)$. The variance estimate $\widehat{\mathbf{Var_0}}\left(\widetilde{\mathbf{Z}}\right)$ is obtained by substituting the parameter estimates $\widetilde{\alpha}_i$ and $\widetilde{\beta}_j$ for α_i and β_j, respectively. This statistic follows a χ^2-distribution with $(r-1)\,(c-1)$ degrees of freedom [Sen and Singer (1993, Theorem 3.4.7)].

31.5　Power Studies

To study the power of the test, we need to assess the behavior of the test statistic under a small departure from the null hypothesis. Consider the local Pitman alternatives.

H_1: the cell counts are independent and $\lambda^{-1}\lambda_{ij} = \alpha_i\beta_j + n^{-1/2}\gamma_{ij}$ with

$$\sum_i \gamma_{ij} = \sum_j \gamma_{ij} = 0.$$

Recall that $\tilde{Z}_{ij} = n^{-1/2}\left(N_{ij} - n\,\widetilde{\alpha}_i\,\widetilde{\beta}_j\right)$, $i = 2, \ldots r$, and $j = 2, \ldots c$. Rewrite this as

$$
\begin{aligned}
\tilde{Z}_{ij} &= \frac{1}{\sqrt{n}}\left(N_{ij} - n\frac{\lambda_{ij}}{\lambda}\right) - \sqrt{n}\left(\widetilde{\alpha}_i\,\widetilde{\beta}_j - \frac{\lambda_{ij}}{\lambda}\right) \\
&= \frac{1}{\sqrt{n}}\left(N_{ij} - n\frac{\lambda_{ij}}{\lambda}\right) - \sqrt{n}\left(\frac{n_{i.}\,n_{.j}}{(n - n_{1.})\,(n - n_{.1})}(1 - \widetilde{\alpha}_1)(1 - \widetilde{\beta}_1) - \frac{\lambda_{ij}}{\lambda}\right).
\end{aligned}
$$

We use the results from the previous sections to linearize this expression. Hence,

$$
\begin{aligned}
E_1\left(\tilde{Z}_{ij}\right) &= E_1\left\{\frac{1}{\sqrt{n}}\left(N_{ij} - n\frac{\lambda_{ij}}{\lambda}\right)\right. \\
&\qquad \left. -\sqrt{n}\left(\frac{n_{i.}\,n_{.j}}{(n - n_{1.})\,(n - n_{.1})}(1 - \widetilde{\alpha}_1)(1 - \widetilde{\beta}_1) - \frac{\lambda_{ij}}{\lambda}\right)\right\} \\
&= E_1\left(-\sqrt{n}\,\alpha_i\beta_j + \kappa_{11}^{ij}Z_{11} + \kappa_{1.}^{ij}Z_{1.} + \kappa_{.1}^{ij}Z_{.1} + \kappa_{i.}^{ij}Z_{i.} + \kappa_{.j}^{ij}Z_{.j}\right) \\
&\qquad + \sqrt{n}\frac{\lambda_{ij}}{\lambda} + O\left(n^{-1/2}\right) \\
&= \gamma_{ij} + \kappa_{11}^{ij}E_1\left(\frac{1}{n^{1/2}}(N_{11} - n\,\alpha_1\beta_1)\right) + O\left(n^{-1/2}\right) \\
&= \gamma_{ij} + \frac{\kappa_{11}^{ij}}{\sqrt{n}}E_1\left(N_{11} - n\frac{\lambda_{11}}{\lambda} - n\,\alpha_1\beta_1 + n\frac{\lambda_{11}}{\lambda}\right) + O\left(n^{-1/2}\right) \\
&= \gamma_{ij} + \kappa_{11}^{ij}\gamma_{11} + O\left(n^{-1/2}\right) \\
&= \gamma_{ij} + \frac{2\,\alpha_i\beta_j}{\alpha_1 + \beta_1 - 2\,\alpha_1\beta_1}\gamma_{11} + O\left(n^{-1/2}\right).
\end{aligned}
$$

Let $\tilde{E}_1\left(\tilde{\mathbf{Z}}\right) \equiv \left[\gamma_{ij} + \dfrac{2\,\alpha_i\beta_j}{\alpha_1 + \beta_1 - 2\,\alpha_1\beta_1}\gamma_{11}\right]_{(r-1)\,(c-1)\times 1} \equiv \boldsymbol{\Gamma} + \boldsymbol{\Delta}$, where

$$\boldsymbol{\Gamma} = [\gamma_{ij}]_{(r-1)\,(c-1)\times 1} \quad \text{and} \quad \boldsymbol{\Delta} = \frac{2\,\alpha_i\beta_j}{\alpha_1 + \beta_1 - 2\,\alpha_1\beta_1}\gamma_{11}\,[1]_{(r-1)\,(c-1)\times 1}.$$

$$
\mathbf{Var_1}\left(\tilde{\mathbf{Z}}\right) \approx \begin{bmatrix} \mathbf{C(22)}^{\tau} \\ \mathbf{C(23)}^{\tau} \\ \vdots \\ \mathbf{C(rc)}^{\tau} \end{bmatrix} \mathbf{Var_1}\left(\mathbf{Z}\right) \begin{bmatrix} \mathbf{C(22)} & \mathbf{C(23)} & \cdots & \mathbf{C(rc)} \end{bmatrix}
$$

$$
\approx \begin{bmatrix} \mathbf{C(22)}^{\tau} \\ \mathbf{C(23)}^{\tau} \\ \vdots \\ \mathbf{C(rc)}^{\tau} \end{bmatrix} \mathbf{Var_0}\left(\mathbf{Z}\right) \begin{bmatrix} \mathbf{C(22)} & \mathbf{C(23)} & \cdots & \mathbf{C(rc)} \end{bmatrix}.
$$

Then, by Theorem 3.4.7 in Sen and Singer (1993),

$$
Q = \tilde{\mathbf{Z}}^{\tau}\mathbf{Var_0}\left(\mathbf{Z}\right)^{-}\tilde{\mathbf{Z}} \sim \chi^2_{rank(\mathbf{Var_0(Z)})}\left(\left(\tilde{E}_1\left(\tilde{\mathbf{Z}}\right)\right)^{\tau}\mathbf{Var_0}\left(\mathbf{Z}\right)^{-}\left(\tilde{E}_1\left(\tilde{\mathbf{Z}}\right)\right)\right)
$$

and the test statistic

$$
\hat{Q} = \tilde{\mathbf{Z}}^{\tau}\widehat{\mathbf{Var_0}}\left(\mathbf{Z}\right)^{-}\tilde{\mathbf{Z}} \sim \chi^2_{rank(\mathbf{Var_0(Z)})}\left(\left(\tilde{E}_1\left(\tilde{\mathbf{Z}}\right)\right)^{\tau}\mathbf{Var_0}\left(\mathbf{Z}\right)^{-}\left(\tilde{E}_1\left(\tilde{\mathbf{Z}}\right)\right)\right)
$$

by Slutsky's theorem because $\hat{Q}/Q$ converges to 1 in probability. If

$$
\boldsymbol{\Gamma}^{\tau}\left(\mathbf{Var_0}\left(\mathbf{Z}\right)\right)^{-}\boldsymbol{\Delta} \neq 0,
$$

the noncentrality parameter will be increased. As the noncentrality parameter becomes larger, the distribution of the test statistics shifts to the right, and the probability that it is greater than a specific value goes to 1, which implies that the power of the test converges to 1.

31.6 Numerical Studies

We present in Tables 31.2 and 31.3 the results of simulations that support the methodological work developed in the previous sections. For a specific sample size and combination of row and column probabilities, a total of 1000 replications was performed. Each simulation proceeds as follows. Given the row and column probability vectors, a contingency table is generated under independence of positions and the multinomial model. The test statistic is then computed under the conditional model. The numbers of such statistics falling above the 90th, 95th, and 99th percentiles of the relevant χ^2-square distribution are entered in the table. It is evident from these tables that the proposed test statistic converges quickly to its asymptotic distribution.

Table 31.2: Percentages of statistics falling above given percentiles of the χ^2-distribution with 4 degrees of freedom. * indicates that an entry is farther than 2 S.D.s away from the expected percentage

Sample	Row Probabilities			Column Probabilities			90	95	99
200	0.80	0.10	0.10	0.80	0.10	0.10	11.8	5.5	2.1 *
	0.70	0.20	0.10	0.70	0.20	0.10	9.6	5.2	1.5
	0.70	0.20	0.10	0.60	0.20	0.20	9.9	5.3	1.1
	0.60	0.20	0.20	0.60	0.20	0.20	9.1	4.5	0.9
	0.50	0.25	0.25	0.50	0.25	0.25	10.0	5.2	1.2
	0.40	0.30	0.30	0.40	0.30	0.30	8.0	4.0	1.4
600	0.80	0.10	0.10	0.80	0.10	0.10	10.1	4.8	1.2
	0.70	0.20	0.10	0.70	0.20	0.10	10.5	6.1	1.5
	0.70	0.20	0.10	0.60	0.20	0.20	9.0	4.8	0.9
	0.60	0.20	0.20	0.60	0.20	0.20	11.1	5.0	0.9
	0.50	0.25	0.25	0.50	0.25	0.25	9.3	3.9	0.7
	0.40	0.30	0.30	0.40	0.30	0.30	9.9	5.3	0.8
1000	0.80	0.10	0.10	0.80	0.10	0.10	9.6	4.0	0.6
	0.70	0.20	0.10	0.70	0.20	0.10	9.7	4.6	1.1
	0.70	0.20	0.10	0.60	0.20	0.20	11.0	6.0	1.6 *
	0.60	0.20	0.20	0.60	0.20	0.20	12.9 *	6.4	1.4
	0.50	0.25	0.25	0.50	0.25	0.25	10.9	5.5	1.4
	0.40	0.30	0.30	0.40	0.30	0.30	10.9	5.3	1.2

Table 31.3: Percentages of statistics falling above given percentile of the χ^2-distribution with 9 degrees of freedom. * indicates that an entry is farther than 2 S.D.s away from the expected percentage

Sample	Row Probabilities	Column Probabilities	90	95	99
200	0.70 0.10 0.10 0.10	0.70 0.10 0.10 0.10	11.2	6.6 *	2.2 *
	0.60 0.20 0.10 0.10	0.60 0.20 0.10 0.10	11.1	5.4	2.1 *
	0.40 0.30 0.20 0.10	0.40 0.30 0.20 0.10	9.1	4.7	0.9
400	0.70 0.10 0.10 0.10	0.70 0.10 0.10 0.10	9.7	5.1	1.0
	0.60 0.20 0.10 0.10	0.60 0.20 0.10 0.10	10.2	6.0	1.1
	0.40 0.30 0.20 0.10	0.40 0.30 0.20 0.10	8.9	4.3	1.0
600	0.70 0.10 0.10 0.10	0.70 0.10 0.10 0.10	10.5	5.6	1.8 *
	0.60 0.20 0.10 0.10	0.60 0.20 0.10 0.10	9.0	5.2	0.8
	0.40 0.30 0.20 0.10	0.40 0.30 0.20 0.10	11.0	4.4	0.8
800	0.70 0.10 0.10 0.10	0.70 0.10 0.10 0.10	10.5	5.9	1.2
	0.60 0.20 0.10 0.10	0.60 0.20 0.10 0.10	10.7	5.3	1.0
	0.40 0.30 0.20 0.10	0.40 0.30 0.20 0.10	9.7	4.3	1.5
1000	0.70 0.10 0.10 0.10	0.70 0.10 0.10 0.10	9.9	5.5	1.4
	0.60 0.20 0.10 0.10	0.60 0.20 0.10 0.10	11.0	5.8	1.1
	0.40 0.30 0.20 0.10	0.40 0.30 0.20 0.10	8.6	4.9	0.8

Table 31.4: Results of analysis with new statistic and other approaches. Q denotes the proposed statistic. Entries are left blank when the test statistic does not reach the 0.99 significance level. * indicates that the test statistic falls above the 99.5 percentile, ** above the 99.9 percentile, and *** outside the support of the reference distribution

Positions	Q	M	G	K
9, 11	20.34 ***	0.05 **	0.03	0.04 **
11, 13	9.30 *		0.07 **	0.07 ***
11, 27	12.76 *	0.03		
12, 18	9.82 *			
14, 16	85.42 ***	0.11 ***	0.11 ***	0.15 ***
14, 20	59.31 ***	0.03 **	0.10 ***	0.04 **
19, 20	83.24 ***	0.02 **	0.08 ***	0.08 ***
29, 32	31.53 ***	0.05 **	0.08 **	0.05 **
32, 34	37.79 ***		0.06 **	0.06 ***

31.7　Data Analysis

The human immunodeficiency virus (HIV) genome evolves rapidly. Indeed, frequent recombination between RNA strands and the high error rate of the reverse transcriptase enzyme give rise to many viral variants. Some of these random changes are advantageous to the virus as they confer a survival advantage. Furthermore, a potentially deleterious mutation at one position may be rescued by a mutation at another position, maintaining the structure of the resulting protein and thus virus viability. These double mutations then become fixed in some subpopulations.

From the Los Alamos database, we have selected 450 amino-acid sequences spanning the V3 loop of the envelope gene *env*. These sequences belong to the so-called clade B, a phylogenetic grouping that comprises North American, Western European, Brazilian, and Thai strains. All have the biological property of not inducing syncitia. We sampled a single sequence from an individual, and to ensure that epidemiological linkage is unlikely we only consider sequences that exhibit at least five different nucleotides in pairwise comparisons.

To take into account possible epidemiological linkages among study subjects as well as the underlying phylogenetic relationships among sequences, we generate the reference distribution on the basis of simulated sequences. In the absence of information on suitable models for within-individual evolution, we resort to a simple evolutionary model, which we now describe. From the sequence data, for each position, we estimate the amino-acid frequencies. In view of structural constraints that block the occurrence of some characters at specific positions, we do not pool the estimates for different sites into overall estimates. We take the observed frequencies as substitution rates. For HIV, this is reasonable as the observed frequencies reflect both structural constraints and immune selection pressures. The event of a mutation at a specific site is a two-step process. First, whether the position undergoes a change is governed by the overall mutation rate. For HIV sequences, this is the error rate for reverse transcriptase, that is, 0.0005 per site per replication [Preston, Poiesz, and Loeb (1988)]. Next, in the case of mutation, the specific substitution is randomly selected according to the following transition matrix,

$$
\begin{array}{c}
\quad\quad\quad\quad\quad\quad \text{time } i+1 \\
\begin{array}{cccccc}
 & & C & NC_1 & NC_2 & NC_3 \\
 & C & \overline{M} & Mp_1 & Mp_2 & Mp_3 \\
\text{time } i & NC_1 & Mp_1 & \overline{M} & Mp_2 & Mp_3 \\
 & NC_2 & Mp_2 & Mp_1 & \overline{M} & Mp_3 \\
 & NC_3 & Mp_3 & Mp_1 & Mp_2 & \overline{M}
\end{array}
\end{array}
$$

where C denotes the consensus character and NC_i a nonconsensus character. M stands for the probability of change $(\overline{M} = 1 - M)$ and p_i for the observed frequency of change from C to NC_i.

The simulation starts with the consensus sequence as seed. It is subjected to the mutation process a random number of times. This random number represents the number of replications before transmission, and is set between 100 and 2400. Indeed, for HIV, mutations occur at the time of replication, and the replication rate is approximately 240 times per year. The original sequence thus gives rise to offspring sequences. In the present application, this branching process mimics HIV transmission: no offspring with probability 0.20 and 1 to 5 offspring with probability 0.16 each [Blower and McLean (1994)]. The tree is grown by repeating this process many times (with the output sequences from the previous generation as seeds). We obtain a total of 150,000 sequences. We sample without replacement as many sequences as there are in the original data set. Sampling is not restricted to the tips of the simulated phylogenetic tree: all generated sequences are candidates for selection. From the sampled sequences we compute the test statistic. The sampling procedure is performed a large number of times (here 100,000) to build up a reference distribution.

The results of our analysis appear in Table 31.4. For the sake of comparison, we also analyzed our data with methodologies that purport to identify corre-lated mutations (Table 31.4). To detect covariation among mutations, Korber *et al.* (1993) utilized an information-theoretic measure computed on the whole data set. Let i denote a position along the genome and a an amino acid appear-ing at that position. If $p_i(a)$ represents the frequency of appearance of amino acid a at position i, the *mutual information* is defined as

$$M(i, j) = H(i) + H(j) - H(i, j),$$

where $H(i)$ denotes the *Shannon entropy* at position i

$$H(i) = - \sum_{a_i} p_i(a_i) \log p_i(a_i)$$

with a_i referring to amino acids appearing at position i, and $H(i, j)$ generalizes this concept to two positions

$$H(i, j) = - \sum_{a_i, b_j} p_{ij}(a_i, b_j) \log p_{ij}(a_i, b_j) .$$

$M(i, j)$ takes its minimum value of 0 when either there is no variation or the positions i and j vary independently. It attains its maximum when the same pairings always occur. To focus on the covariability of a specific pair of residues, define $K_{i,j}(a, b)$ as the $M(i, j)$ statistic obtained by replacing the 20-letter alphabet at site i by $\{a, \bar{a}\}$ (i.e., a and not a) and at site j by $\{b, \bar{b}\}$. Finally,

$$K(i, j) = \max_{a,b} K_{ij}(a, b) \tag{31.1}$$

is reportedly suited to identify linked mutations [Bickel *et al.* (1996)].

To obtain the reference distribution for the statistics $M(i, j)$, the amino acids at each position are permuted independently. A large number B (here 100,000) of pseudo-data sets are created. From each of these pseudo-data sets, the statistics are computed for all pairs of positions. The number b_{ij} of pseudo-statistics for the pair (i, j) that exceeds the observed $M(i, j)$ is computed for all (i, j), which leads to the observed significance level $(b_{ij} + 1)/(B + 1)$. When $b_{ij} = 0$, the observed significance is thus $(B + 1)^{-1}$. Similarly for $K(i, j)$.

Bickel *et al.* (1996) also used the statistic developed by Goodman and Kruskal (1979):

$$G(i, j) = \frac{1}{2} \left\{ \sum_a \hat{p}_{ij}(a, \max) + \sum_b \hat{p}_{ij}(\max, b) - \hat{p}_i(\max) - \hat{p}_j(\max) \right\}$$
$$\bigg/ \left\{ 1 - \frac{1}{2}(\hat{p}_i(\max) + \hat{p}_j(\max)) \right\}, \tag{31.2}$$

where

$$\hat{p}_{ij}(a, \max) = \max_b \hat{p}_{ij}(a, b), \qquad \hat{p}_{ij}(\max, b) = \max_a \hat{p}_{ij}(a, b)$$

$$\hat{p}_i(\max) = \max_a \hat{p}_i(a) .$$

Table 31.5: Data for positions 12 and 18

	R	S	K	G	Q	W	E	A
I	312	26	39	29	14	1	2	1
V	9	4	1	3	2	0	0	1
K	1	0	0	0	0	0	0	0
T	0	0	1	0	0	0	0	0
L	1	0	0	0	1	0	0	0
M	1	0	0	0	0	0	0	0
F	1	0	0	0	0	0	0	0

$G(i, j)$ represents the relative reduction in the probability of guessing incorrectly the amino acid at site j associated with the knowledge of the residue at site i and vice versa. If the two positions are not associated $G(i, j) = 0$. The reference distribution of $G(i, j)$ is generated through the process described above.

31.8 Discussion

With respect to sequence variation, independence has three facets:

- Independence between different sequences

- Independence between positions along a sequence

- Independence of mutations along sequences

This work focuses on the third issue whereas the papers by Korber *et al.* (1993) and Bickel *et al.* (1996) deal with the second issue. It is clear from the above data analysis that these issues are distinct. Indeed, although there is a great deal of agreement between the approaches (Table 31.4), some pairs turn up statistically significant at the chosen threshold but not at the other. For instance, only the statistic Q is highly significant for the pair (12, 28) (Table 31.5). The reverse situation occurs for (14, 19) and (16, 20) (Table 31.6). In the case of (12, 28), the cell with entry 4 drives the significance of the Q statistic. For the other two pairs, the 0 cells along the first row or the first column influence greatly the M, G, and K statistics but are excluded from consideration in the Q statistic (the latter focuses on the inner-table cells).

An alternative explanation for the lack of statistical significance of the Q statistic for the pairs (14, 19) and (16, 20) is the manner in which the reference distributions for the different statistics were generated. The reference

Table 31.6: Data for positions 14 and 19

	A	V	T	S	R	G	N
I	256	7	14	3	0	0	0
M	82	5	6	4	1	0	0
V	8	0	3	1	0	0	1
L	38	1	7	2	0	1	0
F	2	0	2	0	1	0	0
Y	0	1	0	0	0	0	0
T	2	0	0	0	0	0	0
K	0	1	0	0	0	0	0
D	1	0	0	0	0	0	0

distribution for the Q statistic explicitly takes into account the phylogenetic relationships among the analyzed sequences. This ensures that only pairings that occur at several branch tips are declared significant. Otherwise, a chance event that is propagated down a single branch could be found significant. In fact, when a parametric bootstrap procedure is utilized to create the reference distribution (which assumes that the sequences are unrelated), many more pairs are identified than when the phylogenetic approach is adopted (data not shown).

Recall that the proposed methodology is based on the assumption that the probability of the (1,1) cell frequency being greater than all the others is close to 1. In the sequence data we have scrutinized this assumption holds for all pairs of positions but a few. Such an assumption is not tenable when the true probability of the $(1, 1)$ cell is not substantially larger than the others. This situation is usually due to a single highly polymorphic position. Then, it appears that the sample is made up of at least two subpopulations. Each subpopulation should be considered separately.

Yet we need to consider the possibility that the basic assumption is not justified. In this context, we note that it is possible to write the conditional distribution of the cell counts given the $(1, 1)$ cell without assuming anything about maximality. This conditional distribution of the cell counts given N_{11} should be used to obtain the MLEs or similar estimators of the parameters αs and βs. Moreover, estimates of the conditional (given N_{11}) means and variances can be obtained following the same procedures as here. This would give us a parallel test statistic, that would be asymptotically χ^2-distributed. This test, however, does incorporate the information contained in the marginal distribution of N_{11} in the estimation of the parameters. Therefore, the power of this test would be different and might not be as good as the one we obtained earlier where the information in the marginal distribution of N_{11} was incorporated.

In the absence of reliable information about the underlying evolutionary process the simple model, on which the simulation is based, is best. The reference distribution then takes into account an array of possible phylogenetic relationships as generated by this model. The simulation starts with the consensus sequence. However, the ancestral sequence could also be used. Our results indicate that this modification leaves the inferences unchanged.

The test procedure introduced in this paper was constructed for the specific purpose of detecting correlated substitutions. However, it is more widely applicable. For example, it may be used in the investigation of gene or protein networks. There, one wants to assess whether genes or proteins are jointly upregulated or downregulated under specific conditions in a microarray or proteomic experiment.

Acknowledgements. This research was funded in part by the National Science Foundation (DMS-9305588), the American Foundation for AIDS Research (70428-15-RF), and the National Institutes of Health (R29-GM49804, AI47068 and P30-HD37260).

Appendix 31.1

$$P\left(N_{11}\text{ maximum}\right) \approx 1.$$

$P\left(N_{11}\text{ maximum}\right)$
$= P\left(N_{ij} < N_{11} \quad \forall\ (i,j) \neq (1,1)\right)$
$= E\left\{P\left(N_{ij} < N_{11} \quad \forall\ (i,j) \neq (1,1) \mid N_{11}\right)\right\}$
$= E\left\{P\left(N_{12} < N_{11} \mid N_{11}\right) \times P\left(N_{21} < N_{11} \mid N_{11}\right) \times P\left(N_{21} < N_{11} \mid N_{11}\right)\right\}$
$= \displaystyle\prod_{(i,j)\neq(1,1)} E\left\{P\left(\sqrt{N_{ij}} < \sqrt{N_{11}} \mid N_{11}\right)\right\}$
$= \displaystyle\prod_{(i,j)\neq(1,1)} E\left\{P\left\{2\left(\sqrt{N_{ij}} - \sqrt{\lambda_{ij}}\right)\right.\right.$
$$\left.\left. < 2\left(\sqrt{N_{11}} - \sqrt{\lambda_{11}} - \sqrt{\lambda_{ij}} + \sqrt{\lambda_{11}}\right) \mid N_{11}\right\}\right\}$$
$= \displaystyle\prod_{(i,j)\neq(1,1)} E\left\{W_{ij}\right\},$

where

$$W_{ij} = P\left\{2\left(\sqrt{N_{ij}} - \sqrt{\lambda_{ij}}\right) < 2\left(\sqrt{N_{11}} - \sqrt{\lambda_{11}} - \sqrt{\lambda_{ij}} + \sqrt{\lambda_{11}}\right) \mid N_{11}\right\}.$$

Each of these conditional probabilities W_{ij} are bounded and can be approximated by a random variable based on Anscombe's Poisson-normal approximation [Anscombe (1948)]. Hence, the product $W_{12} W_{21} W_{22}$ can be approximated for a given $N_{11} = n_{11}$ by

$$\prod_{(i,j)\neq(1,1)} P\left\{ \mathcal{N}(0,1) < 2 \left(\sqrt{n_{11}} - \sqrt{\lambda_{11}} + \left(\sqrt{\lambda_{11}} - \sqrt{\lambda_{ij}} \right) \right) \right\}.$$

Now, $\sqrt{N_{11}} - \sqrt{\lambda_{11}}$ is bounded in probability and $\lambda_{11} \gg \lambda_{ij}$ for all $(i,j) \neq (1,1)$. Therefore, with probability tending to 1, the above product is close to 1. Because W_{12}, W_{21}, W_{22} are bounded random variables, convergence in probability implies convergence in the first mean and

$$\prod_{(i,j)\neq(1,1)} E\left\{ W_{ij} \right\} \longrightarrow 1,$$

which is what we set out to prove.

Appendix 31.2

$$\frac{n_{i.} n_{.j}}{(n - n_{1.})(n - n_{.1})} = \frac{(n_{i.}/n)(n_{.j}/n)}{\left(1 - \dfrac{n_{1.}}{n}\right)\left(1 - \dfrac{n_{.1}}{n}\right)}$$

$$= f\left(\frac{n_{i.}}{n}, \frac{n_{.j}}{n}, \frac{n_{1.}}{n}, \frac{n_{.1}}{n}\right).$$

We linearize $f = f\left(\dfrac{n_{i.}}{n}, \dfrac{n_{.j}}{n}, \dfrac{n_{1.}}{n}, \dfrac{n_{.1}}{n}\right)$ around $(\alpha_i, \beta_j, \alpha_1, \beta_1)$.

$$\left.\frac{\partial f}{\partial \frac{n_{i.}}{n}}\right|_{\left(\frac{n_{i.}}{n}, \frac{n_{.j}}{n}, \frac{n_{1.}}{n}, \frac{n_{.1}}{n}\right) = (\alpha_i, \beta_j, \alpha_1, \beta_1)} = \frac{\beta_j}{(1 - \alpha_1)(1 - \beta_1)},$$

$$\left.\frac{\partial f}{\partial \frac{n_{.j}}{n}}\right|_{\left(\frac{n_{i.}}{n}, \frac{n_{.j}}{n}, \frac{n_{1.}}{n}, \frac{n_{.1}}{n}\right) = (\alpha_i, \beta_j, \alpha_1, \beta_1)} = \frac{\alpha_i}{(1 - \alpha_1)(1 - \beta_1)},$$

$$\left.\frac{\partial f}{\partial \frac{n_{1.}}{n}}\right|_{\left(\frac{n_{i.}}{n}, \frac{n_{.j}}{n}, \frac{n_{1.}}{n}, \frac{n_{.1}}{n}\right) = (\alpha_i, \beta_j, \alpha_1, \beta_1)} = \frac{\alpha_i \beta_j}{(1 - \alpha_1)^2 (1 - \beta_1)},$$

$$\left.\frac{\partial f}{\partial \frac{n_{.1}}{n}}\right|_{\left(\frac{n_{i.}}{n}, \frac{n_{.j}}{n}, \frac{n_{1.}}{n}, \frac{n_{.1}}{n}\right) = (\alpha_i, \beta_j, \alpha_1, \beta_1)} = \frac{\alpha_i \beta_j}{(1 - \alpha_1)(1 - \beta_1)^2}.$$

$$f = \frac{\alpha_i\,\beta_j}{(1-\alpha_1)\,(1-\beta_1)} + \frac{\beta_j}{(1-\alpha_1)\,(1-\beta_1)}\left(\frac{n_{i.}}{n}-\alpha_i\right)$$

$$+ \frac{\alpha_i}{(1-\alpha_1)\,(1-\beta_1)}\left(\frac{n_{.j}}{n}-\beta_j\right) + \frac{\alpha_i\,\beta_j}{(1-\alpha_1)^2\,(1-\beta_1)}\left(\frac{n_{1.}}{n}-\alpha_1\right)$$

$$+ \frac{\alpha_i\,\beta_j}{(1-\alpha_1)\,(1-\beta_1)^2}\left(\frac{n_{.1}}{n}-\beta_1\right)$$

$$+ o_p\left\|\left(\frac{n_{i.}}{n},\frac{n_{.j}}{n},\frac{n_{1.}}{n},\frac{n_{.1}}{n}\right)-(\alpha_i,\beta_j,\alpha_1,\beta_1)\right\|.$$

$$\widetilde{\alpha_1} = \widetilde{\alpha_1}\left(x,\widehat{\Theta}\right)$$

$$= \frac{1}{2}\left\{1-\frac{n-n_{1.}}{n-n_{.1}}+\sqrt{\left(1-\frac{n-n_{1.}}{n-n_{.1}}\right)^2+4\,\widehat{\Theta}\,\frac{n-n_{1.}}{n-n_{.1}}}\right\}$$

$$= \frac{1}{2}\left\{1-\frac{1-(n_{1.}/n)}{1-(n_{.1}/n)}+\sqrt{\left(1-\frac{1-(n_{1.}/n)}{1-(n_{.1}/n)}\right)^2+4\,\widehat{\Theta}\,\frac{1-(n_{1.}/n)}{1-(n_{.1}/n)}}\right\}$$

$$= \frac{1}{2}\left\{x+\sqrt{x^2+4\,\widehat{\Theta}\,(1-x)}\right\}$$

with $\quad x = 1-\dfrac{1-(n_{1.}/n)}{1-(n_{.1}/n)}$. Expand $\widetilde{\alpha_1}$ around $\left(x,\widehat{\Theta}\right)=\left(1-\dfrac{1-\alpha_1}{1-\beta_1},\Theta\right)$:

$$\widetilde{\alpha_1} = \underbrace{\frac{1}{2}\left\{\left(1-\frac{1-\alpha_1}{1-\beta_1}\right)+\sqrt{\left(1-\frac{1-\alpha_1}{1-\beta_1}\right)^2+4\,\Theta\left(1-\left(1-\frac{1-\alpha_1}{1-\beta_1}\right)\right)}\right\}}_{\alpha_1}$$

$$+ \frac{\partial\widetilde{\alpha_1}\left(x,\widehat{\Theta}\right)}{\partial x}\Big|_{\left(x,\widehat{\Theta}\right)=\left(1-\frac{1-\alpha_1}{1-\beta_1},\Theta\right)}\left(x-\left(1-\frac{1-\alpha_1}{1-\beta_1}\right)\right)$$

$$+ \frac{\partial\widetilde{\alpha_1}\left(x,\widehat{\Theta}\right)}{\partial\widehat{\Theta}}\Big|_{\left(x,\widehat{\Theta}\right)=\left(1-\frac{1-\alpha_1}{1-\beta_1},\Theta\right)}\underbrace{\left(\widehat{\Theta}-\Theta\right)}_{\frac{1}{n}(N_{11}-n\,\alpha_1\,\beta_1)}$$

$$+ o_p\left\|\left(x,\widehat{\Theta}\right)-\left(1-\frac{1-\alpha_1}{1-\beta_1},\Theta\right)\right\|$$

$$= \alpha_1 + \frac{\partial\widetilde{\alpha_1}\left(x,\widehat{\Theta}\right)}{\partial x}\Big|_{\left(x,\widehat{\Theta}\right)=\left(1-\frac{1-\alpha_1}{1-\beta_1},\Theta\right)}\left(\frac{1-\alpha_1}{1-\beta_1}-\frac{1-(n_{1.}/n)}{1-(n_{.1}/n)}\right)$$

$$+ \frac{\partial\widetilde{\alpha_1}\left(x,\widehat{\Theta}\right)}{\partial\widehat{\Theta}}\Big|_{\left(x,\widehat{\Theta}\right)=\left(1-\frac{1-\alpha_1}{1-\beta_1},\Theta\right)}\frac{1}{n^{1/2}}\,Z_{11}$$

$$+ o_p\left\|\left(x,\widehat{\Theta}\right)-\left(1-\frac{1-\alpha_1}{1-\beta_1},\Theta\right)\right\|.$$

$$\frac{\partial \widetilde{\alpha_1}\left(x,\widehat{\Theta}\right)}{\partial x}\Big|_{\left(x,\widehat{\Theta}\right)=\left(1-\frac{1-\alpha_1}{1-\beta_1},\Theta\right)} = \frac{1}{2}\left\{1 + \frac{\alpha_1 - \beta_1 - 2\alpha_1\beta_1(1-\beta_1)}{\sqrt{(\alpha_1 + \beta_1 - 2\alpha_1\beta_1)^2}}\right\}$$

$$= \frac{\alpha_1 - 2\alpha_1\beta_1 + \alpha_1\beta_1^2}{\alpha_1 + \beta_1 - 2\alpha_1\beta_1}$$

because $\alpha_1 + \beta_1 - 2\alpha_1\beta_1 \geq 0$

and $\quad \dfrac{\partial \widetilde{\alpha_1}\left(x,\widehat{\Theta}\right)}{\partial \widehat{\Theta}}\Big|_{\left(x,\widehat{\Theta}\right)=\left(1-\frac{1-\alpha_1}{1-\beta_1},\Theta\right)} = \dfrac{1-\alpha_1}{\alpha_1 + \beta_1 - 2\alpha_1\beta_1}.$

Therefore,

$$\widetilde{\alpha_1} = \alpha_1$$
$$+ \left(\frac{\alpha_1 - 2\alpha_1\beta_1 + \alpha_1\beta_1^2}{\alpha_1 + \beta_1 - 2\alpha_1\beta_1}\right)\left(\frac{1-\alpha_1}{1-\beta_1} - \frac{1-(n_{1.}/n)}{1-(n_{.1}/n)}\right)$$
$$+ \left(\frac{1-\alpha_1}{\alpha_1 + \beta_1 - 2\alpha_1\beta_1}\right)\frac{1}{n^{1/2}}Z_{11}$$
$$+ o_p\left\|\left(1-\frac{1-(n_{1.}/n)}{1-(n_{.1}/n)},\widehat{\Theta}\right) - \left(1-\frac{1-\alpha_1}{1-\beta_1},\Theta\right)\right\|.$$

Linearizing $\dfrac{1-(n_{1.}/n)}{1-(n_{.1}/n)}$ around $\dfrac{1-\alpha_1}{1-\beta_1}$,

$$\frac{1-(n_{1.}/n)}{1-(n_{.1}/n)} = \frac{1-\alpha_1}{1-\beta_1} - \frac{1}{1-\beta_1}\left(\frac{n_{1.}}{n} - \alpha_1\right)$$
$$+ \frac{1-\alpha_1}{(1-\beta_1)^2}\left(\frac{n_{.1}}{n} - \beta_1\right) + o_p\left\|\left(\frac{n_{1.}}{n},\frac{n_{.1}}{n}\right) - (\alpha_1,\beta_1)\right\|$$
$$= \frac{1-\alpha_1}{1-\beta_1} - \frac{1}{1-\beta_1}\frac{1}{n^{1/2}}Z_{1.} + \frac{1-\alpha_1}{(1-\beta_1)^2}\frac{1}{n^{1/2}}Z_{.1}$$
$$+ o_p\left\|\left(\frac{n_{1.}}{n},\frac{n_{.1}}{n}\right) - (\alpha_1,\beta_1)\right\|.$$

Hence,

$$\widetilde{\alpha_1} = \alpha_1 + \left(\frac{\alpha_1 - 2\alpha_1\beta_1 + \alpha_1\beta_1^2}{\alpha_1 + \beta_1 - 2\alpha_1\beta_1}\right)\left(\frac{1}{1-\beta_1}\frac{1}{n^{1/2}}Z_{1.} - \frac{1-\alpha_1}{(1-\beta_1)^2}\frac{1}{n^{1/2}}Z_{.1}\right)$$
$$+ \left(\frac{1-\alpha_1}{\alpha_1 + \beta_1 - 2\alpha_1\beta_1}\right)\frac{1}{n^{1/2}}Z_{11} + o_p\left\|\left(\frac{n_{1.}}{n},\frac{n_{.1}}{n}\right) - (\alpha_1,\beta_1)\right\|$$
$$+ o_p\left\|\left(1-\frac{1-(n_{1.}/n)}{1-(n_{.1}/n)},\widehat{\Theta}\right) - \left(1-\frac{1-\alpha_1}{1-\beta_1},\Theta\right)\right\|.$$

Similarly, linearize $\widetilde{\beta_1} = \widetilde{\beta_1}\left(\widetilde{\alpha_1}, \widehat{\Theta}\right) = \dfrac{\widehat{\Theta}}{\widetilde{\alpha_1}}$ around $\left(\widetilde{\alpha_1}, \widehat{\Theta}\right) = (\alpha_1, \Theta)$.

$$
\begin{aligned}
\widetilde{\beta_1} &= \widetilde{\beta_1}\left(\widetilde{\alpha_1}, \widehat{\Theta}\right) \\[2mm]
&= \beta_1 + \frac{\partial \widetilde{\beta_1}\left(\widetilde{\alpha_1}, \widehat{\Theta}\right)}{\partial \widehat{\Theta}}\bigg|_{\left(\widetilde{\alpha_1}, \widehat{\Theta}\right) = (\alpha_1, \Theta)} \left(\widehat{\Theta} - \Theta\right) \\[2mm]
&\quad + \frac{\partial \widetilde{\beta_1}\left(\widetilde{\alpha_1}, \widehat{\Theta}\right)}{\partial \widetilde{\alpha_1}}\bigg|_{\left(\widetilde{\alpha_1}, \widehat{\Theta}\right) = (\alpha_1, \Theta)} (\widetilde{\alpha_1} - \alpha_1) + o_p \left\|\left(\widetilde{\alpha_1}, \widehat{\Theta}\right) - (\alpha_1, \Theta)\right\| \\[2mm]
&= \beta_1 + \frac{1}{n^{1/2}\alpha_1} Z_{11} - \frac{\Theta}{\alpha_1^2} (\widetilde{\alpha_1} - \alpha_1) + o_p \left\|\left(\widetilde{\alpha_1}, \widehat{\Theta}\right) - (\alpha_1, \Theta)\right\| \\[2mm]
&= \beta_1 + \frac{1}{n^{1/2}\alpha_1} Z_{11} - \frac{\Theta}{\alpha_1^2} \left\{ \left(\frac{\alpha_1 - 2\alpha_1\beta_1 + \alpha_1\beta_1^2}{\alpha_1 + \beta_1 - 2\alpha_1\beta_1}\right) \right. \\[2mm]
&\quad \times \left(\frac{1}{1-\beta_1}\frac{1}{n^{1/2}} Z_{1.} - \frac{1-\alpha_1}{(1-\beta_1)^2}\frac{1}{n^{1/2}} Z_{.1}\right) \\[2mm]
&\quad + \left(\frac{1-\alpha_1}{\alpha_1 + \beta_1 - 2\alpha_1\beta_1}\right)\frac{1}{n^{1/2}} Z_{11} + o_p \left\|\left(\frac{n_{1.}}{n}, \frac{n_{.1}}{n}\right) - (\alpha_1, \beta_1)\right\| \\[2mm]
&\quad + o_p \left\|\left(1 - \frac{1-(n_{1.}/n)}{1-(n_{.1}/n)}, \widehat{\Theta}\right) - \left(1 - \frac{1-\alpha_1}{1-\beta_1}, \Theta\right)\right\| \right\} \\[2mm]
&\quad + o_p \left\|\left(\widetilde{\alpha_1}, \widehat{\Theta}\right) - (\alpha_1, \Theta)\right\| .
\end{aligned}
$$

References

1. Anscombe, F. G. (1948). The transformation of Poisson, binomial and negative binomial data, *Biometrika*, **35**, 246–254.

2. Bickel, P., Cosman, P., Olshen, R., Spector, P., Rodrigo, A., and Mullins, J. (1996). Covariability of V3 loop amino acids, *AIDS Research and Human Retroviruses*, **12**, 1401–1411.

3. Bishop, Y., Fienberg, S., and Holland, P. (1975). *Discrete Multivariate Analysis: Theory and Practice*, MIT Press, Cambridge, Massachusetts.

4. Blower, S. M., and McLean, A. R. (1994). Prophylactic vaccines, risk behavior change, and the probability of eradicating HIV in San Francisco, *Science*, **265**, 1451–54.

5. Felsenstein, J., and Churchill, G. (1996). A hidden Markov approach to variation among sites in rate of evolution, *Molecular Biology and Evolution*, **13**, 93–104.

6. Goodman, L., and Kruskal, W. (1979). *Measures of Association for Cross Classifications*, Springer, New York.

7. Karnoub, M. (1997) Understanding Dependencies among Mutations along the HIV Genome, Ph.D. Thesis, Department of Biostatistics, University of North Carolina at Chapel Hill.

8. Karnoub, M., Seillier-Moiseiwitsch, F., and Sen, P.K. (1999). A conditional approach to the detection of correlated mutations, In *Statistics in Molecular Biology and Genetics* (Ed., F. Seillier-Moiseiwitsch), *Lecture Notes Series*, **13**, pp. 221–235, Institute of Mathematical Statistics and American Mathematical Society.

9. Korber, B. T. M., Farber, R. M., Wolpert, D. H., and Lapedes, A. S. (1993). Covariation of mutations in the V3 loop of the human immunodeficiency virus type 1 envelope protein: An information-theoretic analysis, *Proceedings of the National Academy of Sciences U.S.A.*, **90**, 7176–80.

10. Luenberger, D. (1984). *Linear and Non-Linear Pogramming, Second Edition*, Wiley and Sons, New York.

11. Miedema, F., Meyaard, L., Koot, M., Klein, M. R., Roos, M. T. L., Groenink, M., Fouchier, R. A. M., Van't Wout, A. B., Tersmette, M., Schellekens, P. T. A., and Schuitemaker, H. (1994). Changing virus-host interactions in the course of HIV-1 infection, *Immunological Reviews*, **140**, 35–71.

12. Preston, B. D., Poiesz, B. J., and Loeb, L. A. (1988). Fidelity of HIV-1 reverse transcriptase, *Science*, **242**, 1168–71.

13. Rodrígues, F., Oliver, J. L., Marín, A., and Medina, J. R. (1990). The general stochastic model of nucleotide substitution, *Journal of Theoretical Biology*, **142**, 485–501.

14. Seillier-Moiseiwitsch, F., Margolin, B. H., and Swanstrom, R. (1994). Genetic variability of the human immunodeficiency virus: Statistical and biological issues, *Annual Review of Genetics*, **28**, 559–596.

15. Seillier-Moiseiwitsch, F., Pinheiro, H., Karnoub, M., and Sen, P. K. (1998). Novel methodology for quantifying genomic heterogeneity, In *Proceedings of the Joint Statistical Meetings, Anaheim, California, August 1997*.

16. Sen, P. K., and Singer, J. M. (1993). *Large Sample Methods in Statistics: An Introduction with Applications*, Chapman and Hall, New York.

17. Tavaré, S. (1986). Some probabilistic and statistical problems in the analysis of DNA sequences, *Lectures on Mathematics in the Life Sciences*, **17**, 57–86.

PART X
ANIMAL HEALTH

32

Swiss Federal Veterinary Office Risk Assessments: Advantages and Limitations of The Qualitative Method

R. Hauser, E. Breidenbach, and K. D. C. Stärk

Swiss Federal Veterinary Office, Bern, Switerland

Abstract: The Swiss Federal Veterinary Office (SFVO) applies risk analysis methods in the fields of animal disease control and food safety. Analysis results are used to formulate import regulations for animals and goods, to check the effectiveness of control measures, and to set up monitoring programmes for animal diseases and food contamination. The assessment of the potential health risks to the population from consuming milk and dairy products contaminated with zoonotic agents is used to demonstrate the steps and the advantages of a qualitative risk assessment. The probability of contamination occurring in raw milk, retail milk, and 12 milk products was investigated. The products posing the greatest risk were raw milk and fresh and soft cheeses whereas the risk from pasteurised milk, cream, butter, and hard cheese was seen to be negligible. Based on these results, the first risk-based monitoring of milk products was introduced in Switzerland in 2002. The initial phase of a risk analysis is a qualitative process. Often, while the risk network is being established, it is realised that the required data are unavailable or that data quality is insufficient. Qualitative evaluation of expert opinion is easier than quantitative evaluation. However, assigning risks to qualitative categories is done subjectively and there is no standardised method. Usually the information provided by qualitative assessments is adequate for risk managers for decision making. Management measures in public health are often 'yes' or 'no' decisions. Risk communication between risk managers and stakeholders is simplified when the results of a qualitative assessment are available.

Keywords and phrases: Qualitative risk assessment, milk contamination, risk-based monitoring

32.1 Introduction

The Swiss Federal Veterinary Office (SFVO) is responsible for monitoring the
health and welfare of animals in Switzerland and protecting the public from diseases transmitted by animals or through animal products. Risk analysis methods are used in the fields of disease control and food safety in accordance with
international standards laid out by the Office International des Epizooties (OIE)
[Anonymous (2003)] and in the FAO/WHO's Codex Alimentarius [Anonymous
(2001)].

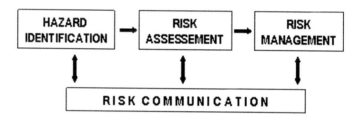

Figure 32.1: The four elements of risk analysis. [Source: OIE, Terrestrial Animal Health Code (2003)]

In accordance with international standards, risk analyses at the FVO are
structured into four elements: Hazard Identification, Risk Assessment, Risk
Management, and Risk Communication.

Hazard Identification involves identifying pathogenic agents that could potentially produce adverse consequences within the use of a defined commodity.

Risk Management is the process of deciding and implementing measures to
achieve the appropriate level of protection, taking into account scientific and
other legitimate factors. The effects of the implemented measures are monitored.

Risk Communication is an important part of a successful risk analysis. It involves the exchange of information and opinions concerning the risk. Risk communication is part of the responsibility of risk management with comprehension
of all participants and communication specialists.

During the *Risk Assessment*, current information is collected, documented, and
assessed according to scientific criteria by means of literature research and expert opinion. Existing knowledge gaps, limitations, and uncertainties are trans-
parently documented. The risk consists of the probability that the undesired

events might happen and the extent of the possible harm. For a qualitative risk analysis, the result is described in words.

Analysis results are used to formulate import regulations for animals and goods, to check the effectiveness of control measures, and to set up monitoring programs for animal diseases and food contamination. Information gained from literature searches and expert opinion is evaluated according to established scientific criteria. Gaps in data, limitations on its use, and uncertainties are identified and documented. Risk is then assessed on the basis of structured information and is expressed in terms of the likelihood of an adverse event occurring and the magnitude of the consequences. Results are usually given in report form (qualitative risk analysis).

32.2 Health Risks from Consumption of Milk and Dairy Products: An Example of a Qualitative Risk Assessment

An analysis of the potential health risks to the population from consuming milk and dairy products is used here to demonstrate the steps involved in qualitative risk analysis and the advantages of the method.

32.2.1 Risk profile

After inspections by the European Union's Food and Veterinary Office in Switzerland, it was recognised that a program of risk-based monitoring of manufactured milk and dairy products, supported by official random sampling, was required to ensure products were fit for export to the EU. In co-operation with risk managers, risk analysts drew up a risk profile establishing the reason for the assessment, identifying the hazards to be investigated, the tolerance values, and a detailed questionnaire. The likelihood of high levels of contamination occurring in raw milk, retail milk, and 12 milk product groups leading to rejection of the products (contamination above tolerance values or above threshold limits) was investigated.

32.2.2 Hazard identification

Hazard identification is an important part of a risk assessment in which all potential hazards are identified including those that will not actually be studied, in this case *Listeria monocytogenes, Salmonella spp., Staphylococcus aureus* and its toxins, *Escherichia coli, Bacillus cereus* and its toxins, and Aflatoxin M_1. No assessment was made of the risk from campylobacter, *Yersinia enterocolitica,*

Vibrio cholerae, and Central European encephalitis. They were assessed to be not relevant for milk products (no or extremely rare evidence). Cattle, goats, and sheep have been officially declared free of *Mycobacterium bovis* and *Brucella spp.* so no assessment was made for these pathogens.

32.2.3 Risk network

After all the potential hazards and their origins were identified, a risk network for milk and dairy products was drawn up, as shown in Figure 32.2.

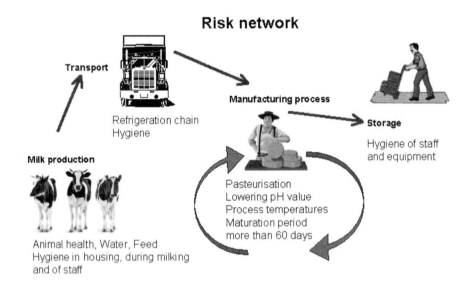

Figure 32.2: Risk network, origin, and identification of hazards in dairy product manufacture

The chain of primary production, manufacturing, and sale of milk and dairy products was divided into four stages. Animal health, water, feed, animal housing, milking hygiene and staff hygiene are all factors that influence the quality of raw milk during primary milk production. Refrigeration and hygiene are crucial during transport. Each manufacturing process used for dairy products has an influence on any potential hazards. During storage and distribution to points of sale, quality is influenced by staff and equipment hygiene.

Potential factors that could have a negative effect on the quality of the end product were identified in the risk network. Expert opinion was obtained to assess the probability of occurrence for each factor and the consequences for the end product. The probability of occurrence was defined as less than 1%, less than 10%, less than 25%, and more than 50%. The consequences were classified qualitatively as 'negligible,' 'low,' 'medium,' and 'high' (see Table 32.1).

Table 32.1: Expert opinion: Factors with negative effects, probability of occurrence, and consequences for the end product

Production Stage	Factor with Detrimental Effect	Probability of Occurrence (%)	Consequences
	Animal health	< 25	Small to medium
	Water quality	< 10	Small
Milk production	Feed contaminated with mycotxin	< 1	Small
	Feed dust	< 10	Small
	Hygiene	> 50	Medium to high
	Break in refrigeration chain	< 10	Small
Transport	Hygiene	< 10	Small
	Water quality	< 1	Negligible
	Contamination during process	< 10	Small
	Water quality	< 10	Negligible to small
	Ineffective pasteurisation	< 1	Negligible
Manufacturing process	Process temperatures low	< 1	Negligible to small
	Lowering pH value	< 1	Small
	Additives	< 10	Medium
	Maturation period too short	< 10	Small to medium
	Contamination of end product	< 10	Medium,
Storage	Hygiene of staff and equipment	< 1	Small

A qualitative assessment was made of each process stage and each was categorised. Pasteurisation and sterilisation completely eliminate pathogens. Lowering the pH value and high processing temperatures reduce contamination risk to 'medium.' Long maturation periods of more than 60 days reduce contamination substantially. Adding water and other supplements during the process may cause pathogens to multiply.

32.2.4 Risk estimation

Various product groups were categorised according to risk, on the basis of the probability of tolerance limits being exceeded. This was an indication of the exposure risk to consumers. For dairy products, the likelihood of contamination occurring was estimated by combining available data and on the basis of expert opinion and was defined as 'negligible,' 'low,' and 'medium' (Figures 32.3 and 32.4).

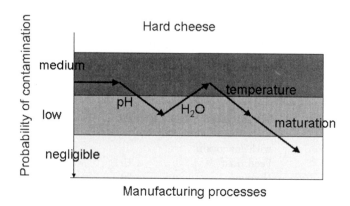

Figure 32.3: Qualitative assessment of hard cheese. The probability of contamination

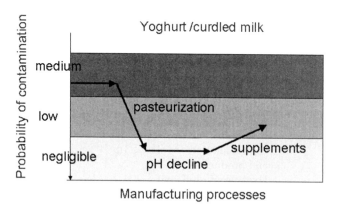

Figure 32.4: Qualitative assessment of yoghurt and curdled milk. The probability of contamination

The products posing the greatest risk were raw milk and fresh and soft cheeses whereas the risk from pasteurised milk, cream, butter, and hard cheese was seen to be negligible.

32.2.5   Recommendations for random sample planning and risk managers

The expected probability of tolerance limits being exceeded was defined as less than 1% for a 'negligible' risk, less than 2.5% for a 'low' risk, and less than 5% for a 'medium' risk.

The number of random samples required was calculated using the usual sample size formulae. Based on the results of the risk assessment and the experience of the authorities, the first risk-based monitoring of end products was introduced throughout Switzerland in the autumn of 2002.

Table 32.2: Probability of contamination above threshold limits

Risk Category	Probability of Contamination over Threshold Limits (%)	Milk Product
Negligible	< 1	Pasteurized milk, cream, butter, hard cheese
Low	< 2.5	Yogurt, dessert, semi-hard cheese
Medium	< 5	Fresh cheese, creamy cheese, raw milk

32.3 Advantages and Disadvantages of Qualitative Risk Assessment

Establishing a risk profile and characterising the hazards in the initial phase of a risk analysis is a qualitative process. A risk network is indispensable to both the qualitative and quantitative methods. Often, while the network is being established, it is seen that the required data are unavailable or data quality is insufficient. Qualitative evaluation of expert opinion is much easier than quantitative evaluation.

Drawing up a qualitative risk assessment to determine whether there is in fact a risk is the first requirement before proceeding with a quantitative risk assessment. If data of sufficiently high quality are available, models can be created and all risk paths can be quantitatively assessed. In practice, risk assessments are comprehensive projects that can keep whole institutes and organisations occupied for years. The qualitative assessment of health hazards in milk and dairy products described in this chapter was completed in less than seven months.

In qualitative risk assessments, the risk can be described in terms such as 'negligible,' 'low,' 'medium,' and 'high.' However, assigning risks to qualitative categories is done subjectively and there is no standardised method. The transition between 'negligible' and 'non-negligible' is defined subjectively by risk managers. International standards could be reached by a broad discussion of terminology leading to more meaningful risk assessments and improved acceptance of the method.

Usually the information provided by qualitative assessments is adequate for risk managers for decision making. In most cases, management measures are general in nature and concern import requirements, monitoring and control regulations, or require 'yes' or 'no' decisions. Often, measures will either be implemented or not, irrespective of the fine shades of risk.

Risk communication between risk managers and stakeholder groups is simplified when the results of a qualitative assessment are available. No special mathematical knowledge is needed to determine the risk paths and to evaluate the data. Complex quantitative models such as dose–effect relationships, simulations, and the like, are usually hard to understand and may be difficult to communicate. They may be perceived as 'black-box' approaches.

32.4   Statistics' Part in Qualitative Risk Assessment

Qualitative risk assessments make use of descriptive statistical evaluations. Probability calculus is used to estimate prevalent risks, their development and the effect of risk reduction measures. It is difficult, if not impossible, to compare risk assessments made in different countries or by different analysts because categorisations are subjective. Statistical methods could help standardise assessments and make comparison possible. Statistics' role is to provide high-quality data resulting in more accurate risk assessments. Inaccuracies are possible in all assessments because of data gaps and variability. High-quality data compensate for lack of knowledge and increase the accuracy of assessments. Well-planned and evaluated studies are needed to obtain such data. Corresponding data from different studies may be combined by means of a meta-analysis.

References

1. Anonymous (2001). Definitions of risk analysis terms related to food safety, In *Codex Alimentarius Commission Procedural Manual*, 12th edition, pp. 43–44, Joint FAO/WHO food standards programme, Food and Agriculture Organization of the United Nations/World Health Organization, Rome.

2. Anonymous (2003). Import risk analysis, In *Office International des Epizooties. Terrestrial Animal Health Code*, Section 1.3, Paris, France.

33

Qualitative Risk Analysis in Animal Health: A Methodological Example

Barbara Dufour and François Moutou

École nationale vétérinaire d'Alfort, Maisons-Alfort, France
AFSSA Lerpaz, Maisons-Alfort, France

Abstract: Risk analysis can be performed following either a quantitative or a qualitative approach. Both methodologies are linked to the same theoretical rules. Once the potential hazard has been identified, the qualitative risk assessment is carried out by combining the probabilities of occurrences of the events (emission and exposition) in the presence of a hazard, and its consequences. The probability of an event can be evaluated by combining the probabilities of the different parameters.

Within the frame of global expertise, the necessity of realizing collegial risk evaluations, sometimes when only few data are available and within a short amount of time, leads us to work on a standardised method for a qualitative approach.

The process of global qualitative risk appreciation is completed by adding support to the rationalisation of the estimation step. It has been proposed that each parameter be evaluated with the help of all available information and that an evaluation of the probability of occurrence of each of these can be realized individually to yield a given level of probability (null, negligible, low, moderate, high) or an interval between two levels (for example: 'negligible to low').

The combination of probabilities and of intervals was carried out using a table that was tested and evaluated through the following risk assessment: qualitative risk evaluations of the transmission of Q fever to humans in France.

Both the advantages and the limitation of this approach are also presented.

Keywords and phrases: Risk analysis, qualitative methodology, Q fever

33.1   Introduction

Risk analysis has undergone rapid development in the whole field of food safety and within a few years become a priority for scientists and decision makers who see in this new tool a way to improve the rationale of their decisions, particularly in animal health expertise.

It is now recognised that risk estimation can be performed following either quantitative or qualitative methodology. Quantitative risk analysis must be fueled by data that are not always available, either easily or rapidly. At the same time, risk analysis needs to be organised around more or less complex models in order to estimate the variables' distributions and occurrence probabilities [Sutmoller and Wrathall (1997) and Gale *et al.* (1998)]. The field of quantitative risk analysis is indeed a rich research domain for scientists. On the other hand, few publications have presented investigations using the qualitative approach, although this may be seen as easier to perform in the absence of some of the basic data. The qualitative approach is nevertheless used by managers [Pharo (2002)] and by expert working groups [Anonymous (2002, 2003, 2004)], especially when time is lacking for a full quantitative analysis or when crude data are missing.

It thus seemed that a methodological approach to quantitative risk analysis could be of some interest. This chapter presents the method used within the collegial scientific expertise of the French food safety agency (AFSSA, *Agence française de sécurité sanitaire des aliments*), following and adapting the work of Zepeda-Sein (1998).

33.2   Global Presentation of the Method

The method to appreciate a risk, as proposed by the Animal World Health Organisation (OIE, Paris), consists of the following five steps [Ahl *et al.* (1993) and OIE (2001)]: (i) hazard identification; (ii) appreciation of the emission (the probability of emission from the source); (iii) appreciation of the exposition (the probability of exposition to the hazard); (iv) appreciation of the consequences (occurrence and severity combined); and (v) estimation of the risk (the combination of the probabilities of occurrence of the emission and of the exposition with its consequences).

Each of the parameters, like emission, exposition, and consequences, may themselves be complex and can be subdivided into simpler elements, each of which contributes to their global occurrence.

As an example to illustrate this, the meanings of these parameters in the field of animal health are presented as follows. The parameter 'emission' is linked to and depends on the sources of virulent materials, the cycle of excretion by the infected animals, as well as the prevalence of the disease in the species of concern. The parameter 'exposition' depends on the characteristics of the exposed populations (density, distribution, sensitivity, etc.) and on the different possible routes of contamination (airborne, foodborne, etc.). The parameter 'consequences' takes into account the sanitary (severity of the disease, morbidity, and lethality rates) and economical costs of the possible outbreak (loss of production, loss of markets, direct slaughtering and destruction of animals) aspects.

For each parameter, the list of all the elements to be taken into account is completed, following the timing and the chronology of the more pertinent event tree, specifically built for the item of concern. Each of these elements is first described; then the available information and data are collected and analysed through the process, to result in an estimation value.

The parameters can be characterized following three modalities: (i) by a *value*: this kind of quantitative analysis is said to be 'punctual' or 'deterministic;' (ii) by a *law of probability*: this kind of quantitative analysis is said to be 'probabilistic' or 'stochastic;' (iii) by a *qualitative appreciation* for which a quantification process will not be used, but instead the level of each parameter will be assessed using descriptive scales or qualifications

Risk can then be evaluated by combining probabilities of each parameter following the rules presented in Figure 33.1. In the case of a quantitative risk appreciation, the laws of probabilities show how to combine the probabilities of each parameter. This chapter proposes a rationalized approach to deal with qualitative risk appreciation (Figure 33.2).

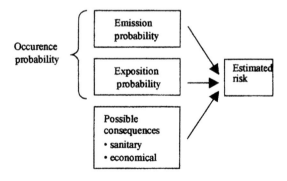

Figure 33.1: The components of risk estimation

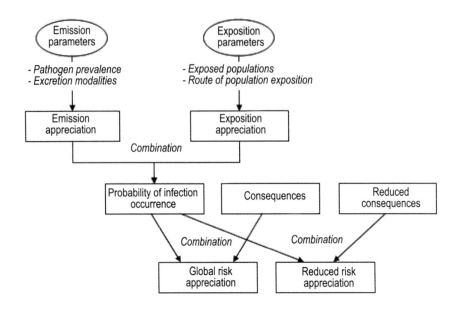

Figure 33.2: Presentation of the global chart of the analysis. [From OIE (2001).]

33.3   Qualitative Appreciation of the Probability of Each Event

The global process of qualitative risk appreciation was completed with the help of the estimation rationalisation adapted from the work of Zepeda-Sein (1998). This author proposes that each of the parameters (emission, exposition, and consequences) can be analysed by using all the available information and that an evaluation of the occurrence probability of each of them can be realised separately to obtain a certain level of probability [five qualifications are then fixed to qualify the occurrence probability of each parameter: *null* (Nu: the occurrence of the event is not possible); *negligible* (N: the occurrence of the event could only be possible under exceptional circumstances); *low* (L: the occurrence of the event is not very high, but is possible under some circumstance); *moderate* (M: the occurrence of the event is clearly possible); or *high* (H: the occurrence of the event is high)] or within a given interval (for instance: between negligible to low).

After each event has been evaluated separately from the others following a qualitative process, the final qualitative appreciation of each parameter is made globally, by combining its event qualifications. The process must be strongly argued and some specific weight can be given to specific events, following the characteristics of each disease. For instance, for the exposition parameter, the event 'contamination route' may or may not be a determinant compared to 'populations of concern,' and its qualification will depend on this.

33.4   Qualitative Risk Appreciation

The combination of the probabilities of two given parameters, as proposed by Zepeda-Sein (1998) has been adapted by Dufour *et al.* (2003) and then used by different working groups organised within the context of the expert specialised groups of the French food safety agency (AFSSA). The method was developed, then tested on different subjects [Anonymous (2003) and Anonymous (2004)], and underwent different adjustments before being validated through an expert consensus of the Animal Health Committee of the French food safety agency in 2004.

For example, the working group on bat rabies and the risk of its transmission played a major role in the realisation and adaptation of this method. Here, the use of the qualitative approach allowed the expert group to characterise the risk of transmission of bat rabies to human beings in France when data on the prevalence of rabies within bat colonies was lacking, making impossible any quantitative analysis [Anonymous (2003)]. However, at the end of this qualitative analysis, the combination table rules were judged to be too severe, quite probably leading to an overestimation of the risk.

Therefore, new adaptations were introduced to take into account the imprecision of some data, the real subjectivity of the evaluation of the different probabilities which are used, and mainly the fact that the combination of two probabilities should result in a lower probability than each of the two original probabilities (as when following this quantitative example: $10^{-4} \times 10^{-4} = 10^{-8}$), which had not been the case in the bat rabies document.

To take this last point into account, the qualification combination rules adopted are as follows.

- Two probabilities with the same qualification combined together give the qualification just below (low × low = negligible),

- Two adjacent probabilities give the lower interval of the lower original probability (low × moderate = negligible to low),

- Two probabilities neither adjacent nor opposed give the lower probability (low × high = low),

- Two opposite probabilities give the higher interval of the lowest probability (negligible × high = negligible to low),

- The combination of probabilities can also be performed by combining one or two interval(s). Table 33.1 shows all these possible combinations.

Using this method, the combination of two 'negligible' qualifications should logically lead to 'null.' However, AFSSA experts estimated that this qualification should be reserved to describe an impossible event, so they decided to use instead the 'null to negligible' interval for all the lowest probability situations.

The combination of these different probabilities for each parameter leads to the probability of occurrence of a hazard, which is therefore also presented using the same five qualifications as seen before (null, negligible, low, moderate, or high) or with the intermediate intervals.

The following remarks are to be taken into account: (i) Table 33.1 gives results that are close to results which could have been obtained through a quantitative analysis, if quantitative data had been available. The multiplication of two probabilities gives a probability lower than each of the two original probabilities; (ii) Table 33.1 gives relative information as opposed to absolute information between the different rows and columns; (iii) the combination of more than two parameters leads to the question of the ordering of the combination. With three parameters, N, M, and H for instance (N × H) × M gives N to L, whereas N × (H × M) yields N. To overcome this difficulty, it is here suggested to return to the event tree and to combine the parameters in the same order every time.

33.5 Qualitative Appreciation Examples

This qualitative approach, after being developed within different working groups, has recently been used by the specialised experts committee on Animal Health of the French food safety agency for an evaluation of Q fever transmission from ruminants to man in France [Anonymous (2004)].

The prevalence of Q fever in domestic ruminants in France is not known. Various surveys, with protocols that are both quite different and difficult to compare, suggested a global serological prevalence somewhere between 5% and 85%, which is not useful in a quantitative evaluation.

Three populations were defined with respect to their degree of risk exposition: people living closely to possibly infected animals, the 'rural' population that could be exposed to airborne contamination, and the global, usually urban, population.

Table 33.1: Results of the combination of the different qualitative appreciations used in the qualitative risk analysis (Nu = Null, N = Negligible, L = Low, M = Moderate, and H = High)

	Nu	Nu to N	N	N to L	L	L to M	M	M to H	H
Nu	Nu	Nu	Nu	Nu	Nu	Nu	Nu	Nu	Nu
Nu to N	Nu	Nu to N	Nu to N	Nu to N	Nu to N	Nu to N	N	N	N
N	Nu	Nu to N	Nu to N	Nu to N	N	N	N	N	N to L
N to L	Nu	Nu to N	Nu to N	Nu to N	N	N	N	N to L	L
L	Nu	Nu to N	N	N	N	N	N to L	L	L
L to M	Nu	Nu to N	N	N	N	N to L	L	L	L
M	Nu	N	N	N	N to L	L	L	L	L to M
M to H	Nu	N	N	N to L	L	L	L	L to M	M
H	Nu	N	N to L	L	L	L	L to M	M	M

The qualitative method used by the working group led to the following points: (i) the risk for the global population, that is, without any known extra risk factor (no pregnancy, valvulopathy, nor immunodepression) could be qualified as very low ('null to negligible'); (ii) globally, the level of risk was higher for populations with extra risk factors, which means that a specific therapy and/or treatment will be of great importance in these subpopulations. Indeed, the global risk is lowered from 'negligible to low' to 'null to negligible' after a therapeutic risk reduction for these subpopulations; (iii) the risk linked to the consumption of contaminated foodstuffs (such as raw milk or milk products from raw milk) was, as a whole, 'null to negligible' except for the populations with extra risk factors, in which it was 'negligible;' (iv) exposure through the airborne route or through close contacts with contaminated animals were the highest risks, so the persons in close contact with infected animals or 'rural persons' were the ones facing the greatest risk; (v) Table 33.2 presents the details of one of the tables obtained in the case of contamination through direct contacts with domestic ruminants issued from the AFSSA report [Anonymous (2004)]. Recommendations could then be established following this risk assessment.

33.6 Discussion

The qualitative approach presented here was built to answer the needs of expert committees of the French food safety agency, who have the obligation to evaluate, within short delays, risks linked to animal health in order to provide advice to risk managers, in this case the Central Veterinary Office (Direction générale de l'alimentation) of the ministry in charge of agriculture. With this background, two items are of specific concern: the method had to be simple, understandable, and easily accessible, both to the experts and to the managers; and it should not overevaluate the risk too much. For the first point, Zepeda-Sein methodology was preferred to semi-quantitative approaches, whose appropriation and understanding by users are more delicate. To prevent any over-estimation of the risk, the combination tables were redrawn from the experience gained in the bat rabies working group [Anonymous (2003)].

The experience of the different AFSSA working groups that have used the method show that the qualitative approach is simpler than the quantitative one and thus open to a wider audience. The experts of these different working groups had no difficulties familiarizing themselves with the method. Another major advantage is to be much less time consuming, and it thus represents a real possibility when there is little time to answer and when the decision behind the assessment is urgent.

This process requires a detailed and organised study of all the parameters that must be taken into account in the decision, including those for which the

Table 33.2: Global and reduced risk appreciation following the contamination route by *Coxiella burnetii* from small domestic ruminants [Anonymous (2004)]

Consequences		Probability of infection occurrence					
		Close Contact Population (*Moderate*)^a		Rural Population (*Moderate*)^a		Global Population (*Low*)^a	
		With extra risks*	Without extra risk	With extra risks	Without extra risk	With extra risks	Without extra risk
Consequences	Global	(*High*)^b Moderate to high	(*Negligible to low*)^b Low	(*High*)^b Moderate to high	(*Low*)^b Low to moderate	(*High*)^b Moderate	(*Low*)^b Low
	Reduced	(*Low to moderate*)^b Moderate	(*Null to negligible*)^b Low	(*Low to moderate*)^b Moderate	(*Null to negligible*)^b Low	(*Low to moderate*)^b Low	(*Null to negligible*)^b Negligible

* Are considered as extra risks: pregnancy, valvulopathies, and immunodepression

Qualifications between brackets are for the corresponding row and column estimations

lack of available data does not allow quantitative analysis to be carried out. This is why the construction of an event tree is so important.

Moreover, the approach points to the data used to obtain the estimation: the whole method is built on the quality of the information used and on the quality of the arguments followed to qualify the parameters. It is then quite easy to judge the pertinence of the analysis and to discuss its results following the quality of the data used to fuel the process. This is quite helpful to prevent spending too much time discussing software, algorithms or distribution laws in the case of quantitative or even semi-quantitative approaches. These discussions may lead one to forget that the real questions are at the data level, not in the computation.

However, the weakness of the qualitative process lies in the important part of subjectivity that is present in it. The attribution of the retained levels of probability (null, negligible, low, moderate, high probabilities) can be seen as arbitrary and thus questionable. A way to decrease the arbitrary part of an individual estimation is to make this process a collective one, by using an expert group to discuss its different steps. In this case, it is important that the experts have a good apprehension of the different proposed probability levels.

It is also necessary to make the process as transparent as possible; for example, the documentation on which the argumentation is built and which leads to each of the qualifications used must be presented in detail.

The quantitative method seems, at a first glance, more rigorous and less arbitrary. It also presents the advantage of permitting a sensitivity analysis of the estimation, compared to the incertitude of the hypothesis. However, this process can be very long and is only possible in a very few situations, as it requires much quantitative information quite often difficult to obtain. When major data are lacking, the evaluators will use hypotheses, which, even if presented with figures, are also arbitrary.

Acknowledgements. The authors are pleased to acknowledge all the colleagues that contributed their participation to the 'bat rabies' and 'Q fever' working groups of the animal health committee of AFSSA. Jayne Ireland is warmly thanked for improving our English. The authors also thank Anne-Marie Hattenberger as well as the two referees who helped improve a first version of the manuscript.

References

1. Ahl, A. S., Acree, J. A., Gipson, P. S., Mc Dowell, R. M., Miller, L., and McElvaine M. D. (1993). Standardisation of nomenclature for animal

health risk analysis, *Revue scientifique et technique (International Office of Epizootics)*, **12**, 1045–1053.

2. Anonymous (2002). *Rapport sur le botulisme d'origine aviaire et bovine*, Rapport réalisé par un groupe de travail du Comité d'experts spécialisé santé animale de l'Agence française de sécurité sanitaire des aliments, 82 p.

3. Anonymous (2003). *Rapport sur la rage des Chiroptères en France métropolitaine*, réalisé par un groupe de travail du Comité d'expert spécialisé "santé animale" de l'Agence française de sécurité sanitaire des aliments, AFSSA, Maisons-Alfort.

4. Anonymous (2004). *Rapport sur l'évaluation des risques pour la santé publique et des outils de gestion des risques en élevage des ruminants*, réalisé par un groupe de travail du Comité d'expert spécialisé " santé animale " de l'Agence française de sécurité sanitaire des aliments, AFSSA, Maisons-Alfort.

5. Dufour, B., Moutou, F., and Hattenberger A. M. (2003). Qualitative and collegial risk analysis method: An example: Bats rabies transmission to man in France, In *Proceedings of ISVEE 10th* (Ed., S. Urcelay), pp. 1–4, ISVEE, Vina del Mar, Chile, November 16–21, 2004.

6. Gale, P., Young, C., Stanfield, G., and Oakes, D. (1998). Development of a risk assessment for BSE in the aquatic environment, *Journal of Applied Microbiology*, **84**, 467–477.

7. Office international des épizooties (2001). *Code zoosanitaire international: mammifères, oiseaux et abeilles*, 10ème édition, OIE, Paris.

8. Pharo, H. J. (2002). Foot-and-mouth disease: An assessment of the risks facing New Zealand, *New Zealand Veterinary Journal*, **50**, 46–55.

9. Sutmoller, P., and Wrathall, A. E. (1997). A quantitative assessment of the risk of transmission of foot-and-mouth disease, bluetongue and vesicular stomatis by embryo transfer in cattle, *Preventive Veterinary Medicine*, **32**, 111–132.

10. Zepeda-Sein, C. (1998). Méthodes d'évaluation des risques zoosanitaires lors des échanges internationaux, In *Séminaire sur la sécurité zoosanitaire des échanges dans les Caraïbes*, 9-11 décembre 1997, Port of Spain, (Trinidad and Tobago), pp. 2–17, OIE, Paris.

Index

Accelerated life 127
Adaptive designs 401
Adverse drug reaction reporting
    systems 75
AIDS clinical trial 289
AIDS incubation time 225
Air pollution 467
Ambient temperature 437

Bayesian credible interval 349
Bayesian hierarchical spatial model 451
Binomial distribution 349
Biosurveillance 437
Breast cancer 151

Cancer 335
Cancer registry 451
Classification on very large
    databases 263
Clayton model 335
Clinical evaluations 323
Clinical trials 109, 335, 361
Clustering 263, 289
Combined response to treatment 387
Complete convergence 211
Computer simulation 75
Conditional autoregressive model 451
Confidence interval 349
Conjoint model 127
Contingency table 491
Correlated frailty model 151
Cross-validation 275

δ-Method 437
Data mining 75
Data monitoring 61
Data reduction 263
Degradation process 127
Disease progression studies 225
Distance model 451

Efficacy 335
Empirical processes 195

Failure time 127
Frailty model 179
Functional estimation 195
Fuzzy system 75

GAM model 467
Generalized linear models 95
Genomic sequences 491
Geometric distribution 349
Gibbs sampler 289
Group sequential plans 61

Hierarchy of experts 239
HIV dynamics 289
Hormesis 179
Hypothesis testing 419

Incidence 451
Independence 491
Individual patient data 3, 39
Isotonic regression estimators 361
Item response theory 109

Kappa coefficient 139
Kernel estimation 195

Latent regression 95
Laws of large numbers 195
Lifetime distributions 195
Longevity 127, 179
Longitudinal data 167, 289
Lung cancer 451

Maximum likelihood estimator 361
Maximum tolerated dose 361
Measure of agreement 139
Measurement error 95
Medical diagnosis 275

Meta-analysis 3, 39
Milk contamination 519
Mixed models 109
Model building 19
Modelling 75
Monte Carlo simulations 361
Multicentre clinical trial 387
Multilevel Gibbs sampling method 305
Multivariate survival analysis 151
MVUE 127

Neural networks 275
Nonlinear mixed-effects 289
Nonparametric estimation 195
Nonparametrics 335
Nuisance parameter 127
Numbers of infectious and
        noninfectious HIV 305

Observation model 305
Optimization 387
Ordinal data 139

Partial credit model 109
Path model 127
Patient safety 323
Phase II/III trials 401
Pilot study 349
Pointwise estimation of variance 225
Prediction trees 239
Predictive marker 39
Predictive process 167
Probabilistic nodes 239
Productively infected CD4$^{(+)}$ T cells 305
Prognosis 39
Prognostic factors 167
Prognostic markers 3, 19
Progressive censoring 61
P-splines 451

Q fever 539
Qualitative methodology 539
Qualitative risk assessment 519
Quality of life 109, 127

Random change points 289
Random effects 95

Random enrolment 387
Rasch models 95
Recruitment time 387
Regression 19
Regression estimation 195
Reliability 127
Right-censored survival data 211
Risk analysis 539
Risk-based monitoring 519
Robustness 361

Safety 61
Salmonella infection 437
Seasonality 437
Select and test designs 401
Semiparametric additive hazard
        model 211
Semiparametric models 467
Sentinel events 61
Sequential adaptive designs 361
Sequential analysis 419
Sequential clinical trials 401
Sequential estimation 211
Sequential tests 109
Shared frailty model 151
Soft failure 127
Statistical test 491
Stochastic equation 305
Survival analysis 127, 167, 179
Survival function 225
Systematic review 3, 39

Time to event analyses 61
Toxicity 335
Traumatic failure 127
Treatment selection 401
Trees 19
Tuberculosis 275
Twins 151

Unbiased estimator 127

Validation 19
Validation studies 75

Weak laws 195

Printed in the United States of America.